KININS—II
Systemic Proteases and Cellular Function

ADVANCES IN EXPERIMENTAL MEDICINE AND BIOLOGY

KININS—II
Systemic Proteases and Cellular Function

Edited by

Setsuro Fujii

Institute for Protein Research
Osaka University
Osaka, Japan

Hiroshi Moriya

Science University of Tokyo
Tokyo, Japan

and

Tomoji Suzuki

Meiji College of Pharmacy
Tokyo, Japan

PLENUM PRESS • NEW YORK AND LONDON

Library of Congress Cataloging in Publication Data

International Symposium on Kinins, Tokyo, 1978.
  Kinins II.

  (Advances in experimental medicine and biology; v. 120)
  Includes index.
  1. Kinins—Congresses. 2. Kallikrein—Congresses. I. Fujii, Setsuro, 1925-
II. Moriya, Hiroshi. III. Suzuki, Tomoji. IV. Title. V. Series.
QP552.K5I55 1978   615.7   79-9079
ISBN 0-306-40197-5 (part B)

Proceedings of the International Symposium on Kinins,
held in Tokyo, Japan, November 6–9, 1978.

© 1979 Plenum Press, New York
A Division of Plenum Publishing Corporation
227 West 17th Street, New York, N.Y. 10011

Preface

In this brief historical retrospect of kinin studies, we
recall the discovery of bradykinin by Professor M. Rocha e Silva
and the pioneer investigations on tissue kallikrein initiated by
Dr. E.K. Frey followed by the work of Professor H. Kraut and
Professor E. Werle who opened the way for the present flourishing
investigations of kinins. The elucidation of the structure of
bradykinin by Dr. F. Elliott in 1960 stimulated further research
of the vasoactive peptides. During the following years, the
physiological and pathological significance of kinins was explored
extensively, resulting in the rapid accumulation of information
regarding their potential importance. Tremendous progress in our
understanding of the involvement of the kallikrein-kinin system
in many physiological phenomena has been facilitated by the
friendly atmosphere among "kininologists" engendered at previous
international kinin symposia. During that time studies were
reported as to the role of kinins in functional vasodilation,
alteration of blood pressure and vascular permeability, shock,
inflammation, and pain production. Thus, through knowledge from
these basic studies, the action of kinins in morbidity is better
understood as are the counter measures for many diseases associated
with kinin formation.

Recent discoveries have focused on abnormally delayed blood
coagulation in the hereditary deficiency of high molecular weight
kininogen together with prekallikrein deficiency. Thus great
strides have been made in elucidating the interrelationships
amongst the blood coagulation, fibrinolysis, and vasopeptide kinin
systems. Moreover, apart from the aforementioned role of bradykinin
as a pharmacologically active substance, other important findings
involving the coordinated actions of prostaglandin and catecholamine
biosynthesis, particularly in the inflammatory process, have
enhanced our appreciation of the complexity of the vasopeptide
kinin system.

The participation of more than 330 scientists from 16 countries
of the world in this International Symposium on Kinins-Kinin '78
Tokyo reflects accurately the interest and research activity in the

diverse and broad implications of the physiological and pathological
functions of the kallikrein-kinin system. A total of 128 papers,
including posters, were presented, attesting to the unquestioned
success of the KININ '78 TOKYO Symposium. This volume in two
sections contains the collective studies presented, studies of
high scientific standard that provoked lively discussions. Also
included in this volume are the two plenary lectures presented
by Dr. K. Austen (USA) and Dr. Hamao Umezawa (JAPAN).

In the future, further closer exchange of information among
investigators from varied bio-medical disciplines will contribute
significantly to our understanding of the important roles played
by the kallikrein-kinin and interrelated systems. Thus will the
scope of the kinin studies be broadened thereby enhancing our
appreciation of cell physiology as well as the possible clinical
impact of the system.

On behalf of the Organizing Committee, the editors of this
volume express their sincere gratitude for the support of the
Ministry of Education, The Scientific Council of Japan, and the
following academic societies in the various branches of medical
sciences: The Japanese Biochemical Society, The Japanese
Pharmacological Society, The Pharmaceutical Society of Japan,
The Japan Hematological Society, Japanese College of Angiology,
The Japanese Rheumatism Association, and the Japanese Society of
Allergology. The editors also express their gratitude for the
generous financial help provided by the Japan World Exposition
Commemorative Fund and other Foundations and Corporations.

The editors deeply appreciate the dedicated assistance of
Professor N. Back (USA) for helping facilitate the publication of
this volume. Appreciation also is extended to Ms. Patricia
Poczkalski of the State University of New York for her skillful
transcription of the manuscripts to uniform type seen in this
volume, and to Mr. Derrick Mancini, Editor of Plenum Press and
his associates for their cooperation in publishing attractively
and speedily this volume. The editors express their indebtedness
to Aaron I. Back for his meticulous proofreading of the manuscripts.

                                        Setsuro Fujii
                                        Hiroshi Moriya
                                        Tomoji Suzuki

Contents

KALLIKREIN-KININ SYSTEMS AND CELLULAR FUNCTION

BLOOD PRESSURE REGULATION: KININ, ANGIOTENSIN AND
PROSTAGLANDIN

Role of Plasma Kallikrein and
Kininogen in Coagulation Fibrinolysis,
and Complement Systems

A MOLECULAR BASIS OF ACTIVATION OF THE ALTERNATIVE PATHWAY OF

HUMAN COMPLEMENT

K. Frank Austen and Douglas T. Fearon

Departments of Medicine, Harvard Medical School and
Robert B. Brigham Division of the Affiliated Hospitals
Center, Inc., Boston, Mass. 02120

ABSTRACT

The fluid phase interaction of native C3, B, $\overline{D}$ and P continuously generates C3b; C3b complexes with B to permit cleavage-
activation by $\overline{D}$, thereby generating C3b,Bb, the amplification C3
convertase. C3b,Bb formed in the fluid phase or on a non-
activating surface for the alternative pathway undergoes decay-
dissociation through release of Bi, and the residual C3b undergoes
cleavage inactivation by the C3b inactivator (C3bINA). The
capacity of P to stabilize C3b,Bb and thereby augment C3 cleavage
is counterbalanced by β1H, which inactivates the convertase by
displacing Bi and facilitates the inactivation of residual C3b by
C3bINA. Transition to amplified C3 cleavage is achieved because
the surface characteristics of an activating particle protect C3b
from inactivation by C3bINA in the presence of β1H, and the
stabilized alternative pathway convertase, P,C3b,Bb, from
extrinsic decay-dissociation by β1H. Natural activating surfaces
such as zymosan (Zy) and rabbit erythrocytes are relatively
deficient in sialic acid residues as compared to non-activating
surfaces such as sheep erythrocytes (E^s). Sialic acid residues
on C3b-bearing particles augment binding of β1H to favor
competition with B, inactivation of C3b and decay-dissociation of
C3b,Bb. The absence of this carbohydrate on the membrane in the
environment of C3b results in low affinity binding of β1H, a
circumstance that permits uptake of B to form the amplification
convertase and impairs extrinsic decay of the C3-cleaving enzyme.
This natural humoral host resistance reaction based on the
relative content of sialic acid on target particles has a cellular

3

counterpart in the capacity of human monocytes to engage in
antibody-independent phagocytosis of sialic acid-deficient cells.
Thus, the non-immune host may respond to such cells by dual
humoral and cellular recognition mechanisms and this response may
represent a primordial basis for protection against microbial
invasion.

INTRODUCTION

A quarter of a century ago, Pillemer and colleagues (Science,
120:279, 1954) described the properdin system as an alternative
route to the utilization of the late stage complement components
and proposed that it had an essential role in the expression of
natural immunity. In the period between 1966 and 1971, the
existence of this alternative pathway of complement utilization
was reconfirmed by several different approaches (Nelson, 1966;
Gewurz et al., 1968a; Marcus et al., 1971; Frank et al., 1971;
Sandberg and Osler, 1971). During the last six years, a molecular
basis has been delineated by which the human alternative pathway
discriminates between activating and non-activating surfaces so as
to direct and amplify its expression (Fearon and Austen, 1977a,
1977b). Studies of the properdin system, now designated as the
alternative complement pathway, are described under four headings:
human alternative complement pathway - amplification; human
alternative complement pathway - activation; human alternative
complement pathway - modulation by non-complement principles; and
direct recognition of alternative complement pathway activating
particles by human monocytes.

THE ALTERNATIVE COMPLEMENT PATHWAY - AMPLIFICATION

Biologic expression of the alternative pathway is dependent
on a positive feedback mechanism in which C3b, the major cleavage
fragment of C3, interacts with B_(Pillemer et al., 1953;
Goodkofsky and Lepow, 1971) and D to generate C3b,Bb, a
C3-cleaving enzyme (Müller-Eberhard and Götze, 1972)(Fig. 1).
This C3b-dependent C3 convertase may amplify C3 cleavage initiated
by proteins of either the alternative or classical activating
pathways and is appropriately termed the amplification C3
convertase (Weiler et al., 1976). In the amplification reaction,
C3b serves as a receptor for B in a Mg^{++}-dependent reversible
interaction to yield C3b,B, a complex in which the proteolytic
site on B is partially revealed (Daha et al., 1976a). D, an enzyme
of the serine esterase class (Fearon et al., 1974) that is present
in its active state in normal serum or plasma (Müller-Eberhard
and Götze, 1972), then cleaves bound B to release the Ba fragment
and uncover fully the C3-cleaving site on the Bb fragment that

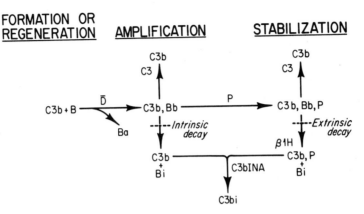

Fig. 1.   Amplification pathway for C3 cleavage. The
amplification C3 convertase, C3b,Bb, is formed from C3b
of any derivation by Mg^{++}-dependent binding of B with
cleavage activation by $\bar{D}$. The active site function of
Bb is stabilized in the complex with C3b by binding of P
and is decayed by intrinsic or extrinsic β1H-mediated
dissociation to yield free Bi. Inactivation of C3b by
C3bINA occurs only when the catalytic unit, Bb, has
decayed from the complex.

remains bound to C3b in the complex, C3b,Bb. This amplification
convertase, prepared on a sheep erythrocyte intermediate, was
labile due to temperature-dependent decay by irreversible
dissociation of Bb to inactive Bi (Fearon et al., 1973). The
convertase can be regenerated on the residual C3b by uptake of
additional B and its cleavage-activation by D. The lability of
the cell-bound C3b,Bb can be overcome by properdin (P) which binds
reversibly to C3b and stabilizes the convertase, P,C3b,Bb, in a
dose-related fashion (Fearon and Austen, 1975b).

        Regulation of the amplification convertase C3b,Bb is essen-
tial for homeostasis of the complement system since C3 cleavage
has a positive feedback action through generation of more
enzyme. Endogenous regulation occurs by four mechanisms:
intrinsic decay-dissociation of the inherently labile C3b,Bb
complex (Fearon et al., 1973); extrinsic decay-dissociation of the
convertase which is mediated by the plasma protein β1H (Weiler et
al., 1976); competition between β1H and B for binding to C3b
(Kazatchkine et al., in press); and inactivation of C3b by C3b
inactivator (C3bINA) (Alper et al., 1972) especially in the
presence of β1H (Whaley and Ruddy, 1976). Intrinsic decay of the
amplification convertase can be circumvented by P stabilization,
thereby necessitating control by extrinsic decay-dissociation

through the action of β1H. Incubation of cell-bound, P-stabilized
amplification convertase, P,C3b,Bb, in the presence of β1H results
in dose-dependent accelerated decay of convertase function and in
release of ^{125}I-Bb from the complex, so that P stabilization
is entirely reversed (Weiler et al., 1976). Because β1H also
accelerates decay of C3b,Bb in the absence of P, and exhibits an
affinity for C3b (Whaley and Ruddy, 1976; Pangburn and
Müller-Eberhard, 1978; Conrad et al., 1978; Kazatchkine et al.,
in press), β1H presumably displaces Bb from its binding site on
C3b. The resultant exposure of C3b permits irreversible cleavage-
inactivation of C3b by C3bINA, a reaction that cannot occur when
protective Bb is complexed to C3b (Daha et al., 1976b). Thus, β1H
and C3bINA act in sequence (Fig. 1), with the former unmasking C3b
by release of Bi from the C3b,Bb complex and the latter inactivating residual C3b to prevent regeneration of the C3b,Bb
convertase. Furthermore, inactivation of C3b by C3bINA is
facilitated by β1H (Whaley and Ruddy, 1976; Pangburn et al., 1978).

The formation of a C5 convertase is essential for the
generation of the C5b,6,7,8,9 cytolytic membrane insertion complex
as well as for the elaboration of other biologic activities
associated with these terminal components of complement. Since
the amplification C3 convertase already contains C3b as a subunit
of the enzyme, a requirement for additional C3b to achieve
C5-cleaving activity was not self-evident. However, the
observation that sheep erythrocytes prepared with relatively
limited amounts of C3b and bearing amplification C3 convertase
sites were lysed by incubation with C3 and C5-C9, but not by C5-C9
alone, suggested that additional cell-bound C3b molecules are
necessary for C5 convertase activity (Fearon et al., 1973).
Quantitative assessment of the different C3b requirements of the
two convertases with ^{125}I-C3 revealed that 60 C3b
molecules/erythrocyte sufficed for generation of amplification C3
convertase sites, whereas at least 200 C3b molecules/cell were
necessary for C5 convertase activity (Daha et al., 1976b).
Cell-bound C3 convertase sites could be transformed into C5
convertase sites by interaction with C3 to increase the number of
C3b molecules/cell without altering the content of C3b,Bb sites.
These newly generated C5 convertases reverted to sites capable of
cleaving only C3 when the additional cell-bound C3b was inactivated with C3bINA. The resistance to C3bINA of C3b forming the C3
convertase, C3b,Bb, as compared to the susceptibility of C3b
necessary for C5 cleavage indicates that the former is protected
by complexed Bb while the latter is exposed. Although differing
in their enzymatic capabilities, the two amplification convertases
share a common proteolytic site which resides in the Bb fragment
complexed to C3b. Both cell-bound convertases exhibit identical
half-lives of 4 min at 30°C, and both decayed enzymes are regenerated to their original specificities upon the introduction of B
in the presence of D̄, indicating that the topographical relation-

ships of membrane-associated C3b which determine C3 or C5
convertase activity are not disturbed by decay and regeneration of
C3b,Bb sites (Daha et al., 1976b). Thus, the composition of a
cell-bound C5 convertase site is C3b,Bb with an additional,
presumably adjacent, C3b which permits interaction of C5 with the
bimolecular complex.

THE ALTERNATIVE COMPLEMENT PATHWAY - ACTIVATION

Activation of the alternative pathway is synonymous with
transition from low grade, continuous C3 cleavage to amplified,
C3b-dependent C3 cleavage. Low grade C3 cleavage by interaction
in the fluid phase of native C3, B, D and P is considered to occur
by mechanisms analogous to those of the amplification reaction.
Native C3 is postulated to interact reversibly with B to form
C3,B, a low affinity complex which D converts to C3,Bb, a convertase capable of acting on C3 to generate initial C3b for the
amplification reaction (Fearon and Austen, 1975c). P enhances the
interaction of the native proteins (Fearon and Austen, 1975a),
presumably in a manner analogous to the stabilizing effect of P on
C3b,Bb (Fearon and Austen, 1975b). This fluid phase mechanism for
the continuous generation of C3b differs from the amplification
reaction in its much slower kinetics and greater dose requirements
for B and D, reflecting the presumed lower affinity of B for C3
than for C3b.

C3b generated by this mechanism can bind to bystander
surfaces or remain in the fluid phase because of rapid decay of
the C3b binding site. C3b molecules remaining in the fluid phase
or bound to a non-activating particle will be rapidly inactivated
by the action of C3bINA and β1H, and amplification by formation of
C3b,Bb will not occur. In contrast, the surface characteristics
of three activating particles of the alternative pathway, zymosan
(Pillemer et al., 1954), rabbit erythrocytes (Platts-Mills and
Ishizaka, 1974) and E. coli (Gewurz et al., 1968a), protect bound
C3b from inactivation by C3bINA/β1H and the stabilized amplification convertase, P,C3b,Bb, from extrinsic decay-dissociation by
β1H (Fearon and Austen, 1977a, 1977b), thereby permitting surface-
directed transition to amplified C3 cleavage. The circumvention
of the regulatory action of endogenous control proteins sustains a
positive feedback in which C3b deposited by the action of
particle-bound P,C3b,Bb on C3 provides further amplification.

Membrane sialic acid was then identified (Fearon, 1978) as
playing a critical role in determining whether or not a particle
would activate the alternative human complement pathway. Natural
activators such as zymosan and rabbit erythrocytes lack (Phaff,
1963) and have diminished (Aminoff et al., 1976) amounts of
surface sialic acid, respectively, relative to the abundance of

this moiety on the surface membrane of a non-activating particle such as the sheep erythrocyte. Both enzymatic removal of the sialic acid residues with sialidase and their conversion to a heptulosonic acid derivative by mild oxidation with periodate and reduction with borohydride, respectively, converted the sheep erythrocyte into an activating particle of the alternative complement pathway in whole human serum. As removal of the C8 and C9 carbon atoms of the polyhydroxylated side chain of sialic acid by chemical treatment was functionally equivalent to deletion of the entire sialic acid moiety, secondary effects of the enzymatic deletion such as diminution in surface charge or exposure of the penultimate galactose residues are not considered to be responsible for the acquisition of activating capacity. In a molecular model system employing C3b,Bb bound to desialated sheep erythrocytes, there proved to be a linear relationship between deletion or chemical modification of membrane sialic acid residues and the decrease in the capacity of the regulatory protein, β1H, to be taken up so as to cause extrinsic decay-dissociation of Bb from C3b,Bb (Fearon, 1978).

The observation that mouse erythrocytes from 21 inbred strains had variable capabilities to activate the human alternative complement pathway permitted the demonstration that natural variation in membrane sialic acid content was inversely related to activating capacity and was regulated by codominant alleles of a single autosomal locus. Linear regression analysis also demonstrated a significant inverse correlation between the sialic acid content of erythrocytes from four inbred mouse strains, and the concentration of β1H required for decay-dissociation of the properdin-stabilized amplification convertase on the erythrocytes. Erythrocytes from F_1 hybrids derived from strains with high and low alternative pathway activating capacities and from their backcrosses exhibited the alternative pathway activating capacities expected if the activity was regulated by alleles of a single autosomal locus. That this same locus predominantly regulated the sialic acid content of the mouse erythrocytes was established by the significant inverse correlation between the sialic acid content and the alternative pathway activating capacity of erythrocytes from mice of the F_1 and backcross generations (Nydegger et al., in press). Although the fluid phase interaction of C3, B and $\overline{D}$ continuously generates C3b (Fearon and Austen, 1975c) in a reaction augmented by properdin (Fearon and Austen, 1975a), it is the covalent attachment of C3b to bystander surfaces deficient in sialic acid (Fearon, 1978) that activates the alternative complement pathway at that site because of impaired binding of β1H to C3b on such surfaces (Fearon and Austen, 1977a, 1977b). Thus, discrimination between activating and non-activating surfaces occurs after C3b deposition, and sialic acid deficiency represents the molecular basis for our initial finding that activating particles circumvent the regulatory actions of the control proteins of the alternative pathway.

The molecular basis for the inverse relationship between sialic acid content of a membrane and the capacity of β1H to decay-dissociate amplification convertases on that membrane has been examined by Scatchard analysis of the uptake of β1H by C3b on native and modified erythrocyte membranes (Kazatchkine et al., in press). The effect of sheep erythrocyte membrane sialic acid residues on the binding of B and β1H to membrane-associated C3b was determined with radiolabeled proteins and a technique for separating bound from free ligand by centrifugation of the erythrocytes through an oil/aqueous interphase. The affinity constants at equilibrium (Kassoc) for the interaction of B and β1H with C3b on normal sheep erythrocytes in the presence of 5 mM Mg^{++} were 2.1×10^6 M^{-1} and 1×10^7 M^{-1}, respectively, indicating an approximately five-fold greater affinity of β1H for the C3b binding sites which were present in approximately equal numbers for the two ligands and in the same range as estimated by the amount of ^{125}I-C3b/cell. The affinity of B for C3b on the sheep erythrocytes from which 80% of the sialic acid had been enzymatically removed or chemically modified and for C3b on the zymosan particles was relatively unchanged, and the number of effective binding sites again corresponded to the independent assessment of ^{125}I-C3b present. In contrast, the number of C3b binding sites having a Kassoc for β1H of approximately 10^7 M^{-1} on the sialic acid-deficient erythrocytes or zymosan particles was only 1/5 to 1/6 the number interacting with B. The presence of additional C3b binding sites for β1H having an affinity so low that they were not revealed by Scatchard analysis because of the dominant effect of the high affinity C3b sites was determined in competitive binding studies that measured the capacity of β1H to inhibit uptake of B by C3b on the sialic acid-deficient surfaces. The Kassoc for the interaction of β1H with these C3b sites is approximately 4×10^5 M^{-1}, an affinity that is between 10 and 100-fold less than that of the sialic acid-dependent high affinity C3b sites. Furthermore, the relative inefficiency of β1H in competing with B for binding to C3b on the sialic acid-deficient particles correlated with the decreased capacity of β1H to decay-dissociate Bb from C3b,Bb convertase sites on such particles (Kazatchkine et al., in press). Thus, the content of sialic acid-containing glycoproteins and glycolipids in the microenvironment of bound C3b regulates its interaction with β1H. The presence of sialic acid augments binding of the regulatory protein to favor competition with B, inactivation of C3b and decay-dissociation of C3b,Bb, whereas the absence of sialic acid residues results in low affinity C3b binding of β1H, a circumstance that permits uptake of B to form the amplification convertase and impairs extrinsic decay of the C3 cleaving enzyme (Fig. 2).

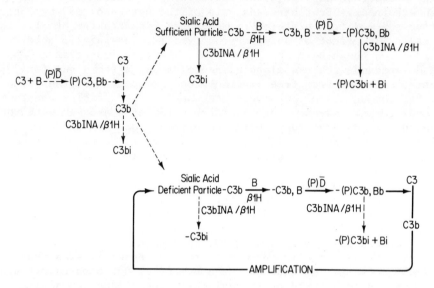

Fig. 2.   Activation of the alternative complement pathway by a
           sialic acid-deficient particle. C3b is slowly generated
           in the fluid phase and may attach to bystander
           surfaces. Those molecules remaining unbound or on
           sialic acid-sufficient particles are rapidly inactivated
           by C3bINA/β1H, and exhibit higher affinities for β1H
           than for B. In contrast, C3b on sialic acid-deficient
           surfaces is relatively resistant to inactivation and
           binding of β1H is impaired, thereby permitting formation
           and function of the amplification convertase (from
           Fearon and Austen, in press).

THE ALTERNATIVE COMPLEMENT PATHWAY – ACTIVATION BY C3 NEPHRITIC
FACTOR (C3NeF), AN AUTOANTIBODY

     Activation of C3 by an alternative pathway occurs in some
patients with membranoproliferative glomerulonephritis who exhibit
marked depressions of C3 but relatively normal levels of C1, C4
and C2 in their sera (Gewurz et al., 1968b). Addition of serum
from these patients to normal serum induced C3 cleavage and this
activity was ascribed to a principle termed C3 nephritic factor
(Spitzer et al., 1969). The action of C3NeF was dependent on the
presence in normal serum of Mg^{++} and B, but not Ca^{++} or C4,
indicating that cleavage of C3 was occurring by the alternative
rather than by the classical pathway (Vallota et al., 1970; Ruley

et al., 1973). A principle with similar characteristics was
subsequently identified in the serum of most patients with partial
lipodystrophy with or without glomerulonephritis (Sissons et al.,
1976).

The capacity of C3NeF to promote C3 cleavage by the
alternative pathway was established as being due to stabilization
of cell-bound or fluid phase C3b,Bb (Daha et al., 1976c) in a
manner such that the convertase was relatively resistant to
decay-dissociation by β1H (Weiler et al., 1976). This in turn
prevented the action of C3bINA since C3bINA cannot inactivate C3b
to which Bb is bound (Daha et al., 1976b). The stabilizing
effects of C3NeF on C3b,Bb permitted isolation of the otherwise
labile complex on sucrose density gradient ultracentrifugation
with the demonstration that the amplification convertase was
indeed a bimolecular complex of C3b,Bb. Stabilization occurs by
the physical association of C3NeF with C3b,Bb (Schreiber et al.,
1976b), and the molecular composition of the stabilized amplification convertase, C3b,Bb(C3NeF), is 1:1:1 (Daha et al., 1976a,
1977).

C3NeF, recognized by its capacity to stabilize the cell-bound
amplification C3 convertase, C3b,Bb, was purified from sera of
three patients with hypocomplementemic glomerulonephritis and of
two patients with partial lipodystrophy by QAE-A50 Sephadex and
sulfopropyl C-25 Sephadex chromatography, affinity for the fluid
phase amplification C3 convertase, and QAE-A50 Sephadex
chromatography (Daha et al., 1977, 1978). Each C3NeF preparation
exhibited heterogeneity during cation exchange chromatography and
the isoelectric points of the eluted fractions ranged from pI 8.3
to 8.9. The chromatographic fractions were incubated with
purified B, $\overline{D}$ and C3 to form fluid phase C3b,Bb(C3NeF), which
sedimented as a 10S complex on sucrose density gradient
ultracentrifugation; the isolated convertase was decayed with
release of C3NeF, which was separated from C3b and Bi by anion
exchange chromatography. Purified preparations of C3NeF that had
been radiolabeled with ^{125}I were bound from 92 to 98% by
erythrocytes bearing C3b,Bb, whereas erythrocytes carrying C3b
bound from 0.6 to 18%, and sensitized erythrocytes alone engaged
in no specific uptake. Analysis of all ^{125}I-C3NeF preparations
by sodium dodecyl sulfate - polyacrylamide gel electrophoresis
demonstrated an apparent m.w. of 150,000. After reduction in the
presence of 8 M urea each ^{125}I-C3NeF preparation revealed
polypeptide chains of 54,000 and 23,500 m.w. which corresponded
with the positions of the heavy and light chains of reduced IgG.
The reaction of ^{125}I-C3NeF from four patients was positive with
Sepharose-bound antisera to IgG, γ1, γ2, κ and λ and negative with
antisera to μ, α, δ , γ3 and γ4. C3NeF from the fifth patient
differed in not reacting with antiserum to κ. These studies
(Daha et al., 1978) indicate that C3NeF is an autoantibody

directed against antigens expressed by the amplification C3
convertase, C3b,Bb, and extend work by others demonstrating
antigenic similarities between C3NeF and IgG (Thompson, 1972;
Davis et al., 1977).

The alternative findings that C3NeF was not an immunoglobulin
because it lacked antigenic identity with IgG on Ouchterlony
analysis with antiserum specific for heavy and light chain
determinants (Vallota et al., 1974) and was composed of two
disulfide-linked polypeptide chains of 85,000 m.w. (Schreiber et
al., 1976b) led to the view that it represented an activated form
of an initiating factor. It is now clear, however, that C3NeF is
an autoantibody to the amplification convertase, C3b,Bb (Daha et
al., 1978). Further, the view that the alternative complement
pathway is comprised of six proteins (Fig. 2) whose interaction is
amplified by surface-dependent deregulation and deposition (Fearon
and Austen, 1977a, 1977b) has been confirmed in studies in which a
previously stated requirement for a postulated initiating factor
(Schreiber et al., 1976a; Medicus et al., 1976) was withdrawn
(Schreiber et al., 1978).

DIRECT RECOGNITION OF ALTERNATIVE COMPLEMENT PATHWAY ACTIVATORS BY
HUMAN MONOCYTES

Zymosan particles and rabbit and mouse erythrocytes were
directly ingested by monolayers of human peripheral blood
monocytes in a serum-free synthetic medium, while sheep and guinea
pig erythrocytes which do not activate the human alternative
complement pathway were not directly ingested by the monocytes
(Czop et al., 1978a). The capacity of human monocytes to ingest
zymosan particles and rabbit erythrocytes was largely diminished
when the monocytes were pretreated with quantities of affinity-
purified trypsin which had no effect on monocyte Fc or C3b
receptor function. This trypsin-sensitive mechanism of monocytes
involved in ingestion of alternative pathway activating particles
was regenerated over 48 hrs during in vitro culture in a serum-
free medium, a result compatible with the restoration of function
of a membrane-associated protein. Thus, the human monocyte
possesses a mechanism for recognition of natural particulate
activators of the alternative complement pathway in the absence of
opsonizing factors such as IgG or C3b that had not previously been
recognized as distinct.

Direct evidence has now been obtained that the monocyte
phagocytic response is initiated by the same surface characteristics that enable a particle to activate the alternative
complement pathway. Sheep erythrocytes, which do not ordinarily
activate the human alternative pathway or initiate a direct monocyte phagocytic response, can be modified to exhibit both func-

tions by deletion or alteration of membrane sialic acid residues
(Fearon, 1978; Czop et al., 1978b). Enzymatic removal of the
sialic acid residues with sialidase or their conversion to
heptulosonic acid derivatives by limited oxidation with $NaIO_4$
and reduction with $NaBH_4$ have equivalent dose-response effects
on the capacity of sheep erythrocytes to initiate directly the
monocyte phagocytic response and to activate the alternative
pathway. The trypsin-sensitive monocyte membrane protein(s)
involved in ingestion of the natural activators, zymosan and
rabbit erythrocytes, and distinct from monocyte Fc and C3b
receptors was also involved in recognition of the altered sheep
erythrocytes. Fixation of C3b to the surface of the desialated
sheep erythrocytes increased the number of monocytes ingesting the
particles, revealing a synergistic interaction between the
monocyte C3b receptor and the trypsin-sensitive receptor for
activators of the alternative pathway. Since such particles would
naturally become coated with C3b in vivo through activation of the
alternative pathway, the synergistic interaction between these two
monocyte receptors would normally be operative for phagocytosis.
The capacity of the non-immune human host to respond to desialated
particles by a dual humoral and cellular recognition mechanism may
represent a primordial biochemical basis for differentiation of
one cell from another or even self from non-self.

REFERENCES

Alper, C.A., Rosen, F.S., and Lachmann, P.J., 1972. Inactivator
      of the third component of complement as an inhibitor in the
      properdin pathway. Proc. Natl. Acad. Sci. USA. 69: 2910.
Aminoff, D., Bell, W.C., Fulton, J., and Ingebrightsen, N., 1976.
      Effect of sialidase on the viability of erythrocytes in
      circulation, Amer. J. Hematol., 1: 419.
Conrad, D.H., Carlo, J.R., and Ruddy, S., 1978. Interaction of
      β1H with cell-bound C3b: Quantitative analysis of binding and
      influence of alternative pathway components on binding. J.
      Exp. Med., 147: 1792.
Czop, J.K., Fearon, D.T., and Austen, K.F., 1978a. Opsonin-inde-
      pendent phagocytosis of activators of the alternative complement
      pathway by human monocytes. J. Immunol., 120: 1132.
Czop, J.K., Fearon, D.T., and Austen, K.F., 1978b. Membrane sialic
      acid on target particles modulates their phagocytosis by a
      trypsin-sensitive mechanism on human monocytes. Proc. Natl.
      Acad. Sci. USA, 75: 3831.

Daha, M.R., Fearon, D.T., and Austen, K.F., 1976a. Isolation of
    alternative pathway C3 convertase containing uncleaved B and
    formed in the presence of C3 nephritic factor (C3NeF). J.
    Immunol., 116: 568.
Daha, M.R., Fearon, D.T., and Austen, K.F., 1976b. C3 requirements
    for formation of alternative pathway C5 convertase, J. Immunol.
    117: 630.
Daha, M.R., Fearon, D.T., and Austen, K.F., 1976c. C3 nephritic
    factor (C3NeF): Stabilization of fluid phase and cell-bound
    alternative pathway convertase. J. Immunol., 116: 1.
Daha, M.R., Austen, K.F., and Fearon, D.T., 1977. The incorporation
    of C3 nephritic factor (C3NeF) into a stabilized C3 convertase,
    C3b,Bb(C3NeF), and its release after decay of convertase
    function. J. Immunool., 119: 812.
Daha, M.R., Austen, K.F., and Fearon, D.T., 1978. Heterogeneity,
    polypeptide chain composition and antigenic reactivity of C3
    nephritic factor. J. Immunol., 120: 1389.
Davis, III, A.E., Ziegler, J.B., Gelfand, E.W., Rosen, F.S., and
    Alper, C.A., 1977. Heterogeneity of nephritic factor and its
    identification as an immunoglobulin. Proc. Natl. Acad. Sci.
    USA. 74: 3980.
Fearon, D.T., 1978. Regulation by membrane sialic acid of β1H-
    dependent decay-dissociation of amplification C3 convertase
    of the alternative complement pathway. Proc. Natl. Acad. Sci.
    USA, 75: 1971.
Fearon, D.T., and Austen, K.F., 1975a. Properdin: Initiation of
    alternative complement pathway. Proc. Natl. Acad. Sci. USA.
    72: 3220.
Fearon, D.T., and Austen, K.F., 1975b. Properdin: Binding to C3b
    and stabilization of the C3b-dependent C3 convertase, J. Exp.
    Med., 142: 856.
Fearon, D.T., and Austen, K.F., 1975c. Initiation of C3 cleavage
    in the alternative complement pathway. J. Immunol., 115: 1357.
Fearon, D.T., and Austen, K.F., 1977a. Activation of the alternative
    complement pathway due to resistance of zymosan-bound amplifi-
    cation convertase to endogenous regulatory mechanisms. Proc.
    Natl. Acad. Sci. USA. 74: 1683.
Fearon, D.T., and Austen, K.F., 1977b. Activation of the alternative
    complement pathway with rabbit erythrocytes by circumvention
    of the regulatory action of endogenous control proteins. J.
    Exp. Med., 146: 22.
Fearon, D.T., and Austen, K.F., in press. Activation mechanisms of
    the alternative complement pathway and amplification step. In:
    "The Physical Chemistry, Molecular Biology and Physiological
    Function of Human Plasma Proteins," Dr. Bing, ed., Pergamon
    Press, Inc., New York.
Fearon, D.T., Austen, K.F., and Ruddy, S., 1973. Formation of a
    hemolytically active cellular intermediate by the interaction
    between properdin factors B and D and the activated third
    component of complement, J. Exp. Med., 138: 1305.

Fearon, D.T., Austen, K.F., and Ruddy, S., 1974. Properdin factor
    D: Characterization of its active site and isolation of the
    precursor form. J. Exp. Med., 139: 355.
Frank, M.M., May, J., Gaither, T., and Ellman, L., 1971. In vitro
    studies of complement function in sera of C4-deficient guinea
    pigs. J. Exp. Med., 134: 176.
Gewurz, H., Shin, H.S., and Mergenhagen, S.E., 1968a. Interactions
    of the complement system with endotoxic lipopolysaccharide:
    Consumption of each of the six terminal complement components.
    J. Exp. Med., 128: 1049.
Gewurz, H., Pickering, R.J., Mergenhagen, S.E., and Good, R.A.,
    1968b. The complement profile in acute glomerulonephritis,
    systemic lupus erythematosus and hypocomplementemic chronic
    glomerulonephritis. Int. Arch. Allergy. 34: 556.
Goodkofsky, I., and Lepow, I.H., 1971. Functional relationship of
    factor B in the properdin system to C3 proactivator of human
    serum. J. Immunol., 107: 1200.
Götze, O., and Müller-Eberhard, H.J., 1971. The C3-activator
    system: An alternate pathway of complement activation. J. Exp.
    Med., 134, Suppl. 90.
Kazatchkine, M.K., Fearon, D.T., and Austen, K.F., in press.
    Human alternative complement pathway: Membrane-associated
    sialic acid regulates the competition between B and β1H for
    cell-bound C3b. J. Immunol.
Marcus, R.L., Shin, H.S., and Mayer, M.M., 1971. An alternate
    complement pathway: C3-cleaving activity, not due to C4b,2a,
    on endotoxic lipopolysaccharide after treatment with guinea
    pig serum. Proc. Natl. Acad. Sci. USA. 68: 1351.
Medicus, R.G., Schreiber, R.D., Götze, O., and Müller-Eberhard,
    H.J., 1976. A molecular concept of the properdin pathway.
    Proc. Natl. Acad. Sci. USA. 73: 612.
Müller-Eberhard, H.J., and Götze, O., 1972. C3 proactivator
    convertase and its mode of action. J. Exp. Med., 135: 1003.
Nelson, R.A. Jr., 1966. A new concept of immunosuppression in
    hypersensitivity reactions and in transplantation immunity.
    Survey Ophthalmol., 11: 498.
Nydegger, U.E., Fearon, D.T., and Austen, K.F., in press. Regulation
    by an autosomal locus of the inverse relationship between
    sialic acid content and the capacity of mouse erythrocytes
    to activate the human alternative complement pathway. Proc.
    Natl. Acad. Sci. USA.
Pangburn, M.K., and Müller-Eberhard, H.J., 1978. Complement C3
    convertase: Cell surface restriction of β1H control and
    generation of restriction on neuraminidase-treated cells.
    Proc. Natl. Acad. Sci. USA. 75: 2416.
Pangburn, M.K., Schreiber, R.D., and Müller-Eberhard, H.J., 1978.
    Molecular interactions of the control proteins, C3b inactivator
    and β1H, with various complement intermediates. J. Immunol.,
    120: 1791.

Phaff, H.J., 1963. Cell wall of yeasts. Ann. Rev. Microbiol., 17: 15.

Pillemer, L., Lepow, I.H., and Blum, L., 1953. The requirement for a hydrazine-sensitive serum factor and heat-labile serum factors in the inactivation of human C3 by zymosan. J. Immunol., 71: 339.

Pillemer, L., Blum, L., Lepow, I.H., Ross, O.A., Todd, E.D., and Wardlaw, A.C., 1954. The properdin system and immunity: I. Demonstration and isolation of a new serum protein, properdin, and its role in immune phenomena. Science. 120: 279.

Platts-Mills, T.A.E., and Ishizaka, K., 1974. Activation of the alternate pathway of human complement by rabbit cells. J. Immunol., 113: 348.

Ruley, E.H., Forristal, J., Davis, N.C., Andres, C., and West, C.D., 1973. Hypocomplementemia of membranoproliferative nephritis: Dependence of the nephritic factor reaction on properdin factor B. J. Clin. Invest. 52: 896.

Sandberg, A.L., and Osler, A.G., 1971. Dual pathways of complement interaction with guinea pig immunoglobulins. J. Immunol., 107: 1268.

Schreiber, R.D., Götze, O., and Müller-Eberhard, H.J., 1976a. Alternative pathway of complement: Demonstration and characterization of initiating factor and its properdin-independent function. J. Exp. Med., 144: 1062.

Schreiber, R.E., Götze, O., and Müller-Eberhard, H.J., 1976b. Nephritic factor: Its structure and function and relationship to initiating factor of the alternative pathway. Scand. J. Immunol., 5: 705.

Schreiber, R.D., Pangburn, M.K., LeSavre, P.H., and Müller-Eberhard, H.J., 1978. Initiation of the alternative pathway of complement: Recognition of activators by bound C3b and assembly of the entire pathway from six isolated proteins. Proc. Natl. Acad. Sci. USA. 75: 3948.

Sissons, J.G.P., West, R.G., Fallows, J., Williams, D.G., Boucher, B.J., Amos, N., and Peters, D.K., 1976. The complement abnormalities of lipodystrophy. New Engl. J. Med., 297: 461.

Spitzer, R.E., Vallota, E.H., Forristal, J., Sudora, E., Stitzel, A., Davis, N.G., and West, C.D., 1969. Serum C3 lytic system in patients with glomerulonephritis. Science. 164: 436.

Thompson, R.A., 1972. C3 inactivating factor in the serum of a patient with chronic hypocomplementemic proliferative glomerulonephritis. Immunology. 22: 147.

Valotta, E.H., Forristal, J., Spitzer, R.E., Davis, N.C., and West, C.D., 1970. Characteristics of a non-complement dependent C3 reactive complex formed from factors in nephritic serum and normal serum. J. Exp. Med., 131: 1306.

Vallota, E.H., Götze, O., Spiegelberg, H.H., Forristal, J., West, C.D., and Müller-Eberhard, H.J., 1974. A serum factor in chronic hypocomplementemic nephritis distinct from immunoglobulin and activating the alternative pathway of complement. J. Exp. Med. 139: 1249.

Weiler, J.M., Daha, M.R., Austen, K.F., and Fearon, D.T., 1976. Control of the amplification convertase of complement by the plasma protein β1H. Proc. Natl. Acad. Sci. USA. 73: 3268.

Whaley, K., and Ruddy, S., 1976. Modulation of the alternative complement pathway by β1H globulin. J. Exp. Med., 144: 1147.

ROLE OF BOVINE HIGH-MOLECULAR-WEIGHT (HMW) KININOGEN IN CONTACT-MEDIATED ACTIVATION OF BOVINE FACTOR XII

H. KATO, T. SUGO, N. IKARI, N. HASHIMOTO, I. MARUYAMA,
Y. N. HAN[*], S. IWANAGA[**] and S. FUJII

Institute for Protein Research, Osaka University
Suita, Osaka 565, Japan

High-molecular-weight (HMW) kininogen is now accepted as an essential factor in the contact-mediated activation of Factor XII (Hageman factor), a precursor protein of a serine protease (activated Factor XII, XIIa), which is activated in contact with many kinds of solid surfaces (Wuepper et al. 1975, Colman et al. 1975, Saito et al. 1975, Kaplan et al. 1976). This activation is a complex reaction which involves the interaction of at least four proteins, viz., Factor XII, HMW kininogen, prekallikrein and Factor XI, triggering intrinsic blood coagulation and kinin liberation (Mandle et al. 1976, Thompson et al. 1977, Revak et al. 1978, Griffin, 1978). HMW kininogen accelerates the reaction by serving as a cofactor (Griffin and Cochrane, 1976, Meier et al. 1977, Lie et al. 1977, Wiggins et al. 1977, Saito, 1977), analogous to Factor V and Factor VIII in the activation of prothrombin and Factor X, respectively. However, the mechanism of action of HMW kininogen as cofactor remains to be established.

In the present work, we studied the effect of bovine HMW kininogen and its fragments on the activation of Factor XII in the presence of prekallikrein and kaolin, in order to elucidate the functional site of HMW kininogen which interacts with kaolin and prekallikrein.

Bovine HMW kininogen is a single-polypeptide glycoprotein with a molecular weight of 76,000, consisting of four domains, heavy chain (M.W. 48,000), the kinin moiety (M.W. 1,000), fragment 1·2 (M.W. 12,000) and light chain (M.W. 16,000) (Kato et al. 1976), as shown in Fig. 1. We have determined the amino acid sequences of

---

[*] Present address: Korea Ginseng Research Institute, Seoul, Korea
[**] Present address: Dept. of Biology, Faculty of Science, Kyushu University, Fukuoka 812, Japan.

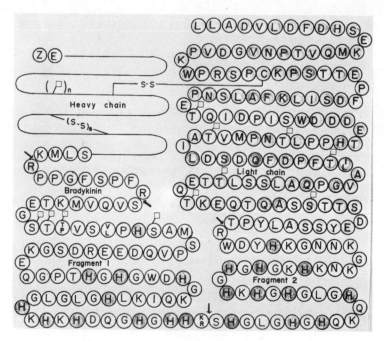

Fig. 1.   Partial amino acid sequence of bovine HMW kininogen.
(Han et al. 1975, 1976, Hashimoto et al. 1977)
↓ Cleaved by plasma kallikrein
Ϙ Carbohydrate chain

fragment 1·2 (Han et al. 1975, Han et al. 1976) and light chain
portion (Hashimoto et al. 1977). Bovine plasma kallikrein liberates
bradykinin and fragment 1·2 (formerly named as histidine-rich peptide) and carbohydrate-free fragment 1·2 (formerly named fragment
X) from HMW kininogen (Han et al. 1978ab). The carbohydrate structure of the fragment 1·2 has also been determined (Endo et al. 1977).
Waldmann et al. (1976) and Matheson et al. (1976) have found in
collaboration with us that bovine HMW kininogen corrects the coagulation abnormality of kininogen deficient plasma, Fitzgerald trait
and Flaujeac trait plasmas. They have also revealed that kinin-
free protein and a polypeptide consisting of fragment 1·2 and light
chain have the correcting activity on the kininogen deficient plasmas, while kinin and fragment 1·2-free protein and light chain did
not show any activity (Waldmann et al. 1977, Wuepper et al. 1978).
Oh-ishi et al. (1977) have found that fragment 1·2 has the strong
inhibitory activity on the activation of Factor XII. These results
suggest that a region containing fragment 1·2 and light chain in
HMW kininogen has the important roles in the surface-mediated activation of Factor XII.

The activation of Factor XII has been assessed by measuring the kallikrein generated from prekallikrein with substrates such as TAME (Cochrane et al. 1973, Chan et al. 1976), Z-Phe-Val-Arg-p-nitroanilide (Meier et al. 1977) or Z-Pro-Phe-Arg-p-nitroanilide (Griffin 1978). We have found that Z-Phe-Arg-4-methylcoumarin amide is a specific and sensitive fluorogenic substrate for plasma kallikrein (Morita et al. 1977). In the work described below, this substrate was used for the quantitative estimation of the effect of HMW kininogen on the activation of Factor XII by measuring the kallikrein generated after mixing Factor XII, HMW kininogen and prekallikrein with kaolin. The results indicate that fragment 1·2 and light chain regions in HMW kininogen plays important roles for the activation of Factor XII, interacting with kaolin and prekallikrein.

MATERIALS AND METHODS

Bovine plasma kallikrein (23.5 TAME units per mg of protein) and bovine plasmin (10 TAME units per mg of protein) were prepared as reported previously (Han et al. 1978b). Human urinary kallikrein (1.7 TAME units per mg of protein) was kindly supplied by Dr. N. Ogawa, Mochida Pharmaceutical Co. Carbobenzyloxy-phenylalanyl-arginyl-4-methylcoumarin amide (Z-Phe-Arg-MCA) was a product of the Protein Research Foundation, Minoh, Osaka. Kaolin (acid washed-American Standard) was purchased from Fisher Scientific Co., Pittsburgh, PA. Derivatives of HMW kininogen were prepared as follows: Kinin-free protein was isolated after the incubation of HMW kininogen with human urinary kallikrein (Han et al. 1978b). Kinin and fragment 1·2-free protein and fragment 1·2 were prepared by the incubation of HMW kininogen with bovine plasma kallikrein (Han et al. 1976). Heavy chain and light chain were obtained by the reduction and carboxymethylation of kinin and fragment 1·2-free protein. A polypeptide consisting of fragment 1·2 and light chain was obtained by the reduction and carboxymethylation of kinin-free protein (Han et al. 1978b). HMW kininogen with a single polypeptide chain was isolated by CM-Sephadex C-50 column chromatography after reduction and carboxymethylation and designated as RCM-HMW kininogen-b (Komiya 1972). Low-molecular-weight (LMW) kininogen was prepared as reported previously (Yano et al. 1967). p-Chlorobenzyl-amine-ε-aminocaproyl-Sepharose (PCB-Sepharose) was made by coupling Sepharose 4B with ε-aminocaproyl-p-chlorobenzylamine (Product of Protein Research Foundation, Minoh, Osaka), using cyanogen bromide, according to the method of Cuatrecasas (1970).

Bioassay of kinin was performed as reported elsewhere (Yano et al. 1971). Polyacrylamide gel electrophoresis in the presence of sodium dodecyl sulfate (SDS) was performed as described by Weber and Osborn (1969). The following proteins were used for the calibration of molecular weight: cytochrome c, myoglobin, chymotrypsinogen A, ovalbumin, bovine serum albumin and phosphorylase b.

Factor XII activity was measured by kaolin-activated partial thromboplastin time, using Factor XII-deficient plasma, which was kindly supplied by Prof. E. W. Davie, University of Washington, Seattle,
and by Dr. T. Kamiya, Nagoya University School of Medicine, Nagoya.
Purification of HMW Kininogen, Factor XII and Prekallikrein
       HMW kininogen (Komiya et al. 1974a), prekallikrein (Takahashi
et al. 1972) and Factor XII (Fujikawa et al. 1977a) were prepared
from bovine plasma by the modification of the previous methods as
described below.
       Bovine plasma (5.2 1) was first applied to a column (23 x 7
cm) of DEAE-Sephadex A-50, which was equilibrated with 0.02 M Tris-
HCl buffer, pH 8.0, containing 0.04 M NaCl, benzamidine (3 mM) and
polybrene (0.5 mg/l). After washing with 18 1 of the same buffer,
gradient elution was performed with each 9 1 of the same buffer and
the buffer containing 0.6 M NaCl. Factor XII and kininogen were
eluted with 0.2 M NaCl and 0.3 M NaCl, respectively. Although prekallikrein was eluted in three fractions, nonadsorbed fraction,
Factor XII fraction and kininogen fraction, about two-thirds of
total prekallikrein was found in the nonadsorbed fraction.
       For further purification of HMW kininogen, kininogen fractions
were pooled and subjected to second DEAE-Sephadex A-50 column chromatography. Prekallikrein, which had been contaminated in the
kininogen fractions in the first step, could not be separated from
kininogen in the second step. However, the contaminating prekallikrein was successfully removed by a PCB-Sepharose 4B column. Kininogen fraction from second DEAE-Sephadex column chromatography was
applied to the PCB-Sepharose column (7 x 20 cm), which had been
equilibrated with 0.02 M Tris-HCl buffer, pH 8.0, containing 0.05 M
NaCl. After washing the column with 1 1 of the buffer, prekallikrein was eluted with the buffer containing 25 % dioxane. Final
purification of HMW kininogen was performed as described in the
previous method (Komiya et al. 1974a), by using CM-Sephadex C-50
column chromatography and gel-filtration on a column of Sephadex
G-150. HMW kininogen thus obtained showed the same patterns on
SDS-polyacrylamide gel electrophoresis as reported previously
(Komiya et al. 1974a) (Fig. 2). The present preparation of HMW
kininogen did not liberate kinin spontaneously by incubating it at
37°C, overnight. The absence of prekallikrein in HMW kininogen was
also confirmed using Factor XIIa. For the purification of Factor
XII, fractions from the first DEAE-Sephadex A-50 column, was subjected to second DEAE-Sephadex A-50 and PCB-Sepharose column chro-
matographies to remove prekallikrein. Further purification of
Factor XII was performed according to the method of Fujikawa et al.
(Fujikawa et al. 1977a). Prekallikrein was purified from the nonadsorbed fraction of the first DEAE-Sephadex A-50 column chromatography (Takahashi et al. 1972), except the use of PCB-Sepharose
instead of Arg-Sepharose. Homogeneity of Factor XII and prekallikrein is shown in Fig. 2.
Iodination of HMW kininogen by [125]Iodine
       In 2.5 ml of 0.1 M phosphate buffer, pH 7.5, containing 0.9

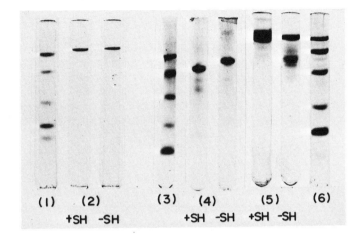

Fig. 2. SDS-polyacrylamide gel electrophoresis of Factor XII, prekallikrein, and HMW kininogen.
(1) Marker proteins: bovine serum albumin, ovalbumin, chymotrypsin-
ogen-A, myoglobin and cytochrome c   (2) Factor XII   (3) Marker
proteins: phosphorylase b, bovine serum albumin, ovalbumin, chymo-
trypsinogen-A and myoglobin   (4) prekallikrein   (5) HMW kininogen
(6) Same as (3).   Electrophoresis was carried out in 8.0 %
polyacrylamide gel at 7 mA/tubr for 4 hr as described in METHODS.
The anode was at the bottom of the gels.

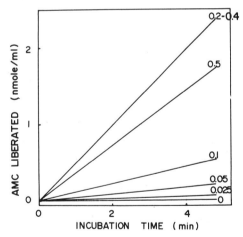

Fig. 3. Accelerating effect of HMW kininogen on the activation of
Factor XII. Activation of Factor XII was performed by mixing HMW
kininogen, Factor XII, kaolin and subsequently adding prekallikrein,
as described in METHODS. Kallikrein generated was estimated by its
initial velocity to hydrolyze Z-Phe-Arg-MCA. The values in the
figure indicate the final concentration (μg/ml) of HMW kininogen in
the reaction mixture.

mC of $Na^{125}I$ (the radiochemical centre, England), 100 µl of HMW
kininogen (2 mg/ml) and 50 µl of chloramine T (1 mg/ml) were added.
After 10 min at 4°C, 50 µl of $Na_2S_2O_5$ solution (1 mg/ml) was added.
DFP was added to the solution to give a final concentration of 50
mM.   After 3 hr at 20°C, the solution was dialyzed three times
against 5 l of 0.02 M Tris-EDTA-0.2 M NaCl buffer, pH 8.0. ^{125}I-
HMW kininogen showed the same patterns on SDS-polyacrylamide gel
electrophoresis and the same acceleration effect on the activation
of Factor XII as that of non-labelled HMW kininogen.

Measurement of Activation of Factor XII

    The system used was as follows: in 0.475 ml of 0.02 M Tris-
HCl buffer, pH 8.0, containing 0.15 M NaCl and bovine serum albumin
(0.1 mg/ml), 5 µl of Factor XII (A_{280}=0.025) was added.   HMW kininogen solution (1 mg/ml) was serially diluted with the above buffer
and each 5 µl was added to the above solution to give final concentration of 0 to 0.5 µg/ml.   To the mixture of Factor XII and HMW
kininogen, 10 µl of kaolin (0.125 % (w/v) in the buffer) was added
and the suspension was incubated at 37°C for 15 min.   Then, 10 µl
of prekallikrein (A_{280}=0.29) was added and the mixture was further
preincubated for 15 min at 37°C.   The kallikrein activity generated
was measured by its initial velocity to hydrolyze Z-Phe-Arg-MCA by
adding 5 µl of 10 mM Z-Phe-Arg-MCA (dissolved in dimethylformamide)
to the reaction mixture.   The amount of 7-amino-5-methylcoumarin
(AMC) liberated within 1 min was estimated fluorometrically (exci-
tation at 380 nm, emission at 460 nm) with a Hitachi fluorescence
spectrophotometer, model MPF-2A (Morita et al. 1977).

Measurement of Prekallikrein

    The activated form of bovine Factor XII (XIIa) was isolated by
the method of Fujikawa et al. (1977b).   Each 5 µl aliquot of prekallikrein was mixed with 0.5 ml of 0.02 M Tris-HCl buffer, pH 8.0
containing 0.15 M NaCl and bovine serum albumin (2 mg/ml).   To the
reaction mixture, 10 µl of Factor XIIa (A_{280}=0.014) was added and
the solution was incubated at 37°C.   After 30 min, 5 µl of 10 mM
Z-Phe-Arg-MCA was added to the reaction mixture and further incubated for 30 min.   The measurement of AMC liberated was performed
as described above.

RESULTS

Accelerating Effects of HMW Kiniogen and Its Fragments on Kaolin-
Mediated Activation of Factor XII

    Fig. 3 shows the initial release of AMC by the kallikrein
generated in a system containing HMW kininogen, Factor XII, kaolin
and prekallikrein.   Kallikrein generation was dependent on the
amount of HMW kininogen in the reaction mixture; only minimal
activity was generated in the absence of HMW kininogen.   In the
presence of 0.2 µg to 0.4 µg of HMW kininogen, the activation of
Factor XII was accelerated 180-fold.   However, under the conditions
used, the activation was less when 0.5 µg of HMW kininogen was
added.   No amidase activity was generated when prekallikrein was
omitted from the reaction mixture.   To exclude the possible con-

tamination of kallikrein or Factor XIIa in the components used, Factor XII, HMW kininogen and prekallikrein were pretreated, respectively, with DFP (final concentration of 10^{-3}M) for 1 hr at room temperature, and dialyzed overnight against 0.02 M Tris-HCl buffer, pH 8.0, containing 0.15 M NaCl. With these preparations, the same kallikrein activity was generated in the complete system. These results show that the activation of Factor XII occurred by the contact of prekallikrein, Factor XII and HMW kininogen with kaolin.

The activation rates of Factor XII with kaolin were very much dependent on the amounts of kaolin. With final concentration of 0.025 % of kaolin, kallikrein activity generated from prekallikrein was dependent on the amounts of Factor XII, when 0.27 µg of HMW kininogen and 2.9 µg of prekallikrein was used. With 0.062 µg of Factor XII, kallikrein activity increased linearly up to 20 min.

Using the optimum conditions described above, the effects of HMW kininogen and its derivatives were examined. The accelerating effect was expressed, comparing with the activation rate of Factor XII in the absence of HMW kininogen. As shown in Fig. 4, the generation of kallikrein was maximum with 1-5 pmole of HMW kininogen. The acceleration effect of HMW kininogen decreased with more than 5 pmole of kininogen and disappeared with 20 pmole or more of HMW kininogen. When HMW kininogen (3 mg) was dissolved in 10 ml of 10 % acetic acid and then lyophilized, the accelerating effect of such acid-treated HMW kininogen was low. The large fragment consisting of fragment 1·2 and light chain (Fl·2-L) showed the same accelerating effect as that of intact HMW kininogen, and the effect did not decrease up to 15 pmole. Although kinin-free protein also showed the same effect, the dose-dependency was quite different from that of HMW kininogen. With 0.25 pmole of kinin-free protein, the maximum activation of Factor XII was observed and the effect disappeared with more than 1 pmole. Kinin and fragment 1·2-free protein, fragment 1·2, light chain, mixture of fragment 1·2 and light chain, heavy chain and LMW kininogen did not show any accelerating effect on the activation of Factor XII, respectively.

The activity of plasma kallikrein to hydrolyze Z-Phe-Arg-MCA was neither accelerated nor inhibited by HMW kininogen and its derivatives within the range of the amounts used in Fig. 4. Since HMW kininogen is a natural substrate for plasma kallikrein, it could inhibit the amidase activity of plasma kallikrein. However, the molar concentration of HMW kininogen (about 10^{-8}M) used in this experiment is far less than that of Z-Phe-Arg-MCA (10^{-4}M).

Fig. 5 summarizes the effects of HMW kininogen and its derivatives on the activation of Factor XII with kaolin. The accelerating effects of these proteins were compared by the minimum amounts of the proteins to show the maximum accelerating effects. The results clearly indicate that only the proteins having both of fragment 1·2 and light chain regions accelerated the kaolin-mediated activation of Factor XII. Among four proteins which showed the accelerating effects, kinin-free protein was the most

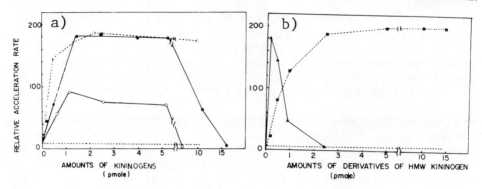

Fig. 4. Acceleration effect of HMW kininogen and its derivatives on the kaolin-mediated activation of Factor XII.
Factor XII was preincubated with kaolin and the various amounts of HMW kininogen and its derivatives, for 15 min and with prekallikrein for 15 min at the same conditions as described in Fig. 2. Relative acceleration rate of HMW kininogen and its derivatives were calculated comparing with the amounts of kallikrein generated in the absence of HMW kininogen.

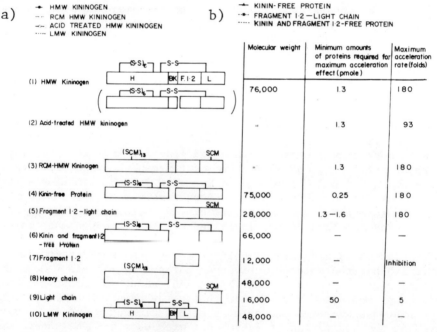

Fig. 5. Summary of the relative acceleration rates of HMW kininogen and its derivatives on the kaolin-mediated activation of Factor XII.
From the data shown in Fig. 2, the acceleration effects of each protein were expressed as the maximum acceleration rates, which were given by minimum amounts of proteins.

efficient for the activation of Factor XII.   However, fragment 1·2 itself inhibited the activation of Factor XII.

As reported previously (Komiya et al. 1974ab), our HMW kininogen preparation contained at least two kinds of molecular species, one of which was nicked at the carboxyl-terminus of the kinin moiety.   Since the separation of these two molecular species is yet unsuccessful, we could not compare their accelerating effects. However, an S-alkylated single chain derivatives of HMW kininogen was separable by CM-Sephadex column chromatography.   The kininogen, called as RCM-HMW kininogen-b, had the same accelerating effect as HMW kininogen.   This result suggests that each HMW kininogen, a single polypeptide chain and two polypeptide chains, has the accelerating effect on the activation of Factor XII.

Changes of the Accelerating Effect of HMW Kininogen during Incubation with Human Urinary Kallikrein, Bovine Plasma Kallikrein or Bovine Plasmin

In the previous studies (Han et al. 1976, Han et al. 1978b) we demonstrated that bovine plasma kallikrein simultaneously liberates fragment 1·2 and bradykinin from bovine HMW kininogen, whereas human urinary kallikrein liberates only kinin.   On the other hand, plasmin liberates kinin slowly, but it rapidly hydrolyzes the portion of HMW kininogen that comprises fragment 1·2 and the light chain, yielding a protein with a molecular weight of 50,000 (Han et al. 1978b).   In the second phase of the present study, we investigated the effect of incubating HMW kininogen with each of these enzymes on its ability to accelerate the activation of Factor XII.

To 0.5 ml of HMW kininogen solution (2 mg/ml of 0.2 M ammonium bicarbonate, pH 8.0), urinary kallikrein, plasma kallikrein or plasmin was added at an enzyme to substrate weight ratio of 1 to 200, 1 to 500 or 1 to 100, respectively.   These enzyme to substrate ratios were chosen to give slow liberation of kinin, referring from the previous report (Han et al. 1978b).   After various periods of incubation at 37°C, 50 μl aliquots were removed and mixed with 5 μl of 50 mM DFP.   After these mixtures had remained at room temperature for 4 hr, 5 μl of each was assayed for kinin with the isolated rat uterus bio-assay, and 25 μl of each was freeze dried and subsequently dissolved in 1.0 ml of 0.02 M Tris-HCl buffer, pH 8.0, containing 0.15 M NaCl and bovine serum albumin (0.1 mg/ml).   Each of the resulting solutions was diluted 20-fold with the same buffer, and 20 μl portions were used to determine their effect on Factor XII activation, as described in METHODS.   In this experiment, the equivalent amount of non-treated HMW kininogen (0.05 μg) accelerated the activation of Factor XII 5-fold. The relative effects of enzyme-treated HMW kininogen were expressed in terms of the accelerating effect of non-treated kininogen, which was taken as 1.0.

As shown in Fig. 6, the accelerating effect of HMW kininogen was markedly enhanced at the early stages of incubation with either plasma kallikrein or urinary kallikrein.   In the former case, the

Fig. 6. Changes of the accelerating effect of HMW kininogen
during incubation with human
urinary kallikrein, bovine
plasma kallikrein or bovine
plasmin.
The experimental procedures
used are described in the text.
The relative effect of enzyme-
treated HMW kininogen at each
stage of incubation was calculated by taking the accelerating effect of HMW kininogen as 1.0. Treated with
urinary kallikrein (——●——),
plasma kallikrein (——▲——) and
plasmin (——■——). Kinin liberated from HMW kininogen with
urinary kallikrein (--○--),
plasma kallikrein (--△--) and
plasmin (--□--). Inset shows
patterns of the digests of HMW
kininogen with urinary kallikrein after 0.5 and 3 hr and with
plasma kallikrein after 1 and 3
hr and of HMW kininogen without
incubation on SDS-polyacrylamide gel electrophoresis in the
presence of 2-mercaptoethanol.

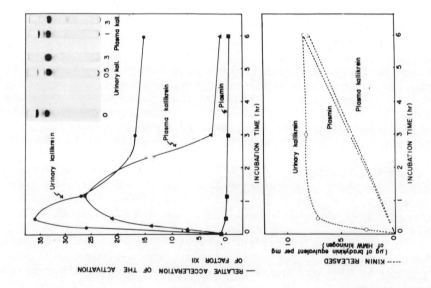

enhancement occurred long before the release of kinin reached a maximum. Whereas the enhancement produced by pretreatment with plasma kallikrein decayed rapidly, that obtained with urinary kallikrein fell to about half its maximal value and remained relatively constant. On the other hand, no amplification was observed with plasmin-treated HMW kininogen; in fact the accelerating effect of intact HMW kininogen appeared to be abolished by plasmin (Fig. 6).

The accelerating effect of HMW kininogen decayed during prolonged incubation with plasma kallikrein. This decay may be due, in part, to the accumulation of fragment 1·2 liberated from the kininogen; isolated fragment 1·2 has been shown to be a potent inhibitor of the contact activation of Factor XII (Oh-ishi et al. 1977). Moreover, a later product of HMW kininogen incubation with plasma kallikrein (viz., the kinin- and fragment 1·2-free protein) has no accelerating effect under the conditions described above. By contrast, a later product of HMW kininogen incubation with urinary kallikrein, kinin-free protein, had a potent accelerating effect. This combination of factors may explain why the enhancement brought about by plasma kallikrein decayed more rapidly than that produced with urinary kallikrein. Furthermore, the complete abolition of HMW kininogen's accelerating effect by treatment with plasmin emphasizes the importance of the fragment 1·2-light chain region of bovine kininogen in the acceleration of Factor XII activation.

The inset of Fig. 6 shows reduced SDS-gel patterns of HMW kininogen incubation with urinary kallikrein and plasma kallikrein for 0.5 hr, 3 hr and 1 hr, 3 hr, respectively. Since our HMW kininogen preparation is a mixture of a single polypeptide protein and a nicked protein, its SDS-gel pattern at zero time shows two bands, which corresponds to a single polypeptide kininogen and a polypeptide consisting of heavy chain and the kinin moiety. After 30 min or 60 min incubation with urinary kallikrein, the single polypeptide kininogen appeared to have been degraded into a two-chains protein, and completely degraded after 3 hr. These results strongly indicate that a nicked form of HMW kininogen has the most potent accelerating effect on kaolin-mediated activation of Factor XII.

Interaction of HMW Kininogen with Prekallikrein and Kaolin

It has been reported that human prekallikrein makes a complex with human HMW kininogen (Mandle et al. 1976). Thus, the role of HMW kininogen has been suggested to concentrate prekallikrein on surface, interacting with prekallikrein and kaolin. As described in the previous section, we have revealed that fragment 1·2 and light chain region in bovine HMW kininogen is essential for the accelerating effect on the activation of Factor XII. In this section, we intended to examine the functional sites of HMW kininogen which are required for the interaction with prekallikrein and kaolin, using ^{125}I-HMW kininogen.

We first tried to find what portion of HMW kininogen contributes to the binding with kaolin. Kaolin was first pretreated with

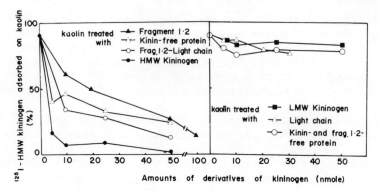

Fig. 7.   Inhibition of adsorption of ^{125}I-HMW kininogen on kaolin
by derivatives of HMW kininogen.
In 0.1 ml of 0.02 M Tris-HCl-0.15 M NaCl buffer, pH 8.0, containing
various amounts of the derivatives of HMW kininogen (0-100 nmole),
100 µl of 0.2 % kaolin was added.   After 20 min at room temperature, supernatant was removed by centrifugation at 3,000 r.p.m.
for 3 min.   The precipitate was suspended in 0.2 ml of 0.02 M Tris-
HCl-0.15 M NaCl buffer, pH 8.0, containing 1 µg of ^{125}I-HMW kininogen, and the radioactivity of the suspension was measured (T).
After 20 min at room temperature, precipitate was removed by centrifugation and 100 µl of the supernatant was subjected to the
measurement of radioactivity (S/2).   The percentage of ^{125}I-HMW
kininogen adsorbed on kaolin was calculated by the equation of
T-S/T x 100.

the various amounts of HMW kininogen and its derivatives.   After
centrifugation, ^{125}I-HMW kininogen was mixed with the precipitate
and HMW kininogen adsorbed on kaolin was quantitated by measuring
the radioactivity of the supernatant.   Fig. 7 shows that fragment
1·2 and the proteins with the fragment 1·2 moiety inhibited the
adsorption of ^{125}I-HMW kininogen on kaolin, while the proteins
without the fragment 1·2 moiety and LMW kininogen did not.
     The results suggest that HMW kininogen binds on kaolin
through fragment 1·2 region.   As previously reported (Oh-ishi et
al. 1977), fragment 1·2 has an inhibitory action on the activation
of Factor XII in rat and human plasmas.   Moreover, fragment 1·2
inhibited the accelerating effect of HMW kininogen on kaolin-
mediated activation of Factor XII, as described in this paper.
Thus, it can be speculated that HMW kininogen accelerates the
activation of Factor XII by binding on kaolin through fragment 1·2
region in a form of complex with prekallikrein.   The inhibitory
activity of fragment 1·2 can be partly explained by its competitive
binding on kaolin with HMW kininogen.
     To confirm a complex formation between prekallikrein and ^{125}I-
HMW kininogen, these were mixed in a various molar ratio and sub-

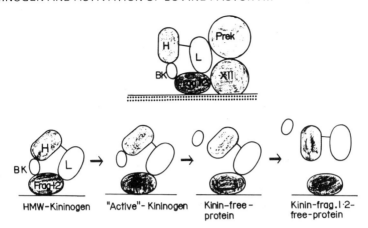

Fig. 8. Tentative scheme for the kaolin-mediated activation of Factor XII with HMW kininogen and prekallikrein in bovine system.

jected to gel-filtration on a column of Sephacryl S-200. Since bovine HMW kininogen alone shows an apparent molecular weight of 200,000-300,000 on gel-filtration, the complex of prekallikrein and HMW kininogen could not be separated from HMW kininogen. However, in a molar ratio of one to one or less than that, all prekallikrein added was co-eluted with HMW kininogen, indicating that bovine prekallikrein and bovine HMW kininogen form a complex consisting of each one mole of proteins. What portion of HMW kininogen is responsible for the interaction with prekallikrein is not known yet. It seems to be a light chain portion, since fragment 1·2 and light chain region is essential for the accelerating effect of HMW kininogen and fragment 1·2 region is required for the binding with kaolin.

DISCUSSION

It has been revealed that the coagulation abnormality of kininogen deficient plasma is corrected not only by human HMW kininogen but also by bovine HMW kininogen (Waldmann et al. 1976, Matheson et al. 1976). In order to examine the role of HMW kininogen in contact phase, it seems to be necessary to examine the effect of HMW kininogen on the activation of Factor XII, using purified components. Before we start these works, we had to dissolve two problems; the preparation of HMW kininogen free from prekallikrein and the development of the sensitive assay method to measure quantitatively Factor XII activity. As described previously (Komiya et al. 1974a), it has been quite difficult to remove a trace amount of prekallikrein contaminated in HMW kininogen preparation. We tried to find the best ligand for affinity chromato-

graphy of prekallikrein, and we found that prekallikrein in HMW
kininogen preparation can be successfully removed by the application of p-chlorobenzylamine-Sepharose. We have previously developed the sensitive fluorogenic substrate for kallikrein, Z-Phe-Arg-
MCA (Morita et al. 1977). Using this substrate, we could follow
quantitatively the activation of Factor XII in the presence of HMW
kininogen, prekallikrein and kaolin by measuring the initial velocity of kallikrein activity generated.

This paper presented unequivocally the evidence that kallikrein was generated by mixing the precursor forms of serine proteases, Factor XII and prekallikrein, in the presence of kaolin
and HMW kininogen. No appreciable contamination of the activated
forms, XIIa and kallikrein, in the above preparations has been
detected. The activation rate of Factor XII was very much dependent on each concentration of kaolin, Factor XII, HMW kininogen and
prekallikrein. We have examined the optimum condition varying
their concentrations and found that the activation of Factor XII
was accelerated 180-fold by the optimum concentration of HMW
kininogen. Since, our assay system does not distinguish the effects on both activations of Factor XII and prekallikrein, the
accelerating effect of HMW kininogen may be due to their effects
on the two reactions. We do not know why the activation was inhibited by the excess amounts of HMW kininogen. It may be due to
the competitive binding of Factor XII and HMW kininogen on the
surface of kaolin.

The activation of Factor XII was accelerated not only by HMW
kininogen, but also by kinin-free protein, which was derived from
HMW kininogen, removing kinin only by urinary kallikrein. The same
accelerating effect as HMW kininogen was observed with kinin-free
protein. It is quite interesting that a polypeptide consisting of
fragment 1·2 and light chain has the same accelerating effect as
HMW kininogen and, fragment 1·2 or light chain itself has no activity. The accelerating effect of HMW kininogen was abolished only
by fragment 1·2. These results indicate that both of fragment 1·2
and light chain regions are required for the accelerating effect
of HMW kininogen, which are consistent with the results obtained
using kininogen deficient plasma (Waldmann et al. 1977, Wuepper et
al. 1978). Moreover, the accelerating effect of HMW kininogen on
the kaolin-mediated activation of Factor XII was strikingly enhanced by brief treatment of HMW kininogen with human urinary kallikrein and bovine plasma kallikrein. Since the enhancement induced
by kallikreins preceeded the liberation of kinin and a single polypeptide kininogen almost disappeared at this stage, it seems likely that the enhancement is due to the action of a kininogen derivative, which has undergone limited proteolysis, possibly the
arginyl-seryl linkage at the COOH-terminus of the kinin moiety.
It is well known that the activities of Factor V and Factor VIII,
which serve as cofactors in the activation of prothrombin and
Factor X, respectively, are enhanced by thrombin (Davie and
Fujikawa, 1975). The result presented here seems to reflect an

analogous phenomenon, inasmuch as a proteolytic change in HMW kininogen was required to develop its maximal activity.

From these resons, we called tentatively "active kininogen" for the nicked HMW kininogen with the most potent accelerating effect on the activation of Factor XII.

It has been speculated that the accelerating effect of HMW kininogen on the contact-mediated activation of Factor XII is due to the binding of HMW kininogen with prekallikrein and thus formation of trimolecular complex of Factor XII on the surface of kaolin (Wiggins et al. 1977, Meier et al. 1977). In this paper, we have proved that HMW kininogen is easily adsorbed on kaolin through fragment 1·2 region. We do not yet have the direct evidence on the functional site of HMW kininogen to bind with prekallikrein, although the complex formation of HMW kininogen with prekallikrein in a molar ratio of one to one has been proved. However, we presume that the light chain region located in the COOH-terminal portion of HMW kininogen must be one of the functional sites, which interacts with prekallikrein, since a polypeptide consisting of fragment 1·2 and light chain accelerated the activation of Factor XII and the role of fragment 1·2 is thought to be the binding with kaolin.

From the evidence presented, we speculate the role of HMW kininogen in the kaolin-mediated activation of Factor XII, as shown in Fig. 8. HMW kininogen is adsorbed on kaolin through fragment 1·2 region (histidine-rich region), making a complex with prekallikrein through probably light chain portion. Since Factor XII is also adsorbed on kaolin, a trimolecular complex must be formed on the kaolin surface. We can not explain why the formation of the complex on kaolin leads to the activation of Factor XII. It has been speculated that a small amount of kallikrein will be generated by the formation of the complex and the kallikrein reciprocally activates Factor XII (Griffin 1978). It has also been established that the functional role of kallikrein in contact phase of blood coagulation is the positive feed back activation of Factor XII by kallikrein (Cochrane et al. 1973). On the other hand, kallikrein cleaves HMW kininogen into "active kininogen", which has the most potent accelerating effect on the activation of Factor XII, and then release kinin. Therefore, we would like to add one more function of plasma kallikrein in contact phase, that is, induction of a derivative of HMW kininogen to enhance the contact-mediated activation of Factor XII.

In bovine system, kallikrein will leave from the surface into fluid phase in a complex form with kinin and fragment 1·2-free protein, which has no site to bind to kaolin. On the contrary, fragment 1·2 remains on the surface, inhibiting further activation of Factor XII.

ACKNOWLEDGEMENTS

We express our thanks to Drs. E. W. Davie and K. Fujikawa for their kind information about the purification of bovine Factor XII. This work was supported in part by grants from the Scientific Research Fund of the Ministry of Education, Science and Culture, of Japan.

REFERENCES

Cochrane, C. G., Revak, S. D. and Wuepper, K. D. (1973): Activation of Hageman Factor in solid and fluid phases. A critical role of kallikrein. J. Exp. Med., 118, 1564-1583.

Colman, R. W., Bagdasarian, A., Talamo, R. C., Scott, C. F., Seavey, M., Guimaraes, J. A., Pierce, J. V. and Kaplan, A. P. (1975): Human kininogen deficiency with diminished levels of plasminogen proactivator and prekallikrein associated with abnormalities of the Hageman factor-dependent pathways. J. Clin. Invest., 56, 1650-1662.

Chan, J. Y. C., Habal, F. M., Burrowes, C. E. and Movat, H. Z. (1976): Interaction between Factor XII (Hageman Factor), high molecular weight kininogen and prekallikrein. Thromb. Research, 9, 423-433.

Cuatrecasas, P. (1970): Protein purification by affinity chromatography. Derivatizations of agarose and polyacrylamide beads. J. Biol. Chem., 245, 3059-3065.

Davie, E. W. and Fujikawa, K. (1975): Basic mechanisms in blood coagulation. Ann. Rev. Biochem., 44, 799-829.

Endo, Y., Yamashita, K., Han, Y. N., Iwanaga, S. and Kobata, A. (1977): The carbohydrate structure of a glycopeptide released by the action of plasma kallikrein on bovine plasma high-molecular-weight kininogen. J. Biochem., 82, 545-550.

Fujikawa, K., Walsh, K. A. and Davie, E. W. (1977a): Isolation and characterization of bovine Factor XII (Hageman Factor). Biochemistry, 16, 2270-2277.

Fujikawa, K., Kurachi, K. and Davie, E. W. (1977b): Characterization of bovine Factor XIIa (Activated Hageman Factor). Biochemistry, 16, 4182-4188.

Griffin, J. H. and Cochrane, C. G. (1976): Mechanisms for the involvement of high molecular weight kininogen in surface-dependent reactions of Hageman factor. Proc. Natl. Acad. Sci., U.S.A., 73, 2554-2558.

Griffin, J. H. (1978): Role of surface in surface-dependent activation of Hageman factor (blood coagulation Factor XII). Proc. Natl. Acad. Sci. U.S.A., 75, 1998-2002.

Han, Y. N., Komiya, M., Iwanaga, S. and Suzuki, T. (1975): Studies on the primary structure of bovine high-molecular-weight kininogen. Amino acid sequence of a fragment ("Histidine-rich peptide) released by plasma kallikrein. J. Biochem., 77, 55-68.

Han, Y. N., Kato, H., Iwanaga, S. and Suzuki, T. (1976): Primary structure of bovine plasma high-molecular-weight kininogen: The amino acid sequence of a glycopeptide portion (Fragment 1) following the C-terminus of the bradykinin moiety. J. Biochem., 79, 1201-1222.

Han, Y. N., Kato, H., Iwanaga, S., Oh-ishi, S. and Katori, M. (1978a): Primary structure of bovine plasma high-molecular-weight kininogen. Characterization of carbohydrate-free fragment 1·2 (Fragment X) released by the action of plasma kallikrein and its biological activity. J. Biochem., 83, 213-221.

Han, Y. N., Kato, H., Iwanaga, S. and Komiya, M. (1978b): Action of urinary kallikrein, plasmin and other kininogenase on bovine plasma high-molecular-weight kininogen. J. Biochem., 83, 223-235.

Hashimoto, N., Han, Y. N., Kato, H. and Iwanaga, S. (1977): Primary structure of bovine HMW kininogen. Limited hydrolysis with various kininogenases. Seikagaku (in Japanese), 49, 896.

Kato, H., Han, Y. N., Iwanaga, S., Suzuki, T. and Komiya, M. (1976): Bovine plasma HMW and LMW kininogens: Structural differences between heavy and light chains derived from their kinin-free proteins. J. Biochem., 80, 1299-1311.

Kaplan, A. P., Meier, H. L. and Mandle, R.Jr. (1976): The Hageman dependent pathways of coagulation, fibrinolysis and kinin generation. Seminars in Thromb and Hemostasis, 3, 1-26.

Komiya, M. (1972): Purification of bovine high molecular weight and low molecular weight kininogen and their biochemical properties. Doctral Thesis of Osaka University

Komiya, M., Kato, H. and Suzuki, T. (1974a): Bovine plasma kininogens. I. Further purification of high molecular weight kininogen and its physicochemical properties. J. Biochem., 76, 811-822.

Komiya, M., Kato, H. and Suzuki, T. (1974b); Bovine plasma kininogens. II. Microheterogeneities of high molecular weight kininogens and their structural relationships. J. Biochem., 76, 823-832.

Lie, C. Y., Scott, C. F., Bagdasarian, A., Pierce, J. V., Kaplan, A. P. and Colman, R. W. (1977): Potentiation of the function of Hageman factor fragments by high molecular weight kininogen. J. Clin. Invest., 60, 7-17.

Mandle, R. J., Colman, R. W. and Kaplan, A. P. (1976): Identification of prekallikrein and high-molecular-weight kininogen as a complex in human plasma. Proc. Natl. Acad. Sci. U.S.A., 73, 4179-4183.

Matheson, R. T., Miller, D. R., Lacombe, M. J., Han, Y. N., Iwanaga, S. Kato, H. and Wuepper, K. D. (1976): Flaujeac factor deficiency: Reconstitution with highly purified bovine HMW kininogen and delineation of a new permeability enhancing peptide released by plasma kallikrein from bovine HMW kininogen. J. Clin. Invest., 58, 1395-1406.

Meier, H. L., Pierce, J. V., Colman, R. W. and Kaplan, A. P. (1977): Activation and function of human Hageman factor. The role of high molecular weight kininogen and prekallikrein. J. Clin. Invest., 60, 18-31.

Morita, T., Kato, H., Iwanaga, S., Takada, K., Kimura, T. and Sakakibara, S. (1977): New fluorogenic substrates for α-thrombin, factor Xa, kallikreins and urokinase. J. Biochem., 82, 1495-1498.

Oh-ishi, S., Katori, M., Han, Y. N., Iwanaga, S., Kato, H. and

Suzuki, T. (1977): Possible physiological role of new peptide fragments released from bovine high-molecular-weight kininogen by plasma kallikrein. Biochem. Pharmacol., 26, 115-120.

Revak, S. D., Cochrane, C. G., Bouma, B. N. and Griffin, J. H. (1978): Surface and fluid phase activities of two forms of activated Hageman factor produced during contact activation of plasma. J. Exp. Med., 147, 719-729.

Saito, H., Ratnoff, O. D., Waldmann, R. and Abraham, J. P. (1975); Fitzgerald trait. Deficiency of a hitherto unrecognized agent, Fitzgerald factor, participating in surface-mediated reactions of clotting, fibrinolysis, generation of kinins, and the property of diluted plasma enhancing vascular permeability (PF/DlL). J. Clin. Invest., 55, 1082-1089.

Saito, H. (1977): Purification of high molecular weight kininogen and the role of this agent in blood coagulation. J. Clin. Invest., 60, 584-594.

Takahashi, H., Nagasawa, S. and Suzuki, T. (1972): Studies on prekallikrein in bovine plasma. I. Purification and properties. J. Biochem., 71, 471-483.

Thompson, R. E., Mandle, R.,Jr. and Kaplan, A. P. (1977): Characterization of human high molecular weight kininogen. Procoagulant activity associated with the light chain of kinin-free high molecular weight kininogen. J. Clin. Invest., 60, 1376-1380.

Waldmann, R., Scicli, A. G., McGregor, R. K., Carretero, O. A., Abraham, J. P., Kato, H., Han, Y. N. and Iwanaga, S. (1976): Effect of bovine high molecular weight kininogen and its fragments on Fitzgerald trait plasma. Thromb. Research, 8, 785-795.

Waldmann, R., Scicli, A. G., Scicli, G. M., Guimaraes, J., Carretero, O. A., Kato, H., Han, Y. N. and Iwanaga, S. (1977): Significant role of fragment 1·2 plus light chain of bovine high molecular weight kininogen in contact mediated coagulation. Thromb. Haemostasis, 38, 14.

Weber, K. and Osborn, M. (1969): The reliability of molecular weight determinations by dodecyl sulfate-polyacrylamide gel electrophoresis. J. Biol. Chem., 244, 4406-4412.

Wiggins, R. C., Bouma, B. N., Cochrane, C. G. and Griffin, J. H. (1977): Role of high molecular weight kininogen in surface-binding and activation of coagulation factor XI and prekallikrein. Proc. Natl. Acad. Sci. U.S.A., 74, 4636-4640.

Wuepper, K. D., Miller, D. R. and Lacombe, M. J. (1975): Flaujeac trait. Deficiency of human plasma kininogen. J. Clin. Invest., 56, 1663-1672.

Wuepper, K. D., Miller, D. R., Han, Y. N., Kato, H. and Iwanaga, S. (1978): HMW-kininogen deficiency: Delineation of a fragment of bovine HMW-kininogen which repairs the defect. Fed. Proc. (U.S.A.) 37 , 1587.

Yano, M., Kato, H., Nagasawa, S. and Suzuki, T. (1967): An improved method for the purification of kininogen-II from bovine plasma. J. Biochem., 62, 386-388.

Yano, M., Nagasawa, S. and Suzuki, T. (1971): Partial purification and some properties of high molecular weight kininogen, bovine kininogen-I. J. Biochem., 69, 471-481.

MOLECULAR MECHANISMS OF SURFACE-DEPENDENT ACTIVATION OF HAGEMAN

FACTOR (FACTOR XII)

John H. Griffin and Gregory Beretta

Department of Immunopathology
Scripps Clinic and Research Foundation
La Jolla, California, 92037

INTRODUCTION

Exposure of human plasma to a variety of negatively charged surfaces initiates the kinin-forming pathway (Margolis, 1958), the intrinsic coagulation pathway (Ratnoff, 1966; Nossel, 1964), and the fibrinolytic pathway (Niewiarowski and Prou-Wartelle, 1959; Iatrides and Ferguson, 1961). Hageman factor (blood coagulation Factor XII) is the enzyme central to these surface-dependent reactions since activated Hageman factor enzymatically converts prekallikrein to kallikrein and Factor XI to activated Factor XI (see review by Davie and Fukikawa, 1975). Activated Hageman factor also can stimulate the extrinsic coagulation pathway by activating Factor VII (Radcliffe et al., 1977; Kisiel et al., 1977; Laake and Østerud, 1974). High MW kininogen has recently been identified as a non-enzymatic cofactor that participates in surface-dependent reactions (see other chapters in this volume by Kerbiriou and Griffin, Kaplan et al., Iwanaga et al.). The molecular event central to contact activation is the surface-dependent activation of Hageman factor. This chapter is concerned with recent studies on the role of negatively charged surfaces in the surface-dependent activation of Hageman factor. The results summarized here have been recently presented in part elsewhere in more detail (Griffin, 1977; Griffin, 1978).

REACTIONS OF HAGEMAN FACTOR WITH DFP. Hageman factor is a serine protease zymogen that is converted to an active proteolytic enzyme when it is activated (Fujikawa et al., 1977; Griffin, 1977; Meier et al., 1977). For many years it was supposed but never proven that Hageman factor is activated simply by binding to negatively charged surfaces in the absence of any proteolytic modification of the protein. This idea was tested using ^{3}H-DFP (diisopropylfluorophosphate) as a quantitative active site titrant since DFP reacts stoichiometrically with a serine residue in the active site of the activated protein.

It was necessary to use reduced SDS polyacrylamide gel electrophoretic analysis to establish the molecular weight of the molecules that react with DFP since, as shown below, Hageman factor on a surface can be very easily cleaved. Figure 1 shows the radioactivity profiles of ^{3}H-DIP-protein on SDS gels. In the bottom profile, the uptake of ^{3}H-DFP by Hageman factor in solution is seen. In this case a small but reproducible amount of radioactivity was taken up by the zymogen at 76,000 MW. In the middle profile in Figure 1, the uptake of ^{3}H-DFP by celite-bound Hageman factor in the absence or presence of high MW kininogen is shown. The binding of Hageman factor to negatively charged celite in the absence or presence of high MW kininogen did not result in a detectable increased uptake of ^{3}H-DFP over the small level seen for Hageman factor in solution. This suggests that surface-binding in itself does not result in the formation of a detectable number (i.e. less than 1%) of new active sites. The upper panel in Figure 1 shows a control experiment in which surface-bound Hageman factor in the presence of high MW kininogen was activated by exposure to a small amount of kallikrein resulting in the limited proteolytic activation of the zymogen. This results in the formation of a 28,000 MW polypeptide fragment of Hageman factor that contains the active site serine. This active site serine reacts stoichiometrically with DFP seen in Figure 1 as a very large peak of tritium at a molecular weight of 28,000.

Table 1. Uptake of ^{3}H-DFP By
Hageman Factor (HF) In 10 Minutes at 37°.
(Taken from Griffin et al., manuscript in preparation)

	mol DFP per mol HF
HF	0.010 to 0.019
HF + Kaolin	0.015
HF + Celite	0.017
HF + 10^{-3}M Ellagic Acid	0.014
HF + Celite + HMW Kininogen	0.013
HF + 10^{-3}M Ellagic Acid + HMW Kininogen	0.012
HF + Celite + HMW Kininogen + Kallikrein	0.65
HF + Trypsin	0.95

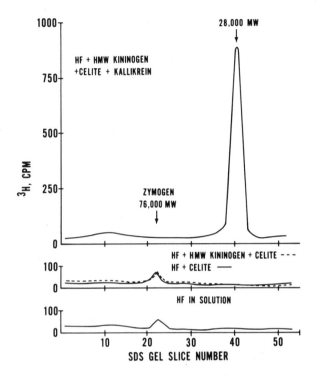

Figure 1.   Reaction of Hageman factor (HF) with the quantitative
            active site titrant, ^{3}H-DFP. For the profiles seen in
            the lower two panels, Hageman factor either in solution
            or bound to celite in the absence or presence of high MW
            kininogen was exposed to ^{3}H-DFP. Following separation
            of excess DFP, samples were analyzed on reduced SDS poly-
            acrylamide gels and the radioactivity profiles shown here
            were obtained. The upper panel shows the radioactivity
            profile obtained when celite-bound Hageman factor in the
            presence of high MW kininogen was activated by traces of
            plasma kallikrein prior to exposure to ^{3}H-DFP. Under these
            conditions the tritium uptake at 28,000 MW in the upper
            panel corresponded to 0.65 moles DFP per mole of Hageman
            factor. In other control experiments not shown here,
            Hageman factor activated by trypsin bound 0.95 moles DFP
            per mole protein. (Taken from Griffin et al., manuscript
            in preparation).

Table 1 summarizes many studies of the uptake of DFP by Hageman factor in the absence or presence of various negatively charged surfaces and high MW kininogen. The binding of Hageman factor to celite, kaolin, or ellagic acid in the absence or presence of high MW kininogen did not result in the binding of increased amounts of DFP over the low levels observed for Hageman factor in solution. From these data it is concluded that surface binding in itself does not result in the formation of a detectable number of new active sites.

The data in Table 1 showing that surface-binding of Hageman factor does not result in enhanced uptake of DFP are in agreement with other studies of bovine and human Hageman factor (Fujikawa et al., 1977; Claeys and Collen, 1977; Meier et al., 1977). However, it should be noted that Ratnoff and Saito (1977) suggested that Sephadex-ellagic acid mixtures do activate Hageman factor zymogen without proteolytic modification.

The time dependence of slow uptake of DFP by Hageman factor in solution is seen in Figure 2. It was observed that there is a progressive binding of DFP to the Hageman factor zymogen. Furthermore, this slow uptake of DFP was not accelerated by the binding of Hageman factor to celite.

The question then arose whether or not this slow uptake of DFP was in any way related to the activity of the molecule? Purified human Hageman factor was incubated in solution at 37° with different concentrations of DFP. At various times, aliquots were withdrawn from the reaction mixture and tested for their clotting activity. In control experiments in the absence of DFP, no loss of coagulant activity was observed. In the presence of DFP at 5.6, 16, and 44 mM, an accelerated loss of clotting activity was observed (Griffin et al., manuscript submitted). These data allowed the calculation of the second order rate constant for the inhibition of the Hageman factor zymogen by DFP at 0.24 $M^{-1}Min^{-1}$. The uptake of ^{3}H-DFP by the Hageman factor zymogen either in solution or bound to celite exhibited the same reaction kinetics. That is, the kinetic data demonstrated that the uptake of DFP by the Hageman factor zymogen was directly responsible for the loss of procoagulant activity.

The reaction of an enzyme with DFP to give an inhibited enzyme is characterized by k, the second order rate constant, according to the following reaction.

$$\text{ENZYME} + \text{DFP} \xrightarrow{\;\;k\;\;} \text{DFP-ENZYME} + F^-$$

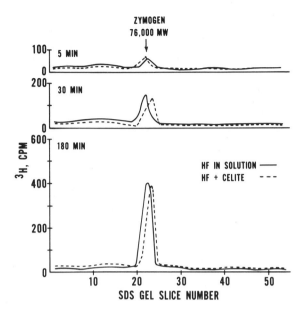

Figure 2. Radioactivity profiles from reduced SDS polyacrylamide gels showing time dependent uptake of ^{3}H–DFP by Hageman factor (HF) either in solution or bound to celite. SDS gel radioactivity profiles from different gels for each time point are superimposed to facilitate comparison of integrated ^{3}H uptake by celite–bound HF with HF in solution. (Taken from Griffin et al., manuscript in preparation).

As seen in Table II, the second order rate constant for the reaction of trypsin with DFP is 300 M^{-1}min^{-1}. Neurath and his colleagues (Morgan et al., 1972) first drew attention to the fact that trypsinogen reacts with DFP at a measurable rate giving a second order rate constant of 0.01 M^{-1}min^{-1}. Moreover, they demonstrated that both trypsinogen and chymotrypsinogen possess weak but detectable activity not only with DFP but also with ester substrates (Gertler et al., 1974; Kerr et al., 1975, 1976). Thus, the idea that serine protease zymogens are totally inactive was challenged and it was suggested that zymogens may exhibit weak enzymatic activity (Kay and Kassell, 1971; Kassell and Kay, 1973). How do these considerations relate to Hageman factor? As seen in Table II, activated Hageman factor reacts with DFP with a second order rate constant of 150 to 170 M^{-1}min^{-1}. And Factor XII reacts with DFP in

Table II
Second Order Rate Constants For the
Reaction of Enzymes with DFP
(Taken from Griffin et al., manuscript in preparation)

ENZYME	k $(M^{-1}min^{-1})$
Trypsinogen[*]	0.04
Trypsin[*]	300.
Factor XII	0.24
Bovine α-XII$_a$	170.
Human β-XII$_a$	150.
Prekallikrein	0.38
Kallikrein	500.

[*]Morgan et al. (1972)

a reaction that results in loss of coagulant activity with a second order rate constant of 0.24 $M^{-1}min^{-1}$ (Griffin et al., manuscript in preparation). Thus, the Hageman factor zymogen reacts with DFP about 1/600 as well as activated Hageman factor. Based on these observations and on the possible analogies with trypsinogen and trypsin, the possibility that surface-bound Hageman factor may function as an active zymogen in the activation of prekallikrein should be considered.

Human plasma prekallikrein was found to react with DFP with a second order rate constant of 0.38 $M^{-1}min^{-1}$, as seen in Table II. Kallikrein reacts with DFP about as well as trypsin does (Table II). Thus, prekallikrein reacts with DFP about 1/1000 as well as kallikrein does. Consequently, it may also be appropriate to consider that prekallikrein might function as a weakly active zymogen. In such a case, the prekallikrein zymogen might activate surface-bound Hageman factor since surface-binding makes Hageman factor very susceptible to proteolytic activation (Griffin, 1978; see below).

SURFACE-DEPENDENT CONFORMATIONAL CHANGES IN HAGEMAN FACTOR.
Negatively charged surfaces are not simply binding sites that serve to achieve high local concentrations of the contact activation proteins. It appears that such surfaces alter the structure of Hageman factor in a critical manner. Experiments such as those shown in Figure 3 demonstrate that surface-binding makes Hageman factor much more susceptible to limited proteolytic activation than is Hageman factor in solution (Griffin, 1978). In these experiments, mixtures of purified ^{125}I-bovine and ^{131}I-human Hageman

factor were incubated either in solution or in the presence of
kallikrein or in the presence of kallikrein and celite. Then each
reaction mixture was analyzed on reduced SDS polyacrylamide gels to
determine the extent of limited proteolysis reflected as cleavage
of the native 76,000 to 80,000 MW polypeptide to give fragments
of 52,000 and 28,000 MW. As shown in the bottom panel of Figure 3,
bovine and human Hageman factors exhibit peaks at their characteristic molecular weight. When Hageman factor was incubated in
solution with 34 nM kallikrein, no detectable cleavage of the
molecules occurred. However, if the human and bovine Hageman
factor molecules were surface-bound to celite, in the presence
of the same low concentration of kallikrein, extensive proteolytic
cleavage of the Hageman factor molecules occurred (Figure 3, upper
panel). Based on many experiments such as these, it was possible
to estimate quantitatively the enhanced susceptibility of Hageman
factor to cleavage by various proteases (Griffin, 1978). The
results for human Hageman factor were essentially the same as those
for bovine Hageman factor (Griffin et al., manuscript in preparation).

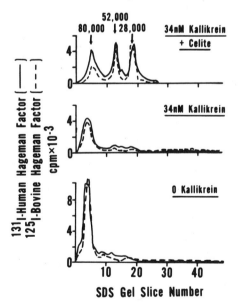

Figure 3. Surface-Dependent Enhancement of the Susceptibility of
           Human and Bovine Hageman factor to Proteolytic Activation.
           See text for discussion. (Taken from Griffin et al.,
           manuscript in preparation).

Celite-bound Hageman factor is 50 times more susceptible to kallikrein than Hageman factor in solution (Griffin, 1978). In addition if high MW kininogen is present, the rate of cleavage of Hageman factor is increased by a factor of 10. These two factors multiply, and thus surface-bound human or bovine Hageman factor in the presence of high MW kininogen is cleaved 500 times more rapidly by kallikrein than is Hageman factor in solution. When plasmin is used, celite-bound Hageman factor is 100 times more susceptible to cleavage than Hageman factor in solution. Interestingly, in this case the presence of high MW kininogen was without effect. Rate enhancements were also observed when activated Factor XI or trypsin were used to cleave Hageman factor (Griffin, 1978). Based on these data, it was suggested that a major role of negatively charged surfaces in the activation of Hageman factor involves an induced conformational change of the surface-bound Hageman factor to give a molecule that is much more susceptible to limited proteolysis by kallikrein or by other proteases. The schematic model in Figure 4 depicts such a conformational distortion of the surface-bound Hageman factor molecule.

Observations of radiolabelled Hageman factor in plasma during contact activation are entirely consistent with this hypothesis. Susan Revak et al. (1977) observed that radiolabelled Hageman factor in plasma during contact activation is rapidly cleaved from its 80,000 MW to give fragments of 52,000 and 28,000 MW. Moreover, they found that Hageman factor molecules that are bound to the negative surface in plasma are cleaved while molecules that are free in solution are not rapidly cleaved. It was also demonstrated that in plasmas deficient in high MW kininogen or prekallikrein, that is, in plasmas deficient in contact activation reactions, surface-bound radiolabelled Hageman factor was not cleaved in a rapid and characteristic manner. Consequently, observations of radiolabelled Hageman factor in human plasma during contact activation are entirely consistent with the hypothesis that surface-binding in itself does not result in the formation of activated Hageman factor. Rather, activation of Hageman factor involves rapid and limited proteolysis of surface-bound molecules that are exquisitely sensitive to proteases such as kallikrein.

In order to see whether bovine Hageman factor behaved like human Hageman factor in plasma during contact activation, mixtures of ^{131}I-human and ^{125}I-bovine Hageman factor were added to bovine or human plasmas that were then subjected to contact activation by kaolin (Griffin et al., manuscript in preparation). These studies demonstrated that bovine Hageman factor in plasma during contact activation behaved very much like the human molecule as reported by Revak et al. (1977). Thus, both in purified reaction mixtures and in human and bovine plasma, bovine Hageman factor, like the human molecule, becomes increasingly susceptible to limited proteolysis when bound to negatively charged surfaces.

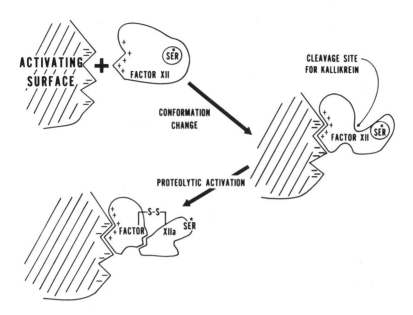

Figure 4.   Schematic model depicting the contribution of surface
            to the activation of Hageman factor (Factor XII).   In
            this drawing, a molecule of Factor XII, which is a serine
            protease zymogen, combines with a negatively charged
            surface, inducing a conformational change in the molecule.
            This conformational change does not per se activate the
            molecule, but rather it renders Factor XII much more
            susceptible to proteolytic activation by kallikrein.
            This results in a surface-bound Factor XII$_a$ molecule of
            80,000-MW containing two polypeptide chains linked by a
            disulfide bond.   Not shown here is the possibility that
            cleavage of Factor XII sometimes also occurs outside the
            disulfide bond and results in the formation of a 28,000
            MW form of Factor XII$_a$ that is free to diffuse away from
            the surface.   Each form of Factor XII$_a$ is a potent
            activator of prekallikrein, while only the surface-
            bound 80,000-MW form of Factor XII$_a$ in the presence of
            high MW kininogen is a potent activator of Factor XI
            (Revak et al., 1978).   (Taken from Griffin, 1978).

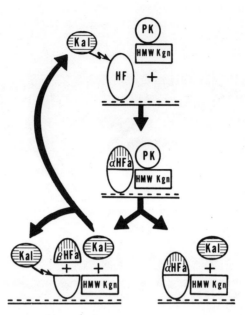

Figure 5.   Reciprocal Proteolytic Activation of Hageman Factor
            and Prekallikrein. See text for discussion. Abbreviations
            are: HF, α-HF$_a$, β-HF$_a$, Hageman factor and the α and β
            forms of activated Hageman factor; PK, Kal, Prekallikrein
            and Kallikrein; HMW Kgn, High MW Kininogen.

INITIATION AND PROPAGATION OF CONTACT ACTIVATION.   Several
events thought to be involved in the reciprocal proteolytic activation
that occurs during surface-dependent activation of the contact system
are depicted in Figure 5. In the upper portion (Figure 5) Hageman
factor is shown bound to a negatively charged surface. Prekallikrein
which circulates in a non-covalent complex with high MW kininogen
(Nagasawa and Nakayasu, 1973; Wendel et al., 1972; Mandle et al.,
1976) is shown binding to the negatively charged surface with high
MW kininogen acting as the surface receptor for prekallikrein
(Wiggins et al., 1977). As depicted, limited proteolytic activation
of surface-bound Hageman factor occurs by the action of kallikrein.
The resulting surface-bound activated Hageman factor can then activate
prekallikrein to give kallikrein shown in the bottom reaction.
Kallikrein can readily dissociate from the surface binding site and
subsequently can do several things. As shown by the arrow, it can
recycle to activate other surface-bound Hageman factor molecules,
hence, participating in a reciprocal proteolytic activation process.

Additionally, as shown by another arrow, it can cleave surface-bound activated Hageman factor (α-HF$_a$) at another site to release a 28,000 MW fragment of activated Hageman factor that is designated β-HF$_a$. This form of activated Hageman factor, β-HF$_a$, has also been described as Hageman factor fragments. The use of the term, Hageman factor fragments, to designate an active form of the enzyme seems unfortunate, and it is suggested that the term β-Factor XII$_a$ or β-HF$_a$ be used to designate the 28,000 MW form of the activated enzyme.

The reciprocal proteolytic relationship depicted here for the activation of Hageman factor and prekallikrein is essential for understanding the molecular mechanisms responsible for contact activation. However the scheme depicted in Figure 5 does not answer the fundamental and basic question of what provides the initial trigger for this reciprocal cycle? There are several potential triggering mechanisms that may provide the initiating proteolytic activity. Based on data summarized above, surface-bound Hageman factor is extremely sensitive to proteolytic activation not only by kallikrein but also by plasmin or other proteases. In addition kallikreins derived from cells such as the one studied by Newball et al. (this volume), may be responsible for activating the first few surface-bound Hageman factor molecules. It is also possible that in the event of vascular injury or inflammatory reactions, small amounts of plasmin or other proteases may be generated that can activate surface-bound Hageman factor. Alternatively, active zymogens may initiate the system. Hageman factor or prekallikrein zymogens may themselves be weakly active enzymes whose activity is expressed because negatively charged surfaces either can make Hageman factor more susceptible to the active prekallikrein zymogen or can provide the assembly site for placing prekallikrein next to the active Hageman factor zymogen, Each of these various possibilities could be responsible for triggering the surface-dependent activation of Hageman factor and prekallikrein. Much further work is needed to explore each of these possibilities.

SUMMARY

Based on studies using ^{3}H-DFP as an active site titrant, it is suggested that surface binding in itself does not result in the formation of new active sites in the Hageman factor molecule. Moreover, it was found that surface-binding of human and bovine Hageman factor renders these molecules 100 to 1000 times more susceptible to proteolytic activation by kallikrein, plasmin, or other proteases. Initiation of contact activation may involve proteolytic activation of surface-bound Hageman factor by a number of different proteases.

Both Hageman factor and prekallikrein react with DFP like weakly
active zymogens. Initiation of contact activation may also involve
the expression of low intrinsic catalytic activity of these zymogens.

REFERENCES

Claeys, H. and D. Collen, 1978, Purification and characterization
    of bovine coagulation Factor XII, Eur. J. Biochem. 87: 69.
Davie, E.W. and K. Fujikawa, 1975. Basic mechanisms in blood
    coagulation. Ann. Rev. Biochem., 44: 799.
Fujikawa, K., K. Kurachi and E.W. Davie, 1977. Characterization of
    bovine Factor XII$_a$ (activated Hageman factor), Biochemistry
    16: 4182.
Gertler, A., K.A. Walsh and H. Neurath. 1974. Catalysis by chymo-
    trypsinogen. Demonstration of an acyl-zymogen intermediate,
    Biochemistry 13: 1302.
Griffin, J.H. 1977. Molecular mechanisms of surface-dependent
    activation of Hageman factor (HF) (coagulation Factor XII).
    Fed. Proc. 36: 329.
Griffin, J.H. 1978. Role of surface in surface-dependent activation
    of Hageman factor (blood coagulation Factor XII), Proc. Natl.
    Acad. Sci. USA 75: 1998.
Iatridis, S.G. and J.H. Ferguson, 1961. Effect of surface and
    Hageman factor on the endogenous or spontaneous activation of
    the fibrinolytic system. Thromb. Diath. Haemorrh. 6: 411.
Kassell, B. and J. Kay. 1973. Zymogens of proteolytic enzymes,
    Science 180: 1022.
Kay, J. and B. Kassell. 1971. The autoactivation of trypsinogen.
    J. Biol. Chem. 21: 6661.
Kerr, M.A., K.A. Walsh and H. Neurath. 1975. Catalysis by serine
    proteases and their zymogens. A study of acyl intermediates
    by circular dichroism. Biochemistry 14: 5088.
Kerr, M.A., K.A. Walsh and H. Neurath. 1976. A proposal for the
    mechanism of chymotrypsinogen activation. Biochemistry 15:
    5566.
Kisiel, W., K. Fujikawa and E.W. Davie. 1977. Activation of bovine
    factor VII (proconvertin) by factor XII$_a$ (activated Hageman
    factor). Biochemistry 16: 4189.
Laake, K. and B. Østerud. 1974. Activation of purified plasma
    factor VII by human plasmin, plasma kallikrein and activated
    components of the human intrinsic blood coagulation system.
    Thromb. Res. 5: 759.
Mandle, R.J., R.W. Colman and A.P. Kaplan. 1976. Identification of
    prekallikrein and high molecular weight kininogen as a complex
    in human plasma. Proc. Natl. Acad. Sci. USA. 73: 4179.
Margolis, J., 1958. Activation of plasma by contact with glass:
    Evidence for a common reaction which releases plasma kinin and
    initiates coagulation. J. Physiol. 144: 1.

Meier, H.L., J.V. Pierce, R.W. Colman and A.P. Kaplan. 1977. Acti-
    vation and function of human Hageman factor. The role of high
    molecular weight kininogen and prekallikrein. J. Clin. Invest.
    60: 18.
Morgan, P.H., N.C. Robinson, K.A. Walsh and H. Neurath. 1972.
    Inactivation of bovine trypsinogen and chymotrypsinogen by
    diisopropylphosphofluoridate. Proc. Natl. Acad. Sci. USA
    69: 3312.
Nagasawa, S. and T. Nakayasu. 1973. Human plasma prekallikrein as
    a protein complex. J. Biochem. (Jap.) 74: 401.
Niewiarowski, S. and P. Prou-Wartell. 1959. Role du facteur contact
    (facteur Hageman) dans la fibrinolyse, Throm. Diath. Haemorrh.
    3: 593.
Nossel, H.L., 1964. The Contact Phase of Blood Coagulation, Blackwell
    Scientific Publishers, Oxford, England.
Radcliffe, R., A. Bagdasarian, R. Colman and Y. Nemerson. 1977.
    Activation of bovine factor VII by Hageman factor fragments,
    Blood 50, 611.
Ratnoff, O.D., 1966. The biology and pathology of the initial stages
    of blood coagulation. Prog. Hematol. 5: 204.
Ratnoff, O.D. and H. Saito, 1977. Activation of Hageman factor
    (Factor XII) by Sephadex-ellagic acid mixtures. Thromb. and
    Haemostasis (abst.) 38: 12.
Revak, S.D., C.G. Cochrane, B.N. Bouma and J.H. Griffin, 1978.
    Surface and fluid phase activities of two forms of activated
    Hageman factor produced during contact activation of plasma,
    J. Exp. Med. 147: 719.
Revak, S.D., C.G. Cochrane and J.H. Griffin, 1977. The binding and
    cleavage characteristics of human Hageman factor during contact
    activation. A comparison of normal plasma with plasmas deficient
    in Factor XI, prekallikrein, or high molecular weight kininogen,
    J. Clin. Invest. 59: 1167.
Wendel, V., W. Vogt and G. Seidel. 1972. Purification and some
    properties of a kininogenase from human plasma activated by
    surface contact, Hoppe Serlers Z. Physiol. Chem. 353: 1591.
Wiggins, R.C., B.N. Bouma, C.G. Cochrane and J.H. Griffin. 1977.
    Role of high molecular weight kininogen in surface-binding and
    activation of coagulation factor XI and prekallikrein. Proc.
    Natl. Acad. Sci. USA 74: 4636.

A NEW PREKALLIKREIN ACTIVATOR IN HUMAN PLASMA WHICH DIFFERS FROM HAGEMAN FACTOR AND ITS FRAGMENTS*

M.E. Webster, R.C.R. Stella, M.L. Villa & O. Toffoletto

Dept. Biochem., Escola Paulista de Medicina

Caixa Postal 20372, 01000 São Paulo, SP, Brasil

It is now well established that Hageman factor adsorbed to a negative particle remains essentially inactive unless two components of the plasma kallikrein-kinin system, prekallikrein (Webster and Pierce, 1973; Wuepper, 1973; Weiss et al., 1974) and its specific substrate high molecular weight (HMW) kininogen (Saito et al.,1975; Colman et al., 1975; Wuepper et al., 1975; Donaldson et al., 1976; Webster et al., 1976) are also present. Thus both prekallikrein and HMW-kininogen are early components of the intrinsic coagulation system.

However, evidence is available that additional factors may be required. As shown in Table 1 (Webster et al., 1976) Hageman factor adsorbed to a negative particle forms no detectable active Hageman factor. Even when prekallikrein is present in amounts equivalent to that found in plasma no active Hageman factor is formed. However, HMW-kininogen at the same concentration can produce a small amount of active Hageman factor and the addition of both prekallikrein and HMW-kininogen results in even more active Hageman factor being formed. Nevertheless, the amount of active Hageman generated was substantially less than that formed by the addition of either Hageman factor deficient plasma or concentrations of HMW-kininogen which are eight times that found in normal human plasma. Therefore, it would appear likely that additional factor(s) are required for the normal rate of activation of Hageman factor on a negative surface.

*Supported by grants from Financiadora de Estudos e Projetos(FINEP), Rio de Janeiro; Fundação de Amparo à Pesquisa do Estado de São Paulo (FAPESP), São Paulo and Conselho Nacional de Desenvolvimento Científico e Tecnológico (CNPq), Rio de Janeiro.

Table 1. HMW-kininogen and prekallikrein as activators of Hageman
        factor*

Plasma Component	Active Hageman factor (cpm)
Hageman factor (520 ng)	164
Hageman factor + Prekallikrein	130
Hageman factor + HMW-kininogen (0.45 µg BK/ml)	1074
Hageman factor + Prekallikrein + HMW-kininogen	4577
Hageman factor + Hageman factor deficient plasma	8792
Hageman factor + HMW-kininogen (3.6 µg BK/ml)	10326
Hageman factor + Kallikrein	164
Hageman factor + Kallikrein + HMW-kininogen (0.45 µg)	3568

* Data taken from Webster et al., 1976

In our present studies (Webster et al., 1979) we were initially
interested in developing a radiochemical method for the detection of
plasma deficient in either prekallikrein, Hageman factor or HMW-
kininogen. We had previously developed a method for their measurement
(Webster and Oh-ishi, 1976; Webster et al., 1976) which involved
adsorption of human plasma on a negatively charged surface, removal
of inibitors by washing and measurement of the active Hageman factor
bound on the surface of the particle by determining the amount of
kallikrein it formed from added prekallikrein using a radiolabeled
substrate (^{3}H-TAME). Using this procedure plasma deficient in either
prekallikrein, Hageman factor or HMW-kininogen failed to form active
Hageman factor. This method, however, required the preparation of
prekallikrein by chromatography on DEAE-cellulose and it was decided
to investigate the possibility that the plasma's own prekallikrein
could be used as substrate. This procedure was based, like the
clotting test, on the addition of celite (10 µg) to 1-2 µl human
plasma and the reaction quantitated by measuring the formation of
active kallikrein using ^{3}H-TAME. Under the conditions chosen seven
normal human plasmas (2 and 1 µl, respectively) formed 7036 ± 479
and 4643 ± 381 cpm ^{3}H-methanol while less than 500 cpm were formed
by plasma deficient in either prekallikrein, Hageman factor or
HMW-kininogen.

It was thought that this radiochemical method could also be
utilized to determine the factor which was deficient in these plasmas.

It was easily shown that addition of 35% of the prekallikrein of
normal plasma to plasma deficient in prekallikrein was sufficient to
form the same amount of kallikrein as that found in equivalent concentrations of normal plasma. Maximum amounts of kallikrein were
formed by replacement of 70% of the normal concentration. However,
when these same concentrations of prekallikrein were added to plasma
deficient in HMW-kininogen kallikrein was also formed although not
as readily as by plasma deficient in prekallikrein. These results
were unexpected since prekallikrein should not have been activated
by Hageman factor in the absence of HMW-kininogen and suggested to
us that still another activator of prekallikrein, provisionally
called Brasil factor, might exist in human plasma.

Further studies have shown that Brasil factor can be partially
separated from other plasma components by chromatography on DEAE-
cellulose. In these experiments prekallikrein is found, as expected,
with the proteins which fail to adsorb to DEAE-cellulose. Hageman
factor elutes shortly after the gradient commences followed by low
molecular weight kininogen. Brasil factor eluted shortly after the
main protein peak and between low and high molecular weight kininogens.
Although a clear separation of activities could not be obtained by
this chromatography, it was possible to select fractions which contained various proportions of Hageman factor and Brasil factor and
to clearly demonstrate that these two prekallikrein activators were
different. In addition Brasil factor, like Hageman factor, adsorbed
readily to celite, but unlike active Hageman factor (Oh-ishi and
Webster, 1975) it was inhibited by hexadimethrine bromide (1-2 µg/ml)
added after its adsorption to the negative particle. These combined
results indicate that Brasil factor is neither Hageman factor nor
active Hageman factor and its fragments.

Brasil factor can readily be quantitated when added to a constant amount of prekallikrein in the presence of celite (30 µg) and,
for example, forms 1271, 2454 and 5420 cpm ^{3}H-methanol when 1,2 and
5 µl of a solution are added, respectively. It is readily inhibited
by sodium chloride giving maximum formation of kallikrein in the
absence of sodium chloride except that furnished by the celite
(0.03 M). Increasing the concentration of NaCl to 0.11, 0.19 and
0.43 M inhibits the activation of prekallikrein by Brasil factor
by 28, 60 and 88%, respectively.

The role of Brasil factor in the intrinsic coagulation system
remains to be determined. Plasma deficient in Hageman factor is
capable of activating Hageman factor at much faster rates than can
be explained by the available amount of prekallikrein, Hageman factor
and HMW-kininogen (Table 1). Brasil factor, therefore might be the
missing factor previously proposed. Our current concept of the
activation of Hageman factor is shown in Fig. 1. Brasil factor,
prekallikrein, HMW-kininogen and Hageman factor are all firmly bound

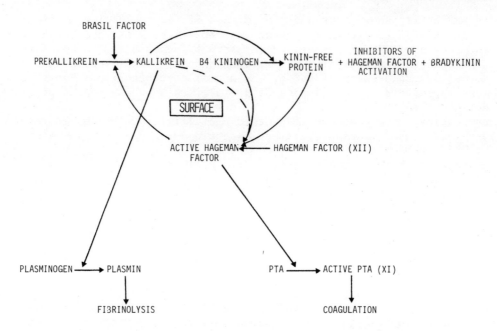

Fig. 1.   Possible role for Brasil factor in the in vitro activation of the intrinsic coagulation system by increasing
the rate of activation of Hageman factor on a negative
surface.

to the negative surface. Brasil factor forms some active kallikrein
from prekallikrein. HMW-kininogen in the presence of this kallikrein
can now partially activate Hageman factor and this active Hageman
factor in turn activates residual prekallikrein which can now form
more active Hageman factor in the presence of HMW-kininogen.   The
active Hageman factor formed in these reactions can then form active
PTA from PTA and thus initiate the intrinsic coagulation system.
The kallikrein formed can also act on plasminogen to form plasmin
and thus induce fibrinolysis.   In the absence of the negative particle it is well known that kallikrein acts on HMW-kininogen to release a kinin-free protein, histidine rich peptides which inhibit
the activation of Hageman factor and bradykinin.   However, whether
these reactions occur on a negative surface has not yet been established.

Another and perhaps more exciting role for Brasil factor is
shown in Fig. 2.   It is well known that patients deficient in prekallikrein, Hageman factor and HMW-kininogen exhibit no in vivo
haemostatic disorder and that patients deficient in PTA have only
a mild bleeding tendency.   Kallikrein has been shown to shorten the

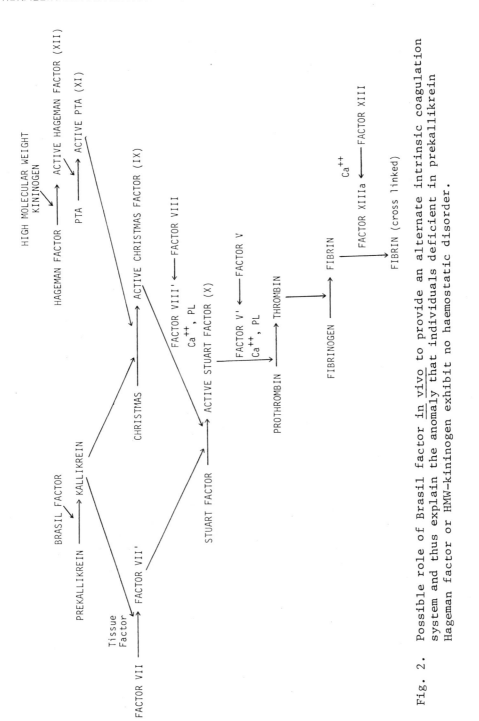

Fig. 2. Possible role of Brasil factor in vivo to provide an alternate intrinsic coagulation system and thus explain the anomaly that individuals deficient in prekallikrein Hageman factor or HMW-kininogen exhibit no haemostatic disorder.

clotting time of normal rabbit plasma (Wuepper and Cochrane, 1972) and to a lesser extent that of human plasma. It has also been reported to activate the extrinsic coagulation system by its ability to activate Factor VII through its action as a plasminogen activator (Laake and Osterud, 1974) and to activate Factor IX directly (Osterud et al., 1975). It is this latter possibility which would provide an alternate mechanism for the activation of the intrinsic coagulation system. Individuals deficient in either Hageman factor or HMW-kininogen could activate their intrinsic coagulation system by Brasil factor forming kallikrein from prekallikrein and the kallikrein in turn activating Factor IX. On the other hand, individuals deficient in prekallikrein can form a small amount of active Hageman factor by utilizing their normal levels of HMW-kininogen. This small amount of Hageman factor may well be sufficient to provide adequate clotting in vivo. Experimental examination of these possibilities is indicated.

REFERENCES

Colman, R.W., A. Bagdasarian, R.C. Talamo, C.F. Scott, M. Seavey, J.A. Guimarães, J.V. Pierce and A.P. Kaplan, 1975, William's trait. Human kininogen deficiency with diminished levels of plasminogen proactivator and prekallikrein associated with abnormalities of the Hageman factor-dependent pathways, J. Clin. Invest. 56, 1650.

Donaldson, V.H., H.I. Glueck, M.A. Miller, H.Z. Movat and F. Habal, 1976, Kininogen deficiency in Fitzgerald trait: role of high molecular weight kininogen in clotting and fibrinolysis, J.Lab. Clin. Med. 87, 327.

Laake, K., and B. Osterud, 1974, Activation of purified plasma factor VII by human plasmin, plasma kallikrein, and activated components of the human intrinsic blood coagulation system, Thrombosis Res. 5, 759.

Oh-ishi, S. and M.E. Webster, 1975, Vascular permeability factors (PF/Nat and PF/Dil): their relationship to Hageman factor and the kallikrein-kinin system, Biochem. Pharmacol. 24, 591.

Osterud, B., K. Laake and H. Prydz, 1975, The activation of human Factor IX, Thrombos. Diathes. haemorrh. (Stuttg.) 33, 553.

Saito, H., O.D. Ratnoff, R. Waldmann and J.P. Abraham, 1975, Fitzgerald trait. Deficiency of a hitherto unrecognized agent, Fitzgerald factor, participating in surface-mediated reactions of clotting, fibrinolysis, generation of kinins and the property of diluted plasma enhancing vascular permeability (PF/Dil), J.Clin. Invest. 55, 1082.

Webster, M.E. and S. Oh-ishi, 1976, Activation of Hageman factor (Factor XII): requirement for activators other than prekallikrein. Fogarty Int. Center Proc. 27, 55.

Webster, M.E. and J.V. Pierce, 1973, Activators of Hageman factor
    (Factor XII): identification and relationship to the kallikrein-
    kinin system, Chem. Abs. 32, 845.
Webster, M.E., J.A. Guimarães, A.P. Kaplan, R.W. Colman and J.V.
    Pierce, 1976, Activation of surface-bound Hageman factor: pre-
    eminent role of high molecular weight kininogen and evidence for
    a new factor, Adv. Exp. Med. Biol. 70, 285.
Webster, M.E., R.C.R. Stella, M.L. Villa and O. Toffoletto, 1979,
    Brasil factor - a new prekallikrein activator in human plasma,
    (Submitted for publication).
Weiss, A.S., I.J. Gallin and A.P. Kaplan, 1974, Fletcher factor de-
    ficiency. A diminshed rate of Hageman factor activation caused by
    absence of prekallikrein with abnormalities of coagulation,fibrin-
    olysis, chemotactic activity, and kinin-generation, J.Clin.Invest.
    53, 622.
Wuepper, K.D., 1973, Prekallikrein deficiency in man, J.Exp. Med.
    138, 1345.
Wuepper, K.D. and C.G. Cochrane, 1972, Effect of plasma kallikrein
    on coagulation in vitro, Proc. Soc. Exp. Biol. Med. 141, 271.
Wuepper, K.D., K.R. Miller, M.J. LaCombe, 1975, Flaujeac trait: de-
    ficiency of human plasma kininogen, J. Clin. Invest. 56, 1663.

INTERACTIONS AMONG HAGEMAN FACTOR (HG, FACTOR XII), PLASMA THROMBO-
PLASTIN ANTECEDENT (PTA, FACTOR XI), PLASMA PREKALLIKREIN (PK,
FLETCHER FACTOR) AND HIGH MOLECULAR WEIGHT KININOGEN (HMW-K,
FITZGERALD FACTOR) IN BLOOD COAGULATION

Hidehiko Saito and Oscar D. Ratnoff*

Department of Medicine, Case Western Reserve University
School of Medicine and University Hospitals of Cleveland
Cleveland, Ohio 44106

ABSTRACT

Studies of plasmas from individuals with Hageman trait (factor
XII deficiency), plasma thromboplastin antecedent (PTA, factor XI)
deficiency, Fletcher trait (plasma prekallikrein deficiency) and
Fitzgerald trait (high molecular weight-kininogen deficiency) have
revealed the importance of these proteins in blood coagulation.
The interactions among them, however, are not fully elucidated.
We have studied these reactions by two different approaches.
(1) In a purified system, high molecular weight kininogen was
absolutely required for activation of PTA by HF and ellagic acid
(EA). The yield of activated PTA was proportional to the amount
of HF, HMW-K, and PTA in the mixtures, suggesting that these three
proteins may form a complex in the presence of EA. (2) In experiments with whole plasma, we took advantage of the adsorption of EA
to Sephadex gels. When normal plasma or plasma deficient in HF,
PK, HMW-K or PTA was exposed to Sephadex-EA and was separated by
centrifugation, each supernatant plasma except that deficient in
HF shortened the prolonged partial thromboplastin time (PTT) of
HF-deficient plasma. Plasma simultaneously depleted of HMW-K, PK
and PTA also shortened the PTT of HF-deficient plasma and of plasma
depleted of HF and PK, but had virtually no procoagulant effect
upon the PTT of plasma depleted of HF and MHW-K. Thus, exposure
of HF in plasma to Sephadex-EA appeared to generate a clot-
promoting form of HF in the absence of other clotting factors,
but its expression required the presence of HMW-K.

*Career Investigator of American Heart Association

INTRODUCTION

Normal human plasma clots rapidly upon contact with certain
negatively charged surfaces such as glass and kaolin, through a
sequence of reactions designated as the intrinsic pathway of
thrombin formation. The initial stages of this pathway are therefore called the contact phase of blood coagulation. The discovery
and studies of patients with various congenital clotting factor
deficiencies have had a major impact upon the development of our
knowledge of blood clotting. Studies of Hageman trait (Ratnoff
and Colopy, 1955) and plasma thromboplastin antecedent deficiency
(Rosenthal et al., 1953) have shown the participation of Hageman
factor (HF, factor XII) and plasma thromboplastin antecedent (PTA,
factor XI) in the contact phase of blood coagulation. Until
recently, only HF and PTA were recognized as contact factors. It
was originally postulated that surfaces activated HF and that
activated HF in turn, activated PTA directly (Soulier and Prou-
Wartelle, 1960; Ratnoff et al., 1961; Nossel, 1964). This is now
known to be an inadequate description of the early events of clotting. Recent studies of plasmas from individuals with Fletcher
trait (Hathaway et al., 1965; Wuepper 1973; Saito et al., 1974a;
Weiss et al., 1974) and Fitzgerald trait (Saito et al., 1975;
Wuepper et al., 1975; Colman et al., 1975; Donaldson et al., 1976)
have established the importance of plasma prekallikrein and high
molecular weight (HMW)-kininogen in the contact phase of blood
coagulation. Without these congenitally deficient plasmas, our
knowledge in this area would still be rudimentary.

Thus, four plasma proteins (HF, PTA, prekallikrein and HMW-
kininogen) are now recognized to participate in the contact phase.
All four proteins have the striking property of being readily
adsorbed to negatively charged surfaces. The interactions among
them, however, appear to be very complicated and are not fully
elucidated. Interactions may occur among agents adsorbed to
surfaces or between adsorbed agents and substances in the fluid
phase. We have studied these reactions by two different approaches:
(1) experiments with purified proteins and (2) experiments in
whole plasma.

MATERIALS AND METHODS

HF, prekallikrein, HMW-kininogen and PTA were prepared as
described (Saito, 1977). The specific activity of the preparations
in coagulant assays used were: HF (59 and 50 u/mg protein), prekallikrein (8 u/mg protein), HMW-kininogen (17 u/mg protein) and
PTA (90 and 200 U/mg protein). One unit of procoagulant activity
was arbitrarily defined as that amount present in 1 ml of a standard pooled plasma (Zimmerman et al., 1971). Procoagulant assays
of HF, prekallikrein, HMW-kininogen and PTA were performed as

reported earlier (Hathaway et al., 1965; Saito et al., 1975).

Monospecific antiserums to HF, PTA, prekallikrein and HMW-kininogen were prepared in rabbits (Saito, et al., 1977) and a crude immunoglobulin fraction was separated. These fractions were used in all experiments. A crude immunoglobulin fraction prepared similarly from normal rabbit serum was used as a control.

Plasmas from patients with congenital clotting factor deficiencies were obtained as reported previously (Zimmerman, et al., 1971). Fitzgerald trait plasma was kindly supplied by Dr. R. Waldmann, Henry Ford Hospital, Detroit, Michigan.

The activation of PTA in a purified system (Fig. 1) was studied by incubating 0.075 ml PTA with 0.025 ml HF, 0.025 ml prekallikrein, 0.025 ml HMW-kininogen and 0.075 ml 0.1 mM ellagic acid (K&K Laboratories, Inc., Plainview, New York) in barbital-saline buffer (pH 7.4) in a 10 x 75 mm polystyrene tube at 37°C. At intervals, 0.05 ml aliquots were transferred to prewarmed 10 x 75 mm polystyrene tubes containing 0.1 crude phospholipid (Centrolex "0", Central Soya Co., Inc., Fort Wayne, Indiana) and 0.1 ml bovine PTA-deficient plasma (Kociba et al., 1969). 0.1 ml of 0.025M $CaCl_2$ was immediately added and the clotting time was measured at 37°C.

Sephadex G10- ellagic acid was prepared by mixing 10 ml of settled volume of Sephadex G10 (Pharmacia Fine Chemicals, Inc., Piscataway, New Jersey) with 30 ml of 0.1 mM ellagic acid (Synthesized by Dr. J.D. Crum) for 5 min. The mixture was allowed to settle and the supernatant fluid was decanted. The Sephadex-ellagic acid was then washed 15 times with 100 ml of buffer, discarding the supernatant fluid each time after the Sephadex-ellagic acid had settled. The fifteenth wash contained less than 10^{-7} M ellagic acid (Ratnoff and Saito, 1977).

Plasmas simultaneously deficient in more than one factor were prepared by absorbing congenitally deficient plasma with appropriate antiserums (Ratnoff and Saito, 1977).

Activation of HF in whole plasma was performed as follows: Plasma containing HF was mixed with 10 volumes of settled Sephadex-ellagic acid in polystyrene tubes, stirred gently with a plastic pipette at RT for 2 min, and allowed to stand for 5 min. Nine volumes of buffer were added and the mixture was again stirred for 2 min and then allowed to settle for 10 min. The supernatant diluted plasma was transferred to a polypropylene tube and centrifuged at 30,000 g for 15 min at 2°C. The supernatant plasma was then tested for clot-promoting activity in 10 x 75 mm polystyrene tubes without kaolin.

RESULTS AND DISCUSSION

Interactions in a purified system

The addition of purified activated PTA (XIa) corrected the abnormal partial thromboplastin time of prekallikrein-deficient and HMW-kininogen deficient plasma (Saito et al., 1974a; Saito et al., 1975). These experiments suggested that both prekallikrein and HMW-kininogen participate in the clotting at a point earlier than that at which activated PTA functions.

Therefore, the role of HF, prekallikrein, HMW-kininogen, PTA and ellagic acid (Ratnoff and Crum, 1964) in the generation of activated PTA was examined in an experimental system as shown in Fig. 1. When all these agents were incubated together at 37°C, clot-promoting activity generated progressively as incubation proceeded (Table I). The clot-promoting activity was identified as activated PTA (XIa) from the following experiments (Saito, 1977). First, when aliquots of the mixture in Fig. 1 were tested on a substrate of Christmas factor (factor IX)-deficient plasma, there was no shortening of the clotting time. This result suggested that the activity generated participated in the sequence of blood clotting before the point at which Christmas factor functions. Second, only antibody directed against activated PTA inactivated the clot-promoting activity, whereas antibodies against HF, pre-kallikrein and HMW-kininogen had no effect.

When either HF, HMW-kininogen, PTA or ellagic acid was deleted from the mixture, the clotting time did not shorten. We previously reported that the presence or absence of prekallikrein did not influence the generation of activated PTA (Saito, 1977). Schiffman and Lee also reported that prekallikrein was not necessary for the activation of PTA (1975). More recently, we have observed a slight accelerating effect of prekallikrein upon the activation of PTA (Table I, B), when a different preparation of HF was used.

```
HF (F XII)        ⎫
PREKALLIKREIN     ⎬  → ALIQUOTS TESTED
HMW-KININOGEN     ⎬    ON PTA-DEFICIENT
PTA (F XI)        ⎪    PLASMA
ELLAGIC ACID      ⎭
```

Fig. 1. Test for PTA Activation.

In any case, prekallikrein was not an absolute requirement for PTA
generation, unlike HF, PTA, HMW-K or ellagic acid. This is consistent with the original observation of Hathaway et al. (1965)
that the abnormally long partial thromboplastin time of patients
with Fletcher trait (prekallikrein deficiency) shortens to normal
if the plasma is exposed for a prolonged period to glass.

Crude kinetic studies were performed by changing the concentration of each agent as noted in Fig. 1, and studying the effect
of these maneuvers upon the generation of activated PTA activity.
Since the system under study was complex and it was difficult to
use conditions in which the substrate (PTA) was saturated, we could
not measure the initial velocity of the reactions. Instead, we
measured the yield of activated PTA. The yield of activated PTA
was related to the concentration of PTA, HF and HMW-kininogen in
the mixtures (Saito, 1977). These results are consistent with the
view that HF, PTA and HMW-kininogen form a complex in the presence
of ellagic acid. Direct evidence of complex formation, however,
remains to be obtained. Other investigators also have reported
the stoichiometric interactions of HF and HMW-kininogen (Griffin
and Cochrane, 1976; Schiffman and Lee, 1975; Meier et al., 1977).

Human HF is known to be fragmented by the action of proteolytic enzymes such as plasmin, kallikrein, or trypsin (Kaplan and
Austen, 1971; Cochrane et al., 1972; Soltay et al., 1971). HF-
fragments of approximately MW 30,000 are potent activators of prekallikrein, but only weakly clot-promoting. When HF-fragments
were tested in the system depicted in Fig. 1, they activated PTA
directly in the absence of HMW-kininogen and ellagic acid (Saito,
1977). This is in good agreement with studies of Schiffman et al.,
(1977). Similarly, Kurachi and Davie (1977) reported that two-
chained species of bovine activated HF activated human PTA in the
absence of HMW-kininogen and kaolin.

Interactions in whole plasma

Although the experiments utilizing purified clotting factors
gave us important information, they have at least two inherent
drawbacks. First, clotting factors may be so altered during purification that their behavior may be different from that in plasma.
For example, preparations of human (Saito et al., 1975) and bovine
HF (Fujikawa et al., 1977) corrected the clotting defect of
Fletcher trait as well as Hageman trait plasma. Second, the experiments were performed in the absence of inhibitors. Human
plasma contains many agents that inhibit the activity of clotting
factors. The activity of human activated PTA, for example, is
inhibited by C1INH (Forbes, et al., 1970), α_1-antitrypsin (Heck
and Kaplan, 1974) or α_2-plasmin inhibitor (Saito et al., 1977).

TABLE I

ACTIVATION OF PTA IN A PURIFIED SYSTEM

Incubation Mixture	Clotting Time (sec)			
	10 sec	10 min	20 min	30 min
A) HF + PTA + Prekallikrein + HMW-K + EA	309	222	194	192
HF + PTA + Prekallikrein + Buffer + EA	312	310	315	309
	10 sec	5 min	10 min	15 min
B) HF + PTA + Prekallikrein + HMW-K + EA	165	145	134	132
HF + PTA + Buffer + HMW-K + EA	166	157	149	137

A) In 10 x 75 mm polystyrene tubes, the following reagents were incubated at 37°C.: 0.075 ml PTA (0.07 U/ml, specific activity 90 U/mg protein), 0.025 ml HF (1.8 U/ml, specific activity 59 U/mg protein), 0.025 ml prekallikrein (0.2 U/ml), 0.025 ml HMW-K (0.4 U/ml) or bovine serum albumin (BSA) and 0.075 ml 0.1 mM ellagic acid (EA). At intervals, 0.05 ml aliquots were tested for activated PTA activity as described in methods. The results are the average of triplicate determination.

B) In 10 x 75 mm polystyrene tubes, the following reagents were incubated at 37°C: 0.075 ml PTA (0.05 U/ml, specific activity 200 U/mg protein), 0.025 ml HF (0.17 U/ml, specific activity 50 U/mg protein), 0.025 ml prekallikrein (0.05 U/ml) or BSA, 0.025 ml HMW-K (0.2 U/ml) and 0.075 ml 0.1 mM ellagic acid (EA). At intervals, aliquots were tested as above. The results are the average of triplicate determination.

Furthermore, normal plasma contains substances which interact with negatively charged surfaces so as to block their clot-promoting property (Nossel et al., 1968; Saito et al., 1974b).

We therefore attempted to study the interactions of HF, pre-kallikrein, HMW-kininogen and PTA in whole plasma. We took advantage of the adsorption of ellagic acid to Sephadex gels, observed some years ago (Ratnoff and Crum, 1964). Human or bovine PTA-deficient plasma, mixed with Sephadex G10-ellagic acid and then separated from the gel, corrected the clotting defect of HF-deficient plasma, but not that of PTA-deficient or Christmas factor-deficient plasma, as if the HF in PTA-deficient plasma that had been exposed to the gel had been activated. Suitable experiments ruled out the possibility that the clot-promoting action of Sephadex-ellagic acid-treated plasma was due to elution of sufficient ellagic acid from the gel to influence the assay system used. Similar results were obtained when prekallikrein-deficient or HMW-kininogen-deficient plasma was mixed with Sephadex G10-ellagic acid and then tested upon HF-deficient plasma. Clot-promoting activity also generated in plasmas that were simultaneously deficient in PTA, prekallikrein and HMW-kininogen, as tested upon HF-deficient plasma. These results suggest that exposure of HF in plasma to Sephadex-ellagic acid generated a clot-promoting form of HF in the absence of other contact factors (Ratnoff and Saito, 1977).

Prekallikrein and HMW-kininogen are present in the HF-deficient plasma used as a substrate in the experiments just described. When plasmas simultaneously deficient in PTA, prekallikrein and HMW-kininogen were exposed to Sephadex-ellagic acid and tested upon substrates deficient in HF and prekallikrein, clot-promoting activity generated more slowly. In contrast, no clot-promoting activity could be measured when the substrate was deficient in HF and HMW-kininogen. These results imply that HMW-kininogen is absolutely required for the expression of clot-promoting properties by Sephadex-ellagic acid-treated HF (Ratnoff and Saito, 1977).

Finally, it is important to point out that all these findings came from in vitro experiments. Curiously, individuals with HF deficiency, prekallikrein deficiency or HMW-kininogen deficiency have no bleeding tendency at all in the face of grossly abnormal laboratory tests. We must admit that there is a big discrepancy between our in vitro experiments and in vivo phenomenon.

ACNOWLEDGEMENTS

Ms. Laura Stith and Ms. Ellen Strecker provided invaluable technical help.

This work was supported in part by research grant HL 01661 from the National Heart, Lung and Blood Institute of the National

Institutes of Health, U.S. Public Health Service and in part by
grants from the American Heart Association and its Northeast Ohio
affiliate.

REFERENCES

Cochrane, C.G., S.D. Revak, B.S. Aikin and K.D. Wuepper. 1972.
    Structural characteristics and activation of Hageman factor.
    In: Inflammation: Mechanisms and Controls. Lepow, I.H. and
    Ward, P.A. (Academic Press, Inc., New York p. 119).

Colman, R.W., A. Bagdasarian, R.C. Talamo, C.F. Scott, M. Seavey,
    J.A. Guimaraes, J.V. Pierce and A.P. Kaplan. 1975. Williams
    Trait. Human kininogen deficiency with diminished levels of
    plasminogen proactivator and prekallikrein associated with
    abnormalities of the Hageman factor-dependent pathways. J.
    Clin. Invest. 56: 1650.

Donaldson, V.H., H.I. Glueck, M.A. Miller, H.Z. Movat and F. Habal.
    1976. Kininogen deficiency in Fitzgerald trait: role of high
    molecular weight kininogen in clotting and fibrinolysis. J.
    Lab. Clin. Med. 87: 327.

Forbes, C.D., J. Pensky and O.D. Ratnoff. 1970. Inhibition of
    activated Hageman factor and activated plasma thromboplastin
    antecendent by purified serum $C\overline{1}$ inactivator. J. Lab. Clin.
    Med. 76: 809.

Fujikawa, K., K.A. Walsh and E.W. Davie. 1977. Isolation and
    characterization of bovine factor XII (Hageman factor).
    Biochemistry 16: 2270.

Griffin, J.H. and C.G. Cochrane. 1976. Mechanisms for the involve-
    ment of high M.W. kininogen in surface dependent reaction of
    Hageman factor. Proc. Nat'l. Acad. Sci., U.S.A. 73: 2554.

Hathaway, W.E., L.P. Belhasen, and H.S. Hathaway. 1965. Evidence
    for a new plasma thromboplastin factor. I. Case report, co-
    agulation studies and physico-chemical properties. Blood
    26: 521.

Heck, L.W. and A.P. Kaplan. 1974. Substrates of Hageman factor I.
    Isolation and characterization of human factor XI (PTA) and
    inhibition of the activated enzyme by α_1-antitrypsin. J.
    Exp. Med. 140: 1615.

Kaplan, A.P. and K.F. Austen, 1971. A prealbumin activator of
    prekallikrein II. Derivation of activators of prekallikrein
    from active Hageman factor by digestion with plasmin. J. Exp.
    Med. 133: 696.

Kociba, G.J., O.D. Ratnoff, W.F. Loeb, R.L. Wall and L. E. Heider.
    1969. Bovine plasma thromboplastin antecedent (Factor XI)
    deficiency. J. Lab. Clin. Med. 74: 37.

Kurachi, K. and E.W. Davie. 1977. Activation of human Factor XI
    (plasma thromboplastin antecedent) by Factor XIIa (activated
    Hageman factor). Biochemistry 16: 5831.

Meier, H.L., J.V. Pierce, R.W. Colman and A.P. Kaplan, 1977.
    Activation and Function of human Hageman Factor. The role of
    high molecular weight kininogen and prekallikrein. J. Clin.
    Invest. 60: 18.
Nossel, H.L., 1964. Contact phase of blood coagulation. (Blackwell
    Scientific Publications, Ltd. Oxford).
Nossel, H.L., H. Rubin, M. Drillings and R. Hsieh, 1968. Inhi-
    bition of Hageman factor activation. J. Clin. Invest. 47: 1172.
Ratnoff, O.D. and J.E. Colopy, 1955. A familial hemorrhagic trait
    associated with a deficiency of a clot-promoting fraction of
    plasma. J. Clin. Invest. 34: 602.
Ratnoff, O.D., E.W. Davie and D.L. Mallet, 1961. Studies on the
    action of Hageman factor. Evidence that activated Hageman
    factor in turn activates plasma thromboplastin antecedent.
    J. Clin. Invest. 40: 803.
Ratnoff, O.D. and J.D. Crum, 1964. Activation of Hageman factor
    by solutions of ellagic acid. J. Lab. Clin. Med. 63: 359.
Ratnoff, O.D. and H. Saito, 1977. Activation of Hageman factor
    (HF, Factor XII) by Sephadex-Ellagic acid mixtures. Throm-
    bosis and Hemostasis, 38: 12.
Rosenthal, R.L., O.H. Dreskin and N. Rosenthal, 1953. New hemo-
    philia-like disease caused by deficiency of a third plasma
    thromboplastin factor. Proc. Soc. Exp. Biol. Med. 82: 171.
Saito, H., 1977. Purification of high molecular weight kininogen
    and the role of this agent in blood coagulation. J. Clin.
    Invest. 60: 584.
Saito, H., O.D. Ratnoff and V.H. Donaldson, 1974a. Defective
    activation of clotting, fibrinolytic, and permeability-
    enhancing systems in human Fletcher-trait plasma. Circ. Res.
    34: 641.
Saito, H., O.D. Ratnoff, V.H. Donaldson, G. Haney and J. Pensky,
    1974b. Inhibition of the adsorption of Hageman factor (factor
    XII) to glass by normal human plasma. J. Lab. Clin. Med.
    84: 62.
Saito, H., O.D. Ratnoff, R. Waldmann and J.P. Abraham, 1975.
    Fitzgerald trait. Deficiency of a hitherto unrecognized agent,
    Fitzgerald factor, participating in surface-mediated reactions
    of clotting, fibrinolysis, and generation of kinins and PF/Dil.
    J. Clin. Invest. 55: 1082.
Saito, H., G.H. Goldsmith, M. Moroi and N. Aoki, 1977. The spectrum
    of α_2-plasmin inhibitor. Blood 50: 282 (Abstract).
Schiffman, S. and P. Lee, 1975. Partial purification and charac-
    terization of contact activation cofactor. J. Clin. Invest.
    56: 1082.
Schiffman, S., R. Pecci and P. Lee, 1977. Contact activation of
    Factor XI: Evidence that the primary role of contact activation
    cofactor (CAC) is to facilitate the activation of factor XII.
    Throm. Res. 10: 319.

Soltay, M.I., H.Z. Movat and A.H. Özge-Anwar. The kinin system
     of human plasma V. The probable derivation of prekallikrein
     activator from activated Hageman factor (XIIa). Proc. Soc.
     Exp. Med. 138: 952.
Soulier, J.P. and O. Prou-Wartelle, 1960. New data on Hageman
     factor and plasma thromboplastin antecedent: the role of
     'contact' in the initial phase of blood coagulation. Brit.
     J. Haemat. 6: 88.
Weiss, A.S., J.I. Gallin and A.P. Kaplan, 1974. Fletcher factor
     deficiency. A diminished rate of Hageman factor activation
     caused by absence of prekallikrein with abnormalities of
     coagulation, fibrinolysis, chemotactic activity, and kinin
     generation. J. Clin. Invest. 53: 622.
Wuepper, K.S., 1973. Prekallikrein deficiency in man. J. Exp.
     Med. 138: 1345.
Wuepper, K.D., D.R. Miller and M.J. Lacombe, 1975. Flaujeac
     trait: deficiency of kininogen in man. J. Clin. Invest.
     56: 1663.
Zimmerman, T.S., O.D. Ratnoff and A.E. Powell, 1971. Immunologic
     differentiation of classic hemophilia (factor VIII deficiency)
     and von Willebrand's disease. J. Clin. Invest. 50: 244.

THE ROLE OF HIGH MOLECULAR WEIGHT KININOGEN IN CONTACT ACTIVATION

OF COAGULATION, FIBRINOLYSIS AND KININ GENERATION

Allen P. Kaplan

Division of Allergy, Rheumatology and Clinical
Immunology
State University of New York, Stony Brook, N.Y. 11794

During the past decade, considerable progress has been made
in understanding the mechanism by which the intrinsic coagulation
and fibrinolytic pathways are activated and defining their relationship to the generation of the vasoactive peptide, bradykinin. In
fact, the three proteins of the plasma kinin-forming system; namely,
Hageman factor (Ratnoff and Rosenblum, 1958), prekallikrein (Wuepper,
1973; Weiss et al., 1974; Saito et al., 1974) and high molecular
weight (HMW kininogen (Colman et al., 1975; Wuepper et al., 1975)
have been shown to be the major factors required for contact activation of plasma. In this review I will present a detailed analysis
of our present concept of the early events of these pathways.
Emphasis will be placed upon the role of HMW-kininogen as a cofactor
that is essential for surface dependent activation of coagulation
and fibrinolysis and the molecular mechanisms by which this function
is accomplished.

Interaction of Prekallikrein, Factor XI and HMW-kininogen in Plasma

Reports suggesting that kallikrein can be purified as a complex
with another plasma protein (Wendel, et al., 1972) and that prekallikrein appears to circulate in plasma as a complex (Nagasawa
and Nakayasu, 1973) prompted the studies of Mandle Jr. et al. (1976)
and Thompson et al. (1977) in which prekallikrein and factor XI
were each shown to circulate bound to HMW-kininogen. When normal
human plasma was fractionated on Sephadex G-200, the apparent
molecular weight of each of the above proteins could be determined.
Factor XI was found at a molecular weight of 380,000, prekallikrein
was found at 260,000, Hageman factor fractionated at 115,000, and

plasminogen was located at 95,000. However, when the molecular
weights of purified factor XI and prekallikrein were assessed by
gel filtration, values of 175,000 and 100,000 respectively were
obtained, a discrepancy of approximately 200,000. Purified Hageman
factor and plasminogen fractionated at the same position as they
did when whole plasma was assessed, and therefore, did not appear
to circulate as part of a complex. When the molecular weight of
prekallikrein and factor XI was determined in plasma that is
deficient in HMW-kininogen, factor XI was found at 175,000 and prekallikrein was found at 100,000 suggesting that each protein normally
circulates bound to HMW-kininogen. Reconstitution of HMW-kininogen
deficient plasma with purified HMW-kininogen followed by fractionation
by Sephadex G-200 gel filtration reproduced the chromatographic
pattern of factor XI and prekallikrein in normal plasma. In
addition, direct binding of purified prekallikrein to HMW-kininogen
(Mandle, Jr. et al., 1976) and direct binding of partially purified
factor XI to HMW-kininogen (Thompson, et al., 1977) have been
demonstrated.

Normal plasma contains approximately twice the concentration
of HMW-kininogen as the sum of the factor XI and prekallikrein
concentrations, thus complete binding of factor XI and prekallikrein results. No complex has been observed containing prekallikrein, factor XI, and HMW-kininogen as a single entity; prekallikrein and factor XI appears to circulate bound to different molecules of HMW-kininogen. Binding to HMW-kininogen also appears to
be a specific property of the Hageman factor substrates and the
complexes of prekallikrein-HMW-kininogen and factor XI-HMW-kini-
nogen are each adsorbed to surfaces where they then interact with
surface-bound Hageman factor. A schematic diagram showing the
critical constituents bound to the surface is shown in Figure 1.

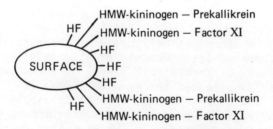

Figure 1.   Binding of Hageman factor and complexes of HMW
            kininogen with prekallikrein and factor XI to a surface.

Activation and Fragmentation of Hageman Factor: The Role of
the Surface, HMW-Kininogen, and Prekallikrein

The activation of Hageman factor, to be described herein, may
occur by at least two different mechanisms. The first consists of
a cleavage without obvious fragmentation in which the active enzyme
consists of chains linked by disulfide bonds, and the second, a
cleavage which liberates one òr more active fragments. The discovery of the active fragments of Hageman factor by Kaplan and
Austen (1970) provided the first evidence that activation could be
performed enzymatically (Kaplan and Austen, 1971). The final
product, a prealbumin fragment observed as two closely migrating
bands upon alkaline disc gel electrophoresis, functioned as a
potent prekallikrein activator but retained only 2 to 5 percent of
the coagulant activity of the unfragmented Hageman factor. Subsequently, plasmin was shown to be capable of directly digesting
Hageman factor to yield these fragments (Kaplan and Austen, 1971).
Similar prealbumin activities described in the rabbit (Wuepper et
al., 1970), guinea pig (Treloar and Movat, 1970) and man (Movat et
al., 1971; Wuepper and Cochrane, 1971) were subsequently shown to
be derived from Hageman factor (Cochrane and Wuepper, 1971; Soltay
et al., 1972) and the ability of plasmin to activate and fragment
Hageman factor was confirmed (Burrowes et al., 1972). Although
not purified, an activated preparation of Hageman factor was also
described whose molecular weight upon gel filtration (115,000) was
identical to that of unactivated Hageman factor, yet it readily
clotted Hageman factor deficient plasma in the absence of kaolin.
This preparation was designated intact activated Hageman factor
(Kaplan and Austen, 1971). In addition, at least two active fragments were described whose molecular weight was intermediate between
that of the prealbumin fragments and the unfragmented active
molecule. Thus by gel filtration, active species were detected at
molecular weights of 115,000, 90,000, 60,000 and 40,000 (Kaplan
et al., 1971) and each of the first three species could be converted
to the 40,000 mol. wt. prealbumin fragment (Kaplan and Austen, 1971;
Kaplan, et al., 1971).

The discovery of prekallikrein deficient plasma lead to an
examination of the ability of kallikrein to activate and fragment
Hageman factor. Kallikrein was found to function in a similar
manner to plasmin, however, it was approximately 10 times as effective (Cochrane et al., 1973) and could act upon either surface
bound or fluid phase Hageman factor. When Hageman factor was
iodinated, digested, and examined by SDS gel electrophoresis,
trypsin plasmin, and kallikrein were found to yield similar patterns
(Revak, et al., 1974). The molecular weight of Hageman factor was
90,000 in unreduced gels and 80,000 after reduction; upon digestion
it was converted to a 28,000 active fragment which corresponded to
the stable prealbumin fragment previously described, and a 50,000
dalton fragment remained. Further digestion converted the 50,000

dalton fragment to fragments of 40,000 and 10,000. However, the
formation of an active, unfragmented form of Hageman factor was
not detected. The 50,000 dalton fragment was subsequently shown
to be the portion of the molecule that binds to surfaces (Revak
et al., 1976).

With the discovery of HMW kininogen deficiency, it became
clear that the proposed reciprocal mechanism in which activated
Hageman factor converts prekallikrein, and kallikrein in turn
activates the Hageman factor was incomplete. Thus, when the role
of HMW kininogen was further examined it was found to enhance both
the function of activated Hageman factor and the formation of activated Hageman factor. For a fixed quantity of surface bound
Hageman factor, the subsequent activation of each Hageman factor
substrate appeared proportional to the quantity of HMW kininogen
added (Griffin and Cochrane, 1976; Meier et al., 1977a). Such an
experiment demonstrates the effect of HMW kininogen upon the system
but does not distinguish an effect upon the function of activated
Hageman factor from the formation of activated Hageman factor.
However, augmentation of the ability of Hageman factor fragments
to convert prekallikrein to kallikrein in the absence of a surface
has been reported (Meier et al., 1977a; Liu et al., 1977). In
this case the Hageman factor utilized is already active thus the
effect observed is upon its function. Furthermore, addition of
Hageman factor fragments to HMW-kininogen deficient plasma failed
to yield the predicted activation of either prekallikrein or factor
XI and this abnormality was corrected upon reconstitution with HMW-
kininogen (Liu et al., 1977). Alternatively, limited trypsin
treatment of surface-bound Hageman factor could be utilized to
achieve activation, and the enhancing effect of HMW kininogen upon
the subsequent activation of prekallikrein or factor XI could then
be observed (Griffin and Cochrane, 1976). The reaction appeared
stoichiometric in that the activity observed was proportional to
the HMW kininogen input; however there appeared to be an optimal
concentration of HMW kininogen that could be used and excess HMW
kininogen was inhibitory (Meier et al., 1977a). The same profile
has been reported for the effect of HMW kininogen upon the function
of the Hageman factor fragments (Liu et al., 1977), however, the
cause of this inhibition is not known. Critical to the interpretation of these experiments is a determination of whether HMW
kininogen affects binding of Hageman factor to surfaces. When
this was examined no effect was found (Meier et al., 1977a).
Furthermore, any activated Hageman factor detected was firmly
adsorbed to the surface suggesting that the molecular form of
activated Hageman factor was not the prealbumin fragments since
these fragments lack the binding site for the surface.

Although these data demonstrate an effect of HMW kininogen
upon the function of activated Hageman factor, they do not pre-
clude an effect upon the activation of Hageman factor. Griffin

and Cochrane (1976) reported that the rate of cleavage of Hageman factor by kallikrein appeared to be enhanced by HMW kininogen suggesting an effect upon Hageman factor activation. Meier et al. (1977a) assessed this reaction functionally and demonstrated that the ability of kallikrein to activate Hageman factor was markedly augmented by HMW kininogen. Figure 2 is a demonstration of the ability of kallikrein to activate Hageman factor as assessed in the same two-stage assay described above. Unactivated Hageman factor and kallikrein were adsorbed to the surface in the presence or absence of HMW kininogen. The mixture was centrifuged, the pellet was washed and the washed pellet was assayed for its ability to convert prekallikrein to kallikrein. Activation of Hageman factor during the initial incubation with kallikrein was observed only in the presence of HMW kininogen and the active moiety generated was bound to the surface. When the incorporation of ^{3}H-DFP into the surface-bound reactants was examined, incorporation of ^{3}H-DFP into Hageman factor was not enhanced by the surface alone or the surface plus HMW-kininogen. However, incorporation of ^{3}H-DFP into Hageman factor occured upon incubation with kallikrein and a marked augmentation of ^{3}H-DFP uptake occurred upon addition of kallikrein plus HMW-kininogen (Meier et al., 1977a). Figure 3 is a schematic diagram of this reciprocal interaction of surface-bound Hageman factor and prekallikrein indicating that the reaction rate in each direction is augmented by HMW kininogen.

It should be emphasized that the surface and the active site of kallikrein were required for this activation of Hageman factor to proceed. Thus kallikrein did not correct prekallikrein deficient plasma in the absence of a surface (Kaplan et al., 1974), DFP-kallikrein did not correct prekallikrein deficient plasma in the presence of a surface (Meier et al., 1977a) and DFP-kallikrein would not activate purified surface-bound Hageman factor (Meier et al., 1977a). The surface has been estimated to augment the rate of cleavage of Hageman factor by kallikrein by as much as 50-fold (Griffin, 1978) and, when activation of Hageman factor was examined by incorporation of ^{3}H-DFP, no activation of Hageman factor by the surface was observed in the absence of prekallikrein and HMW kininogen. Thus the surface appears to augment the rate of interaction of the reactants, and, in particular, render the Hageman factor a better substrate for plasma kallikrein. The ability of HMW kininogen to augment the function of activated Hageman factor has been estimated to be 3-4 fold while its effect upon the activation of Hageman factor yields a 40 fold enhancement, (Meier, et al., 1977a). When combined with the surface, the rate is augmented 6000 fold. The major theoretical consideration that is not yet resolved is whether some combination of the surface, Hageman factor, prekallikrein and HMW kininogen generates an active site or whether trace quantities of one of the enzymes normally circulates in an active form. In the latter case, binding to the surface in the presence of HMW kininogen might augment the reaction rate sufficient-

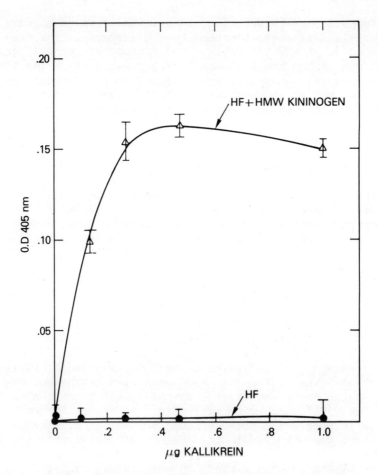

Figure 2.   Dose-response of the activation and function of
bound Hageman factor by kallikrein in the presence
and absence of HMW kininogen.

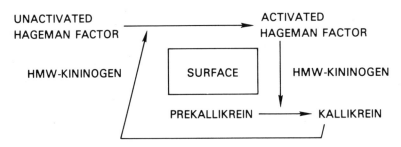

Figure 3.   Schematic diagram of the reciprocal activation
of surface-bound Hageman factor and prekallikrein
that is catalyzed by HMW kininogen.

ly to initiate the cascade. It is possible that changes observed
upon binding of Hageman factor to surfaces or ellagic acid, (Mc
Millan, et al., 1974) may relate to the increased rate of cleavage
of Hageman factor rather than the generation of a new active site
in the Hageman factor. The initial cleavage of human Hageman
factor has been reported to occur within a disulfide bridge such
that the product was the same size as the starting material (Revak
et al., 1977; Revak, et al., 1978) and remained bound to the surface.
A second cleavage external to the disulfide bond liberates the
28,000 dalton Hageman factor fragment.

Alternative Mechanisms of Hageman Factor Activation

Since the major activator of Hageman factor is kallikrein,
it is likely that one or more alternative enzymes account for the
gradual activation of Hageman factor observed in prekallikrein
deficient plasma. Both plasmin and factor XIa have been shown to
be capable of activating and cleaving Hageman factor in the fluid
phase, (Kaplan et al., 1971; Bagdasarian, et al., 1973; Cochrane
et al., 1973) and the ability of both of these enzymes to activate
surface-bound Hageman factor has been investigated, (Meier, et al.,
1977b; Griffin, 1978). At ratios of enzyme/Hageman factor of 1:50,
both plasmin and factor XIa activated Hageman factor as assessed
by the subsequent ability of the surface bound Hageman factor to
convert prekallikrein to kallikrein. Plasmin was approximately
one-tenth as effective an activator as kallikrein, and, in contrast
to kallikrein, no augmentation by HMW kininogen was evident. When
factor XIa was assayed, it was also about one-tenth as potent a
Hageman factor activator as kallikrein, however, Hageman factor
activation, as assessed by the subsequent conversion of prekallikrein to kallikrein, was augmented 2-3 fold in the presence of HMW
kininogen (HMW kininogen augmented the ability of kallikrein to

activate Hageman factor 40-fold). When the effect of HMW kininogen
upon the rate of cleavage of Hageman factor was assessed, no
augmentation was seen when plasmin was used as the activator,
however no significant effect was seen when factor XIa was the
activator, (Griffin, 1978). It is possible that the small functional
augmentation seen when factor XIa is the activator represents an
effect upon prekallikrein activation, which is utilized to assay
for HFa. Nevertheless, it is clear that the major effect of HMW
kininogen upon Hageman factor activation occurs when kallikrein
is used as the activator. In all cases, the presence of the
surface augmented the rate of cleavage of Hageman factor by each
of the enzymes tested (Griffin, 1978).

The main effect of HMW kininogen is to place the Hageman
factor substrates on the surface in an optimal position for their
subsequent interaction with Hageman factor (Mandle, Jr., et al.,
1976; Thompson, et al, 1977). In the absence of HMW kininogen,
less prekallikrein or Factor XI is bound to the surface (Wiggins,
et al., 1977) and neither activation of Hageman factor, nor activation of prekallikrein or Factor XI proceed at a normal rate.
The augmentation of the rate of activation and cleavage of prekallikrein and Factor XI by activated Hageman factor observed in
the presence of HMW kininogen may therefore, reflect an effect
upon the Hageman factor substrates. However, it is also possible
that HMW kininogen directly augments the function of the active
site of Hageman factor. Evidence to suggest this possibility is
the observation that the rate of cleavage of acetyl-glycyl-lysyl-
methyl ester by Hageman factor fragments is augmented by HMW
kininogen, (Liu et al., 1977).

Prekallikrein

Human prekallikrein has been purified by Mandle and Kaplan
(1977) utilizing fractionation on QAE Sephadex SP Sephadex, and
Sephadex G150 gel filtration followed by passage over a combined
immunoadsorbent to IgG and B_2 glycoprotein I.

The molecular weights reported for human prekallikrein as
assessed by gel filtration have ranged from 100,000 to 127,000.
However, when purified prekallikrein was examined by SDS gel
electrophoresis, two molecular variants were identified at 88,000
and 85,000 daltons respectively which have been designated prekallikreins I and II. Upon immunoelectrophoresis, in 1% agar at
pH 8.3, prekallikrein migrated as a fast γ globulin and its isoelectric point was determined to be between 8.5 and 9.0 (peak
value at 8.7) utilizing ampholytes that ranged from pH 7 to 10.

The Mechanism of Activation of Human Prekallikrein

Activation of human prekallikrein by HFa proceeds by limited

proteolytic digestion. Each of the molecular forms of prekallikrein seen at 88,000 and 85,000 daltons is cleaved and upon reduction
a two-chain disulfide linked enzyme results. A heavy chain of
52,000 daltons is linked to a light chain of either 36,000 or
33,000 daltons corresponding to the two forms of the starting
material. Figure 4 shows a preparation of ^{125}I prekallikrein which
was partially activated so that approximately 50 percent was converted to kallikrein. The mixture was then reduced, subjected to
SDS gel electrophoresis, and an autoradiogram of the gel was made.
One can readily visualize the undigested prekallikrein, the kallikrein heavy chain and the two kallikrein light chains. On the
same figure is shown an identical experiment in which non-radio-
labeled prekallikrein was activated, incubated with ^{3}H-DFP, reduced,
and subjected to SDS gel electrophoresis and autoradiography. All
of the ^{3}H-DFP was seen in the light chains indicating that this
portion of the molecule contains the active site of kallikrein,
(Mandle and Kaplan, 1977). A time course of cleavage of 15 ug
prekallikrein with 0.5 ug Hageman factor fragments as assessed
after reduction and SDS gel electrophoresis is shown in Figure 5.
As the two forms of prekallikrein were cleaved, there was a gradual
formation of the kallikrein heavy chain and the two light chains.
The evolution of functional activity has been shown to parallel
the percent conversion to the cleaved form. In the absence of
reducing agents, the molecular weight of prekallikrein and kallikrein were the same, thus there was no evidence of release of any
peptide during activation, and activation occurred by cleavage
within a disulfide bridge. The difference in molecular weight of
prekallikreins I and II was reflected in the light chains. The
evidence that both bands represent prekallikrein included: 1) both
were cleaved by Hageman factor fragments and yielded similar
activation patterns, 2) they were not interconvertible upon activation by Hageman factor or incubation of prekallikrein with
kallikrein, 3) they contained the same antigenic determinants,
4) DFP was incorporated into the light chains of each molecular
form of the active enzymes and, 5) neither band was seen when
prekallikrein deficient plasma was fractionated, (Mandle and Kaplan,
1977).

Purification and Characterization of Human HMW Kininogen

Thompson et al. (1978) have utilized a modification of the
procedure of Habal, et al. (1974) and Habal and Movat (1974) to
isolate human HMW kininogen. The purified material had a molecular
weight of 210,000 upon Sephadex G-200 gel filtration, an isoelectric point of 4.3 and a molecular weight of 120,000 when
assessed by SDS gel electrophoresis. Over 90 percent of the
material remained at 120,000 daltons after reduction indicating
that the HMW kininogen isolated was a single chain. It, therefore,
appears likely that two-chain forms of human or bovine HMW kininogen that have been isolated were partially cleaved during the

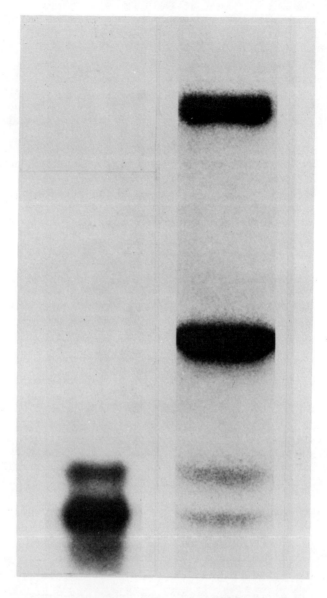

Figure 4. Autoradiogram of a mixture of ^{125}I-labeled
kallikrein and prekallikrein showing the prekallikrein, the kallikrein heavy chain and the
two kallikrein light chains (right gel). The
left gel is an autoradiogram of a reduced SDS-
polyacrylamide gel electrophoresis of ^{3}H-DFP
treated kallikrein showing incorporative of
^{3}H-DFP into both kallikrein light chains.

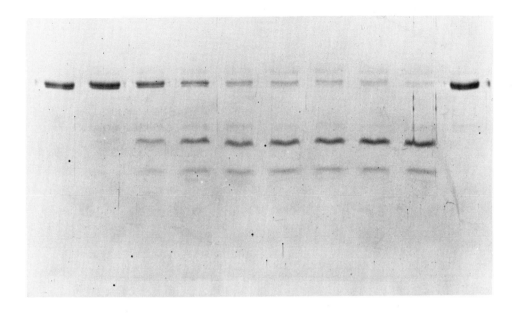

Figure 5. Kinetics of prekallikrein activation by Hageman
           factor fragments. From left to right the gel
           contains the starting material followed by time
           0, 2, 5, 10, 15, 25, 40, and 60 minute time-points
           after addition of Hageman factor. The final
           sample is a premixed control of SDS-buffer plus
           starting material and Hageman factor fragments
           incubated at 37°C for 60 minutes.

purification.

Digestion of HMW Kininogen by Plasma Kallikrein

When human HMW kininogen was digested by plasma kallikrein
and examined by SDS gel electrophoresis, an apparent loss of
approximately 15,000 daltons was seen. The peptides released,
have not been isolated (other than bradykinin) however, release
of a fragment analogous to bovine fragment 1.2 has not been observed. When a time course of digestion of human HMW kininogen
by plasma kallikrein was performed, the mixture reduced, and then
examined by SDS gel electrophoresis, the pattern shown in Figure
6 was seen. A heavy chain represented by two closely spaced bands
at approximately 66,000 and 56,000 daltons, and a light chain

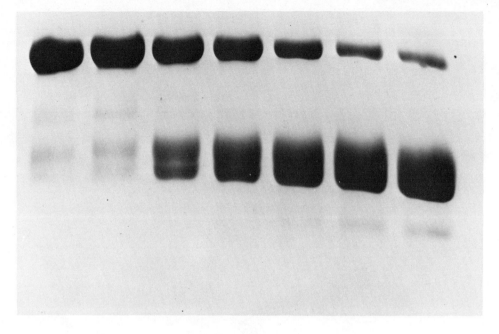

Figure 6.   Time course of interaction of 500 ug of HMW
             kininogen with 5 ug plasma kallikrein at 37°C.
             SDS polyacrylamide gel electrophoresis of 30 ug
             of reduced protein is shown after digestion for
             0, 1, 5, 10, 20, 30, and 40 minutes. Two heavy
             chain bands at 66,000 and 56,000 daltons are seen
             as well as the light chain band at 37,000 daltons.

seen at 37,000 daltons, were progressively formed as the starting
HMW kininogen was cleaved. The reason for the heavy chain heterogeneity is not clear; it was present in the small amount of cleaved
HMW kininogen in the starting material and conversion of the 66,000
dalton band to the 56,000 dalton band was not observed. When
human HMW kininogen was cleaved by plasma kallikrein, there was
no apparent loss in coagulant activity; furthermore, a combination
of kallikrein cleavage, reduction and alkylation, and treatment
with 6M quanidine hydrochloride did not inactivate it. Thus the
individual chains could be isolated and tested for coagulant
activity. As shown in Figure 7, all of the coagulant activity was
associated with the HMW kininogen light chain (Thompson et al.,
1978).

    Antibody to HMW kininogen has been prepared and used to deter-
mine the distinguishing features of HMW kininogen and LMW kininogen.
A sheep was immunized with kininogen and the sheep plasma adsorbed

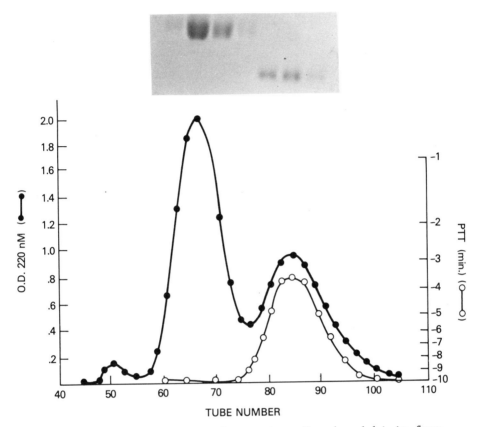

Figure 7. Sephadex G-200 gel filtration of reduced kinin-free
           HMW kininogen. The absorbance at 220 nm is shown
           as well as the ability of aliquots to correct the
           partial thromboplastin time of HMW kininogen deficient
           plasma. Above is shown the SDS-polyacrylamide gel
           electrophoretic pattern obtained after electrophoresis
           of 100 ul of tubes 60, 65, 70, and 75 (heavy chain)
           followed by electrophoresis of 100 ul of 10-fold
           concentration of tubes 80, 85, and 90 (light chain).

with Williams trait plasma to yield an antibody that reacts with
both high and low molecular weight kininogens. When the sheep
antiserum was adsorbed with Fitzgerald trait plasma (which has
significant quantities of LMW kininogen) an antiserum that was
monospecific for HMW kininogen resulted.

Factor XI

Activation of Human Factor XI

Purified preparations of human factor XI have a molecular
weight of 155,000 to 160,000 upon SDS gel electrophoresis, however
upon reduction, the molecular weight is 80,000 to 82,000 and only
a single band is seen (Wuepper, 1973; Kaplan et al., 1974).
Thus it appears that factor XI is a two chain molecule and the
two constituent chanis are virtually the same size. A similar
observation has been made when highly purified bovine factor XI
was examined (Kaode, et al., 1977) and thus far, incorporation of
high concentrations of benzamidine and DFP into the isolation procedure has not resulted in the formation of a single chain form
of factor XI.

Cleavage of human factor XI by trypsin (Wuepper, 1972; Saito
et al., 1973), Hageman factor fragments (Kaplan, et al., 1974;
Heck and Kaplan, 1974; Kaplan et al., 1976) or surface bound activated Hageman factor (Bouma and Griffin, 1977a; Kurachi and Davie,
1977) resulted in cleavage of the 80,000 daltons chains within a
disulfide bridge. Thus in the absence of reduction, the molecular
weight of factor XI and factor XIa were essentially the same.
However, upon reduction the two 80,000 chains of the starting
material appeared to be cleaved to chains of 50,000 and 30,000.
When factor XI was activated by Hageman factor, inactivated by
^{3}H-DFP, and reduced, ^{3}H-DFP was incorporated into the 30,000 dalton
light chain (Bouma and Griffin, 1977a). When binding of antithrombin III heparin by factor XIa was quantitated, two moles of
antithrombin III appeared to be bound by each mole of factor XIa
suggesting that there are two active sites in factor XIa, one for
each light chain present, (Kurachi and Davie, 1977).

Factor XI circulates as a complex with HMW kininogen, (Thompson
et al., 1977), the rate of conversion of factor XI to factor XIa
is augmented by HMW kininogen and the rate of formation of activated
Hageman factor (and factor XIa) are dependent upon prekallikrein.
Yet prekallikrein circulates to different HMW kininogen molecules
than does factor XI thus a mechanism must exist in which Hageman
factor that is activated by kallikrein can interact with the factor
XI-HMW kininogen complex. This may require movement of either
kallikrein or activated Hageman factor along the surface or release
and readsorption of activated molecules at the surface-fluid phase
interface. The ability of factor XIa-HMW kininogen to activate
Hageman factor may, in part, account for the gradual correction
of prekallikrein deficient plasma as the time of incubation with
the surface is increased. The ability of factor XIa to completely
correct the coagulation of defect of Hageman factor, prekallikrein,
or HMW kininogen deficient plasmas, and the normal rate of generation
of plasmin and bradykinin upon activation of factor XI deficient

plasma indicate that in a practical sense, activation of factor XIa represents the second step in the intrinsic coagulation pathway. It may, however, play an alternative role in the initial step when prekallikrein is absent.

The Role of the Early Steps of the Intrinsic Coagulation Pathway in Fibrinolysis

Hageman factor dependent conversion of plasminogen to plasmin is readily demonstrable in whole plasma (Niewiarowski and Prow-Wartelle, 1959; Iatridis and Ferguson, 1962; McDonagh and Ferguson, 1970). Since prekallikrein and HMW kininogen are required for optimal activation and function of Hageman factor, they are also required for activation of the Hageman factor dependent fibrinolytic pathway. However, identification of the molecule or molecules that directly convert plasminogen to plasmin has been the subject of numerous investigations and the results have not been clear. Colman (1969) first reported that incubation of kallikrein with plasminogen leads to the generation of plasmin and the kinetics of the reaction appeared to be stoichiometric. Ogston et al., (1969) demonstrated a cofactor required for Hageman factor dependent fibrinolysis that appeared to be distinguishable from kallikrein and factor XIa. However, it was clearly present in plasma fractions containing these factors. The assay for this protein was dependent upon reconstitution of glass-adsorbed plasma from which the fibrinolytic factor had been depleted. This "Hageman factor co-factor" had a molecular weight of 160,000 and it migrated with the γ globulins. Kaplan and Austen (1972) subsequently demonstrated a Hageman factor-activatable plasma factor called plasminogen proactivator, which upon activation, was able to directly convert plasminogen to plasmin. These authors proposed that the plasminogen activator derived was responsible for the plasminogen-converting activity in kallikrein preparations. The demonstration of plasminogen proactivator activity in the γglobulin fraction of prekallikrein deficient plasma appeared to confirm their interpretation (Kaplan et al., 1973). Subsequently, Laake and Vennerod (1974) reported their inability to separate prekallikrein from plasminogen proactivator and concluded that kallikrein and plasminogen-activating activities are functions of the same molecule. When these authors examined the γ globulin effluent obtained from prekallikrein-deficient plasma, no plasminogen activator or proactivator activity was observed (Vennerod and Laake, 1976).

The successful purification of human prekallikrein has shed further light upon this question. First, when human prekallikrein was isolated in the presence of proteolytic inhibitors, the prekallikrein and plasminogen proactivator activates coincided and the two-banded pattern was shown to represent prekallikrein heterogeneity rather than two separate Hageman factor substrates, (Mandle and Kaplan, 1977). Second, kallikrein was shown to cleave

prekallikrein and decrease its molecular weight by 10,000 daltons;
this difference in size corresponded to the previously reported
difference in size between prekallikrein and plasminogen proactivator. Finally, fractionation of prekallikrein deficient plasma
demonstrated that the plasminogen proactivator activity seen
associated with prekallikrein was absent, (Mandle and Kaplan, 1977).
Hence the conclusion was reached that prekallikrein is a plasminogen
proactivator and that the previous reported activity was a property
of prekallikrein and/or the prekallikrein degradation product.
However, plasminogen activating activity was again found in the
γ globulin fraction of normal plasma (Mandle and Kaplan, 1977)
which was not attributable to prekallikrein and this same activity
was found in prekallikrein-deficient plasma. Further fractionation
of this material demonstrated that the activity was superimposed
upon factor XI. In addition, two plasminogen proactivator peaks
have been reported upon subsequent chromatography of the γ globulin
fraction obtained from normal plasma (Kaplan et al., 1976) suggesting that factor XI may be a second proactivator. The observation
that plasminogen activating activity does indeed reside in the γ
globulin effluent of prekallikrein deficient plasma has been confirmed (Bouma and Griffin, 1977b); however, these authors did not
demonstrate that the activity was Hageman factor activatable and

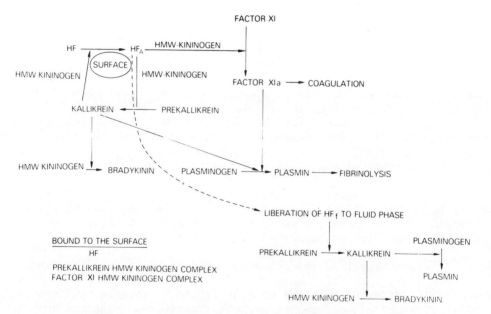

Figure 8. Diagram of the known interactions leading to
            Hageman factor dependent coagulation, fibrinolysis,
            and the generation of bradykinin.

considered prekallikrein to be the only plasminogen proactivator.
Clearly, the gradual conversion of plasminogen to plasmin observed
in prekallikrein deficient plasma is secondary to a Hageman factor
dependent enzyme that is not kallikrein. Recently, Goldsmith
et al., 1977, have presented evidence that activated Hageman factor
itself can function as a plasminogen activator. However, when
experiments are performed in which the fibrinolytic capacity of
prekallikrein is assessed, the concentration of HFf incubated with
plasminogen was less than 5 percent of the activity seen with
kallikrein. Thus larger quantities of activated Hageman factor
may be required for this effect to reach significant levels. It
appears clear that prekallikrein is a plasminogen proactivator,
factor XI may function as a second proactivator, and HFa or HFf
may directly contribute to plamsinogen activation.

Further studies in whole plasma are needed to distinguish
the effect of kallikrein upon fibrinolysis via its ability to
activate Hageman factor from its ability to convert plasminogen
to plasmin. It is of interest that one estimate of the direct
contribution of kallikrein to the conversion of plasminogen was
approximately 50 percent of the total Hageman factor dependent
fibrinolytic activity present in plasma. (Kluft, 1977).

A summary of the known interactions leading to coagulation,
fibrinolysis and kinin-formation is shown in Figure 8.

REFERENCES

Bagdasarian, A., Lahiri, B., and Colman, R.W. 1973. Origin of
        the high molecular weight activator of prekallikrein. J.
        Biol. Chem. 248: 7742-7747.
Bouma, B.N. and Griffin, J.H. 1977a. Human blood coagulation factor
        XI: Purification, properties and mechanism of activation.
        J. Biol. Chem. 252: 6432-6437.
Bouma, B.N. and Griffin, J.H., 1977b. Human prekallikrein (plas-
        minogen proactivator): Purification, characterization and
        activation by activated factor XII. Thromb. and Haemostasis.
        38: 136.
Burrowes, C.E., Movat, H.Z., and Soltay, M.J. 1972. The kinin
        system of human plasma VI. The action of plasmin. Proc. Soc.
        Exp. Biol. Med. 135: 959-966.
Cochrane, C.G., Revak, S.D., and Wuepper. K.D. 1973. Activation
        of Hageman factor in solid and fluid phases. J. Exp. Med.
        138: 1564-1583.

Cochrane, C.G. and Wuepper, K.D. 1971. The first component of the
    kinin-forming system in human and rabbit plasma. Its relation-
    ship to clotting factor XII (Hageman factor). J. Exp. Med.
    134: 896-1004.
Colman, R.W. 1969. Activation of plasminogen by human plasms kalli-
    krein. Biochem. Biophys. Res. Commun. 351: 273-279.
Colman, R.W., Bagdasarian, A., Talamo, R.C., Scott, C.F. Seavey, M.
    Guimares, J.A., Pierce, J.V., and Kaplan, A.P., 1975. Williams
    trait. Human kininogen deficiency with diminished levels of
    plasminogen proactivator and prekallikrein associated with
    abnormalities of the Hageman factor-dependent pathways. J.
    Clin. Invest. 56: 1650-1662.
Goldsmith, G.H., Saito, H., and Ratnoff, O.D., 1978. The activa-
    tion of plasminogen by Hageman factor (factor XII) and Hageman
    factor fragments. J. Clin. Invest. 62: 54-60.
Griffin, J.H., 1978. Role of surface in surface-dependent activa-
    tion of Hageman factor (Blood coagulation factor XII). Proc.
    Natl. Acad. Sci. 75: 1998-2002.
Griffin, J.H. and Cochrane, C.G., 1976. Mechanisms for the involve-
    ment of high molecular weight kininogen in surface-dependent
    reactions of Hageman factor. Proc. Nat. Acad. Sci., 8: 2554-2558.
Habal, F.M. and Movat, H.Z., 1974. Some physico chemical and func-
    tional differences between low and high molecular weight
    kininogens of human plasma. In: The chemistry and biology of
    the kallikrein-kinin system in health and disease. John J.
    Pisano and K. Frank Austen, eds. Fogarty International Center
    Proceedings No. 27, U.S. Government Printing Office, Washington
    D.C. pp. 129-131.
Habal, F.M., Movat, H.Z. and Burrowes, C.E., 1974. Isolation of
    two functionally different kininogens from human plasma -
    separation from proteinase inhibitors and interaction with
    plasma kallikrein. Biochem. Pharmacol. 23: 2291-2302.
Heck, L.W., and Kaplan, A.P., 1974. Substrates of human factor I.
    Isolation and characterization of PTA (Factor XI) and its
    inhibition by α_1 antitrypsin. J. Exp. Med. 140: 1615-1630.
Iatridis, S.G. and Ferguson, J.H., 1962. Active Hageman factor.
    A plasma lysokinase of the human fibrinolytic system. J.
    Clin. Invest. 41: 1277-1287.
Johnson, A.R., Ulevitch, R.J., and Ryan, K., 1976. Biochemical
    and biological properties of rabbit prekallikrein. Fed. Proc.
    35: 693.
Kaode, T., Hermodson, M.A., and Davie, E.W., 1977. Active site of
    bovine Hageman factor XI (plasma thromboplastin antecedent).
    Nature 266: 729-731.
Kaplan, A.P. and Austen, K.F., 1970. A prealbumin activator of
    prekallikrein. J. Immunol. 105: 802-811.
Kaplan, A.P. and Austen, K.F., 1971. A prealbumin activator of pre-
    kallikrein II. Derivation of activators of prekallikrein from
    active Hageman factor by digestion with plasmin. J. Exp.
    Med. 133: 672-712.

Kaplan, A.P. and Austen, K.F., 1972. The fibrinolytic pathway of human plasma. Isolation and characterization of the plasminogen proactivator. J. Exp. Med. 136: 1378-1393.

Kaplan, A.P., Goetzl, E.J., and Austen, K.F., 1973. The fibrinolytic pathway of human plasma II. Generation of chemotactic activity by activation of plasminogen proactivator. J. Clin. Invest. 52: 2591-2597.

Kaplan, A.P., Meier, H.W., and Mandle Jr., R., 1976. The Hageman factor dependent pathways of coagulation, fibrinolysis, and kinin-generation. Seminars Thrombosis Haemostasis 3: 1-26.

Kaplan, A.P., Meier, H.S., Yecies, L.D., and Heck, L.W., 1974. Hageman factor and its substrates: the role of factor XI (PTA), prekallikrein, and plasminogen proactivator in coagulation, fibrinolysis and kinin-generation. In: Chemistry and biology of the kallikrein-kinin system in health and disease. J.J. Pisano and K.F. Austen (eds) Fogarty International Center Proceedings No. 27, U.S. Government Printing Office, Washington, D.C., pp. 237-254.

Kaplan, A.P., Spragg, J., and Austen, K.F., 1971. The bradykinin-forming system in man. In: Biochemistry of the acute allergic reaction. K.F. Austen and E.L. Becker, eds. Oxford, Blackwell Scientific Publications Ltd., pp. 279-298.

Kato, H., Han, Y.N., Iwanaga, S., Suzuki, T., and Komiya, M., 1966. Bovine plasma HMW and LMW kininogens. Structural differences between heavy and light chains derived from the kinin-free proteins. J. Biochem. 80: 1299-1311.

Kluft, C., 1977. An inventory of plasminogen activators in human plasma. Thromb. and Haemostasis 38: 134.

Kurachi, K. and Davie, E.W., 1977. Activation of human factor XI (Plasma Thromboplastin Antecedent) by factor XIIa (Activated Hageman Factor). Biochem. 5831-5839.

Laake, K. and Vennerod, A.M., 1974. Factor XII-induced fibrinolysis. Studies on the separation of prekallikrein, plasminogen proactivator, and factor XI in human plasma. Thromb. Res. 4: 285-302.

Liu, C.Y., Scott, C.F., Bagdasarian, A., Pierce, J.V., Kaplan, A.P., and Colman, R.W. 1977. Potentiation of the function of Hageman factor fragments by high molecular weight kininogen. J. Clin. Invest. 60: 7-17.

Mandle, Jr., R., Colman, R.W., and Kaplan, A.P., 1976. Identification of prekallikrein and HMW-kininogen as a circulating complex in human plasma. Proc. Natl. Acad. Sci. U.S.A. 73: 4179-4183.

Mandle, Jr., R. and Kaplan, A.P., 1977. Hageman factor substrates. Human plasma prekallikrein: mechanism of activation by Hageman factor and participation in Hageman factor-dependent fibrinolysis. J. Biol. Chem. 252: 6097-6104.

McDonagh, K.S. and Ferguson, J.H., 1970. Studies on the participation of Hageman factor in fibrinolysis. Throm. et. Diath. Haemorrh. 24: 9.

McMillin, C.R., Saito, H., Ratnoff, O.D., and Walton, A.G., 1974.
    The secondary structure of human Hageman factor (Factor XII)
    and its alteration by activating agents. J. Clin. Invest.
    54: 1312–1322.
Meier, H.S., Pierce, J.V., Colman, R.W., and Kaplan, A.P., 1977a.
    Activation and function of human Hageman factor. The role
    of high molecular weight kininogen and prekallikrein. J. Clin.
    Invest. 60: 18–31.
Meier, H.L., Thompson, R.E., and Kaplan, A.P. Activation of Hageman
    factor by factor XIa–HMW–kininogen. Thromb. and Haemostasis
    38: 14, 1977b.
Movat, H.Z., Poon, M.C., and Tukeuchi, Y. 1971. The kinin system
    of human plasma I. Isolation of a low molecular weight
    activator of prekallikrein. Int. Arch. Allergy Appl. Immunol.
    40: 89–112.
Nagasawa, S. and Nakayasu, T., 1973. Human plasma prekallikrein
    as a protein complex. J. Biochem. 74: 401–403.
Niewiarowski, S. and Prow-Wartelle, O., 1959. Role du facteur
    contact (Facteur Hageman) dans la fibrinolyse. Thromb.
    Diath. Haemorrhag. 3: 593–603.
Ogston, D., Ogston, C.M., Ratnoff, O.D., and Forbes, C.O., 1969.
    Studies on a complex mechanism for the activation of plasmino-
    gen by kaolin and by chloroform: the participation of Hageman
    factor and additional cofactors. J. Clin. Invest. 48: 1786–
    1801.
Ratnoff, O.D. and Rosenblum, J.M., 1958. Role of Hageman factor in
    the initiation of clotting by glass: evidence that glass
    frees Hageman factor from inhibition. Am. J. Med. 25: 160–168.
Revak, S.D., Cochrane, C.G., Johnston, A., and Hugli, T., 1974.
    Structural changes accompanying enzymatic activation of
    Hageman factor. J. Clin. Invest. 54: 619–627.
Revak, S.D. and Cochrane, C.G., 1976. The relationship of structure
    and function in human Hageman factor. The association of
    enzymatic and binding activities with separate regions of
    the molecule. J. Clin. Invest. 57: 852–860.
Revak, S.D., Cochrane, C.G., Bouma, B.N., and Griffin, J.H., 1978.
    Surface and Fluid Phase Activities of Two Form of Activated
    Hageman Factor Produced During Contact Activation of Plasma.
    J. Exp. Med. 147: 719–229.
Revak, S.D., Cochrane, C.G., and Griffin, J.H., 1977. The binding
    and cleavage characteristics of human Hageman factor during
    contact activation. A comparison of normal plasma with
    plasmas deficient in factor XI, prekallikrein, or high mole-
    cular weight kininogen. J. Clin. Invest. 59: 1167–1176.
Saito, H., Ratnoff, O.D., and Donaldson, V.H., 1974. Defective
    activation of clotting, fibrinolytic and permeability enhan-
    cing systems in human Fletcher trait plasma. Circ. Res. 34:
    641–651.

Saito, H., Ratnoff, O.D., Marshall, J.S. and Pensky, J., 1973.
    Partial purification of plasma thromboplastin antecedent
    (factor XI) and its activation by trypsin. J. Clin. Invest.
    52: 850-861.
Soltay, M.J., Movat, H.Z. and Ozge-Anwar, A.H., 1972. The kinin
    system of human plasma V. The probable derivative of pre-
    kallikrein activator from activated Hageman factor. Proc.
    Soc. Exp. Biol. Med. 138: 952-958.
Thompson, R.E., Mandle, Jr., R., and Kaplan, A.P., 1977. Associa-
    tion of factor XI and High Molecular weight kininogen in
    human plasma. J. Clin. Invest. 60: 1376-1380.
Thompson, R.E., Mandle, Jr., R., and Kaplan, A.P., 1978. Charac-
    terization of Human High Molecular Weight Kininogen. Pro-
    coagulant activity associated with the light chain of
    Kinin-Free High Molecular Weight Kininogen. J. Exp. Med.
    147: 488-499.
Treloar, M.P. and Movat, H.Z., 1970. Isolation of two small mole-
    cular activators of the plasma kinin system in the guinea
    pig. Fed. Proc. 59: 576.
Vennerod, A.M. and Laake, K., 1976. Prekallikrein and plasminogen
    proactivator: Absence of plasminogen proactivator in
    Fletcher factor deficient plasma. Thromb. Res. 8: 519-522.
Weiss, A.S., Gallin, J.I., and Kaplan, A.P., 1974. Fletcher factor
    deficiency. Abnormalities of coagulation, fibrinolysis,
    chemotactic activity, and kinin generation attributable to
    absence of prekallikrein. J. Clin. Invest. 53: 622-633.
Wendel, U., Vogt, W., and Seidel, G., 1972. Purification and some
    properties of a kininogenase from human plasma activated by
    surface contact. Hoppe Seylers Z. Physiol. Chem. 353:
    1591-1606.
Wiggins, R.C., Bouma, B.N., Cochrane, C.G. and Griffin, J.H., 1977.
    Role of High Molecular Weight Kininogen in surface-binding
    and activation of coagulation factor XI and prekallikrein.
    Proc. Natl. Acad. Sci. 77-: 4636-4640.
Wuepper, K.D., Biochemistry and biology of components of the
    plasma kinin-forming system. In: Inflammation: Mechanism and
    Control.
Wuepper, K.D., 1973. Prekallikrein deficiency in man. J. Exp. Med.
    138:1345-1355.
Wuepper, L.D. and Cochrane, C.G., 1971. Isolation and mechanism
    of activation of components of the plasma kinin-forming
    system. In: The biochemistry of the acute allergic reactions-
    Second International Symposium. K.F. Austen and E.L. Becker,
    eds. Blackwell Scientific Publication, Ltd. pp. 299-320.
Wuepper, K.D., Miller, D.R., and LaCombe, M.J., Flaujeac trait.
    Deficiency of human plasma kininogen. J. Clin. Invest. 56:
    1663-1672, 1975.
Wuepper, K.D., Tucker, III, E.S., and Cochrane, C.G. 1970. Plasma
    kinin system: proenzyme components. J. Immunol. 105: 1307-1311.

FUJIWARA TRAIT: THE FIRST CASE OF KININOGEN DEFICIENCY IN JAPAN

Sachiko Oh-Ishi, Akinori Ueno, Yasuhiro Uchida, Makoto
Katori, Hisatomo Hayashi*, Hiromichi Koya*, Koichi
Kitajima*, and Ikuro Kimura*

Department of Pharmacology, Kitasato University School
of Medicine, Sagamihara, Kanagawa 228 and *2nd Department, Internal Medicine, Okayama University, Medical
School, Shikadacho, Okayama, Japan

ABSTRACT

Asymptomatic identical twins were found to show the prolonged
activated partial thromboplastin time, which was corrected by addition of normal, Hageman factor deficient or Fletcher trait plasma
but not corrected by Fitzgerald or Williams plasma. The prolonged
activated partial thromboplastin time was also corrected by addition
of highly purified bovine high molecular weight kininogen but not by
low molecular weight kininogen. When total kininogen was measured
as the amount of bradykinin released by trypsin on acid treated
plasma, only trace amount was detected in Fujiwara and Williams
plasmas, although Fitzgerald plasma showed approximately 50% of the
total kininogen of normal plasma level. Acetone-kaolin activated
amidase activity of plasma kallikrein was not generated by Fujiwara
plasma. Substitution with normal plasma in various ratios showed
plasma kallikrein activity proportionally to the normal plasma contents. Extrapolation with the values at 120 min after activation
gave the prekallikrein content of Fujiwara plasma as 30% of the
normal value.

INTRODUCTION

Asymptomatic identical twins showing the prolonged activated
partial thromboplastin time (APTT) were found at Okayama University
Hospital (Hayashi et al, 1978). Coagulation factors, I, II, V, VII,
VIII and IX were examined to be normal and factor XII was functionally
normal, when assayed with the deficient plasma. The prolonged APTT

was corrected by factor XII deficient, factor XI deficient or Fletcher
factor deficient plasma. Further, bovine high molecular weight
(HMW) kininogen corrected the prolonged APTT of Fujiwara plasma,
but low molecular weight (LMW) kininogen did not. The deficient
was designated as Fujiwara trait and a part of above results was
reported at 40th General Meeting of the Japan Hematological Society
(Hayashi et al, 1978; Oh-ishi et al, 1978) and at Congress of the
International Society of Hematology (Paris) (Hayashi et al, 1978).

In this report, plasma kallikrein-kinin system and its components in Fujiwara trait plasma were examined and discussed in comparison with similar deficient plasma already reported, such as
Fitzgerald (Saito et al, 1975) and Williams (Colman et al, 1975).

MATERIALS AND METHODS

Kaolin (k-5, Fisher Sci. Co., Fair Lawn, N.J.), Thrombofax reagent (Ortho Diagnostics Inc., Raritan, N.J.), factor XII deficient
plasma (Dade Division American Hospital Supply Co., Miami, Florida),
and Carbobenzoxy-L-phenylalanyl-L-arginine 4-methylcoumarinyl-7-
amide (Z-Phe-Arg-MCA, Peptide Institute Inc., Osaka) were purchased.

Authors are indepted to Drs. H. Kato and S. Iwanaga, Protein
Research Institute, Osaka University, for highly purified bovine HMW
and LMW kininogens, to Drs. H. Saito and O.D. Ratnoff, Case Western
Reserve University, for Fitzgerald trait and Fletcher trait plasmas, to Dr. R.W. Colman, University of Pennsylvania and Dr. A.P.
Kaplan, National Institutes of Health, for Williams trait and Fletcher trait plasmas, and to Drs. J.V. Pierce and J.J. Pisano, National Institutes of Health, for highly purified human HMW and LMW
kininogens and antisera to kininogens.

Assay procedure of APTT. 25 µl of the deficient or normal
plasma, 25 µl of kininogen solution in 0.15 M NaCl, or heated plasma
(60°C for 1 hr), 50 µl of Thrombofax reagent were mixed and then
50 µl kaolin suspension (5 mg/ml in 0.15 M NaCl) was added. The
mixture was preincubated at 37°C for exactly 2 min, and then 50 µl
of 0.025 M CaCl2 solution was added and clotting time was measured.

Assay method for total kininogen. The method was previously
reported (Uchida and Katori, 1978). Briefly, acid treated plasma
(pH 2.0) was incubated with trypsin and the released bradykinin was
assayed on rat uterus.

Assay method for prekallikrein. This was also previously
reported (Oh-ishi and Katori). Briefly, the plasma kallikrein activity, generated by a acetone-kaolin activation, was assayed by
peptidylfluorogenic substrate, Z-Phe-Arg-MCA. One unit of the
activity was defined as the enzyme activity that releases 10^{-7} M

aminomethylcoumarin in 10 min under the described condition (Oh-ishi and Katori).

Immunodiffusion. This was performed overnight at room temperature using 1% agarose in 0.02 M tris-HCl buffer, pH 8.0, containing 0.15 M NaCl.

RESULTS AND DISCUSSION

Correction of APTT. Fujiwara trait plasma showed the prolonged APTT, 700 - 800 sec, whereas normal plasma showed 64 sec. Normal, Fletcher (370 sec) and factor XII deficient (1000 sec) corrected the APTT of Fujiwara trait, but Fitzgerald and Williams plasmas did not correct it. Addition of heated plasma (60°C for 30 min) corrected APTT of Fujiwara trait proportionally to the added amounts, and the complete correction to the normal value was observed by addition of 10% of the heated plasma. Bovine highly purified HMW kininogen also corrected the APTT of Fujiwara trait and Fitzgerald trait plasmas, but bovine LMW kininogen did not.

Kinin formation of Fujiwara trait plasma. By kaolin activation (100 µl plasma, 1 mg kaolin in the final volume of 1 ml in 0.1 M tris - 0.15 M NaCl - buffer, pH 8.0, incubated for 1 hr), Fujiwara plasmas of twin patients generated less amount than 0.03 µg bradykinin/ml plasma, whereas normal citrated plasma generated 0.7 µg bradykinin/ml plasma.

Kinin formation was again tested after addition of 100 µl of the heated plasma. Fujiwara trait plasmas, generated kinin, 0.8 and 1.0 µg bradykinin/ml plasma, respectively, which corresponded to the kininogen amounts in the heated plasma added. Normal plasma generated 2.0 µg bradykinin/ml plasma under the same condition, which is the sum of the kininogen contents in normal plasma and heated plasma. This result strongly indicates the kinin-forming enzyme is present in Fujiwara trait plasmas.

Further, when Fujiwara trait plasmas were treated at 60°C for 30 min, and then partially purified plasma kallikrein (Oh-ishi and Katori) was added and incubated for 1 hr, kinin was hardly detected in Fujiwara trait plasmas, whereas normal plasma under the same condition showed 1.1 µg bradykinin/ml plasma.

Total kininogen content of Fujiwara trait plasma. Total kininogen was measured as reported (Uchida and Katori, 1978), and expressed as bradykinin equivalent/ml plasma. The levels in Fletcher and factor XII deficient plasmas were 3.06 and 3.61 µg bradykinin/ml plasma, respectively, but Fujiwara and Williams plasmas were 0.05 and 0.02, respectively. Fitzgerald plasma showed 1.84, about a half of the normal level.

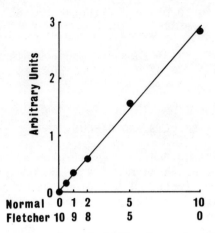

Fig 1. Standard curve of prekallikrein using Fletcher trait plasma.
     Abscissa indicates the ratios of the mixtures of normal and
Fletcher plasmas. The values of activities at 60 min after the
kaolin addition were plotted.

     Prekallikrein content of Fujiwara trait plasma. As reported
previously (Oh-ishi and Katori), kaolin-activation of prekallikrein
requires 10% of factor XII and also 10% of HMW kininogen. Prekallikrein content also affected the activation rate of prekallikrein
by a positive feedback. The prekallikrein content in the mixture
of Fletcher plasma and normal plasma was assayed. Activation rates
were proportional to the normal plasma content, and 100% normal
plasma reached the plateau in 30 min, but the mixtures reached them
in 60 min. Fig 1. shows the prekallikrein activity in the mixtures
of various ratios of normal plasma in Fletcher plasma. A linear
relationship was observed between the content of prekallikrein in
normal plasma and hydrolysis of Z-Phe-Arg-MCA.

     HMW kininogen was reported to be essential to the activation
of factor XII (Saito et al, 1975; Colman et al, 1975), and so this
prekallikrein assay could be affected by the content of HMW kininogen. As shown in Fig 2., Fujiwara trait plasma itself did not show
any kallikrein activity by this method. However, Fujiwara plasma
substituted by varying amounts of normal plasma showed the prekallikrein activity, which would be the sum of the prekallikrein contents
of normal and Fujiwara plasmas. Addition of more than 10% of normal
plasma showed the full activation of prekallikrein in 120 min, but
when the mixture contained less than 5% of normal plasma it did not
reach the plateau even in 180 min later. Then the peak values of
the mixtures containing more than 10% of normal plasma were replotted as shown in Fig 3. The prekallikrein levels of the mixtures
showed a linear relationship to the concentration of normal plasma
in percent. Hundred % of Fujiwara or Fitzgerald plasma itself showed

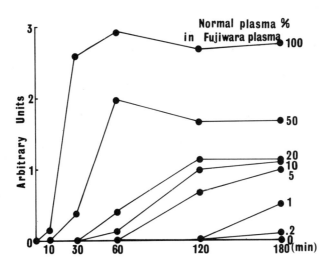

Fig. 2. Plasma kallikrein activities in the mixtures of Fujiwara trait and normal Plasma after kaolin activation. Ordinate indicates the arbitrary units of kallikrein activity. Abscissa shows the time after addition of kaolin (min).

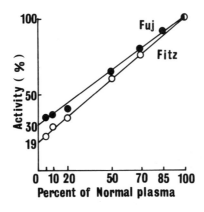

Fig. 3. Plasma kallikrein activity in percent, in the mixtures of normal and HMW kininogen deficient plasmas. The peak activities in Fig. 2 were replotted in percent of 100% normal plasma (Fuji) and in the same manner for Fitzgerald plasma (Fitz). Extrapolation at the ordinate shows the prekallikrein contents of 30% for Fujiwara and 19% for Fitzgerald plasma.

no activity. But extrapolation of the lines gave the prekallikrein
contents of 30% for Fujiwara trait and 19% for Fitzgerald trait
plasma. Williams plasma was estimated as 23% in the same way.

Immunodiffusion of deficient plasma. Against anti-HMW kininogen antiserum (goat), Fujiwara, Williams and Fitzgerald plasma
showed no precipitin line, but normal plasma and human HMW kininogen showed precipitin lines. Against anti-LMW kininogen antiserum
(goat), Fujiwara and Williams plasmas did not show any precipitin
line, but normal and Fitzgerald plasmas, HMW kininogen and LMW
kininogen showed the precipitin lines. The result indicates Fitzgerald plasma contains immunoreactive LMW kininogen protein, but
Fujiwara as well as Williams plasma did not contain either that of
HMW or LMW kininogen.

CONCLUSION

Plasma kallikrein-kinin system of Fujiwara twins, with no
clinical symptom, were examined in comparison with the available
plasmas of similar deficiency. Contents of kininogen and prekallikrein were assayed using previously reported methods. The immunoreactive kininogens were also examined. Those results showed that
Fujiwara trait is the deficiency of HMW kininogen, which participates in the contact activation of the intrinsic coagulation system
as well as plasma kallikrein-kinin system. Further Fujiwara trait
closely resembles Williams trait, in that both traits are deficient
in LMW kininogen also. As for the prekallikrein content all plasmas
from Fujiwara, Williams and Fitzgerald traits showed low levels by
the acetone-kaolin assay. These facts may concern with the proposal
that prekallikrein is present as complex with HMW kininogen in circulating blood (Mandle et al, 1976).

ACKNOWLEDGEMENTS

This work was supported partly by Scientific Research Grants
from the Ministry of Education, Sciences and Culture (310507).

REFERENCES

Colman, R.W., A. Bagdasarian, R.C. Talamo, C.F. Scott, M. Seavey,
J.A. Guimaraes, J.V. Pierce and A.P. Kaplan, 1975. Williams trait.
Human kininogen deficiency with diminished levels of plasminogen
proactivator and prekallikrein associated with abnormalities of the
Hageman factor-dependent pathways. J. Clin. Invest. 56, 1650.

Hayashi, H., H. Koya, K. Kitajima and I. Kimura, 1978. Coagulation
factor deficiency apparently related to the Fitzgerald trait: The
first case in Japan. Acta Med. Okayama 32, 81.

Hayashi, H., H. Koya, K. Kitajima, I. Kimura, S. Oh-ishi, A. Ueno, Y. Uchida and M. Katori, 1978. Fujiwara trait: The first case of a possible kininogen deficiency in Japan, Part I. Proceedings of the 40th General Meeting of the Japan Hematological Society. Acta Haematol. Jap. 41, 243. (in Japanese)

Hayashi, H., H. Koya, K. Kitajima, I. Kimura, M. Katori and S. Oh-ishi, 1978. Fujiwara trait: Kininogen deficiency in identical Japanese female twins. Proceedings of 17th Congress of the International Society of Hematology (July 26-29, Paris) 517.

Oh-ishi, S., A. Ueno, Y. Uchida, M. Katori, H. Hayashi, H. Koya, K. Kitajima and I. Kimura, 1978. Fujiwara trait: The first case of a possible kininogen deficiency in Japan, Part II. Proceedings of the 40th General Meeting of the Japan Hematological Society. Acta Haematol. Jap. 41, 243. (in Japanese)

Oh-ishi, S. and M. Katori, Fluorometric assay for plasma prekallikrein using peptidylmethylcoumarinylamide as a substrate. Thrombosis Res. (in press).

Mandle, R.J., R.W. Colman and A.P. Kaplan, 1976. Identification of prekallikrein and high-molecular-weight kininogen as a complex in human plasma. Proc. Natl. Acad. Sci. USA 73, 4179.

Saito, H., O.D. Ratnoff, R. Waldmann and J.P. Abraham, 1975. Fitzgerald trait: Deficiency of a hitherto unrecognized agent, Fitzgerald factor, participating in surface-mediated reactions of clotting, fibrinolysis, generation of kinins, and the property of diluted plasma enhancing vascular permeability (PF/DIL). J. Clin. Invest. 55, 1082.

Uchida, Y. and M. Katori, 1978. An improved method for determination of the total kininogen in rabbit and human plasma. Biochem. Pharmacol. 27, 1463.

DEXTRAN-INDUCED LOWERING OF PARAMETERS OF THE KALLIKREIN-KININ

SYSTEM IN RAT PLASMA

Kjell Briseid, Rolf Johansen and Liv Rustenberg

Department of Pharmacology, Institute of Pharmacy

University of Oslo, Blindern, Oslo 3, Norway

Pretreatment of rats with tranexamic acid inhibited the rapid lowering of the plasma levels of acetone/kaolin-activated prekallikrein proactivator and prekallikrein caused by the intravenous injection of dextran, but did not inhibit the reduction in the level of plasminogen, and potentiated the lowering of high molecular weight kininogen. By acetone/kaolin activation of normal rat plasma a mixture of surface-bound factor XII_a and unbound XII_f was obtained, and a BAEe-esterase (MW about 47,000) possessing weak kininogenase activity was present in addition to kallikrein. In activated plasma from dextran-treated rats the cleavage of XII_a was strongly reduced, and the second esterase was almost absent. It is suggested that dextran induces the loss of a plasma factor which is important for the cleavage of factor XII_a in the adopted procedure. This factor was not high molecular weight kininogen, and the lowering of plasminogen was too small to account for the reduction in PKA-activity.

INTRODUCTION

The intravenous injection of dextran into rats causes a marked and lasting hypotension. The mechanism initiating this reaction is not known. In a recent paper Briseid et al. (1978) showed that dextran induced rapid and significant reductions in the plasma levels of prekallikrein proactivator (pro-PKA), prekallikrein (PK) and high molecular weight kininogen (HMWK). They also found that pretreatment of the rats with an inhibitor of plasminogen (PG) activation, ε-aminocaproic acid, provided some protection against the hypotensive effect of dextran, and abolished the decreases in the plasma levels of pro-PKA and PK.

In the present investigation the early effect of intravenously injected dextran on factors of the kallikrein-kinin system and
the fibrinolytic system in rat plasma was further investigated,
to acquire information on the probable interference between the two
systems. We decided to assay HMWK, pro-PKA, PK, PG and factor XII
(as kaolin-activated PKA, Laake and Vennerød, 1973 a,b) both in rat
citrated plasma (RCPL) and in plasma from which PG had been removed
by chromatography on lysine-Sepharose (RCPL-P). By using RCPL-P in
their experiments Briseid et al. (1978) eliminated any interference
from plasmin in the BAEe-esterase assay of kallikrein. It was noticed, however, that the chromatography of RCPL on lysine-Sepharose,
as opposed to what was observed for human plasma, regularly reduced
the yields of pro-PKA and PK (unpublished experiments), and the investigation in parallel of RCPL and RCPL-P seemed relevant.

MATERIALS AND METHODS

The materials and methods were as described recently (Briseid
et al. 1978) with some additions: Fibrinolytic activity was assayed
by the fibrin plate method in the modification of Haverkate and
Brakman (1975), using plasminogen-containing or plasminogen-free fibrinogen. No effect was obtained with urokinase (0.10 - 1.10 Ploug
units/ml) on the plasminogen-free plates, while the effect of plasmin
was about the same on both types of plates. Thirty μl samples of
column fractions or acetone-activated plasma samples were applied
on the plates and incubated at $37^{O}C$ for 20 hours. A standard curve
for plasmin was constructed by using dilutions of human plasmin in
gelatin buffer. A linear log concentration effect curve was obtained for lysis zone diameters of 12-30 mm (0.02 - 1.25 CU/ml). To assay for plasminogen activator 50 μl of the sample to be tested was
diluted with 100 μl 0.22 M phosphate buffer (pH 7.4) and incubated
with 50 μl rat plasminogen (0.3 mg/ml) for 30 minutes at $37^{O}C$. Thirty μl samples from the incubate were applied to plasminogen-free
fibrin plates and incubated at $37^{O}C$ for 20 hours.

Plasmin, human plasmin 15 CU/mg protein, AB, Kabi, Stockholm,
Sweden. Test-Fibrinogen ORPH and plasminogen-free fibrinogen, bo-
vine fibrinogen, Behring-Werke A.G., Marburg, Germany. Bovine throm-
bin and Urokinase reagent, Leo Pharmaceutical Products, Ballerup,
Denmark. Tranexamic acid for injections was a gift from AB, Kabi,
Stockholm, Sweden.

RESULTS

Lowering of High Molecular Weight Kininogen by Dextran and by
Chromatography on Lysine-Sepharose.

Table 1 shows that a dextran injection of 30 mg/100 g caused

TABLE 1

Lowering of high molecular weight kininogen (HMWK) by dextran and
by chromatography on lysine-Sepharose.

Dextran was injected intravenously and tranexamic acid (AMCHA) intraperitoneally respectively 3-5 and 45 min before blood collection.
In each experiment the pooled plasma from 6-10 rats was assayed together with control plasma, and all data given are average values
from two parallels corrected to the same level on the basis of the
control plasma. The results are calculated as bradykinin equivalents
of free kinin and kinin released in rat citrated plasma (RCPL) or in
plasminogen-free rat citrated plasma (RCPL-P) by an excess amount of
rat plasma kallikrein.

Plasma batch	Rats treated with mg/100 g	HMWK and kinin µg/ml RCPL	RCPL-P
1	Saline	1.01 - 0.16	0.94 - 0.16
2	Saline	0.85 - 0.04	0.73 - 0.10
3	Saline	0.84 - 0.02	0.73 - 0.11
4	Dextran 10	1.08 - 0.07	0.69 - 0.09
5	Dextran 15	0.92 - 0.06	0.73 - 0.13
6	Dextran 30	0.66 - 0.07	0.40 - 0.17
7	AMCHA 40	0.90 - 0.02	0.53 - 0.19
8	AMCHA 10 Dextran 10	0.75 - 0.03	0.74 - 0.05
9	AMCHA 20 Dextran 10	0.71 - 0.04	0.61 - 0.12
10	AMCHA 40 Dextran 15	0.58 - 0.23	0.52 - 0.29

a strong reduction of the plasma level of HMWK, while no effect
was observed after doses of 10 or 15 mg/100 g. No loss of HMWK
took place during chromatography on lysine-Sepharose of normal RCPL,
while a significant lowering of HMWK was noticed for RCPL collected from dextran-treated rats. The highest dose of AMCHA used (40 mg/
100 g) had alone no effect on the plasma level of HMWK, but doses

TABLE 2

Lowering of prekallikrein proactivator (pro-PKA), prekallikrein (PK) and plasminogen (PG) by dextran and by chromatography on lysine-Sepharose.

Enzyme preparations were obtained by incubation of RCPL or RCPL-P with acetone 23% v/v for about 17 hours at 20-22°C, evaporation of the acetone at low pressure, and further activation with kaolin. The amount of pro-PKA present is given in PKA-U per ml plasma, one PKA-U being the amount of activator which activates one BAEe-esterase unit of PK per minute at 25°C. The amount present of PK is given in BAEe-esterase units per ml plasma, one BAEe-U being the amount of esterase which splits 1 µmol ester per min at 25°C. PG was assayed in acid-treated plasma incubated with casein and urokinase. Undigested casein was precipitated after 0 and 30 min with perchloric acid and the optical density read at 275 mµ. For other details see text to table 1.

Plasma batch	Rats treated with mg/100g	pro-PKA PKA-U/ml		PK BAEe-U/ml		PG $\Delta OD \times 10^2$/ml	
		RCPL	RCPL-P	RCPL	RCPL-P	RCPL	RCPL-P
1	Saline	3.7	2.2	1.05	0.77	304	16
2	Saline	3.5	2.2	0.96	0.77	304	8
3	Saline	3.6	2.1	0.99	0.74	304	0
4	Dextran 10	2.6	1.6	0.86	0.64	232	0
5	Dextran 15	2.2	1.7	0.72	0.55	280	0
6	Dextran 30	2.2	1.9	0.89	0.62	264	16
7	AMCHA 40	2.9	1.9	0.93	0.77	256	56
8	AMCHA 10 Dextran 10	2.8	2.1	0.84	0.62	248	0
9	AMCHA 20 Dextran 10	3.1	2.0	0.95	0.70	232	56
10	AMCHA 40 Dextran 15	3.3	2.6	0.86	0.73	224	96

of 10-40 mg/100 g potentiated the reductions induced by dextran.
Most of the free kinin assayed in RCPL must have been released after
blood collection, and the figures for free kinin were added to the
HMWK-values in table 1 to give a more correct estimation of the in
vivo effects of the different treatments. The amounts of free kinin
were generally higher in RCPL-P than in RCPL, and became still higher if the concentration of EDTA during chromatography was increased
from 0.003 M (Deutsch and Mertz, 1970) to 0.04 M. For plasma batch
9 the kinin assayed was increased from 0.12 µg/ml (table 1) to
0.41 µg/ml.

Lowering of Prekallikrein by Dextran and by Chromatography on Lysine-Sepharose.

    Small reductions in the PK-level of rat plasma were induced by
dextran injection and also by affinity chromatography on lysine-Sepharose (table 2). By gel filtration of acetone-activated normal
RCPL on Sephadex G-100, two peaks of BAEe-esterase activity regularly
appeared, one more high molecular corresponding to kallikrein (K 1),
and the other (K2) eluting later (MW 47,000) and amounting to about
one third of the total activity (fig. 1, lower panel). By gel filtration of acetone-activated RCPL-P the K 2 esterase peak was not
detectable (Berstad, manuscript in preparation), while experiments
in the present work showed that the K 2 peak present in acetone-
activated RCPL was not removed by chromatography on lysine-Sepharose.
When RCPL from rats injected with dextran (15 mg/100 g) was acetone-
activated and filtered through Sephadex G-100, the K 2 esterase peak
was almost absent, while the amount of kallikrein present was about
the same as in acetone-activated RCPL from control rats (fig. 1,
upper panel).

    The crude peak fractions of K 2 which eluted just ahead of
XII_f (MW 32,000), and which contained traces of XII_f, were concentrated by dialysis in vacuo against 0.22 M phosphate buffer (pH 7.4)
to a BAEe-esterase activity of 0.33 U/ml, and submitted to a preliminary study. The esterase showed no caseinolytic activity (method
limit of detection of plasmin corresponding to about 0.03 BAEe-U/ml),
but had a weak fibrinolytic activity (0.30 CU/BAEe-U), which was
lost after 15 minutes at 60°C. Urokinase-activated rat plasmin retained about 50% of its fibrinolytic activity after 60 minutes at
60°C. The K 2 peak had also a weak kininogenase activity (0.30 KU/
BAEe-U), and about the same ratio was obtained whether the kininogen
substrate was 60°C-heated human plasma or highly purified human high
molecular weight kininogen (Briseid et al. 1978). No effect was registered against human low molecular weight kininogen. Fractions
from the K 1 peak yielded a KU/BAEe-U ratio of about 3 when tested
against 60°-heated human plasma, which was close to the ratio of 2.7
reported by Briseid et al. (1978) for the total activity in acetone-
activated RCPL-P, and supposed to reflect the kallikrein present.

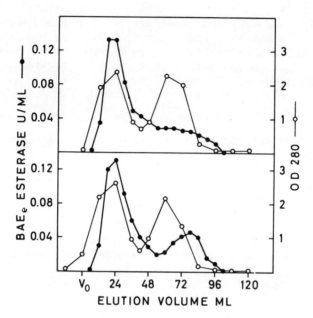

Fig. 1.   Sephadex G-100 gel filtration of acetone-activated normal
rat citrated plasma (lower panel) and plasma from rats injected
intravenously with dextran 15 mg/100 g 3 min before blood collection
(upper panel).   The plasma was incubated with 23% acetone v/v for
17 hours at 20-22°C.   The acetone was removed at low pressure and
the plasma then centrifuged for 30 min at 40,000 x g.   5 ml of the
supernatant (1.02 and 0.85 BAEe-U/ml) were applied to the column
(2.6 x 92 cm) which was developed with tris buffer 50 mM pH 7.4.
The flow rate was 6 ml/hr and the fractions were 6 ml. V_0 represents
void volume (192 ml) which was estimated with Blue Dextran 2000.

Lowering of Prekallikrein Proactivator by Dextran and by Chromatography on Lysine-Sepharose.

     The level of acetone- and kaolin-activated pro-PKA was strong-
ly reduced in plasma from rats injected with dextran, and the passage of RCPL through a column with lysine-Sepharose caused a still
more extensive reduction (table 2).   Assays of the PKA-activity in
fractions from chromatography on Sephadex G-100 of acetone-activated

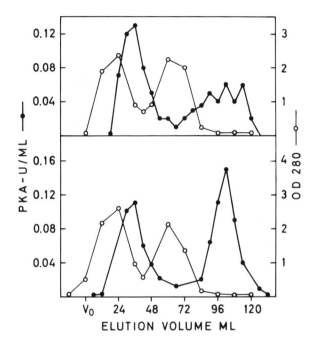

Fig. 2. Sephadex G-100 gel filtration of acetone-activated normal
rat citrated plasma (lower panel) and plasma from rats injected
intravenously with dextran 15 mg/100 g (upper panel). For details
see text to fig. 1.

RCPL or RCPL-P demonstrated two peaks of activity, one more
high molecular peak probably corresponding to XII_a, and a later
eluting larger peak (MW 32,000) corresponding to XII_f (Berstad,
manuscript in preparation). By kaolin treatment the bulk of XII_a
in acetone-activated RCPL-P was rapidly converted to XII_f and recovered in the fluid phase, while XII_a in acetone-activated RCPL
was adsorbed to kaolin without significant cleavage. By gel filtration of acetone-activated RCPL from rats injected with dextran,
it was found (fig. 2, upper panel) that the conversion of XII_a to
XII_f was less extensive than the conversion taking place in acetone-
activated RCPL from control rats (fig. 2, lower panel).

TABLE 3

Assay of kaolin-activated prekallikrein proactivator (pro-PKA) in
rat citrated plasma (RCPL) and in plasminogen-free rat citrated
plasma (RCPL-P).

The activation was carried out at 0°C according to the method developed by Laake and Vennerød (1973 a,b) for the determination in
human plasma of factor XII as prekallikrein activator. For details
see text to tables 1 and 2.

Plasma batch	Rats treated with mg/100 g	pro-PKA - U/ml RCPL	RCPL-P
1	Saline	1.4	1.5
2	Saline	1.3	1.5
3	Saline	1.4	1.4
6	Dextran 30	1.4	1.2
7	AMCHA 40	1.2	1.4
10	AMCHA 40 Dextran 30	1.3	1.3

Factor XII in rat plasma was also assayed as kaolin-activated
prekallikrein activator at 0°C by a method developed for the assay
of factor XII in human plasma by Laake and Vennerød (1973 a,b).
Table 3 shows that no differences were observed between plasma specimens from dextran-injected rats and from control rats, and that
the highest doses of dextran and of AMCHA used, 30 and 40 mg/100 g
respectively, did not alter the plasma level of pro-PKA. The same
result was obtained when dextran was used after pretreatment with
AMCHA. No differences were detectable between RCPL and RCPL-P.
The data do not provide any evidence that the reductions in pro-
PKA registered by the acetone activation procedure were due to a
lowering of the level of the precursor of PKA.

Protection of Prekallikrein Proactivator against Dextran by Pretreatment of the Rats with Tranexamic Acid.

The dextran-induced lowering of pro-PKA was strongly reduced
by pretreatment of the rats with AMCHA, while a protection of the
PK-level was not clearly demonstrable (table 2). Dextran caused
minor reductions in the plasma level of PG. The reductions were of
the same order of size (10-24%) in rats pretreated with AMCHA. The
presence of some PG in RCPL-P from rats given the two highest doses
of AMCHA can probably be ascribed to PG eluted from the lysine-
Sepharose column by AMCHA still present in plasma at the point in
time of blood collection.

When rat PG isolated by chromatography on lysine-Sepharose was
added to RCPL-P before acetone activation, an amount of PG corresponding to about 1/4 of the normal plasma level was found to increase the pro-PKA value assayed to a level which was about 80% of
that obtained in RCPL. The addition of higher amounts of PG caused
no further increase. If an amount of PG corresponding to less than
about 1/8 of the normal plasma level was added to RCPL-P, no effect
on the pro-PKA assay value was detectable. The addition of PG did
not yield higher PK-values than those observed for RCPL-P alone
(Berstad, manuscript in preparation). The mentioned results provide
evidence that the reduced level of pro-PKA registered after dextran
injection could not be due to the relatively small reductions in the
level of PG, and only part of the lowering of pro-PKA by lysine-
Sepharose chromatography could be directly accounted for by the removal of PG (table 2).

DISCUSSION

In accordance with the results of previous experiments (Briseid
et al. 1978) rapid reductions in the plasma levels of pro-PKA, PK
and HMWK were registered after the intravenous injection of dextran
into rats. The results in the present work together with other experimental data referred to (Berstad, manuscript in preparation),
indicate that the dextran-induced lowering of PK was mainly due to
a reduction of the amount present in acetone-activated RCPL of a
BAEe-esterase (K 2), which during Sephadex G-100 gel chromatography
eluted after kallikrein (K 1), and before XII_f. The molecular weight
was roughly estimated to 47,000. The development of K 2 activity
seemed to depend on the presence in plasma of PG, but also another
factor was needed. No K 2 esterase peak appeared on gel filtration
of acetone-activated RCPL-P, but the addition to RCPL-P of PG before
acetone activation did not increase the yield of esterase activity,
and the K 2 peak was almost absent when RCPL from dextran-injected
rats was activated with acetone and gel filtered. The results indicate that dextran induces a reduction of the amount present of the
precursor of K 2 or a factor of significance for the activation of
K 2.

Acetone-activated RCPL-P prepared from normal rat plasma as well as from plasma collected from rats injected with dextran, contained a mixture of more high molecular PKA, probably corresponding to XII_a, and low molecular PKA (MW 32,000) corresponding to XII_f. By kaolin activation XII_a was rapidly converted to XII_f. Also acetone-activated RCPL from control rats and from dextran-injected rats contained a mixture of XII_a and XII_f, but the extent of cleavage of XII_a was lower in the preparation of dextran-plasma, and by activation with kaolin no further cleavage took place in that preparation while part of XII_a was converted to XII_f in the preparation of normal plasma. The remaining XII_a was adsorbed onto kaolin in both preparations, but the PKA activity of surface-bound XII_a in plasma from dextran-treated rats was significantly lower than in the corresponding preparation from control rats. The mentioned results might indicate that dextran injected intravenously into rats causes the loss of a factor of significance for the extent of cleavage of XII_a to XII_f, and possibly of significance for the PKA-activity of surface-bound XII_a. It was shown by Briseid et al. (1978) that the addition of human HMWK before the acetone activation procedure, significantly increased the PKA activity of the final enzyme preparation. The low yield of PKA-activity obtained in plasma from dextran-treated rats could, however, not be due to a loss of HMWK. Firstly, the lowering of HMWK in the present work required larger doses of dextran than those causing a clear reduction of the yield of PKA-activity. Secondly, a pretreatment of the rats with AMCHA potentiated the dextran-induced loss of HMWK, but protected the plasma level of pro-PKA. Dextran-treatment was found to reduce the amount of a BAEe-esterase (K 2) in acetone-activated RCPL, which had a low, but distinct kininogenase activity. Experiments carried out to see if K 2 added before kaolin potentiated the PKA-activity of acetone-activated RCPL or RCPL-P from dextran treated rats provided no evidence of such an effect.

The PKA-activity of a mixture of surface-bound XII_a and unbound XII_f in acetone- and kaolin-activated normal RCPL was much higher than the activity of XII_f after total conversion of XII_a in the corresponding preparation prepared from RCPL-P. The addition of PG isolated by chromatography on lysine-Sepharose to RCPL-P before activation significantly increased the yield of PKA-activity, probably by reducing the extent of cleavage of XII_a. The level of PKA did not, however, reach the level obtained for RCPL, indicating the loss by affinity chromatography on lysine-Sepharose of a factor of significance for the assayed PKA-activity, as was observed also after dextran injection. It is known that lysine-Sepharose chromatography might remove plasma factors in addition to PG. Recently Radcliffe and Heinze (1978) reported on the isolation by such chromatography of a PG activator from human plasma. In our experiments no evidence for the presence of an activator for PG in acetone- and kaolin-activated RCPL was provided, but pretreatment of the rats with an inhibitor of PG activation, AMCHA, inhibited the dextran-induced lowering of pro-PKA, and at the same time potentiated the loss of HMWK. The mechanism of AMCHA is very complex, because the substance not only reacts with PG and plasmin, forming reversible complexes, but also with plasminogen activator and fibrin. In addition the turnover rate of PG in vivo has been reported to increase in the presence of AMCHA (Collen et al. 1972). The affinity for PG of AMCHA is much higher than for activators and fibrin, and therapeutic concentration is around 10^{-4} M (Thorsen 1978), and definitely higher than the dissociation constants for plasminogen or plasmin and the amino acid (Abiko et al. 1969; Brockway and Castellino 1972; Iwamoto 1975). The amounts of AMCHA used in the present work probably provide higher plasma concentrations in the rat than that mentioned, and the inhibition of activation of plasminogen is possibly the most important consequence of its presence in plasma. The higher yield of PKA-activity in RCPL from rats given AMCHA before the dextran treatment could well be due to a reduced fragmentation. According to Kaplan et al. (1971) the addition of ε-aminocaproic acid to a crude mixture of unactivated Hageman factor, prekallikrein and PG permitted glass activation of Hageman factor, but suppressed its fragmentation. As mentioned above the PKA-effect of the mixture of XII_a adsorbed to kaolin and XII_f present in acetone- and kaolin-activated RCPL was found to be higher than the effect of the corresponding preparation from RCPL-P, containing XII_f only. At the present time, however, no explanation can be given for the increased loss of HMWK after dextran taking place in rats pretreated with AMCHA.

REFERENCES

Abiko, Y., M. Iwamoto and M. Tomikawa, 1969, Plasminogen-plasmin system. V. A stoichiometric equilibrium complex of plasminogen and a synthetic inhibitor, Biochim. Biophys. Acta, 185, 424.

Briseid, G., K. Briseid, E.-L. Toverud and J. Kristoffersen, 1978, Dextran-induced lowering of prekallikrein proactivator and prekallikrein in rat plasma, Acta pharmacol. et toxicol., 42, 93.

Brockway, W.J. and F.J. Castellino, 1972, Measurements of the binding of antifibrinolytic amino acids to various plasminogens, Arch. Biochim. Biophys., 151, 194.

Collen, D., G. Tytgat, H. Claeys, M. Verstraete and P. Wallén, 1972, Metabolism of plasminogen in healthy subjects: Effect of tranexamic acid, J. Clin. Invest., 51, 1310.

Deutsch, D.G. and E.T. Mertz, 1970, Plasminogen: Purification from human plasma by affinity chromatography, Science, 170, 1095.

Haverkate, F. and P. Brakman, Fibrin plate assay, 1975, in: Progress in Chemical Fibrinolysis and Thrombolysis, Vol. 1, eds. J. F. Davidson, M.M. Samama and P.C. Desnoyers (Raven Press, New York) p. 151.

Iwamoto, M., 1975, Plasminogen-plasmin system IX. Specific binding of tranexamic acid to plasmin, Thromb. Diath. Haemorrh., 33, 573.

Kaplan, A.P., J. Spragg and K.F. Austen, The bradykinin forming
    system of man, 1971, in: Biochemistry of the Acute Allergic React-
    ions, Second International Symposium, eds. K.F. Austen and E.L.
    Becker (Blackwell, Oxford) p. 279.
Laake, K. and A.M. Vennerød, 1973 a, Determination of factor XII in
    human plasma with arginine proesterase (prekallikrein). I. Pre-
    paration and properties of the substrate, Thrombosis Research, 2,
    393.
Laake, K. and A.M. Vennerød, 1973 b, Determination of factor XII in
    human plasma with arginine proesterase (prekallikrein). II.
    Studies on the method, Thrombosis Research, 2, 409.
Radcliffe, R. and T. Heinze, 1978, Isolation of plasminogen activa-
    tor from human plasma by chromatography on lysine-Sepharose, Arch.
    Biochim. Biophys., 189, 185.
Thorsen, S., 1978, Influence of fibrin on the effect of 6-amino-
    hexanoic acid on fibrinolysis caused by tissue plasminogen acti-
    vator or urokinase, in: Progress in Chemical Fibrinolysis and
    Thrombolysis, Vol. 3, eds. J.F. Davidson, R.M. Rowan, M.M. Samama
    and P.C. Desnoyers (Raven Press, New York) p. 269.

EFFECTS OF SOME CLINICAL PROCEDURES ON COMPLEMENT

S.G. Binysh, V. Eisen and R.S. Tedder

Middlesex Hospital Medical School

London W1P 9PG, England

In common with blood clotting, fibrinolysis and possibly kinin formation, complement is important for survival but may also contribute to harmful, or at least unpleasant pathological processes. The activation or inhibition of complement by clinical procedures may therefore have beneficial and/or untoward effects. An activating or depressing action on complement is attributed to a growing number of clinical procedures. In the case of some drugs, this action is regarded as an important factor in their clinical effectiveness.

This present study examines the effects on complement of the following clinical procedures: 1. extra-corporeal circulation as used in cardio-pulmonary bypass (CPB) surgery; 2. gold salts used in the treatment of rheumatoid arthritis.

METHODS

The methods used to measure or purify complement factors and other plasma constituents are given in brackets: total complement measured as $CH50$ titres or by the kinetic method (Lachmann et al., 1973); haemolytic plate method for measuring C4 (Lachmann et al., 1973); Cobra venom factor haemolytic titre for measuring factor B (Brai and Osler, 1972); purification of C1q (Yonemasu and Stroud, 1971); C3 conversion (Laurell, 1965); solid phase radioimmunoassay of immunoglobulin aggregates (Hay et al., 1976); gold levels were measured by atomic absorption spectrophotometry; antigenic levels of complement components (Mancini et al., 1965).

CPB surgery involves a temporary diversion of the circulation away from the heart and lungs, which are replaced by a mechanical pump and oxygenator. During such extracorporeal circulation, plasma proteins may be denatured and blood cells damaged by exposure to oxygen bubbles and to the foreign surfaces of tubing and of the oxygenator, by turbulence and other flow disturbances, and by cooling. Nagaoka and Katori (1975) reported that in CPB lower kininogen and higher kinin levels were found in plasma within 20 minutes; both changes continued to increase until the end of the CPB. Denaturation of immunoglobulins and the release of proteolytic enzymes from leucocytes could cause activation of complement. Indeed Hairston et al. (1969) and Parket et al. (1972) reported that complement levels were reduced after CPB surgery. Parker et al. (1975) also found C3 conversion after CPB. Activation or consumption of complement may contribute to post-operative pulmonary oedema (Ratcliffe et al., 1973; Robin et al., 1972), infection (Goodman et al., 1968), haemolysis (Keith et al., 1961) and pulmonary infiltration of polymorphs (Wilson, 1972).

Hahn-Pedersen et al. (1978) reported that complement is activated during surgery without CPB.

In the present work, the changes in complement have been studied in some detail in an attempt to clarify the mechanism(s) of activation, the involvement of the alternative pathway, and the role of haemodilution. Twenty one male and five female patients undergoing CPB surgery were studied. Seven were operated for mitral valve disease, three for aortic stenosis and incompetence, eleven for coronary artery disease, one for left ventricular aneurysm, and two for Fallots tetralogy. Anaesthesia was carried out with thiopentone, pancuronium, omnopon, and N_2O/O_2/halothane mixtures. Heparin was administered before the CPB was started; after CPB, it was neutralized with protamine sulphate.

In this work, the levels of complement and its components were expressed per mg protein, as recommended by Nagaoka and Katori (1975) for kininogen. Fig. 1 shows just how important this mode of expressing levels is in the case of CPB. Although in this way the effects of haemodilution by electrolyte solutions could be excluded, the possibility that low complement levels were due to the admixture of transfusion blood remained. However, in 8 citrated plasmas obtained from blood transfusion used in these patients, the titre of total haemolytic complement was 1679 ± 571 (m ± s.d.) CH50 units (normal 1352 ± 304). It seemed therefore unlikely that blood transfusion was responsible for low complement levels.

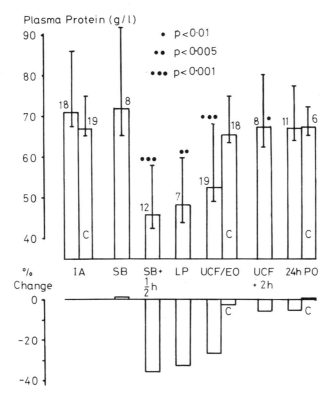

Fig. 1.   Concentrations of plasma protein (upper graph; mean + s.d.,
          -s.e. shown) and its mean percentage change (lower graph)
          during CPB and during surgery without CPB (columns marked
          C). Number of patients given on top of columns. Times
          of blood collection along abscissa: IA - induction of
          anaesthesia; SB = start of bypass; LP = lung perfusion;
          UCF = unassisted cardiac function restored; EO = end of
          operation; PO = post operation. P values refer to
          differences from measurements at IA.

        Nagaoka and Katori (1975) provided evidence that kinin
formation occurred during the passage through the heart lung
machine, particularly when extracorporeal circulation lasted 60
or more minutes. In the present work, there were no significant
differences between paired arterial and venous samples in their
CH50 titres and C4 and C3 levels, at any stage of CPB operations.

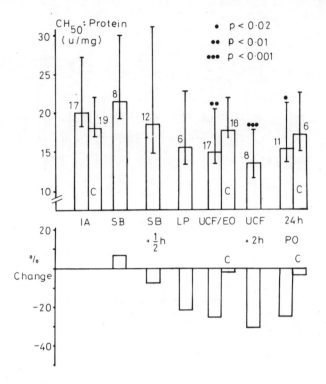

Fig. 2.   Changes in total haemolytic complement during CPB. Upper
graph gives CH50 units per mg plasma protein, and lower
graph percentage change from value at IA. Other information as in Fig. 1.

Total haemolytic complement (CH50 units per mg protein) fell
only gradually during CPB (Fig. 2). Titres were significantly
reduced when unassisted cardiac function (UCF) was reestablished
and remained low for the next 24 hours. When titres in individual
patients were followed, 13/17 patients showed at UCF a fall (−30.1
± 6 per cent), and 4/17 a slight rise (4 per cent). No comparable
falls were found in patients undergoing surgery without CPB
(Fig. 2, C).

Next, the changes in several individual complement components
were examined. Subcomponent Clq was reduced by some 40 per cent
(p < 0.005) within 30 minutes of starting the CPB (Fig. 3.). It
was slightly higher at UCF (−20 per cent), and again at −40 per
cent), and again at −40 per cent 24 h after the operation.

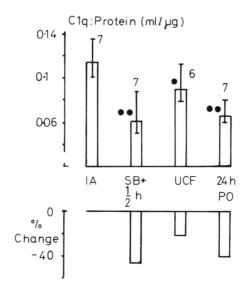

Fig. 3.   Changes in antigenic Clq during CPB. Upper graph shows
          Clq level (as % of level in pooled normal serum per µg
          plasma protein x 10^{-1}). Lower graph gives percentage
          change from value at IA. IA, SB, UCF and PO as in Fig. 1.
          ● = $p < 0.05$;   ●● = $p < 0.001$.

          C4, the next component in the classical sequence, showed a
curious pattern (Fig. 4). The ratio of antigenic C4 to protein
rose very promptly and was 30 minutes after the start of CPB 26
per cent higher than at IA ($p < 0.005$). After that C4 decreased
in similar fashion as did CH50. When C4 was measured by a functional haemolytic method, the changes in its ratio to protein also
showed an early rise and subsequent fall, which unlike the changes
in antigenic C4 were not statistically significant.

          The plasma levels of C3, the bulk component of complement,
were at the beginning of the operation (IA) higher in CPB patients
than in control surgical patients (19.6 ± 6.9 µg and 14.6 ± 4.6 µg
per mg protein, respectively). The difference was statistically
significant but both means were within the normal range in our
laboratory. During CPB, the changes in C3 were smaller (12 per
cent) and occurred later than the changes in CH50 and C4. Only at
UCF did the fall in C3 become significant ($p < 0.01$); the largest
drop was found 2 hours later (21 per cent).

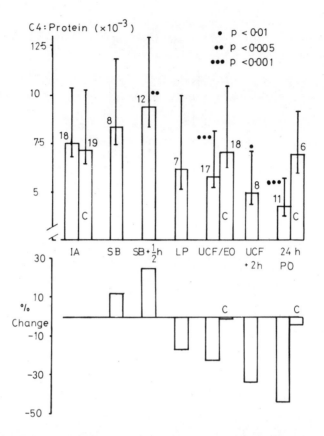

Fig. 4.   Changes in antigenic C4 during CPB. Upper graph gives
         mg C4 per mg protein x 10^{-3}, and lower graph percent
         change from value at IA. Other information as in Fig. 1.

Conversion of C3 to C3b, and subsequent C3c and C3d, is one
of the more direct proofs of complement activation. Evidence for
in vivo conversion was found in 9 out of 15 CPB operations. It
developed gradually, was extensive at UCF, and remained so or even
progressed further in the next 24 hours. No C3 conversion was
found at any stage of the operations without CPB.

The demonstrated changes strongly suggest that complement is
activated during CPB surgery, and that this activation involves the
classical pathway. To assess whether the alternative pathway is
also triggered by CPB, factor B in plasma was measured by

activating and complexing it with excess Cobra venom factor and
then establishing the haemolytic titre in a system deficient in
Ca^{++} (Brai and Osler, 1972). Although the factor B : protein
ratios fell during CPB by 25 percent, the changes were not significant. One-dimensional immunoelectrophoresis also failed to
reveal any conversion of factor B.

Late effects of CPB   Extracorporeal circulation in CPB
appears to influence the turnover of complement components, in
particular of C3, in a way that ordinary surgery does not. The
ratios of CH50, C4 and C3 to protein were higher 5 to 6 days after
operation than at IA, but only the increase in C3 was statistically
significant (p < 0.005).

Possible mechanisms of complement activation in CPB   Several
factors could lead to enhanced use and possibly consumption of Cl
esterase inhibitors (CllNA). Unlike other proteolytic inhibitors,
CllNA is not present in large excess so that its engagement by any
of the numerous enzymes it inhibits could quickly lead to a deficiency. In 8 patients, the CllNA : protein ratio rose between IA
and the start of CPB, but was lower at and after the end of the
operation. None of the observed changes was statistically significant.

Another possibility was that the exposure of blood to foreign
surfaces and to oxygen bubbles led to denaturation and aggregation
of immunoglobulins. These aggregates would then bind to Clq and
thereby trigger the classical pathway. Sera from CPB patients
were therefore tested for aggregated IgG, IgA and IgM by a solid
phase Clq binding assay developed for immune complexes (Hay et al.,
1976). No evidence for aggregation was detected.

Fibrinolytic activity is enhanced in most types of surgery
(Mansfield, 1972). Plasmin of course may activate the complement
sequence at several stages. We assessed fibrinolysis by measuring
fibrinogen degradation products in plasma (FDP). The levels
changed little during the operation, but rose well above the normal
range (0 - 10 μg/ml) 24 hours after the operation. This meant
that the rise in FDP developed later than the complement changes.

This was also true of C-reactive protein (CRP), an acute
phase protein which potently activates complement (Siegel and
Gewurtz, 1974).

There was no correlation between the extent of change in
complement and the change in FDP or CRP. It seemed therefore
unlikely that either of these factors was responsible for
complement activation.

In order to obtain some information on the pathological significance of complement changes during and after CPB surgery, the patients were divided according to their post-operative clinical course into those with an uncomplicated recovery and those who developed moderate to severe complications. The patients who had uncomplicated recoveries showed the following mean percentage changes between the times of IA and UCF and between IA and 24 hr after operation, respectively: CH50= -7.58 and -7.47; C4= -16.8 and -40.1; C3= -10.4 and -11.9. In the group with moderate to severe pulmonary complications the corresponding figures were as follows: CH50 = -29.8 and -35.9; C4 = -19.0 and -44.9; C3 = -22.1 and -23.6. It is clear that CH50 and C3, but not C4, decreased in patients who developed postoperative complications much more than in those whose recovery was free of complications.

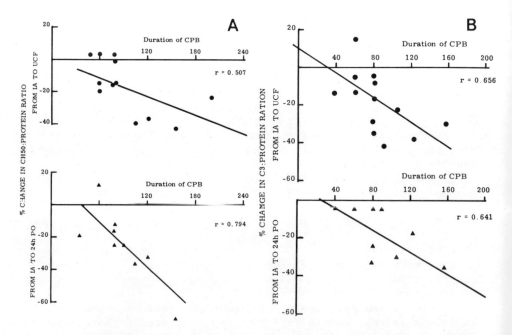

Fig. 5. Duration of CPB (minutes) and percentage change in CH50 titres (Fig. 5A) and in C3 levels (Fig. 5B) between IA and UCF and between IA and 24 hr after the operation (PO).

The data suggest that during CPB complement is activated to an extent which makes it likely that this process contributes to pulmonary edema and other complications. The findings that the main changes occur at the end and after CPB, and that there are no consistent arterio-venous differences, are difficult to reconcile with a direct activation of complement during passage of blood through the pump and oxygenator. Yet, the extent to which CH50 and C3 were reduced was definitely influenced by the duration of the CPB (Fig. 5). (The fall in C4 was not dependent on the length of the bypass.) In recirculation experiments in which the exposure of blood to the pump surfaces and to oxygen bubbles was mimicked, it was seen that the gas bubbles, but not the pump tubing, induced considerable complement activation including C3 conversion. A hypothesis compatible with the present findings would be that an activating factor is generated which persists in the circulation for some time after the CPB. Conceivably, such a factor could be derived from red blood cells, leucocytes or platelets which are damaged during oxygenation by the vigorous agitation and gas bubbles. The activation of the pathways triggered by Hageman factor, implied by the work of Nagaoka and Katori (1975), could also generate a complement activator.

Pruitt et al. (1971) found that oxygenation of pure gamma-globulin solutions induced aggregation. However, no aggregates of IgG, IgA or IgM were detected in the present work in whole plasma from patients.

Gold salts. Gold salts are effective drugs in rheumatoid arthritis. They probably suppress this chronic inflammation by several mechanisms. Schultz et al. (1974) reported that gold salts inhibit complement in synovial exudates, and suggested that this may be an important factor in their clinical effect. We examined the action of sodium aurothiomalate on several stages of complement, and found that only the highest clinically relevant concentrations of gold (0.2 mM) depressed complement. The interaction between C1 and C4 was particularly sensitive, as described by Schultz et al. (1974). However, the action of C1 esterase on synthetic esters was not affected.

Now in most complement assays, serum is highly diluted, a factor which distorts the avid binding of gold (and many other drugs) on to albumin and other plasma proteins. The effect of high protein concentrations on the inhibition by gold was therefore examined. Neither albumin (12.5 mg/ml final concentration) nor serum (20%) depleted of complement interfered with the inhibitory action of gold. On the other hand, the effectiveness of gold decreased as the concentration of gold in complement increased. Extrapolation showed that gold would not inhibit the normally circulating complement concentrations.

Unlike dialysis (Schultz et al., 1974), addition of penicillamine in stoichiometric proportions, completely reverses the inhibition by gold. Surprisingly, the chelating agent penicillamine did not detectably affect the binding of gold on to total plasma proteins. Preliminary data suggest that the affinity of gold is for albumin > penicillamine > complement.

The findings do not support the view that inhibition of complement plays an important part in the therapeutic effects of gold salts.

ACKNOWLEDGEMENTS

We are grateful to Mr. M.F. Sturridge, FRCS and Dr. P.J. Bennett for their interest and for providing the blood samples from CPB patients.

REFERENCES

Brai, M. and Osler, A.G. (1972) Proc. Soc. exp. Biol. Med., 140: 1116-1121.

Goodman, J.S., Schaffner, W., Collins, H.A., Battersby, E.J. and Koening, M.G. (1968) New Engl. J. Med., 278: 117.

Hahn-Pedersen, J., Sorensen, H. and Kehlet, H. (1978) Surgery, Gynacology & Obstetrics, 146: 66-68.

Hairston, P., Manos, J.P., Graber, C.D. and Lee, W.M. (1969) J. surg. Res., 9: 567-593.

Hay, F.C., Nineham, L.J. and Roitt, I.M. (1976) Clin. exp. Immunol., 24: 396.

Kaplan, M.H. and Volanakis, J.E. (1974) J. Immunol., 112: 2135-2147.

Keith, M.B., Ginn, E., Williams, G.R. (1961) J. Thorac. Cardiovasc. Surg., 41: 404-407.

Lachmann, P.J., Hobart, M.J. and Aston, W.P. (1973) Complement Technology In: Handbook of Immunology, Ed. D.M. Weir, Oxford, Blackwell Scientific Publications.

Laurell, C.B. (1965) Analyt. Biochem. 10: 358.

Mancini, G., Carbonara, A.O. and Heremans, J.F. (1965) Immuno-chemistry, 2: 235.

Mansfiel, A.O. (1972) Br. J. Surg., 59: 754.

Nagaoka, H. and Katori, M. (1975) Circulation, 52: 325-332.

Parker, D.J., Cantrell, J.W., Karp, R.B., Stroud, R.M. and Digerness, S.B. (1972) Surgery, 71: 824-827.

Parker, D.J., Cook, S., Turner-Warwick, M. (1975) In: "Lung Metabolism", Ed. A.E. Junod & R. de Haller, Academic Press London, pp. 481-491.

Pruitt, K.M., Stroud, R.M. and Scott, J.W. (1971) Proc. Soc. Exp.
    Biol. Med., 173: 714-718.
Ratliff, N.B., Young, W.G., Hackel, D.B., Mikat, E. and Wilson,
    J.W. (1973) J. Thorac. Cardiovasc. Surg., 65: 425.
Robin, E.D., Carey, L.C., Grenvik, A., Glauser, F. and Gaudio, R.
    (1972) Arch. Int. Med., 130 : 66.
Schultz, D.R., Volanakis, J.E., Arnold, P.I., Gottleib, N.L.,
    Sakai, K. and Stroud R.M. (1974) Clin. exp. Immunol., 17:
    395-406.
Siegel, J., Rent, R. and Gewurz, H. (1974) J. exp. Med., 140:
    631-647.
Wilson, J.W. (1972) Surg. Gynecol. Obstet., 134: 675.
Yonemasu, K. and Stroud, R.M. (1971) J. Immunol., 106: 304-313.

SUBSTRATE MODULATION AS A CONTROL MECHANISM IN THE ACTIVATION OF PLASMA MULTIENZYME SYSTEMS

Walther Vogt

Department of Biochemical Pharmacology
Max-Planck-Institut für experimentelle Medizin
3400 Göttingen, Hermann-Rein-Str. 3, Germany

Besides acting as a vehicle for the transport of cells and dissolved material, plasma contains several biochemical systems with various significant biological functions, e.g., in circulation control, haemostasis, defense reactions and exchange of solutes between blood and tissues. All these systems consist of enzymes and substrates which are dissolved and freely mobile in the same medium.

While biochemical systems in cells are well controlled through compartmentalization in organelles separated by barriers, or by fixation in insoluble membranes, the unlimited contact of soluble constituents in plasma requires other control mechanisms for blood-borne reactions. Most plasma systems, e.g. the Hageman factor-dependent kallikrein and clotting systems, and complement are multi-enzyme systems consisting of pre-enzymes which are activated in sequence when started by a trigger event; the sequential activation has a multiplying effect and leads to a rapid, cascade-like build-up of high activity. The extent and duration of activation is controlled by inhibitors and enzymic inactivators which block the enzymes or destroy co-factors once formed. Further, in the complement system, the activity of some complex enzymes is limited by spontaneous decay due to dissociation of the complexes.

Still another principle has turned out in the last few years to control activation processes, in the complement system as well as in the Hageman factor-dependent systems, namely, a modulation of substrates produced by their interaction with specific partners; without such interactions even the active enzymes would not recognize or attack their specific substrate. Four examples will be presented,

three from the complement system, and one significant in Hageman
factor-dependent reactions.

Activation of Factor B

Factor B is a pre-enzyme in plasma, which upon activation
yields the key enzyme of the alternative pathway of the complement
sequence, a C3 (and C5) convertase. Activation is effected by
specific hydrolytic cleavage of a peptide bond which generates a
major fragment Bb and a minor one, Ba. The natural B cleaving
enzyme in plasma is factor $\bar{D}$* (also termed C3 proactivator convertase, Müller-Eberhard and Götze, 1972), an already active enzyme
(Fearon et al., 1974; Vogt et al., 1974). $\bar{D}$ does, however, not
cleave B directly, the activation proceeds only in the presence of
C3b (the activated fragment of C3) and Mg^{++} ions (Müller-Eberhard
and Götze, 1972). Trypsin is capable of cleaving B into its two
fragments but again, an active C3 convertase does not form unless
C3b and Mg^{++} are also present (Vogt et al., 1975). Together with
two further observations, namely that the free Bb fragment is
inactive and that native B forms a reversible Mg^{++}-dependent
complex with C3b, these findings have led to the reaction scheme
shown in fig. 1 and experimentally supported by sequential assembly
of the constituents (Vogt et al., 1975; 1977): Factor $\bar{D}$ cleaves
B only when this is bound to C3b, the resulting Bb fragment remains
bound, and the complex C3bBb then represents the active C3/C5
convertase. It decays spontaneously by dissociation, preformed
free Bb fragment does not (re)combine with C3b. Obviously, factor
B is altered in its conformation when complexed with C3b and is
thereby made accessible to $\bar{D}$. The necessity for C3b prevents the
unlimited consumption of B by $\bar{D}$.

Generation of the C3/C5 Convertase, $C\overline{42}$

In the classical complement reaction activation of C3 and C5
is effected by the complex of activated C4 (C4b fragment) with
activated C2 (C2a fragment), C4b2a. Both fragments are released
through peptide cleavage by $C\bar{1}$. The C3 convertase activity proper
of the complex resides in the C2a fragment but free C2a is inactive.
It has hitherto been assumed that C2a is bound to C4b immediately
after its release (Müller-Eberhard, 1969) which means that $C\bar{1}$ would
first directly cleave free C2. An enhancing effect of C4 on the
activation of C2 by $C\bar{1}$ has been explained as a removal, by C4b,
of some steric hindrance in $C\bar{1}$ (which is a complex of three proteins,
one of them, $C1\bar{s}$, being the C2 cleaving enzyme) (Gigli and Austen,
1969).

---

* A bar over the letters or numbers indicates an active (activated)
   component.

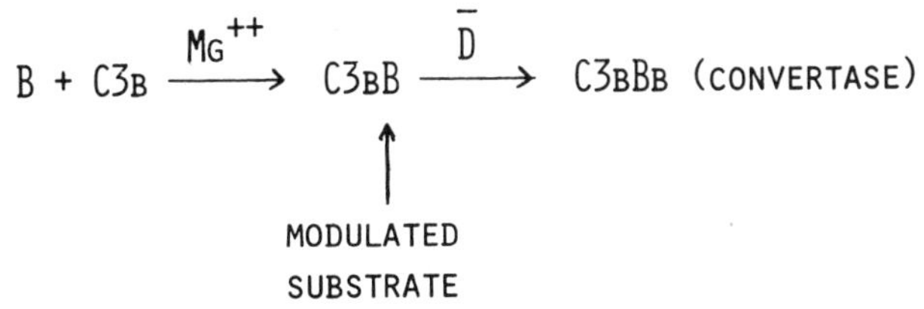

$$B + C3b \xrightarrow{\text{Mg}^{++}} C3bB \xrightarrow{\bar{D}} C3bBb \text{ (CONVERTASE)}$$

$$\uparrow$$

MODULATED

SUBSTRATE

Figure 1.   Activation of factor B of the alternative complement
pathway. First, B forms a reversible, Mg^{++}-dependent
complex with C3b. In this state B is obviously altered
in its structural configuration since only then can it
be cleaved by factor $\bar{D}$, an active serine esterase of
plasma. The cleaved fragment, Bb, remains attached to
C3b, this complex represents the active C3 convertase
of the alternative pathway.

Recent experiments, however, rather indicate that - in analogy to
the activation of factor B - C2 must first be bound to C4b in order
to be efficiently cleaved and capable of forming the $C\overline{42}$ complex.
At first site this sequence is not as obvious as the one of B
activation, since in a fluid system soluble $\overline{C1}$ is indeed capable of
cleaving C2 directly, C4(b) exerting only an enhancing effect.
However, when fixed to a surface in amounts as present e.g. on
sensitized red cells in the state $EAC\overline{1}$, $C\overline{1}$ is virtually devoid of
any direct C2 cleaving potency, and only in the presence of C4b,
i.e. on $EAC\overline{14}$ cells does it effectively cleave C2 (fig. 2). The
effect of C4b is directed to C2 rather than to $C\overline{1}$ since it is completely abolished by elimination of Mg^{++}. This ion is, however,
necessary only for reversible complex formation between native C2
and C4b, not for the esterolytic and C2 cleaving potency of $C\overline{1s}$.
Further, C2a is incapable of combining with preformed C4b, even
immediately after its release by trypsin. These findings indicate
that the reaction of C2 activation proceeds as depicted in fig. 3.

Activation of C5

     The fifth component of complement is activated through cleavage
of a peptide bond by the same convertases which also cleave C3:
$C\overline{42}$ and C3bBb. However, neither of the two enzymes attacks C5
directly, both need additional, surface-fixed C3b. In the classical
pathway the C3b fragment has been envisaged as a modulator of $C\overline{42}$;
by formation of a complex $C\overline{423}$ the enzyme proper (the C2a fragment)
is thought to acquire an affinity for C5 (Müller-Eberhard, 1969).

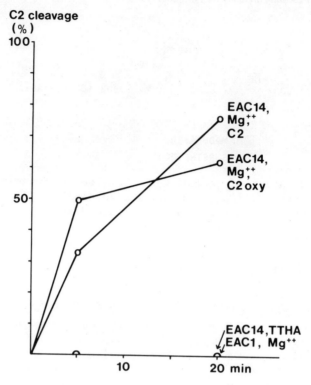

Figure 2.   Cleavage of human C2 in its natural or oxidized (stabilized)
            form (C2oxy), by cell intermediates EAC$\overline{1}$ and EAC$\overline{14}$. EAC$\overline{1}$
            cells do not cleave either of the two C2 species, only
            EAC$\overline{14}$ (bearing the same amount of C$\overline{1}$, and in addition
            activated C4) are active. The effect of C$\overline{4}$ is abolished
            when Mg^{++} is withdrawn by addition of the Mg^{++}-chelator,
            thriethylene tetramine hexaacetic acid (TTHA).

In the alternative pathway aggregates of C3b have been considered
necessary to convey C5 cleaving activity to the activated factor B
in C3bBb (Daha et al., 1976; Medicus et al., 1976). We have not
found indications for an interaction of C3b with either of the
convertases. However, surface-fixed C3b does interact with the
substrate C5. Further, whenever the opportunity for C5 to bind to
surface-fixed C3b is given - and only then -, are the C3 convertases
capable of cleaving it, even soluble C3bBb (Vogt et al., 1978).
Other proteins which also bind to C3b such as factor B and properdin
can interfere with C5 binding and activation. A further indication
for the essential interaction between C3b and C5 comes from the
observation of incompatibilities between heterologous C5 and C3 in
complement haemolysis (von Zabern et al., 1979). The scheme in
fig. 4 shows the reaction sequence of C5 activation deduced from
and compatible with the findings mentioned above.

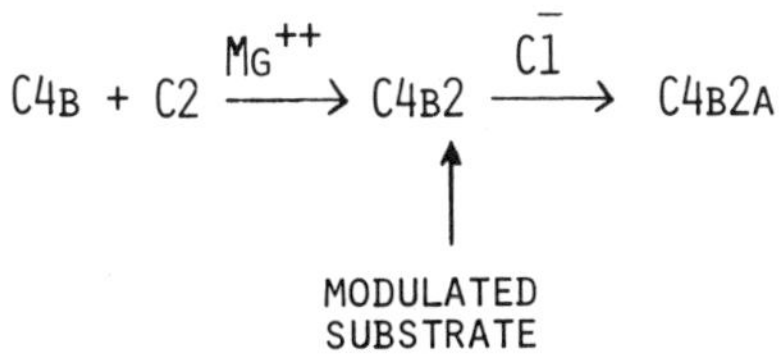

$$C4B + C2 \xrightarrow{Mg^{++}} C4B2 \xrightarrow{\bar{C1}} C4B2A$$

$$\uparrow$$

MODULATED
SUBSTRATE

Figure 3.   Activation of C2. Subsequent to the generation of C4b,
by $\bar{C1}$-induced cleavage of C4 (not shown), C2 forms a
Mg^{++}-dependent reversible complex with the C4 fragment.
In this combination C2 probably acquires a configuration
favourable if not essential for its cleavage by $\bar{C1}$. The
resulting fragment, C2a, remains attached to C4b, and
represents the C3 convertase of the classical pathway
of complement.

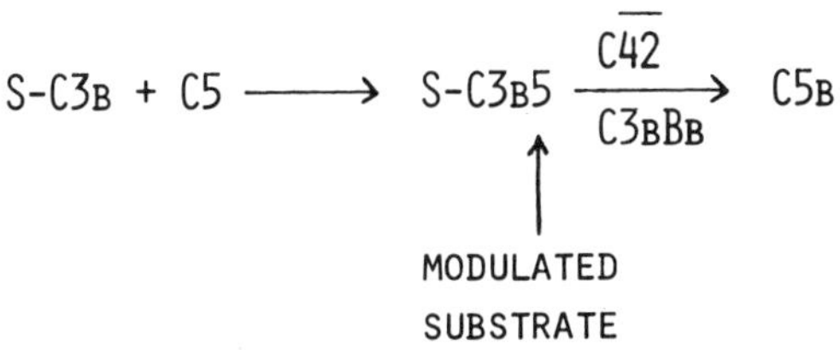

$$S-C3B + C5 \longrightarrow S-C3B5 \xrightarrow[C3BBB]{\bar{C42}} C5B$$

$$\uparrow$$

MODULATED

SUBSTRATE

Figure 4.   Activation of C5. Surface-fixed C3b (S-C3b) binds C5
reversibly. In this combination C5 obviously acquires
a conformation which exposes the critical peptide bond
to be cleaved, to the convertase ($\bar{C42}$ or C3bBb).
Without binding cleavage, and hence activation, of C5
does not proceed.

Activation of Hageman Factor

Hageman Factor (HF) can be activated by contact with suitable
surfaces, e.g. collagen or silica. Active HF (HF_a) then activates
plasma pre-kallikrein and the clotting system. The activation of
HF by contact is, however, a reaction with poor efficiency only, it
is greatly enhanced by a feed-back mechanism: kallikrein activates
HG (Cochrane et al., 1973). This is again not an efficient direct
reaction involving the two partners, enzyme and substrate (HF),
alone. Rather a third constituent is essential, namely high
molecular weight kininogen (HMW-K) (Schiffman and Lee, 1975; Chan
et al., 1976). This kinin precursor appears to have several effects
in its interaction with HF, pre-kallikrein, and factor XI. Griffin
and Cochrane (1976) proposed that HMW-K by forming a complex with
HF renders the latter much more susceptible, as a substrate, to
hydrolytic activation by the enzyme, kallikrein. On the other hand,
Mandle et al. (1976) found that in human plasma HMW-K complexes with
pre-kallikrein and suggested that after being bound to a surface

with the aid of the kininogen pre-kallikrein acquires a configuration
favourable for its hydrolytic activation by active HF. Both
reactions would represent an example of substrate modulation. In
addition HMW-K may, however, also act as a co-factor of the
activated enzyme(s), kallikrein and/or HF_a, to enhance their hydrolytic activity.

SUMMARY

Since plasma is a homogenous fluid its biochemical systems
need special control mechanisms to prevent their unlimited and
continuous activity. In general, enzymic activity is not preformed
but generated by trigger processes. Activation is then enhanced by
cascade reactions. It can be controlled by enzyme inhibitors, by
enzymes which destroy co-factors, or by spontaneous decay of enzyme
complexes involved in the system. In addition, in some reactions of
the complement and Hageman factor-dependent systems the necessity
of substrate modulation controls the extent of activation. Thus,
factor B of the properdin system is activatable by factor $\bar{D}$ only
when bound to the activated third component of complement, and C3b
fragment; similarly C2 is activated and forms the C3 converting
complex, C42, only when bound to C4b prior to its cleavage by Cl;
C5 can be activated by either of the two convertases only when
bound to surface-fixed C3b; and the mutual activation of Hageman
factor and pre-kallikrein on surfaces proceeds efficiently only
when HMW-kininogen is present which complexes with pre-kallikrein
and possibly with Hageman factor.

REFERENCES

Chan, J.Y.C., F.M. Habal, C.E. Burrowes and H.Z. Movat, 1976.
    Interaction between factor XII (Hageman factor), high molecular
    weight kininogen and prekallikrein. Thromb. Res. 9: 423.
Cochrane, C.G., S.D. Revak and K.D. Wuepper, 1973. Activation of
    Hageman factor in solid and fluid phases. A critical role of
    kallikrein. J. exp. Med. 138: 1564.
Daha, M.R., D.T. Fearon and K.F. Austen, 1976. C3 requirements
    for formation of alternative pathway C5 convertase. J. Immunol.
    117: 630.
Fearon, D.T., K.F. Austen and S. Ruddy, 1973. Formation of a hemo-
    lytically active cellular intermediate by the interaction
    between properdin factors B and D and the third component of
    complement. J. exp. Med. 138: 1305.
Gigli, I., and K.F. Austen, 1969. Fluid phase destruction of $C2^{hu}$
    by $C1^{hu}$. II. Unmasking by $C4b^{hu}$ of $\overline{C1}^{hu}$ specificity for C2hu.
    J. exp. Med. 130: 833.

Griffin, J.H., and C.G. Cochrane, 1976. Mechanisms for the involve-
     ment of high molecular weight kininogen in surface-dependent
     reactions of Hageman factor. Proc. Natl. Acad. Sci. USA 73:
     2554.
Mandle, R.J., R.W. Colman and A.P. Kaplan, 1976. Identification of
     prekallikrein and high-molecular-weight kininogen as a complex
     in human plasma. Proc. Natl. Acad. Sci. USA 73: 4179.
Medicus, R.G., O. Götze and H.J. Müller-Eberhard, 1976. Alternative
     pathway of complement: recruitment of precursor properdin
     by labile C3/C5 convertase and the potentiation of the path-
     way. J. exp. Med. 144: 1076.
Müller-Eberhard, H.J., 1969. Complement. Ann. Rev. Biochemistry
     38: 389.
Müller-Eberhard, H.J., and O. Götze, 1972. C3 proactivator convertase
     and its mode of action. J. exp. Med. 135: 1003.
Schiffman, S., and P. Lee, 1975. Partial purification and character-
     ization of contact activation cofactor. J. clin. Invest.
     56: 1082.
Vogt, W., L. Dieminger, R. Lynen and G. Schmidt, 1974. Alternate
     pathway to complement activation in human serum: formation and
     composition of the complex with cobra venom factor which cleaves
     the third component of complement. Hoppe-Seylers Z. physiol.
     Chem. 355: 171.
Vogt, W., G. Schmidt, L. Dieminger and R. Lynen, 1975. Formation
     and composition of the C3 activating enzyme complex of the ˙
     properdin system. Sequential assembly of its components on
     solid-phase trypsin-agarose. Z. Immun.-Forsch. 149: 440.
Vogt, W., W. Dames, G. Schmidt and L. Dieminger, 1977. Complement
     activation by the properdin system: formation of a stoichio-
     metric, C3 cleaving complex of properdin factor B with C3b,
     Immunochemistry 14: 201.
Vogt, W., G. Schmidt, B. von Buttlar and L. Dieminger, 1978. A new
     function of the activated third component of complement:
     binding to C5, an essential step for C5 activation.
     Immunology 34: 29.
von Zabern, I., R. Nolte and W. Vogt, 1979. Incompatibility between
     complement components C3 and C5 of guinea pig and man, an
     indication of their interaction in C5 activation by classical
     and alternative C5 convertases. Scand. J. Immunol., in press.

COLD ACTIVATION OF COMPLEMENT AND KININ

Motoharu Kondo, Shuhei Takemura, Toshikazu Yoshikawa,
Haruki Kato, Nobuyoshi Yokoe, Minoru Ikezaki, Keimei
Hosokawa and Masasuke Masuda

Department of Medicine, Kyoto Prefectural University
of Medicine, Kyoto 602, Japan

Differences between serum and plasma complement, which now
is called as the cold activation of complement, was investigated
in relation with the phenomenon reported as the cold promoted activation of factor VII, to which kallikrein and Hageman factor are
known to participate. Despite the presence of several similarities
in these two phenomena, it is concluded that the cold activation
of complement is not related to the coagulation nor the kinin
system. Evidence that tranexamic acid, a potent antiplasmin compound, provided an inhibitory effect on the cold activation of
complement, suggested that the phenomenon could not be explained
by a single mechanism, and plasmin might be involved in the phenomenon in a limited case.

INTRODUCTION

It has been reported that the activation of coagulation factor
VII measured by Thrombotest was shortened in certain females taking
oral contraceptives when their plasma were exposed to the cold
(Gjønnaess, 1972). This phenomenon has been called as "the cold
promoted activation of factor VII", and Hageman factor-derived
activation of kallikrein has been thought to play a role in the
mechanism (Saito & Ratnoff, 1975).

On the other hand, recent investigation of complement has
shown that in some patients with chronic liver diseases complement
level is markedly decreased in serum while it is maintained at a normal
level in their plasma. This phenomenon was initially called "the
differences between plasma and serum complement" (Inai et al., 1976),

133

and was considered as a result of the activation of coagulation system since serum underwent clotting mechanism. It was found later that the reduction of complement was due to exposure of the sample to a cold environment, and Kondo et al (1976) have called the phenomenon as "the cold activation of complement".

MATERIALS AND METHODS

Titration of hemolytic complement activity was carried out by the lysis of sensitized sheep erythrocytes(EA) described by Mayer (1965). Thrombotest was performed according to the method of Owren (1959). Determination of prekallikrein and plasminogen was performed using chromogenic substrates S2302 (H-D-Pro-Phe-Arg-pNA) and S2251 (H-D-Val-Leu-Lys-pNA) respectively.

A patient KN, a 47-year-old man with periodic edema with chronic inactive hepatitis, who had normal $\overline{C1}$ inhibitor, α1-antitrypsin, α2-macroglobulin and normal coagulation study, was used as the source of serum otherwise stated. Blood was incubated at $37^{\circ}C$ for 1 hr, allowed to clot, and the serum was separated by centrifugation at $37^{\circ}C$.

Trasylol (Bayer, Leverkusen), soybean trypsin inhibitor (SBTI; Sigma Chem. Co., St. Louis) and tranexamic acid (trans-AMCHA; trans-4-aminomethyl cyclohexane carboxylic acid; Daiichi Pharm. Co., Tokyo) were used as inhibitors.

RESULTS

Estimation of Complement in Serum and Plasma in Patients with Chronic Liver Disease.

Hemolytic complement activity (CH50) was investigated in patients with chronic liver diseases, and 24 out of 195 patients revealed decreased serum CH50 while normal in plasma. Classification of these 24 patients were; 13 chronic hepatitis and 11 liver cirrhosis. No specific laboratory examination nor the symptoms were found to relate to the phenomenon. Cryoglobulin was detected in 12 patients, and hepatitis B antigen in 3 cases.

Changes of Serum and Plasma Complement at $4^{\circ}C$.

A patients' KN serum separated at $37^{\circ}C$, and his heparinized plasma, were incubated at $37^{\circ}C$ or $4^{\circ}C$, and the change of complement activity was investigated for 24 hr. Serum complement incubated at $4^{\circ}C$ showed a rapid reduction within 2 hr, while plasma started to decrease at 5 hr and then gradually fell down, indicating that

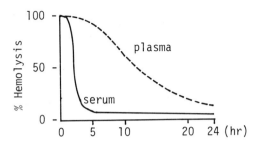

Figure 1.   Complement activity of KN's serum and heparinized
            plasma at 4°C.

both serum and plasma complement is susceptible to the effect of
cold and finally they were fully inactivated (Fig. 1).

Comparison of the Cold Activation of Complement with Cold Promoted
Activation of Factor VII.

     Aliquots of patient's serum separated at 37°C were incubated
at different temperatures for 4 hr and the residual hemolytic
activity was determined. Fig. 2a shows that the cold activation
of complement occurred between 0°C to 11°C. Fig. 2b shows that the
cold promoted activation of factor VII reported by Gjønnaess (1972)
in which activation appeared between -5°C to 5°C. Thrombotest in
KN's plasma revealed no cold promoted activation of factor VII.

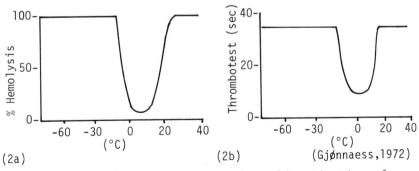

Figure 2.   Effect of temperature on the cold activation of
            complement (2a) and on the cold promoted activation
            of factor VII (2b).

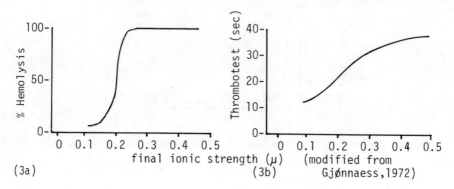

Figure 3.   Effect of ionic strength on the cold activation of
             complement (3a) and on the cold promoted activation
             of factor VII (3b).

When different concentrations of NaCl solution were mixed
with patient's serum and incubated at 4°C for 4 hr, the cold activation of complement was prevented at higher ionic strength over
$\mu=0.025$ (Fig. 3a).   Fig. 3b shows that the cold promoted activation
of factor VII was prevented by the increase of ionic strength over
$\mu= 0.3$ (Gjønnaess, 1972).

Effect of Anticoagulants on the Cold Activation of Complement

Addition of different concentrations of anticoagulants heparin,
citrate or EDTA resulted in the prevention of serum complement from
the cold activation as shown in Table 1.   The same result was observed in plasma treated by the same concentration of anticoagulants.
Therefore, it is suggested that blood coagulation might not be
related to the cold activation of complement.   Anticoagulants acted
on the prolongation of the cold activation, and only a high concentration of EDTA inhibited the cold activation during the observation
for 24 hr.

Effect of Trasylol, SBTI, Trans-AMCHA on the Cold Activation of
Complement.

Trasylol, SBTI or trans-AMCHA was mixed with aliquots of serum
and incubated at 4°C for 4 hr.   It was found that Trasylol and SBTI
failed to prevent the complement from the cold activation, indicating
that the phenomenon might not be related to factor VII nor kallikrein which is inhibitable by these agents.   Trans-AMCHA showed an
inhibitory effect only in some patients and the participation of
plasmin in the mechanism is suggested.

Table 1. Effect of anticoagulants on the cold activation of complement.

	Final Concentration	Residual C activity (%)			
		Before	2	4	24 hr
Buffer		100	12	3	0
Heparin	88 u/ml	100	100	96	30
	44	100	92	80	13
	8.7	100	90	69	5
Citrate	3.8 mg/ml	100	94	78	0
	1.9	100	47	4	0
	0.9	100	31	0	0
EDTA	18.0 mMol	100	100	100	89
	3.6	100	100	96	51
	1.0	100	65	8	0

Plasminogen and Prekallikrein During the Course of the Cold Activation of Complement

KN's plasma was investigated for the change of plasminogen and prekallikrein during the incubation at 4°C for 6 hr. There was no significant difference of the behaviour of both plasminogen and prekallikrein when compared with normal human plasma.

DISCUSSION

Decreased serum complement in man is explained by (i) impaired synthesis of complement protein(s), (ii) increased activation or consumption of complement through the classical or the alternative pathway, or (iii) the presence of anticomplementary factor which interferes the estimation of hemolytic complement assay. Recent knowledge of complement clarified that serum complement in some patients with chronic liver diseases is activated in vitro through its classical pathway in the cold environment. Since complement was believed to be relatively stable in the cold, the phenomenon left us confused in the understanding of complement in the clinical field. Inai et al., (1976) described the phenomenon as "the differences of complement between serum and plasma", and Kondo et al., (1976) reported that the phenomenon should be called "the cold activation of complement" since even plasma complement could be activated in the cold unless high concentration of anticoagulants were used.

In the beginning of our investigation, attention was focused on the participation of blood coagulation in the phenomenon because serum underwent clotting mechanism, and in addition coagulation factor VII is sometimes activated in the cold (Gjønnaess, 1972). Several similarities were observed between the cold activation of complement and the cold promoted activation of factor VII, for example, temperature and ionic strength. Evidence that Trasylol or SBTI could not prevent the cold activation of complement indicated that the phenomenon might not be related to factor VII nor kallikrein. It was also demonstrated that patient's plasma did not generate plasmin or kallikrein during the cold activation. Anticoagulants were effective in reducing the cold activation of complement, but did not provide crucial significance that clotting mechanism played a role. However, the evidence that trans-AMCHA, a potent antiplasmin agent, inhibited the cold activation of complement in some cases, suggested that plasmin might be involved in the mechanism, although how plasmin reacts in the cold is not known.

It is recommended that for the hemolytic complement assay, freshly separated serum at 37°C or EDTA-treated plasma should be used. For the analysis of low serum complement especially in patients with liver diseases, determination of complement protein, for example C4, should be followed to exclude the phenomenon since the antigenicity of C4 protein is not affected by the cold activation.

REFERENCES

Gjønnaess, H., 1972. Cold promoted activation of factor VII. I. Evidence for the existence of an activator. Thrombos. Diathes. Haemorrh. 28: 155.

Inai, S., et al., 1975. Differences between plasma and serum complement in patients with chronic liver disease. Clin. Exp. Immunol. 25: 403.

Kondo, M. et al., 1976. Cold activation of complement. I. Presence of coagulation-related activator. J. Immunol. 117: 486.

Mayer, M.M. 1965. Mechanism of hemolysis by complement. In Ciba Foundation Symposium on Complement. G.E.W. Wolstenholm and J. Knight eds., J. & A. Churchill Ltd., London, p. 4.

Owren, P.A. 1959. Thrombotest. A new method for controlling anticoagulant therapy. Lancet II: 754.

Saito, H. and Ratnoff, O.D., 1975. Alteration of factor VII activity by activated Fletcher factor (a plasma kallikrein): a potential link between the intrinsic and extrinsic blood-clotting systems. J. Lab. Clin. Med. 85: 405.

ACTIVATION OF HUMAN HAGEMAN FACTOR BY A LEUKOCYTIC PROTEASE

Harold H. Newball, Susan D. Revak, Charles G. Cochrane,
John H. Griffin, Lawrence M. Lichtenstein

The Johns Hopkins University School of Medicine
Baltimore, Maryland & Scripps Clinic and Research
Foundation, La Jolla, California

ABSTRACT

We earlier reported the IgE-mediated release of a basophil
kallikrein of anaphylaxis (BK-A) which, like plasma kallikrein, is
an arginine esterase and cleaves human plasma kininogen generating
immunoreactive kinin. We herein report that, like plasma kallikrein,
preparations rich in this basophil protease also activate human
Hageman Factor by proteolytic cleavage of the zymogen molecule into
light and heavy chains. These fragments of 28,000 and 52,000 daltons
are similar in size to those produced during activation of Hageman
Factor by plasma kallikrein. Exposure of Hageman Factor (bound to
a negatively charged surface) to BK-A led to the proteolytic cleavage of Hageman Factor producing a 28,000 molecular weight fragment
(HF_a) which is functionally active and capable of activating prekallikrein to kallikrein. We conclude that, during anaphylaxis,
basophils may release a protease that is capable of cleaving and
activating Hageman Factor, thus providing a mechanism for initiating
the in vivo activation of the Hageman Factor dependent systems.

INTRODUCTION

The surface-dependent activation of Hageman Factor (HF) by plasma kallikrein is associated with the proteolytic cleavage of the
zymogen Hageman Factor molecule (11,15-19). Activated human Hageman
Factor (HF_a) participates in a series of reactions including those
associated with activation of the intrinsic blood coagulation cascade, the kinin-generating system, and the plasma fibrinolytic system (4).

Hageman Factor is activated during its proteolytic cleavage by plasma kallikrein, yielding a functionally active molecule of 80,000 molecular weight, consisting of two polypeptide chains, the heavier of 52,000 molecular weight and the lighter of 28,000 molecular weight, bound by a disulfide linkage. A second cleavage of the HF molecule by kallikrein can occur very close to the first site, but outside of the disulfide linkage. Cleavage at this site results in the release of a 28,000 M.W. fragment that dissociates from the surface. HF_a is, itself, a potent activator of prekallikrein. Thus, once HF is activated, there is a reciprocal activation of pre-kallikrein to kallikrein, and HF to HF_a. The mechanism by which the above sequence is initiated is unknown.

We earlier reported the IgE-mediated release of a basophil kal-likrein of anaphylaxis (BK-A) which, like plasma kallikrein, is an arginine esterase and cleaves human plasma kininogen generating immunoreactive kinin (12-13). We report herein that, like the plas-ma kallikrein described above, preparations rich in BK-A also acti-vate human Hageman Factor by proteolytic cleavage of the zymogen molecule into light and heavy chains. This report, therefore, de-scribes a mechanism whereby a product of IgE-mediated immediate hy-persensitivity reactions may activate the Hageman Factor dependent systems. The IgE-mediated release of this protease provides a po-tential mechanism for the in vivo activation of Hageman Factor, which may be responsible in part for the symptom complex observed during human anaphylaxis, and provides a potential link between IgE-medi-ated events and inflammatory processes.

MATERIALS AND METHODS

Materials. The ^3H - TAMe (210 mCi/mmol) was purchased from Biochemical and Nuclear Corp., Burbank, Calif. Tris buffers used in the release of the arginine esterase from peripheral leukocytes were made of 0.025 M pre-set Tris, pH 7.35 at 37° C (Sigma Chemical Co., St. Louis, Mo.), 0.12 M sodium chloride, 5 mM potassium chlor-ide, and 0.03% human serum albumin (HSA) (Behring Werke, Marburg, Germany). The above constitutes Tris-A; Tris-ACM contains, in addi-tion, calcium 0.06 mM and magnesium 1.0 mM (7). Sepharose 6B, pre-swollen DEAE-Sephacel, Sephadex G-200 and Ficoll were purchased from Pharmacia Fine Chemicals, Inc., Piscataway, N.J. Antigen E was kindly provided by Dr. T.P. King of the Rockefeller University, New York, and anti-IgE by Dr. K. Ishizaka. Tris-buffered saline (TBS) was made by the addition of 0.15M NaCl to 0.01M Tris, pH 7.6. TBS/ BSA refers to a 1 mg/ml solution of bovine serum albumin (BSA, Reheis Chemical Company, Chicago, Illinois) in TBS. Sodium dodecyl sulfate (SDS)was purchased from BioRad Laboratories, Richmond, California.

Leukocyte preparations. Human leukocytes from donors allergic to ragweed or grass and from normal volunteers were separated from

the other formed elements of blood by sedimentation for 60 to 90
minutes in a mixture of dextran-EDTA and dextrose. The cells were
washed twice in Tris-A buffer, then resuspended in a serum-free
Tris-ACM buffer at a concentration of 10^7 cell per ml, as previously
described (7). The immunologic reaction was initiated by the addition of anti-IgE to the cell preparations and the reaction allowed
to proceed for 30 or 45 minutes in the dose-response studies, or
for periods of 90 minutes when generating large quantities of BK-A.
At the completion of the reaction, the cells were centrifuged and
the amount of BK-A released into the supernatant as well as that
present in an aliquot of untreated cells was determined by the radiochemical technique of Beaven et al. (1), as previously described (13).

Arginine esterase activity. Arginine esterase activity of the
supernatant was determined by a radiochemical technique employing
p-toluenesulfonyl-L-arginine ^{3}H --methyl ester (^{3}H -- TAMe) (13)
which was devised by Beaven et al. (1) for the measurement of human
urinary kallikrein and modified for the determination of arginine
esterase activity in supernatants (21). The experimental tubes with
leukocytes were run in duplicate, while the determinations of arginine esterase activity were run in quadruplicate. The total cellular
arginine esterase activity was determined using sonicated aliquots
of untreated cells.

Definition of TAMe unit. A TAMe unit is defined as that quantity of BK-A which hydrolyses one picomole (pmol) of the substrate
^{3}H - TAMe per minute. The activity of a sample is expressed as units
per ml of the sample, or pmol per minute per ml of sample. The specific activity of the ^{3}H-TAMe used in these studies is such that
cpm per 10 μl of sample reported in this manuscript may be converted
to units per ml by simply dividing cpm by 10,000.

Plasma proteins. HF was isolated from human plasma as previously described (2). The purification of prekallikrein employed sequential chromatography on DEAE-, QAE-, and SP-Sephadex, followed
by concanavalin A-Sepharose (B.N. Bouma and J. H. Griffin, 1978.
Manuscript in preparation). Kallikrein, having an activity in a
coagulation assay of 33 u/ml, was obtained by the spontaneous activation of a preparation of prekallikrein following the final step
of purification. Purified HF was radiolabeled with ^{125}I utilizing
the chloramine T method (10).

Cleavage of surface-bound Hageman Factor. For assays of the
ability of various enzymes to cleave HF, the HF was first adsorbed
onto a glass surface. 2 μl (.024 μg) of ^{125}I-HF were added to a
12 x 75 mm borosilicate glass tube containing 20 μl of TBS/BSA and
incubated with shaking at room temperature for 5 min. The fluid
was then aspirated out and the surface-bound HF washed twice with
200 μl of TBS. 10 μl of a solution of 1 mg/ml BSA in 0.2M Tris
pH 8.0 were added and the tube incubated with shaking for 2 min

after which, 20 µl of the enzyme to be tested were added and the incubation continued for the desired time period (usually 20 min). To terminate the reaction, 50 µl of 4% SDS in 0.01M sodium phosphate buffer, pH 7.0 containing 2% β-mercaptoethanol were added and the tubes immediately placed in a boiling water bath for 3 min. This procedure resulted in the elution of greater than 90% of the HF from the surface. The samples were then assayed by electrophoresis on SDS-polyacrylamide gels for the percent of HF cleavage.

SDS-polyacrylamide gel electrophoresis (PAGE). Samples were prepared for electrophoresis as described above. Sucrose was added to a final concentration of 10% and a trace of bromophenol blue was added as a tracking dye. The samples were layered on top of 4.5 x 80 mm 7% polyacrylamide gels containing 0.1% SDS. Electrophoresis was carried out according to the method of Weber and Osborn (20) until the tracking dye was near the bottom of the gels. The gels were removed from the tubes, sliced into 1.2 mm sections and counted for radioactivity.

RESULTS

IgE-mediated release of BK-A. We earlier reported that BK-A is released by IgE-mediated mechanisms (12-13). Figure 1 shows a dose-response curve in which human peripheral leukocytes were challenged with highly specific anti-IgE (3), leading to the release of BK-A. Similar dose-response relationships have been obtained when leukocyte preparations were challenged with purified protein antigens from ragweed (AgE) (6) or grass (Group I) (9).

Purification of BK-A. To generate large quantities of BK-A, leukocytes from 200 to 400 ml of blood were challenged with anti-IgE. The supernatants from these preparations were concentrated tenfold by vacuum dialysis at 4° C using Collodiun bags, No. 100, and stored at -70° C until used for chromatographic studies. BK-A obtained by challenge with anti-IgE was sequentially chromatographed on Sephadex G-200, DEAE-Sephacel, and Sepharose 6B.

Sephadex G-200. A 2.6-X 40-cm column was packed with Sephadex G-200 to a height of 35 cm, and equilibrated with 0.02M PO_4 buffer, pH 6.8 at 4° C. Fifteen ml of supernatant was applied to the column and the pattern developed by upward flow of 10 ml/hr using a peristaltic pump. Eighty 3-ml fractions were collected and assayed for arginine esterase activity. At the completion of the chromatographic study, absorbance of the collected fractions was determined using a spectrophotometer (Model 26, Beckman Instruments). Only one area of esterase activity was observed when the supernatant was chromatographed on Sephadex G-200 (Fig. 2). The esterase-active area eluted with the void volume in the first O.D. peak. The esterase-active fractions from the Sephadex G-200 were further purified by ion

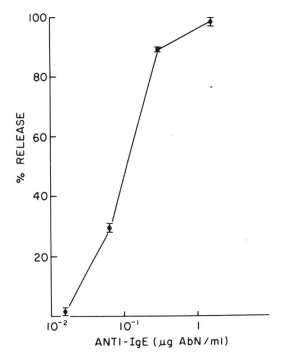

Figure 1.   Kallikrein Release from Human Leukocytes
            IgE-mediated release of BK-A

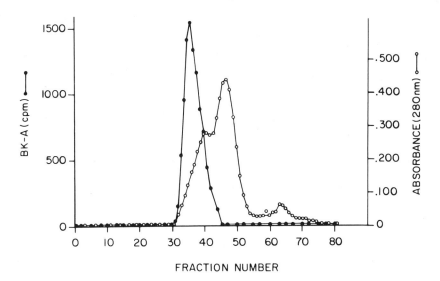

Figure 2.   Sephadex G-200 Chromatography of BK-A
            Sephadex G-200 chromatography of preparations rich
            in BK-A.

exchange chromatography (DEAE-Sephacel).

DEAE-Sephacel. A 1.6-X 20-cm column was packed with Sephacel to a height of 10 cm, and equilibrated with 0.02 M PO_4 buffer, pH 6.8 at 4° C. Forty to 60 ml of esterase-active eluate of the Sephadex G-200 were applied to the column and the pattern developed by downward flow of 30 ml/hr using a peristaltic pump. The column was washed with 200 ml of the equilibrating buffer and eluted with a linear salt gradient of 30 ml of equilibrating buffer and 30 ml of 0.02 M PO_4 buffer, pH 6.8 containing 0.50 M NaCl. A second-step salt gradient was developed with 30 ml of equilibrating buffer containing 0.50 M NaCl and 30 ml of 0.02 M PO_4, pH 6.8 containing 1 M NaCl. Thirty 2-ml fractions were collected from each salt gradient and we determined arginine esterase activity, conductivity, and absorbance (280 nm). Only one esterase-active area was observed (Fig. 3). This eluted with the first NaCl gradient, and coincided with an O.D. peak. A second O.D. peak eluted with the second gradient, however, it had no esterase activity. The esterase-active fractions eluted with a conductivity of 10 mMhos, corresponding to a salt concentration of 0.1 M NaCl. The esterase-active fractions from DEAE-Sephacel were further purified by molecular sieve chromatography (Sepharose 6B).

Sepharose 6B. A 1.6-X 100-cm column of Sepharose 6B was equilibrated with 0.02 M PO_4 buffer, pH 6.8 at 4° C and calibrated with blue dextran, thyroglobulin, ferritin, catalase, and HSA (Mannheim-Boehringer). Six to 8 ml of concentrated esterase-active fractions from DEAE-Sephacel were applied to the column and the pattern developed by upward flow of 10 ml/hr using a peristaltic pump. One hundred 3-ml fractions were collected and we determined arginine esterase activity and absorbance (280 nm). One major esterase-active area was observed (Fig. 4). This esterase-active area coincided with the first O.D. peak and eluted with an estimated molecular weight of 1.2 million. A second arginine esterase-active area is usually present, and is quantitatively of smaller magnitude and of smaller molecular weight (approximately 400,000). A third arginine esterase-active area is variably present, and is quantitatively of smaller magnitude than the 1.2 million or the 400,000 forms. This third form also has the smallest molecular weight (approximately 80,000). The three esterase-active fractions were used for studies of HF cleavage.

Relationship of BK-A and HF cleaving activities. In an effort to determine whether the BK-A arginine esterase and the HF cleaving activities might be subserved by the same protease (s), we determined whether the two activities co-chromatographed during the purification of BK-A. BK-A was sequentially chromatographed on Sephadex G-200, DEAE-Sephacel, and Sepharose 6B, and all fractions were assayed for arginine esterase activity while selected fractions were assayed for HF cleaving activity. The two activities were found

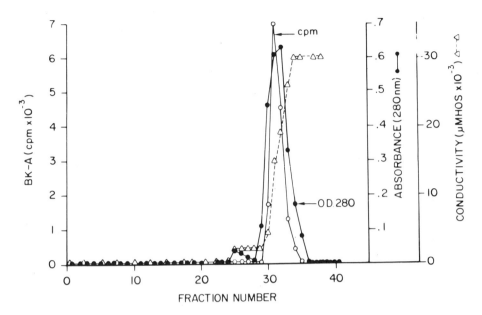

Figure 3.   DEAE-Sephacel chromatography of arginine esterase
            active fractions from Sephadex G-200.

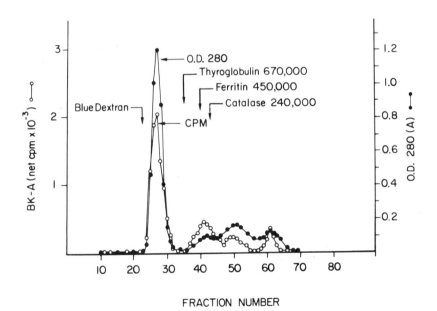

Figure 4.   Sepharose 6B chromatography of arginine esterase active
            fractions from DEAE-Sephacel.

to co-chromatograph on the first two columns. The Sepharose 6B column, however, presented a more complex profile. As shown in Fig. 4,
three protein peaks were observed, corresponding to molecular weights
of approximately 1.2 million, 400,000, and 80,000 daltons. There
is arginine esterase activity clearly associated with the first two
peaks, but little present in the last peak. Fractions from the last
peak were, however, the most potent in cleaving HF. HF-cleaving
capacity was associated with the 400,000 M.W. peak, while the 1.2
million M.W. material was a good activator of HF. The relative a-
amounts of arginine-esterase activity eluting at the three positions
was found to vary from experiment to experiment, but the 80,000 M.W.
peak was consistently found to have the least esterase activity and
most potent HF cleaving activity.

     Cleavage of HF by BK-A. Like plasma kallikrein, preparations
rich in BK-A also activate HF by proteolytic cleavage of HF into
light and heavy chains. These fragments of approximately 28,000
and 52,000 daltons are similar in size to those produced during
activation of HF by plasma kallikrein. Figure 5 shows the proteolytic cleavage of purified HF by purified plasma kallikrein and
preparations rich in BK-A, that were sequentially chromatographed
on Sephadex G-200, DEAE-Sephacel and Sepharose 6B. Radiolabeled HF
was adsorbed to a glass surface after which it was cleaved by either
plasma kallikrein or BK-A. After cleavage, samples were analyzed by
electrophoresis on SDS-PAGE as earlier described (19). The top panel
shows the control in which HF was exposed to buffer. Virtually all
of the radiolabel is at a position corresponding to the molecular
weight of uncleaved HF, namely 80,000. The middle panel shows the
cleavage of HF by plasma kallikrein. Part of the radiolabeled HF
remains uncleaved at the 80,000 M.W. position, while part is cleaved
into fragments of approximately 28,000 and 52,000 daltons. The lower
panel shows the cleavage of HF by BK-A. As with plasma kallikrein,
part of the radiolabeled HF remains uncleaved at a M.W. of 80,000.

     Hageman Factor as a substrate for BK-A. Kinetic studies were
designed in an attempt to determine the relative potency of BK-A
and plasma kallikrein in cleaving Hageman Factor. Optimally, we
would have used equivalent molar quantities of the two proteases to
determine their relative potency on the HF substrate. However, because it was not known whether the BK-A preparations were pure (they
had been sequentially chromatographed on Sephadex G-200, DEAE-Sephacel, and Sepharose 6B) we, instead, used arginine esterase activity
of the two proteases as a standard for comparison in the kinetic
studies. Purified radiolabeled HF was adsorbed to a glass surface
and then exposed to aliquots of purified plasma kallikrein and the
1.2 million M.W. form of BK-A. After cleavage. samples were analyzed by electrophoresis on SDS-PAGE (19). Figure 6 shows that
0.014 units of BK-A led to much greater cleavage of HF than a four-
fold greater quantity of plasma kallikrein. For equivalent arginine
esterase activity, BK-A of 1.2 million M.W. is 16-fold more active

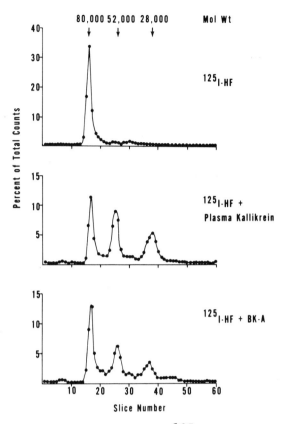

Figure 5.   Cleavage of Surface-Bound ^{125}I-Hageman Factor (HF)
by Plasma Kallikrein and Basophil Kallikrein of
Anaphylaxis (BK-A).

than plasma kallikrein in cleaving HF. Similar experiments suggest
that the 80,000 M.W. form of BK-A has far more HF cleaving activity
than the 1.2 million M.W. form per unit of TAMe activity, while the
400,000 M.W. form is less active.

Activation of Hageman Factor by BK-A. The above data showed
that BK-A cleaves HF producing fragments of approximately 28,000
M.W. We then determined whether the generated fragments possessed
functional activity as assessed by their capacity to activate prekallikrein to kallikrein. Figure 7 illustrates a study in which
purified surface-bound HF was exposed to BK-A at 22° C for 20 minutes (Tube A) resulting in the cleavage of the HF molecule and generation of the 28,000 M.W. fragment β-HF$_a$ (19). Purified human prekallikrein was then exposed to the β-HF$_a$ (Tube B) at 37° for 40 minutes. Prekallikrein was activated to kallikrein by the β-HF$_a$, and

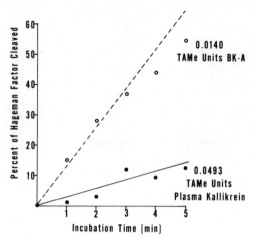

Figure 6.   Comparative Rates of Cleavage of Surface-Bound ^{125}I-
            Hageman Factor by Plasma Kallikrein and Basophil
            Kallikrein of Anaphylaxis (BK-A)

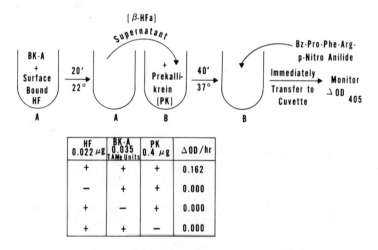

Figure 7.   Measurement of the Activity of the Hageman Factor (HF)
            Fragment Released from the Surface by the Cleavage
            of HF by a Basophil Kallikrein of Anaphylaxis (BK-A).

detected by an assay that utilizes the tripeptide Bz-Pro-Phe-Arg-
p-nitro anilide as a substrate. BK-A, alone, does not cleave the
tripeptide in the concentrations used in these experiments. The
hydrolysis of Bz-Pro-Phe-Arg-pNA by kallikrein results in the release
of free paranitroaniline with an increase in absorbance at 405 nm.

The table (Fig. 7) shows that the interaction of HF and BK-A resulted in the generation of HF_a, which activated prekallikrein to kallikrein and led to a change in absorbance. BK-A was found not to activate prekallikrein to kallikrein in the absence of HF. The data indicate that at least some of the HF_a fragments resulting from the cleavage of HF by BK-A are functionally active in that they are capable of activating prekallikrein to kallikrein.

DISCUSSION

BK-A is released from human peripheral leukocytes during challenge with anti-IgE or specific antigens (Fig. 1). Thus, the release process is initiated by the interaction of antigen or anti-IgE with cell bound IgE, and appears to be similar in mechanism to the release of histamine and other mediators of the immediate hypersensitivity reaction (8).

Our earlier studies with BK-A showed that it had many characteristics in common with plasma kallikrein. Like plasma kallikrein, BK-A is an arginine esterase, generates immunoreactive kinin from human plasma kininogen, and is inhibited by plasma (presumably Cl inhibitor), DFP, and Trasylol. It was these shared characteristics of BK-A and plasma kallikrein that led us to study the ability of BK-A to activate Hageman Factor.

We have shown that, during the purification of BK-A, fractions rich in arginine esterase activity are capable of activating HF. Separation on Sepharose 6B yields an additional peak of HF-cleaving material with little associated esterase activity. Thus, while a correspondence between esterase and HF-cleaving activities is clear for the 1.2 million and 400,000 M.W. enzymes, this is not the case for the enzyme at 80,000 M.W. We, therefore, conclude that either different enzymes elute from the Sepharose 6B column in the regions of 1.2 million, 400,000 and 80,000 M.W. or that the specific activities of three forms of a single enzyme vary in terms of esterase and HF-cleaving properties.

The data show that, like plasma kallikrein, BK-A cleaves HF by proteolytic cleavage of the molecule into light and heavy chains (Fig. 5). These fragments of approximately 28,000 and 52,000 daltons are similar in size to those produced during activation of HF by plasma kallikrein. Figure 7 shows that BK-A not only cleaves but also activates HF in that the interaction of BK-A and HF results in the generation of HF_a which is capable of activating prekallikrein to kallikrein. The kinetic studies (Fig. 6) show that, for equivalent arginine esterase activity, the 1.2 million M.W. form of BK-A is far more active than plasma kallikrein in cleaving HF. Thus, HF appears to be a good substrate for the proteolytic action of BK-A.

There are important potential consequences of the activation of the HF dependent systems by BK-A. The activation of HF by BK-A results in the generation of the functionally active fragment HF_a. HF_a activates prekallikrein to kallikrein and thereby activates the fibrinolytic system. Both plasma kallikrein and BK-A may cleave plasma kininogen and generate kinins, which are potentially putative in the inflammatory response.

There have been reports of the consumption of coagulation factors during human and rabbit anaphylaxis (5,14). The precise mechanism for the in vivo anaphylactic activation of HF is unknown. We have now, however, described a mechanism which may initiate the in vivo activation of HF. BK-A may initiate mechanisms that are responsible in part for the symptom complex observed during human anaphylaxis, and may further provide a potential link between IgE-mediated events and inflammatory processes. The release of this protease and its subsequent activation of the components of the Hageman Factor dependent systems could result in a potentiation of the IgE-mediated allergic response.

ACKNOWLEDGEMENTS

This work was supported in part by Grants Nos. HL18526, HL14153, AI07290, and AI07007 from the National Heart, Lung and Blood Institute and National Institute of Allergy and Infectious Diseases, National Institutes of Health. The authors thank Ms. Judy Mason for her technical assistance.

REFERENCES

1. Beaven, V .H., J.V. Pierce and J.J. Pisano, 1971, A sensitive isotopic procedure for the assay of esterase activity: Measurement of human urinary kallikrein, Clin. Chim. Acta. 32, 67.
2. Griffin, J.H. and C.G. Cochrane, Human Factor XII, 1976, in: Methods in Enzymology, Vol. VL, part B, ed. L. Lorand (Academic Press, N.Y.) p. 56.
3. Ishizaka, T., C.S. Sotta and K. Ishizaka, 1973, Mechanisms of passive sensitization III. Number of IgE molecules and their receptor sites on human basophil granulocytes, J. Immunol. 3, 500.
4. Kaplan, A.P., H.L. Meier and R. Mandle, 1976, The Hageman Factor dependent pathways of coagulation, fibrinolysis, and kinin-generation, Seminars in Thrombosis and Hemostasis 3, 1.
5. Kaplan, A.P., et al., 1977, Human anaphylaxis: A study of mediator systems, Clinical Research 25, 361A.
6. King, T.P., P.S. Norman and J.T. Connell, 1964, Isolation and characterization of allergens from ragweed pollen, Biochem, 3, 458.

7. Lichtenstein, L.M. and A.G. Osler, 1964, Studies on the mechanisms of hypersensitivity phenomena, J. Exp. Med. 120,507.

8. Lichtenstein, L.M., Mechanism of allergic histamine .release from human leukocytes, 1968, in: Biochemistry of the Acute Allergic Reactions, Vol. 153, eds. K.F. Austen and E.L. Becker (Blackwell, Oxford) p. 174.

9. Marsh, D.G., F.H. Milner and P. Johnson, 1966, The allergenic activity and stability of purified allergens from the pollen of common rye grass (Lolium perenne), Int. Arch. Allergy 29, 521.

10. McConahey, P.J. and Dixon, F.J., 1966, A method of trace iodination of proteins for immunologic studies, Int. Arch. Allergy Appl. Immunol. 29, 185.

11. Meier, H.L., et al., 1977, Activation and function of human Hageman Factor: The role of high molecular weight kininogen and prekallikrein, J. Clin. Invest. 60, 18.

12. Newball, H.H., R.C. Talamo and L.M. Lichtenstein, 1975, Release of leukocyte kallikrein mediated by IgE, Nature 254, 635.

13. Newball, H.H., et al., Basophil kallikrein of anaphylaxis, 1978, in: Proceedings of the International Symposium on Kinins, eds. T. Suzuki and H. Moriya. (Plenum Press, N.Y., N.Y.)

14. Pinckard, R.N., C. Tanigawa and M. Halonen, 1975, IgE-induced blood coagulation alterations in the rabbit: Consumption of coagulation factors XII, XI, and IX in vivo, J. Immunol. 115, 525.

15. Revak, S.D., et al., 1974, Structural changes accompanying enzymatic activation of human Hageman Factor, J. Clin. Invest. 54, 619.

16. Revak, S.D. and C.G. Cochrane, 1976, The relationship of structure and function in human Hageman Factor, J. Clin. Invest. 57, 852.

17. Revak, S.D. and C.G. Cohrane, 1976, Hageman Factor: its structure and modes of activation, Thrombosis and Haemostasis 35, 570.

18. Revak, S.D., C.G. Cochrane and J.H. Griffin, 1977, The binding and cleavage characteristics of human Hageman Factor during contact activation, J. Clin. Invest. 59, 1167.

19. Revak, S.D., et al., 1978, Surface and fluid phase activities of two forms of activated Hageman Factor produced during contact activation of plasma, J. Exper. Med. 147, 719.

20. Weber, K. and Osborn, M., 1969, The reliability of molecular weight determination by dodecyl sulfate-polyacrylamide gel electrophoresis, J. Biol. Chem. 244, 4406.

21. Webster, M.E., et al., 1974, Release of histamine and arginine-esterase activity from passively sensitized human lung by ragweed antigen, Ciencia E Cultura 26, 372.

CONTACT ACTIVATION OF PLASMA: STRUCTURE-ACTIVITY RELATIONSHIPS OF

HUMAN HIGH MOLECULAR WEIGHT KININOGEN

Daniele Kerbiriou and John H. Griffin

Department of Immunopathology
Scripps Clinic and Research Foundation
La Jolla, California 92037

INTRODUCTION

Human plasmas deficient in high molecular weight kininogen exhibit abnormalities in contact activation reactions including the kinin-forming, intrinsic coagulation, and fibrinolytic pathways (Wuepper et al., 1975; Saito et al., 1975; Colman et al., 1975; Donaldson et al., 1976). The functional role of high MW kininogen as a non-enzymatic cofactor in the activation of surface-bound Factor XII by kallikrein as well as in the activation of Factor XI or of prekallikrein by surface-bound activated Factor XII has been demonstrated (Griffin and Cochrane, 1976; Schiffman and Lee, 1975; Chan et al., 1976; Meier et al., 1977; Revak et al., 1977). More-over, it has been shown that high molecular weight kininogen associates non-covalently with Factor XI or with prekallikrein in plasma (Nagasawa and Nakayasu, 1973; Wendel et al., 1972; Mandle et al., 1976; Thompson et al., 1977), and it has been suggested that high MW kininogen actually bridges the binding of Factor XI and of prekallikrein to negatively charged surfaces where contact activation reactions occur (Wiggins et al., 1977). Thus, high MW kininogen appears to play the role of surface-bound receptor for either prekallikrein or Factor XI and thereby serves as the focal point for assembling proteins of the contact activation system on negatively charged surfaces. The experiments summarized in this chapter are concerned with two major questions. First, what has been learned about the relationship between structure and function for human high MW kininogen? Second, what happens to human high MW kininogen in plasma during contact activation? The results summarized here have been presented elsewhere (Kerbiriou and Griffin, 1978) and they will be published separately in full detail (Kerbiriou and Griffin, manuscript in preparation).

STRUCTURE-FUNCTION RELATIONSHIPS FOR HUMAN HIGH MW KININOGEN

New methods were developed for the isolation of human high MW kininogen in the form of a single polypeptide chain. The steps employed in the isolation of the protein are listed in Figure 1 which also shows the purified protein on SDS gels. The purified single chain protein exhibits an apparent molecular weight of 110,000 on SDS gels. Previous reports have described the isolation of human high MW kininogen in the form of a two chain molecule or a single chain molecule of similar molecular weight (Habal et al., 1974; Nagasawa and Nakayasu, 1976; Wiggins et al., 1977; Saito, 1977; Thompson et al., 1978).

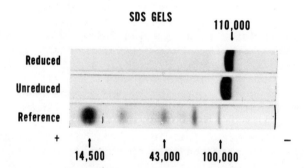

Figure 1.   Purification of human high MW kininogen. The protein was isolated using the sequence of steps described here. The purified protein was analyzed on 7.5% polyacrylamide gels in the presence of sodium dodecyl sulfate, in the presence and absence of mercaptoethanol, shown here as reduced and unreduced gels. The mobility of the protein indicated an apparent molecular weight of 110,000. (Taken from Kerbiriou and Griffin, 1978).

The relationships between structure and activity of human high MW kininogen and of some of its polypeptide fragments are summarized in data presented in Figure 2. In this figure, the native molecule at a molecular weight of 110,000 exhibits a specific clotting activity of 13 units/ml which can also be expressed as 1.4 units/nmol. Incubation of the native molecule with purified human plasma kallikrein liberates bradykinin, as measured in bioassays of rat uterus contractions, and gives a kinin-free two-chain molecule as seen in Figure 2 on the second reduced SDS gel. This molecule containing disulfide-linked chains of 65,000 and 44,000 MW retains full coagulant activity when tested for its ability to correct the activated partial thromboplastin time of plasma deficient in high MW kininogen. Following reduction and carboxymethylation of the kinin-free, two chain molecule, the light chain and heavy chain species can be isolated using SP-Sephadex chromatography at pH 5.8 under conditions where the heavy chain passes through the column and the light chain is subsequently eluted at higher ionic strengths. As seen in Figure 2, the isolated light chain possesses a clotting activity of 31 units/mg or 1.4 units/ nmol.

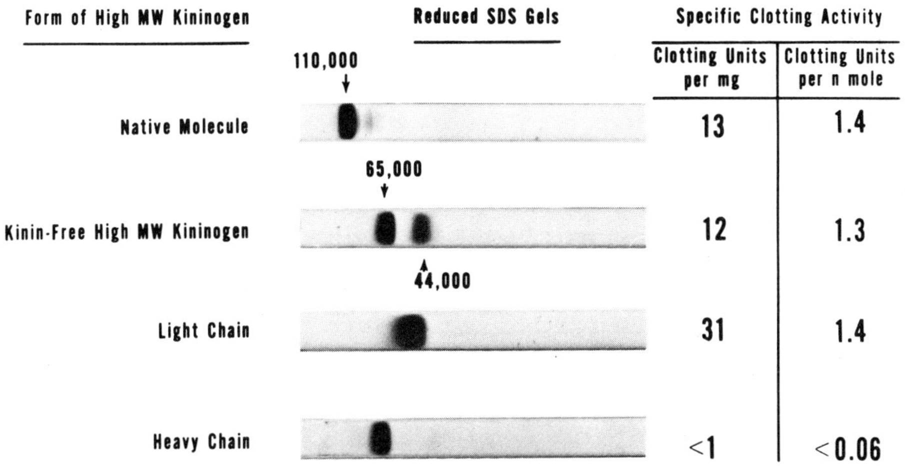

Form of High MW Kininogen	Reduced SDS Gels	Specific Clotting Activity	
		Clotting Units per mg	Clotting Units per n mole
Native Molecule	110,000	13	1.4
Kinin-Free High MW Kininogen	65,000 44,000	12	1.3
Light Chain		31	1.4
Heavy Chain		<1	<0.06

Figure 2. Structure-function relationships for human high MW kininogen. Purified human high MW kininogen or fragments of the molecule were characterized on reduced SDS gels and the specific clotting activity of each preparation was determined using the activated partial thromboplastin time clotting assay with human plasma deficient in high MW kininogen. (Taken from Kerbiriou and Griffin, 1978).

The isolated heavy chain shown on the bottom gel in Figure 2 exhibits no measurable clotting activities. Thus, the isolated light chain quantitatively retains the full clotting activity of the native molecule and must therefore contain all of the structural information necessary for the procoagulant activity of human high MW kininogen.

The amino acid composition of the different molecular species of human high MW kininogen and its fragments was determined and compared to the amino acid compositions of the corresponding species of the bovine molecule (Kerbiriou and Griffin, 1978, manuscript in preparation; Han et al., 1978). In general, the compositions of the human polypeptide chains are very similar to those of the bovine polypeptide chains. It is particularly noteworthy that the histidine content of the isolated human light chain depicted in Figure 2 was 10.8% and reflects most of the histidine content of the native molecule. This proportion of histidine is the same as that observed in the bovine light chain obtained by cleavage of that molecule by human urinary kallikrein (Han et al., 1978). Based on this comparison, it is suggested that the active human light chain that was purified contains the unusual histidine-rich region of the molecule that was demonstrated in sequence data for bovine high MW kininogen (Han et al., 1976).

A model to describe the relationship between structure and function of human high MW kininogen is given in Figure 3. In this model the single polypeptide chain of 110,000 MW is cleaved at arrows designated 1 and 2 by human plasma kallikrein to generate kinin and a two chain kinin-free molecule. The kinin-free molecule is fully active in correcting the coagulation defect of plasma deficient in the native molecule. After reduction and carboxymethylation two kinds of protein can be obtained: an histidine-rich light chain that retains the full clotting activity of the native molecule and an inactive heavy chain. This model in Figure 3 is consistent with the work of Thompson et al. (1978) who showed that a reduced, carboxymethylated light chain derived from the human molecule shortened the clotting time of high MW kininogen-deficient plasma. A similar model was presented for the structure-activity relationships of bovine high MW kininogen with the additional feature that bovine plasma kallikrein cleaved the molecule at a position designated as arrow 3 in Figure 3 (Waldman et al., 1977; Matheson et al., 1977). Cleavage of bovine high MW kininogen at arrow 3 resulted in loss of procoagulant activity of the bovine molecule. It appears that cleavage at arrow 3 is a property of the bovine kininogen and bovine plasma kallikrein but is not a property of the human kininogen and human plasma kallikrein system.

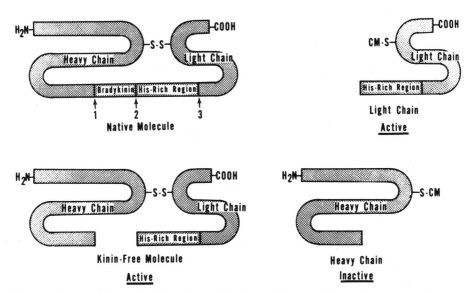

Figure 3.   Schematic drawing of the polypeptide structure of
             human high MW kininogen and of its fragments. See
             text for discussion. (Taken from Kerbiriou and
             Griffin, 1978).

KININ FORMATION AND CLEAVAGE OF HIGH MOLECULAR WEIGHT KININOGEN
DURING CONTACT ACTIVATION IN PLASMA

        Since plasma prekallikrein is activated during contact acti-
vation by Factor XII$_a$, studies were undertaken to determine if this
newly generated kallikrein cleaves the single chain high MW kininogen during contact activation of plasma. To examine if such a
specific cleavage occurs, ^{125}I-high MW kininogen was added to
normal plasma or to plasmas deficient in prekallikrein or Factor
XII. Then contact activation was induced by addition of kaolin to
the plasma. Aliquots were withdrawn from the reaction mixture at
various times and the samples were analyzed either on reduced SDS
gels or in kinin bioassays employing the rat uterus. Results of
such studies are summarized in Figure 4. The single chain high
MW kininogen was progressively and rapidly cleaved with the maximum
cleavage being reached in less than 100 sec after kaolin was added
to plasma. The kinetics of cleavage seen in Figure 4 indicate that,
following an initial lag period, half of the high MW kininogen

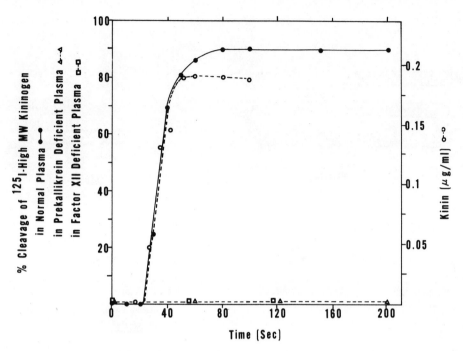

Figure 4. Kinetics of kinin formation and of cleavage of ^{125}I-high
MW kininogen in plasma during contact activation. The
percent of cleavage of ^{125}I-high MW kininogen in normal
and in deficient plasmas following addition of kaolin
was determined using SDS gel electrophoretic analysis.
Kinin formation was assessed using bioassays employing
rat uterine contractions. (Taken from Kerbiriou and
Griffin, 1978).

molecules were cleaved at 35 sec. Furthermore, the kinetics of
kinin appearance very closely paralled the kinetics of cleavage of
high MW kininogen. The total amount of kinin released corresponded
to the maximum amount of kinin available in the high MW kininogen
present in the reaction mixture. As seen in Figure 4, in prekallikrein-deficient or Factor XII-deficient plasma, no cleavage
of high MW kininogen was observed. Addition of purified plasma
kallikrein to plasmas deficient in either prekallikrein or Factor
XII resulted in cleavage of the ^{125}I-high MW kininogen and in the
release of kinin. Thus, it appears that plasma kallikrein is responsible for the rapid cleavage of high MW kininogen in plasma
during contact activation and for the appearance of kinin in such
reaction mixtures. Since purified kinin-free human high MW

kininogen retains full procoagulant activity after exposure to
plasma kallikrein, cleavage of human high MW kininogen in human
plasma during contact activation probably does not result in any
loss of activity as had been previously discussed for the bovine
high MW kininogen (Oh-Ishi et al., 1977; Han et al., 1978).

SUMMARY

Human high MW kininogen can be isolated as a single polypeptide chain of 110,000 MW. Purified human plasma kallikrein
cleaves this molecule to give a disulfide-linked, two chain
molecule, free of kinin, that retains full clotting activity.
Following reduction and carboxymethylation of the two chain
molecule, a light chain can be isolated that quantitatively retains
the full coagulant activity of the native molecule. During contact
activation in normal human plasma a rapid cleavage of high MW
kininogen along with kinin liberation occurs in a reaction that
is dependent upon the presence of prekallikrein and Factor XII
(Hageman factor).

REFERENCES

Chan, J.Y.C., F.M. Habal, C.E. Burrowes and H.Z. Movat, 1976.
    Interaction between Factor XII (Hageman factor), high molecular
    weight kininogen and prekallikrein, Thromb. Res. 9, 423.
Colman, R.W., A. Bagdasarian, R.C. Talamo, C.F. Scott, M. Seavey,
    J.A. Guimaraes, J.V. Pierce, A.P. Kaplan and L. Weinstein,
    1975. Williams Trait. Human kininogen deficiency with dimi-
    nished levels of plasminogen proactivator and prekallikrein
    associated with abnormalities of the Hageman factor-dependent
    pathways, J. Clin. Invest. 56, 1650.
Donaldson, V.H., H.I. Glueck, M.A. Miller, H.Z. Movat and F. Habal,
    1976. Kininogen deficiency in Fitzgerald trait: Role of high
    molecular weight kininogen in clotting and fibrinolysis, J.
    Lab. Clin. Med. 87, 327.
Griffin, J.H. and C.G. Cochrane, 1976. Mechanisms for the involve-
    ment of high molecular weight kininogen in surface-dependent
    reactions of Hageman factor, Proc. Natl. Acad. Sci. USA 73,
    2554.
Habal, F.M., H.Z. Movat and C.E. Burrowes, 1974. Isolation of two
    functionally different kininogens from human plasma. Separat-
    ion from proteinase inhibitors and interaction with plasma
    kallikrein, Biochem. Pharmacol. 23, 2291.
Han, Y.N., H. Kato, S. Iwanaga and M. Komiya, 1978. Action of
    urinary kallikrein, plasmin, and other kininogenases on bovine
    plasma high molecular weight kininogen, J. Biochem. (Jap.)
    83, 223.
Han, Y.N., H. Kato, S. Iwanaga and T. Suzuki, 1976. Primary
    structure of bovine plasma high molecular weight kininogen.

The amino acid sequence of a glycopeptide portion (Fragment
     I) following the C-terminus of the bradykinin moiety, J.
     Biochem. (Jap.) 79, 1201.
Kerbiriou, D.M. and J.H. Griffin, 1978. Structural changes of
     human high molecular weight kininogen during contact activation
     of plasma, Fed. Proc. 37, 1587.
Mandle, R.J., R.W. Colman and A.P. Kaplan, 1976. Identification of
     prekallikrein and high molecular weight kininogen as a complex
     in human plasma, Proc. Natl. Acad. Sci. USA 73, 4179.
Matheson, R.T., D.R. Miller, M.J. Lacombe, Y.N. Han, S. Iwanaga,
     H. Kato and K.D. Wuepper, 1977. Flaujeac factor deficiency.
     Reconstitution with highly purified bovine high molecular
     weight kininogen and delineation of a new permeability-
     enhancing peptide released by plasma kallikrein from bovine
     high molecular weight kininogen, J. Clin. Invest. 58, 1395.
Meier, H.L., J.V. Pierce, R.W. Colman and A.P. Kaplan, 1977.
     Activation and function of human Hageman factor. The role of
     high molecular weight kininogen and prekallikrein, J. Clin.
     Invest. 60, 18.
Nagasawa, S. and T. Nakayasu, 1973. Human plasma prekallikrein as
     a protein complex, J. Biochem. (Jap.) 74, 401.
Nagasawa, S. and T. Nakayasu, Enzymatic and chemical cleavages of
     human kininogens, 1976. In: Chemistry and Biology of the
     Kallikrein-Kinin System in Health and Disease, Fogarty
     International Center Proceedings, No. 27, eds. J.J. Pisano
     and K.F. Austen, p. 139.
Oh-Ishi, S., M. Katori, Y.N. Han, S. Iwanaga, H. Kato and T. Suzuki,
     1977. Possible physiological role of new peptide fragments
     released from bovine high molecular weight kininogen by
     plasma kallikrein, Biochem. Pharmacol. 25, 115.
Revak, S.D., C.G. Cochrane and J.H. Griffin, 1977. The binding and
     cleavage characteristics of human Hageman factor during
     contact activation. A comparison of normal plasma with plasmas
     deficient in Factor XI, prekallikrein, or high molecular weight
     kininogen, J. Clin. Invest. 59, 1167.
Saito, H., 1977. Purification of high molecular weight kininogen
     and the role of this agent in blood coagulation, J. Clin.
     Invest. 60, 584.
Saito, H., O.D. Ratnoff, R. Waldmann and J.P. Abraham, 1975.
     Fitzgerald trait. Deficiency of a hitherto unrecognized agent,
     Fitzgerald factor, participating in surface-mediated reactions
     of clotting, fibrinolysis, generation of kinins, and the pro-
     perty of diluted plasma enhancing vascular permeability (PF/
     dil), J. Clin. Invest. 55, 1082.
Schiffman, S. and P. Lee, 1975. Partial purification and charac-
     terization of contact activation cofactor, J. Clin. Invest.
     56, 1082.
Thompson, R.E., R. Mandle, Jr. and A.P. Kaplan, 1977. Association
     of Factor XI and high molecular weight kininogen in human
     plasma, J. Clin. Invest. 60, 1376.

Thompson, R.E., R. Mandle, Jr. and A.P. Kaplan, 1978. Characteri-
    zation of human high molecular weight kininogen. Procoagulant
    activity associated with the light chain of kinin-free high
    molecular weight kininogen, J. Exp. Med. 147, 488.
Waldmann, R., A.G. Scicli, G.M. Scicli, J.A. Guimaraes, O.A.
    Carretero, H. Kato, Y.N. Han and S. Iwanaga, 1977. Significant
    role of fragment 1·2 plus light chain of bovine high molecular
    weight kininogen in contact mediated coagulation, Thromb.
    Haemostasis 38, 14.
Wendel, V., W. Vogt and G. Seidel, 1972. Purification and some
    properties of a kininogenase from human plasma activated by
    surface contact, Hoppe Seylers Z. Physiol. Chem. 353, 1591.
Wiggins, R.C., B.N. Bouma, C.G. Cochrane and J.H. Griffin, 1977.
    Role of high molecular weight kininogen in surface-binding
    and activation of coagulation Factor XI and prekallikrein,
    Proc. Natl. Acad. Sci. USA 74, 4636.
Wuepper, K.D., D.R. Miller and M.J. Lacombe, 1975. Flaujeac trait:
    Deficiency of human plasma kininogen, J. Clin. Invest. 56,
    1663.

CLEAVAGE OF HUMAN HIGH MOLECULAR WEIGHT KININOGEN BY HUMAN

PLASMA KALLIKREIN

S. Nagasawa and T. Nakayasu

Faculty of Pharmaceutical Sciences, Hokkaido University, Sapporo, and Research Institute of Daiichi Pharmaceutical Company, Tokyo, Japan

Mammalian plasmas contain at least two kininogens which differ in molecular weight and reactivity to kallikrein; the high molecular weight (HMW) form of kininogen is the substrate for plasma kallikrein while the low molecular weight (LMW)-kininogen is the substrate for glandular kallikrein.

Recently, it was found that HMW-kininogen plays an important role in the initiation of Hageman factor-dependent pathways of blood coagulation and fibrinolysis (Saito et al., 1975).

Han et al. (1975) have recently found that several fragments were released together with bradykinin from bovine HMW-kininogen upon prolonged incubation with bovine plasma kallikrein. The fragments, named fragments 1-2, and 2 are extremely rich in histidine and glycine and have an ability to inhibit strongly the surface-dependent activation of Hageman factor (Oh-ishi et al. 1977).

Thus, it is of interest to determine whether such histidine-rich fragments might have been released from human HMW-kininogen and act as a feedback inhibitor for the Hageman factor-dependent pathways in human blood.

The authors (Nagawawa and Nakaysu, 1974) and Thompson et al. (1978) have reported that human HMW-kininogen, which consists of a single polypeptide chain is cleaved by human plasma kallikrein into a kinin-free protein consisting of two polypeptide chains cross-linked by disulfide bonds. Thompson et al. (1978) have also raised the possibility that some fragments might be released

163

together with bradykinin from human HMW-kininogen by human plasma kallikrein.

In the present study, we attempted to isolate the fragment and to characterize its chemical property.

MATERIALS AND METHODS

HMW-kininogen was purified from human plasma by a modification (Nakayasu and Nagasawa, 1979) of the previous method (Nagasawa and Nakayasu, 1974). The specific activity, 15 μg bradykinin/A280 nm unit, of the purified HMW-kininogen means that almost one mole of bradykinin is released from one mole of the HMW-kininogen, assuming the molecular weight of HMW-kininogen to be 120,000 (Nakayasu and Nagasawa, 1979). LMW-kininogen was purified by affinity chromatography using anti-HMW-kininogen antiserum coupled to CNBr-activated Sepharose (unpublished).

Human plasma kallikrein was partially purified as described (Nakayasu and Nagasawa, 1979). The specific activity of plasma kallikrein was 7.21 μmoles Tos-Arg-OMe/A280 unit/min at 37°C. Bovine plasma kallikrein was kindly donated by Dr. Kato, Osaka University.

SDS-polyacrylamide gel electrophoresis (SDS-PAGE) was performed as described by Weber and Osborn (1969). Reduction of the sample was performed with 1% 2-mercaptoethanol in 1% SDS at 90°C for 5 min. The gel was stained with coomassie blue R-250.

RESULTS

Characterization of human HMW-kininogen

Human HMW-kininogen is consisted of two components, the major component of a single polypeptide chain with blocked NH_2-terminal and the minor component of disulfide-linked two chains.[2] The isoelectric point of human HMW-kininogen was estimated to be pH 4.7 (Nakayasu and Nagasawa, 1979).

The amino acid composition of human HMW-kininogen is given in Table 1, which also shows for comparison the values obtained for human LMW-kininogen and bovine HMW-kininogen reported by Komiya et al. (1974).

The amino acid compositions of human HMW- and LMW-kininogens are similar except that HMW-kininogen is rich in histidine and poor in alanine and valine, compared to LMW-kininogen. A high degree of similarity of amino acid composition was observed between human and bovine HMW-kininogens. Human HMW-kininogen is relatively rich in glutamic acid and arginine, but poor in half-cystine and valine, compared to bovine HMW-kininogen.

Table 1.   Amino acid compositions of human kininogens[1]

Amino acids	Human		Bovine HMW-Kininogen[2]
	HMW-	LMW-	
	(mole per cent)		
Asp	11.57	9.79	10.78
Thr	7.84	8.44	7.10
Ser	7.35	8.66	8.48
Glu	13.67	14.40	11.06
Pro	6.43	5.64	6.64
Gly	7.19	6.42	6.67
Ala	4.60	7.01	5.35
1/2 Cys	2.21	2.75	3.51
Val	4.47	6.08	6.57
Met	0.92	0.73	1.37
Ile	4.81	4.63	3.77
Leu	5.16	5.75	6.17
Tyr	3.11	3.55	3.30
Phe	3.89	4.27	3.49
His	4.81	1.37	4.87
Lys	7.33	6.84	7.34
Arg[3]	3.22	3.66	2.27
Trp	1.22	ND[4]	1.29

1)   Calculated from hydrolysates for 24,48, and 72 hr.
     Values of serine and threonine were obtained by extrapolation
     to zero time of hydrolysis.
2)   Taken from the data reported by Komiya et al. (1974).
3)   Estimated from the absorbance at 280 nm and 294 nm.
4)   Not determined.

Cleavage by human plasma kallikrein

     Fig. 1 shows progressive cleavage of HMW-kininogen by human plasma kallikrein. Referring to the paper by Thompson et al. (1978), the two bands of 78,000 and 58,000 daltons seemed to be the heavy chain and its further cleavage product, respectively, and the faint band of 48,000 daltons seemed to be the light chain of kinin-free human protein. After prolonged incubation with human plasma kallikrein, the band of 78,000 daltons was completely converted into the band of 58,000 daltons.

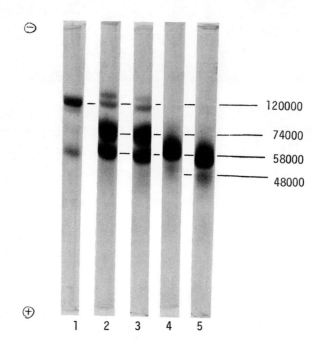

Fig. 1. SDS-PAGE of human HMW-kininogen after incubation with
human plasma kallikrein. Samples were reduced and electrophoresed. (1), control HMW-kininogen; (2) incubated
with 0.08 ml of human plasma kallikrein for 4 hr; (3) with
0.1 ml for 10 hr; (4) with 0.1 ml for 24 hr; and (5) with
0.2 ml for 24 hr at 37°C.

Separation of kinin-free protein, fragment, and kinin

In order to test whether histidine-rich fragment is released
from human HMW-kininogen by human plasma kallikrein, the prolonged
incubation mixture of HMW-kininogen and plasma kallikrein was
applied to a column of Sephadex G-50. The effluent was analyzed
for ultraviolet absorption at 280 nm and contraction of rat uterus.

As shown in Fig. 2, two fragments with absorbance at 280 nm
and one fragment having kinin activity were separated. The large
fragment eluted in the void volume of the column was a kinin-free
protein, from which no more kinin was released upon prolonged
incubation with plasma kallikrein.

The small fragment gave a broad single band on SDS-PAGE and
its molecular weight was estimated to be 8,000 from its electrophoretic mobility in 10% acrylamide gel.

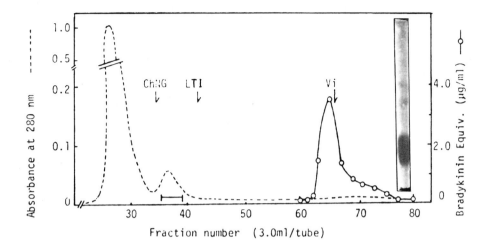

Fig. 2.   Gel filtration of HMW-kininogen after prolonged incubation
          with human plasma kallikrein. 12 mg of HMW-kininogen and
          1.3 units (esterase units) of human plasma kallikrein were
          incubated in 30 ml of 0.002M Tris buffer, pH 8.0 at 37°C
          for 24 hr and lyophilized. The lyophilized material was
          dissolved in 2 ml of 1% acetic acid and gel-filtered on
          a column (2.5 x 44 cm) of Sephadex G-50 equilibrated with
          1% acetic acid. The activity of kinin was determined by
          bioassay using isolated rat uterus.

     SDS-PAGE of the reduced kinin-free protein fraction gave two
stained bands as in Fig. 1 #5 gel.

     The kinin-free protein fractions were pooled, lyophilized, and
reduced with 2-mercaptoethanol. The reduced sample was then gel-
filtered on a column of Sephadex G-100.

     Fig. 3 showed the separation of the heavy and light chains of
human kinin-free protein.

     Table II showed the amino acid compositions of the heavy and
light chains, the fragment, and kinin-like fragment.

     Interestingly enough, the contents of histidine and glycine
in the human fragment was not as high as those in bovine fragments.
Rather, the contents of histidine and glycine were found to be
high in the light chain portion of the kinin-free protein.

     These results suggested that there is a histidine-rich sequence
in human HMW-kininogen and that the histidine-rich sequence in

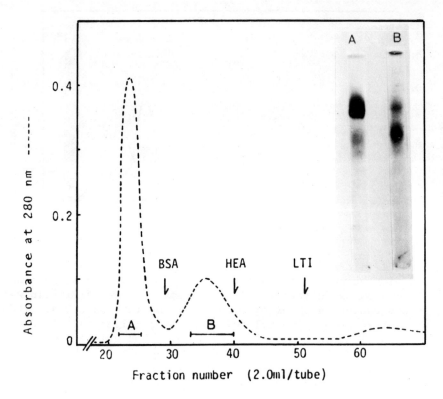

Fig. 3.   Separation of two polypeptide chains of kinin-free
protein. Fractions from 25 to 30 in Fig. 2 were pooled,
lyophilized, and reduced. The reduced fraction was gel-
filtered on a column (1.7 x 57 cm) of Sephadex G-100
equilibrated with 10% acetic acid.

human HMW-kininogen is not released by the action of human plasma
kallikrein but remains bound to the light chain of kinin-free
protein.

The amino acid composition of the kinin-like fragment was
identical to that of bradykinin, and arginine was identified as
the amino-terminal of the kinin by dansyl method. These results
indicated that bradykinin was released from human HMW-kininogen
by the action of human plasma kallikrein.

The sum of the amino acid compositions of the kinin-free
protein, and two fragments was very close to the amino acid composition of native HMW-kininogen.

Cleavage of human HMW-kininogen by bovine plasma kallikrein

Next, we examined a possibility that bovine plasma kallikrein might cleave human HMW-kininogen in a similar manner as reported with bovine HMW-kininogen (Han et al., 1975).

Then, human HMW-kininogen was incubated with bovine plasma kallikrein for 24 hr at 37°C and analyzed by SDS-PAGE.

As shown in Fig. 4, unreduced kinin-free protein migrated slightly faster than native HMW-kininogen. SDS-PAGE of reduced sample revealed three chains. The molecular weights of these polypeptide chains were the same as those of three chains prepared by digestion with human plasma kallikrein.

These results suggested that the possible histidine-rich sequence in human HMW-kininogen is unsusceptible not only to human plasma kallikrein but also to bovine plasma kallikrein.

Table II. Amino acid compositions of HMW-kininogen, kinin-free protein, fragment, and kinin

Amino acids	HMW-kininogen	Kinin-free protein H-chain	L-chain	Fragment	Kinin
Asp	75	40	28	5	0
Thr	51	27	18	4	0
Ser	48	26	20	4	1
Glu	89	52	31	10	0
Pro	42	22	19	4	3
Gly	47	20	23	5	1
Ala	30	20	10	3	0
1/2 Cys	14	9	2	1	0
Val	29	18	9	2	0
Met	6	3	3	1	0
Ile	31	18	10	2	0
Leu	34	19	14	3	0
Tyr	20	11	5	1	0
Phe	25	16	8	1	2
His	31	7	17	3	0
Lys	48	26	20	3	0
Arg	21	10	5	4	2
Total[1]	641	344	242	56	9

[1] Values estimated by assuming the numbers of Arg residues of HMW-kininogen, H-chain, L-chain, fragment, and kinin to be 21,10,5,4, and 2, respectively.

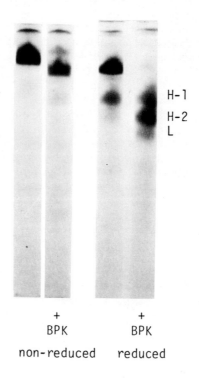

Fig. 4. Cleavage of human HMW-kininogen by bovine plasma kallikrein. Human HMW-kininogen was digested with 1% bovine
plasma kallikrein at 37°C for 24 hr. Left, SDS-PAGE
of unreduced sample; Right; SDS-PAGE of reduced sample.
BPK, bovine plasma kallikrein.

DISCUSSION

There is no direct evidence indicating that human HMW-kininogen contains a histidine-rich sequence which is responsible for
the coagulant activity as Fitzgerald factor. Thompson et al.
(1978) have shown that the light chain of human kinin-free protein
did have the coagulant activity. The light chain prepared by us
was also shown to have the Fitzgerald factor activity by Dr.
Saito, Case Western Reserve University. Thus, our result that the
light chain of human kinin-free protein is rich in histidine may
support a possibility that human HMW-kininogen contains histidine-
rich sequence which is responsible for the coagulant activity, as
in the case of bovine HMW-kininogen.

In contrast to bovine HMW-kininogen, the histidine-rich

sequence in human HMW-kininogen was not released by the action of human and bovine plasma kallikreins.

Although a fragment was released from human HMW-kininogen together with bradykinin by the action of human plasma kallikrein, this fragment is characteristically different from bovine fragments in the amino acid composition. The fragment appears to be released from a region independent of coagulation activity, since the kinin-free protein has full coagulant activity. Judging from SDS-PAGE, this human fragment seemed to be released by the further cleavage of the heavy chain.

Thus, it still remains to be elucidated whether histidine-rich portion is released together with bradykinin and is implicated in the control of Hageman factor-dependent pathways in human blood.

REFERENCES

Han, Y.N., M. Komiya, S. Iwanaga, and T. Suzuki, 1975. Studies on the primary structure of bovine high molecular weight kininoten. Amino acid sequence of a fragment ("histidine-rich peptide") released by plasma kallikrein. J. Biochem. 77, 55.

Komiya, M., H. Kato, and T. Suzuki, 1974. Bovine plasma kininogens II. Microheterogeneities of high molecular weight kininogens and their structure relationship. J. Biochem. 76, 823.

Nagasawa, S. and T. Nakayasu, 1974. Enzymatic and chemical cleavages of human kininogens, In: "Chemistry and Biology of the Kallikrein-kinin System in Health and Disease" eds. J.J. Pisano and F.K. Austen, Fogarty International Center Proceedings No. 27, p. 139.

Nakayasu, T. and S. Nagasawa, 1979. Studies on human kininogens I. Isolation, characterization, and cleavage by plasma kallikrein of high molecular weight (HMW)-kininogen, J. Biochem. in press.

Oh-ishi, S., M. Katori, Y.N. Han, S. Iwanaga, H. Kato, and T. Suzuki, 1977. Possible physiological role of new peptide fragments released from bovine high molecular weight kininogen by plasma kallikrein, Biochem. Pharmacol. 26, 115.

Saito, H., O.D. Ratnoff, R. Waldmann, and J.P. Abraham, 1975. Fitzgerald trait. Deficiency of a hitherto unrecognized agent, Fitzgerald factor, participating in surface-mediated reactions of clotting, fibrinolysis, generation of kinin, and the property of diluted plasma enhancing vascular permeability (PF/Dil), J. Clin. Invest. 55, 1082.

Thompson, R.E., R. Mandle, Jr., and A.P. Kaplan, 1978. Characterization of human high molecular weight kininogen, Procoagulant activity associated with the light chain of kinin-free high molecular weight kininogen, J. Exp. Med. 147, 488.

Weber, K. and M. Osborn, 1969. The reliability of molecular weight determinations by dodecyl sulfate-polycrylamide gel electrophoresis, J. Biol. Chem. 244, 4406.

HUMAN KININOGEN FROM COHNS FRACTION IV: COMPARISONS OF ANTIGENICITY AND MULTIPLE FORMS

Ulla Hamberg, Ann-Christine Syvanen and Tytti Karkkainen

Department of Biochemistry, University of Helsinki

Unioninkatu 35, SF-00170 Helsinki 17, Finland

ABSTRACT

Kininogen was isolated from Cohns fraction IV by DEAE-chromatography, gel filtration and ammonium sulphate precipitation. Immunologically pure kininogen was prepared by removal of protein impurities using specific immunoadsorbents with Sepharose-bound antibody. Anti-kininogen serum was raised in rabbits against the pure antigen. Comparison with anti-kininogen sera prepared with the biologically active LMW antigen from whole plasma suggested antigenic identity by double immunodiffusion analysis. The Cohn-kininogen was shown to contain mainly two components (85%) in about equal amounts focusing with peaks at pI 4.2 (42%) and pI 4.3 (43%). These represent apparently structurally altered forms of the native plasma kininogen focusing at pI 4.5-4.6 (54%), which occurred as a minor component (13%).

INTRODUCTION

The high (HMW) and low molecular weight (LMW) kininogens have been extensively studied as concerns their functional activities in releasing the active kinin segment and the role of HMW kininogen in coagulation (Colman et al., 1975; Bagdasarian et al., 1973; Mandle et al., 1976; Neurath & Walsh, 1976; Griffin & Cochrane, 1976; Thompson et al., 1978). Reports with human plasma (Sharma et al., 1976) and synovial fluid (Hamberg et al., 1978) in acute rheumatoid arthritis suggested that kininogen is an acute phase plasma protein increasing during inflammation. This was confirmed in recent studies with plasma from patients with acute myocardial infarction and immunologically induced inflammation in connection

173

with active immunotherapy of patients suffering from renal-cell
carcinoma (Hamberg & Torstila, 1978; Tallberg & Hamberg, being
published). Considerable increase of the immunoreactive kininogen
in plasma could be shown by single radial immunodiffusion using
monospecific anti-human kininogen serum. On the other hand the
increased heterogeneity shown with isolated LMW-kininogen (Turpeinen
& Hamberg, 1978a,b) may interfere with the immunochemical kininogen
determination. The present study aims to investigate the antigenicity of kininogen isolated from Cohns fraction IV and the antiserum produced against it.

MATERIALS AND METHODS

Crude kininogen from Cohns fraction IV. Freshly precipitated
Cohns fraction IV material (Krijnen et al., 1970)was obtained from
the Finnish Red Cross Blood Transfusion Service, suspended in
distilled water by homogenization in a Waring Blender (approximately
5 kg/7-10 l) and dialysed against running tap water. Kininogen
was absorbed from the supernatant on DEAE-cellulose at pH 5.5 and
the eluate (0.5 M NaCl) was chromatographed on DEAE-Sephadex
according to the method described in detail in an earlier publication (Hamberg et al., 1975). Salt was removed on Sephadex G-25
and the preparation was lyophilized.

Preparation of immunoadsorbents. Specific antisera against
albumin (AB Kabi, Stockholm), α_2 HS-glycoprotein (Behringwerke AG,
Marburg/Lahn), and ceruloplasmin were raised in rabbits. The
ceruloplasmin was isolated from the ceruloplasmin fractions collected after DEAE-Sephadex chromatography of crude kininogen and
further purified with immunoadsorbents using Sepharose-bound
specific antibody columns to remove impurities. The antigen binding
capacity was estimated by single radial immunodiffusion according
to Becker (1969)(SRI-titer). The twice precipitated immunoglobulin
fraction of the respective antisera (50% and 40% ammonium sulphate)
was dialysed against distilled water and 0.1 M $NaHCO_3$, 0.5 M NaCl
pH 8.0, and bound to Sepharose 4 B (Pharmacia) according to Axen
et al., (1967).

Double immunodiffuison analysis was performed according to
Ouchterlony (1948) using 7.5 ml 1% purified agar (Agar Purified,
Difco) on 5 x 7.5 cm glass plates, at pH 7.6 with 0.04 M sodium
diaethylbarbiturate, 0.2 M glycine, 0.15 M NaCl, 0.01% merthiolate.

Single radial immunodiffusion according to Mancini et al. (1965)
was used for the quantitative determination of immunoreactive proteins, using glass plates (5 x 7.5 cm), 1.5% agar gel (Special
Agar Noble, Difco) in 0.04 M sodium diaethylbarbiturate buffer pH
8.6. The amount of specific antisera in the gel (4 ml) was 1-10%

depending on the titer. In some cases commercial M-Partigen plates were used.

Immunological kininogen determination was performed by single radial immunodiffusion using a standard of human pooled blood bank plasma as described in detail before (Hamberg et al., 1978) and containing averagely 0.26 biologically active kininogen per ml determined as bradykinin-equivalents by bioassay on the isolated guinea pig ileum. Monospecific anti-human kininogen serum (Hamberg et al., 1975), SRI-titer 0.46 mg/ml (Becker, 1969) was applied 5% in the agar gel.

Biologically active kininogen was estimated as described in detail before (Hamberg et al., 1975).

Isoelectric focusing was performed in an LKB 8101 column (110 ml) with 1% Ampholine (LKB Products, Bromma Sweden) in a linear sucrose concentration gradient (Vestergerg * Svensson, 1966) at +4°C (KT 33 Refrigerating Bath Circulator, Haake) and pH 3.5-5 with 0.1% Ampholine pH 5-8 added. Samples were mixed uniformly through the pH gradient. Fractions 1.0 ± 0.1 ml were collected (in ice) using an LKB peristaltic pump Zero-Max (Stalprodukter, Uppsala) at a rate approximately 34 ml/hr. The pH was measured (within 2 hr) at +3-4°C using the Radiometer PHM 62 Standard pH Meter. Protein was determined by UV-adsorption at $A^{1\%}_{280nm}$=10, and by the Folin-Lowry method (1951).

RESULTS

Preparation of the pure kininogen antigen. The crude kininogen was rechromatographed on DEAE-Sephadex. The homogenous protein fraction(containing 55% kininogen) was collected between 0.23-0.25 M NaCl (Fig. 1). It contained albumin, α_1-acid glycoprotein. Albumin and part of the α_1-acid glycoprotein were removed by gel filtration (Fig. 2). The kininogen pool was lyophilized after removal of salt (Sephadex G-25 column), the recovery was 84% (58 mg). The preparation (75% kininogen) contained 15% α_1-acid glycoprotein, 7.4% α_2HS-glycoprotein, 2.2% ceruloplasmin and 1.4% albumin.

Removal of α_1-acid glycoprotein was achieved by 1.9 M ammonium sulphate precipitation using 49 mg of the protein dissolved (1%) in distilled water. The precipitate containing 62% of the kininogen was collected by centrifugation and dissolved in distilled water; it was dialysed 24 hr against distilled water and 24 hr against 0.1 M Tris-HCl, 0.5 ml NaCl, 10 KIU/ml Trasylol^R, pH 8.0. The supernatant containing 92% of the α_1-acid glycoprotein was rejected. The further purification was performed applying specific Sepharose-antibody columns for the removal of the respective impurities.

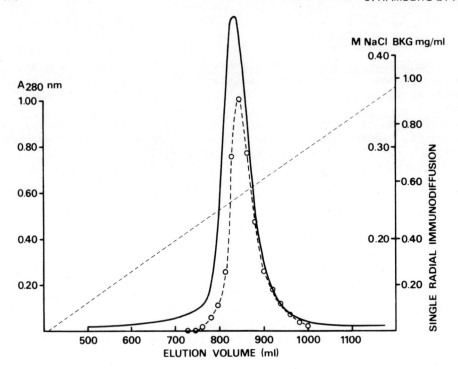

Figure 1.   DEAE-Sephadex chromatography in the linear gradient
             0.06-0.40 M NaCl, 0.2 M EACA and Trasylol[R] 100 KIU
             per ml, pH 5.5 (2.5 cm x 57 cm, 18 ml/hr, +4°C) of
             73 mg kininogen/177 mg protein (41% kininogen).
             The protein profile (——) was obtained by measuring
             the UV-absorption at A_{280nm} kininogen (o---o) was
             determined by single radial immunodiffusion
             (recovery 104%). The salt gradient (---) was
             measured by conductivity (Philips PR 9500).

        Albumin and α_2HS were removed by passing the dialysed kininogen
solution through a mixed antibody column containing Sepharose-anti-
albumin (8.9 ml) and Sepharose-anti-α_2HS (7.3 ml), total bed volume
16.2 ml (0.9 cm x 25.5 cm, 16 ml/hr, +4°C) in 0.1 M Tris-HCl,0.5 M
NaCl, 50 KIU/ml Trasylol[R], pH 8.0. The combined effluent fractions
(10.3 mg protein/10 ml) were subsequently passed through the
Sepharose-anti-ceruloplasmin column (0.9 cm x 22 cm, 12 ml/hr,
+4°C). The pooled effluent (9 mg protein/23 ml) was lyophilized
after the removal of salt.

        Preparation of monospecific antiserum. Immunization was
performed in rabbits by injecting (i.d. or s.c.) approximately 200

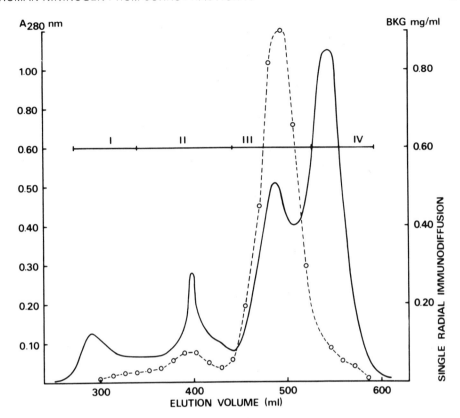

Figure 2.   Sephadex G-200 gel filtration of 68 mg kininogen
(Pharmacia, 2.5 cm x 177 cm, V = 294 ml, 9 ml/hr,
+4°C) in 0.1 M ammonium acetate, 0.2 M EACA, 0.5 M
NaCl, 100 KIU Trasylol^R per ml, pH 6.0. Kininogen
was collected in pool III as indicated (K$_{av}$ 0.34).
Symbols as in Fig. 1. Pools I-II contained α_2HS,
albumin and ceruloplasmin, pool IV α_1-acid glycoprotein and albumin, by Ouchterlony analysis.

µg kininogen antigen in Complete Freunds Adjuvant (Difco Laboratories)
every two weeks. The production of antibody was followed by immunodiffusion analysis of the antiserum showing that the dilution titer
was about 1:32 after 4 weeks. After 6 weeks the titer was 0.83 mg/ml
determined according to Becker (1969).

   Comparison of the antiserum with corresponding antisera prepared with different kininogen antigens. The result is shown in
Figure 3 demonstrating antigenic identity towards the Cohn-antigen
of different antisera applied as well as towards the antibody in
anti-normal human serum.

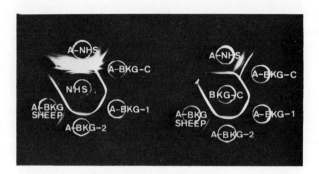

Figure 3.   Immunodiffusion analysis comparing the precipitin
            reaction between the kininogen antigen (Cohn) and its
            antiserum A-BKG-Cohn, titer 0.82 mg/ml with antisera
            raised in rabbits and sheep against the antigen pre-
            pared from different sources: A-BKG-1, titer 0.46
            mg/ml, A-BKG-2, titer 0.19 mg/ml. To the left, same
            antisera with 30 µl (NHS) normal human serum batch
            1001 W (Behringwerke AG). The sheep anti-human kini-
            nogen serum (A-BKG-sheep) was obtained from Dr. J.V.
            Pierce. Anti-normal human serum (A-NHS) was from
            Organon Teknika. In all wells 30 µl; in the right
            center well 10 µg kininogen. (photographed after 45
            hr diffusion at room temperature).

The similar result was obtained compared with normal human serum,
presumed to contain the native form of plasma kininogen. The
respective monospecific antisera used for comparison were raised
in rabbits with the pure antigen prepared from whole plasma (A-BKG-1)
by purification using adsorption-desorption on a whole serum anti-
kininogen polymer (Hamberg et al., 1975), and (A-BKG-2) by removal
of immunoreactive impurities according to Hamberg and Tallberg
(1972).

     Heterogeneity by isoelectric focusing. The results obtained
after focusing of the immunologically pure kininogen is shown in
Figure 4. The distribution of the immunoreactive kininogen was:
42% between pH 4.03-4.25 (peak pI 4.2), 43% between pH 4.27-4.41
(peak pI 4.3), 13% between pH 4.44-4.60 (peak 4.5-4.6), and 2%
4.66-4.69 (peak pI 4.7).

This clearly differs from the focusing pattern obtained with freshly
taken single donor human ACD-plasma (anticoagulant content 0.245%
dextrose, 0.08% citric acid, 0.22% trisodium citrate) shown in
Figure 5.: pI 4.2, 0%, between pH 4.29-4.34 (peak pI 4.3) 14%,
between pH 4.35-4.44 (peak pI 4.4) 27%, between pH 4.47-4.62 (peak
4.5-4.6) 54%, and 4% at pH 4.68 (pI 4.7).

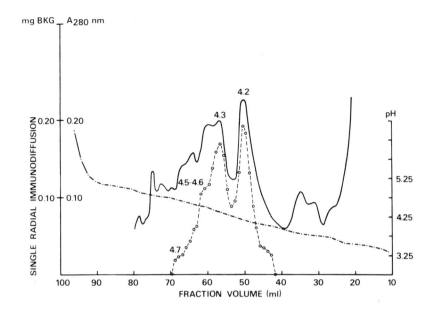

Figure 4.   Isoelectric Heterogeneity of Kininogen Antigen
            Purified from Cohn's Fraction IV.
            Isoelectric focusing of 3.2 mg kininogen in the
            pH gradient 3.5-5 (-·-), 72 hr at 400-1000 V,
            +4°C (recovery 75%). Protein profile at A_{280nm}
            (--); kininogen mg/ml (o--o), fraction volume
            1 ml.

The kinin content of the Cohn-kininogen was determined by bioassay
using 40 μg and 100 μg 84% pure kininogen for the release of the
active segment with trypsin. The protein solutions were adjusted
to pH 2 with 0.5 N HCl and kept for 3 min in a boiling water bath.
The pH was brought to 7.8 with 0.5 N NaOH and 0.1 M Tris-HCl buffer
pH 7.8 and incubated with 50 μg trypsin (EC 3.4,21.4, Worthington,
TRTPCK 33J812) for 30 min at 37°C (Waterbath with shaking). After
addition of 2 volumes of boiling ethanol the samples were dried
under reduced pressure (Rotavapor, Buchi), redissolved in 1 ml
0.15M NaCl and tested for activity on the isolated rat uterus. A
3-point assay was performed using dose between 0.8 to 20 μg protein
(84% immunoreactive kininogen) in the linear dose range 0.25 to
0.38 ng standard synthetic bradykinin (Ragnarsson et al., 1975)
per ml (sensitivity 0.19 ng per ml). No response of the uterus
was obtained with the protein doses. This result indicates that
17 μg kininogen (maximal dose) contained less than 0.2 ng active
(bradykinin) segment. The lineary range checked at the end of the
bioassay experiment was unchanged (sensitivity 0.16 ng per ml).

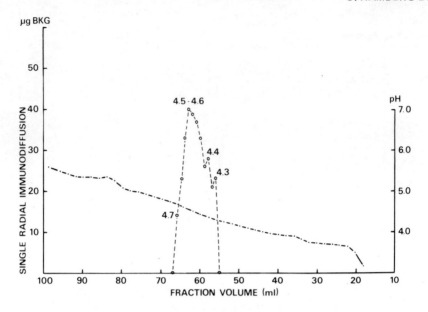

Figure 5.   pI of Native Plasma Kininogen (Single Donor)
            Isoelectric focusing of 2 ml single donor plasma
            between pH 3.5-5, 71 hr, 400-1000 V, +4°C, fraction
            volume 1.0 ± 0.1 ml.
            Symbols as in Fig. 4.

DISCUSSION

The results presented suggest that kininogen antigen from
Cohns fraction IV is immunologically identical with the LMW
kininogen antigen from plasma (Hamberg et al., 1975), although it
differs physico-chemically shown by the changed focusing pattern
(Fig. 4, 5). The reaction of identity shown by the fusion of
precipitin lines in Fig. 3 also indicates that the antigen (BKC-
Cohn) may be immunologically identical with the native plasma
kininogen in normal serum (NHS). The results are still preliminary
and do not exclude the possibility that the antisera may lack
antibodies to different determinants and contain only the antibodies to shared determinants. The possibility to use the Cohns
fraction IV would simplify the preparation of the antigen.

The shift of the pI.s of the heterogenous protein towards the
acid range (85%) may be the result of proteolytic cleavage which
may not have affected the antigenic determinant(s) responsible
for the identical precipitin patterns in Fig. 3. As indicated
by the present findings the active kinin segment apparently is

not connected with the antigenicity.   Further studies are needed
to explain the heterogeneity of the Cohn-kininogen (BKG-C).

The new physiological function of kininogen as an acute phase
plasma protein opens aspects for an evaluation of the activation
of the kinin system in inflammation.   As applied in our studies
the comparison between the immunoreactive and biologically active
kininogen (Hamberg et al., 1978; Hamberg & Torstila, 1978)
provides information about the kinin release.   By using the monospecific antikininogen serum the total kininogen may be estimated
by single radial immunodiffusion regardless of its content of
active kinin segment.   It is suggested that the method may be a
valuable asset particularly in cases where the released kinin
peptide escapes detection by the degradation with enzymes and
rapid destruction of its biological activity.

ACKNOWLEDGEMENTS

Supported by grants from the Academy of Finland, and Societas
Scientiarum Fennica (to U.H.).   Thanks are due to Professor Gert
Haberland, Bayer AG, Dr. Norbert Heimburger,Behringwerke AG and
Dr. Ragnar Lunden, AB Kabi, for the generous gifts of Trasylol[R],
α_2HS-glycoprotein and albumin to Dr. J.V. Pierce, NIH, USA, for
a sample of sheep anti-human kininogen serum, and to Mr. Erkki
Nissinen FL and Mr. Kari Suoranta FK, for preparing crude kininogen.
Valuable technical assistance was given by Miss Maritta Kangas FK.
The bioassay was performed by Miss Leena Laitinen FK.

REFERENCES

Axen, R., J. Porath and S. Ernback, 1967. Chemical coupling of
     peptides and proteins to polysaccharides by means of cyanogen
     halides. Nature 214: 1302-1304.
Bagdasarian, A., B. Lahiri and R.W. Colman, 1973. Origin of the
     high molecular weight activator of prekallikrein. J. Biol.
     Chem. 248: 7742-7747.
Becker, W. 1969. Determination of antisera titres using the single
     radial immunodiffusion method. Immunochemistry 6: 539-546.
Cohn, E.J., L.E. Strong, W.L. Hughes, D.J. Mulford, J.N. Ashwort,
     M. Melin and H.L. Taylor. 1946. Preparation and properties of
     serum and plasma proteins. IV. A system for the separation
     into fractions of the protein and lipoprotein components of
     biological tissues and fluids. J. Amer. Chem. Soc. 68: 459-475.
Colman, R.W., A. Bagdasarian, R.C. Talamo, C.F. Scott, M. Seavey
     Guimares, J.V. Pierce and A.P. Kaplan. 1975. Human kininogen
     deficiency with diminished levels of plasminogen proactivator
     and prekallikrein associated with abnormalities of the Hageman
     factor-dependent pathways. J. Clin. Invest. 56: 1650-1662.

Griffin, J.H. and C.G. Cochrane, 1976. Mechanisms for the involve-
    ment of high molecular weight kininogen in surface-dependent
    reactions of Hageman factor. Proc. Natl. Acad. Sci. USA
    73: 2554-2558.
Hamberg, U., P. Elg, E. Nissinen and P. Stelwagen, 1975.
    Purification and heterogeneity of human kininogen. Use of
    DEAE-chromatography, molecular sieving and antibody specific
    immunosorbents. Int. J. Peptide Protein Res. 7: 261-280.
Hamberg, U., E. Vahtera and L. Moilanen, 1978. Functionally active
    α_2-macroglobulin and kinin release in synovial fluids of
    rheumatoid arthritis. Agents and Actions. 8: 50-56.
Hamberg, U. and I. Torstila, 1978. Immunoreactive kininogen in
    acute myocardial infarction determined by single radial immuno-
    diffusion using monospecific anti-kininogen serum, In:
    Proceedings of the Satellite Symposium "Current Concepts in
    Kinin Research", eds. G.L. Haberland and U. Hamberg (Pergamon
    Press Ltd.), in press.
Krijnen, H.W., 1970. Chemie en bloed. Het optimaal gerbruik van
    menselijk bloed. Chemie en Technick 25: 193-196.
Lowry, O.H., N.J. Rosebrough, A.L. Farr and R.J. Randall, 1951.
    Protein measurement with the Folin phenol reagent. J. Biol.
    Chem. 193: 265-275.
Mancini, G., A.O. Carbonara and J.F. Heremans, 1965. Immunochemical
    quantitation of antigens by single radial immunodiffusion.
    Immunochemistry 2: 235-254.
Mandle, R.J., R.W. Colman and A.P. Kaplan. 1976. Identification of
    prekallikrein and high-molecular-weight kininogen as a complex
    in human plasma. Proc. Natl. Acad. Sci. USA 73: 4179-4183.
Neurath, H. and K.A. Walsh. 1976. Role of proteolytic enzymes in
    biological regulation (A Review). Proc. Natl. Acad. Sci. USA
    73: 3825-3832.
Ouchterlony, O. 1948. Antigen-antibody reactions in gels. Arkiv.
    Mineral. Geol. 26B: No. 14, 1-9.
Pierce, J.V. and J.A. Guimares. Further characterization of highly
    purified human plasma kininogens. 1976. In: Chemistry and
    Biology of the Kallikrein-Kinin System in Health and Disease.
    eds. J.J. Pisano and K.F. Austen (Fogarty International Center
    Proceedings No. 27. U.S. Government Printing Office, Washington)
    pp. 121-127.
Ragnarsson, U., S.M. Karlsson and U. Hamberg, 1975. Synthesis of
    peptides by fragment condensation on a solid support. I.
    Application in preparation of bradykinin. Int. J. Peptide
    Protein Res. 7: 307-312.
Thompson, R.E., R. Mandle, Jr. and A.P. Kaplan, 1978. Characteri-
    zation of human high molecular weight kininogen. Procoagulant
    activity associated with the light chain of kinin-free high
    molecular weight kininogen, J. Exp. Med. 147: 488-499.
Turpeinen U. and U. Hamberg, 1978a. Microheterogeneity of human
    kininogen by isoelectric focusing and crossed immunoelectro-
    phoresis. Int. J. Peptide Protein Res., in press.

Turpeinen, U. and U. Hamberg, 1978b. Heterogeneity of native and
    isolated human plasma kininogens. In: Proceedings of the
    Satellite Symposium "Current Concepts in Kinin Research",
    eds. G.L. Haberland and U. Hamberg (Pergamon Press Ltd.),
    in press.
Webster, M.E., J.A. Guimaraes, A.P. Kaplan, R.W. Colman and J.V.
    Pierce, 1975. Activation of surface-bound Hageman factor: Pre-
    eminent role of high molecular weight kininogen and evidence
    for a new factor, Personal communication.
Vesterberg, O. and H. Svensson, 1966. Isoelectric fractionation,
    analysis, and characterization of ampholytes in natural pH
    gradients. IV. Further studies on the resolving power in
    connection with separation of myoglobins. Acta Chem. Scand.
    20: 820-834.

CHANGES OF PREKALLIKREIN IN THE CASES WITH DISSEMINATED

INTRAVASCULAR COAGULATION SYNDROME

Nobuo Sakuragawa, Kaoru Takahashi and Akira Shibata

1st Dept. of Internal Medicine, Niigata Univ. School

of Medicine, Niigata, 951 Japan

INTRODUCTION

Disseminated intravascular coagulation syndrome (DIC) occurs as a complication of the basic diseases which have definite trigger substances of the activation of the coagulation and fibrinolytic mechanism. The trigger substances show characteristics of both thromboplastic and fibrinolystic substances (1,2). Factor XIIa activates prekallikrein, and kallikrein activates the fibrinolysis, complement, bradykinin systems, and factor VII. Therefore, prekallikrein activation is the important point in the mechanism of the blood coagulation.

In this paper, prekallikrein changes in the blood of cases with DIC was investigated from the point of serine proteases which appears in the blood and makes proteolytic effects on the coagulation factors.

MATERIALS AND METHODS

(1)The lysate of the pathologic cells from a case with acute promyelocytic leukemia was prepared by the method of Sakuragawa et al's (3). The pathologic cells were collected by the Matsuoka's method (4), and the cells were freeze-thawed three times, and centrifuged at 4°C at 3,000 rpm for 15 min to obtain the supernatant as the lysate. The lysate of the cultured well differentiated adenocarcinoma cells was also prepared by the method of Sakuragawa et al's (3). The cultured adenocarcinoma cells (MKN 74) were offered by Prof. S. Ohboshi, Department of Pathology, Niigata University School of Medicine.
(2) Endotoxin (E. coli, Difco Co.) was used.

(3) Serine proteases (factor Xa, thrombin and plasmin) were purified by the methods (5, 6, 7) in our laboratory. The estimation methods were as follows: Factor Xa: Cole-Marciniak's method (8), thrombin: Ware-Seegers' method (9), and plasmin: fibrin plate method (10). The purified prekallikrein was offered by Prof. S. Iwanaga, Department of Chemistry, Kyushu University. The assay method of prekallikrein was that using chromogenic substrate (11). Trypsin (Worthington Biochemical Co.) was used. These materials were dissolved and diluted with saline.

(4) Antithrombin III was purified by our method (12), and assayed by our method (13).

(5) The activation rate and the inhibition rate of the prekallikrein were calculated by our methods (11). The citrated plasma was collected from the blood mixed one part of 3.8% sodium citrate solution to nine parts of the whole blood by centrifugation at 3,000 rpm at 4°C for 15 min. 0.25 ml of the citrated plasma or 0.1 ml of the purified bovine prekallikrein (1 μg) was used in the assay method. When using plasma, prekallikrein was activated by the addition of kaolin solution, and the activation rate was shown by percentage compared with normal plasma prekallikrein. In the case using the purified prekallikrein, the prekallikrein was activated by the addition of trypsin solution to obtain full activation. The activation rate of the specimen was revealed also as percentage compared with activation by the trypsin. The inhibitory rate for the prekallikrein activation was calculated as follows: (Control − Specimen)/ Control X 100 (%).

(6) The inhibitors : Aprotinin (Trasylol, Bayer Co., West Germany), FOY (Methane sulfonic acid salt of ethyl-p-(6- guanidinohexanoyloxy) benzoate , Ono-Yakuhin Co., Japan), and the antithrombin III purified by our method (12) were used.

(7) The normal plasma was collected by use of silicone coated tubes and pipets to avoid factor XII activation.

RESULTS

(1) Prekallikrein activation by the leukemic cells and the cultured cells: 0.1 ml of the lysates of the specimens mentioned above were mixed with 0.25 ml of the citrated plasma, and incubated at 37°C for 10 min. Then the kallikrein was assayed by the addition of the chromogenic substrate. The activation rate of the specimens were calculated by comparing them with normal plasma activated by the addition of kaolin. The leukemic cells (6 X 10^4/cmm) showed 20%, and that of the cultured cells (6 X 10^4/cmm) showed 17% as shown in Fig.1. Then, the purified prekallikrein solutions were added with 0.1 ml of the lysates or trypsin solution (0.03 mg/ml) respectively for activation. As shown in Fig. 2, the leukemic cells did not show clear activation, but that of the cultured cells showed 30% activation.

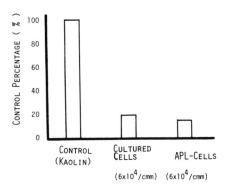

Figure 1. Prekallikrein activating activity of the cultured well differentiated cells and the pathologic cells of acute promyelocytic leukemia. Prekallikrein was assayed by our method (11) using citrated plasma.

(2) Changes of silicone partial thromboplastin time (PTT) and prekallikrein activation by the addition of endotoxin solution: 0.1 ml of the citrated plasma was added to the silicone tube, and incubated at 37°C for one min. Then, 0.1 ml of the phospholipid solution using Trostin (Chugai-Seiyaku Co., Japan, diluted one fiftieth with saline solution) and 0.1 ml of 1/40 mol calcium solution were added to the plasma to obtain the clotting time. Simultaneously, prekallikrein assays were performed using the same reaction mixtures. As shown in Fig. 3, the silicone PTT were shortened depending on endotoxin concentrations compared with the control experiments using saline solution. Prekallikrein was also activated by the factor XIIa induced by the action

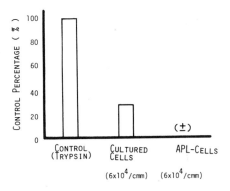

Figure 2. Prekallikrein activating activity of the cultured well differentiated cells and the pathologic cells of acute promyelocytic leukemia using the purified bovine prekallikrein.

of endotoxin to show the decreased values depending on the dosage.
Therefore, in the cases with endotoxin shock, prekallikrein
activation was induced via the factor XII activation by endotoxin
directly.

(3) Prekallikrein activation by serine proteases: A large amount
of factor Xa, thrombin and trypsin made the plasma clot in the test
tube. Therefore, the prekallikrein activation using the chromogenic substrate was performed with the minimum of the serine proteases mentioned above. 0.1 ml of the serine proteases (2 units/ml of
factor Xa, one unit/ml of thrombin, 20 units/ml of plasmin and
0.03 mg/ml of trypsin) were added to 0.2 ml of the plasma, and
incubated at 37°C for 1, 5, 10 and 20 min.   At those incubation
times, trypsin inhibitor of egg white origin (Sigma Co., 0.1 mg/
ml in the saline solution) were added to the reaction mixture to
stop the proteolytic action of these serine proteases without any
effects on the activity of kallikrein (14).

     The rate of prekallikrein activation by thrombin was 5%, by
plasmin: 13%, by factor Xa: 25%, and by trypsin: 41% as shown on
Table 1.   Trypsin and plasmin have the activity of prekallikrein
activation (15, 16).   But thrombin action on prekallikrein
continued at 5% for the whole incubation times.   Therefore, it is
not clear whether thrombin has the propensity to activate prekallikrein.   Factor Xa activated prekallikrein, but it was not clear
to what extent factor XIIa was contaminated in the factor Xa solution.   If factor XIIa was contaminated in the factor Xa solution,
factor XIIa activated the prekallikrein.

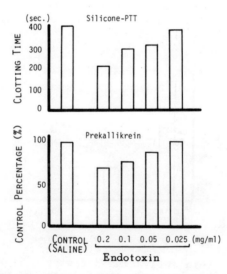

Figure 3.   Changes of silicone PTT and prekallikrein by the influence
of endotoxin.

Then, the purified prekallikrein was activated by the serine proteases. 0.1 ml of the purified prekallikrein (1 μg) was mixed with 0.1 ml of the serine proteases solution mentioned above, and incubated at 37°C for 10 min.   Then, the kallikrein assay was performed by the same technique in the experiments of the cases using plasma.   Control study was performed using trypsin to activate the purified prekallikrein. As shown on Table 2, thrombin showed 10% activation, plasmin: 25 %, and factor Xa: 85%.   From these results, when the serine proteases appear in the blood of the cases with DIC, these proteases activated prekallikrein, and through the activation of factor XII by the kallikrein, the coagulation system will be activated promptly.

(4) The influences of the inhibitors on prekallikrein activation:
      The physiological inhibitors in the blood are antithrombin III α1-antitrypsin, α2-macroglobulin and α-2 antiplasmin.   Antithrombin III is the most important of these inhibitors.   Antithrombin III is a heparin–cofactor, and makes a complex with heparin to become an immediate inhibitor to the serine proteases (12).

Table 1:   Prekallikrein activation by serine proteases using plasma

Incubation time (min) / Serine proteases	1	5	1 0	2 0
Factor Xa (2 U/ml)	8%	20%	25%	24%
Thrombin (1 U/ml)	0	5	5	5
Plasmin (2 0 U/ml)	0	1 0	1 3	1 3
Trypsin (0. 0 3 mg/ml)	7	2 3	4 1	3 2

Table 2:   Prekallikrein activation by serine proteases using the purified bovine prekallikrein.

proteases	Activation rate of prekallikrein (%)
Factor Xa (2u/ml)	8 3%
Thrombin (1u/ml)	1 0%
Plasmin (20u/ml)	2 5%
Trypsin (0.03mg/ml)	1 0 0%

Table 3:   Influence of antithrombin III on prekallikrein activation

Antithrombin III (mg/ml)	Inhibition rate of prekallikrein activation (%)	a−PTT(Sec)
2	100	95.4
1	50	54.2
0.5	37	47.4
0.25	22	45.0
Control(saline)	0	42.0

0.1 ml of the antithrombin III solution (2, 1, 0.5 and 0.25 mg/ml) was added to 0.9 ml of the plasma, and PTT and prekallikrein assay were determined. As shown on Table 3, in the case of using 2 mg/ml of antithrombin III solution, PTT showed 95.4 sec (control clotting time was 42.0 sec), and prekallikrein showed 100 % inhibition.   The inhibitory effects of antithrombin III were depending on the dosage.

Next, the plasma kallikrein solution which was obtained by addition of kaolin solution was added to 0.1 ml of antithrombin III solution (1 mg/ml), and heparin solution (5 units/ml), and antithrombin (1 mg/ml)- heparin (5 units/ml) solution respectively to investigate their inhibitory effects. As shown in Fig. 4, plasma kallikrein activity was only slightly inhibited by heparin alone, and in another instance by antithrombin III alone respectively, but was remarkably inhibited by heparin-antithrombin III solution.   Therefore, heparin showed that it promoted the inhibitory activity of antithrombin III on kallikrein.

(5) Inhibitory effects of aprotinin and FOY on prekallikrein activation: Aprotinin was used for the therapeutic purpose in the cases with DIC (17). Naturally aprotinin inhibits prekallikrein activation as shown on Table 4.   500 units/ml in the final concentration of aprotinin inhibited 85%, 50 units/ml: 70%, and 5 units/ml: 8%.

In the cases using FOY, 0.2 mg/ml in the final concentration showed 68% inhibition, 0.02 mg/ml: 43%, and 0.002 mg/ml: 7%. Additionally, FOY showed the inhibitory effect on prothrombin activation (18).

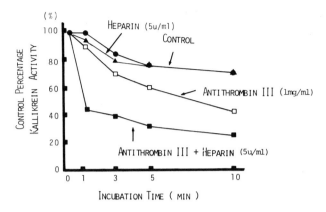

Figure 4.   Inhibitory effects of antithrombin III and heparin on kallikrein.

Table 4:   Inhibitory effects of aprotinin on prekallikrein activation.

Aprotinin (U/ML)	500	50	5	Control
ACTIVATION RATE (%)	15	30	92	100
INHIBITION RATE (%)	85	70	8	0

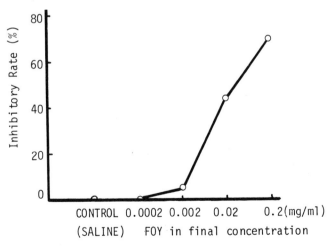

Figure 5:   Inhibitory effects of FOY on prekallikrein activation.

DISCUSSION

Many kinds of serine proteases will appear in the blood of cases with DIC induced by the activation of the coagulation system by trigger substances.   In the cases with disseminated metastasis of gastric cancer and acute promyelocytic leukemia, the trigger substances will activate prekallikrein and coagulation-fibrinolysis simultaneously.   In the cases with endotoxin shock, prekallikrein activation will be induced via factor XII activation by endotoxin.

In this paper, prekallikrein activation in the cases with DIC was investigated.   In DIC, the trigger substances will induce the occurrence of coagulation disorders from activation coagulation-fibrinolysis.   But, from our results, prekallikrein was activated directly by the trigger substances.   Kallikrein activates factor VII to promote the extrinsic coagulation pathway (19).

Antithrombin III inhibits coagulation-fibrinolysis and kallikrein.   Therefore, antithrombin III will be effective in normalizing the coagulation disorders from the viewpoint of enzymology. But, when the serine proteases appear in the blood, antithrombin III is consumed to neutralize the serine proteases to decrease its value.   In this state of under 50% of antithrombin III, administration of heparin which is usually used for the therapeutic purpose in the cases with DIC will not be effective (3). Aprotinin and FOY are the broad spectrum inhibitors, and the former is the natural, and the latter is the synthetised.   In our laboratory, 80 X 10^4 to 100 X 10^4 units of aprotinin, and 200 to 300 mg of FOY a day are administered in the cases with DIC.

SUMMARY

Changes of prekallikrein in the cases with DIC were investigated, i.e., DIC cases including disseminated metastasis of gastric cancer, acute promyelocytic leukemia and endotoxin shock.   Therefore,the trigger substances for this paper were the pathologic cells of the leukemia, the cultured well differentiated adenocarcinoma cells and endotoxin.
(1)   The lysates of the pathologic cells of the leukemia and the cultured cells showed prekallikrein activation.   Endotoxin showed prekallikrein activation via factor XII.
(2)   Serine proteases (factor Xa, thrombin, plasmin and trypsin) activated prekallikrein in the plasma and the purified prekallikrein.
(3)   Antithrombin III, aprotinin and FOY inhibited prekallikrein activation.   Antithrombin III was promoted by heparin in its inhibitory effect.

REFERENCES

(1) Sakuragawa, N., T. Koide, M. Matsuoka et al, 1975, Purification and some characterizations of human thrombin, Acta Med.Biol
(Niigata).23,65.

(2) Sakuragawa, N., T. Takahashi, M. Matsuoka, et al,1973, Cha-
acteristics of thrombin which activates coagulation and fibrinolysis simultaneously, The report of 13th Plasmin Research (Dai-
ich-Seiyaku Co.), p73

(3) Sakuragawa, N., 1978,Pathophysiology of Disseminated Intravascular coagulation syndrome,Acta Haem Jap. 41,744.

(4) Matsuoka,M. and N.Sakuragawa, 1969,Studies on fibrinolytic
activities in normal human leukocytes, 16,91.

(5) Matsuoka, M., T.Takahashi,N.Sakuaragawa,et al, 1977,Purifi-
cation and characteristics of factor VII,IX and X, The Saishin-
Igaku, 32, 593.

(6) Sakuragawa,N.,K.Takahashi and M.Matsuoaka, 1977,Purification
and characteristics of plasmin which is made by using urokinase
Sepharose column chromatography, J.Enzymology 2,202.

(7) Sakuragawa,N.,T.Koide and M.Matsuoka,1975,Activation of human
prothrombin by various procoagulant,Acta Med.Biol.(Niigata)23,57

(8) Cole, E.R., E.Marciniak and W.H.Seegers, 1962, Procedure for
the quantitative determination of autoprothrombin C,Thromb.
Diath.haemorrh. 8,434.

(9) Ware,A.G. and W.H.Seegers, 1949,Two stage procedure for the
quantitative determination of prothrombin concentration, Amer.
J.Clin.Path. 19,471.

(10) Sakuragawa,N.and M.Matsuoka, 1975,Studies on the fibrin
plate method,Jap.J.Clin.Invest.19,980.

(11) Sakuragawa,N.,K.Takahashi and A.Shibata, Studies on the
prekallikrein assay method, The Saishin-Igaku, to be published.

(12) Sakuragawa,N., K.Takahashi and M.Matsuoka, 1977, Disseminated intravascular coagulation syndrome and inhibitors, Acta
Haem.Jap. 40,218.

(13) Sakuragawa,N.,1976,Antithrombin assay method, Jap.J.Clin.
Invest. 20,1009.

(14) Back, N. and R.Steger, 1968,Effect of inhibitor on kinin-
releasing activity of proteases, Fed.Proc.27,96.

(15) Webster,M.E. and D.D.Ratnoff, 1961, Role of Hageman factor
in the activation of vasodilator activity in human plasma,
Nature 192,180.

(16) Mandle, R. and A.P.Kaplan, 1977,Hageman factor substrate,J.
Biol.Chem. 252,6097.

(17) Sakuragawa,N.,1976, Pathophysiology of disseminated intravascular coagulation syndrome, Jap.J.Med.15,43.

(18) Sakuragawa,N. Preparing for publication.

(19) Sakuragawa, N., K.Takahashi and A.Shibata, 1978,Changes of
prekallikrein in the cases with DIC, reported on the 7th meeting
of Japanese Society on Thrombosis and Hemostasis (Tokyo).

THE SIGNIFICANT REDUCTION OF HIGH MOLECULAR WEIGHT-KININOGEN IN

SYNOVIAL FLUID OF PATIENTS WITH ACTIVE RHEUMATOID ARTHRITIS

Kazuhiko Sawai, Shigeo Niwa and Makoto Katori*

Department of Orthopaedic Surgery, Aichi Medical
University, Nagakute, Aichi 480-11, Japan and
*Department of Pharmacology, Kitasato University
School of Medicine, Sagamihara 228, Japan

ABSTRACT

It has been proposed that kinin system was implicated in inflammatory joint diseases such as rheumatoid arthritis. Our present
work provides further support on the involvement of the kinin
system. In osteoarthritis patients, the total, high molecular
weight (HMW)-, and low molecular weight (LMW)- kininogen levels in
synovial fluid were not different from those in plasma. On the
contrary, in rheumatoid patients, HMW-kininogen level in synovial
fluid was significantly lower than that in plasma, whereas LMW-
kininogen level in synovial fluid was not different from that in
plasma. The reduction of HMW-kininogen level in synovial fluid
was much more marked in active cases of those who showed high blood
sedimentation rate and high C-reactive protein value. Furthermore,
the reduction was closely related to the clinical severity. In
active rheumatoid patients, HMW-kininogen level was further reduced
in the synovial fluid after withdrawal of indomethacin.

INTRODUCTION

Pharmacological actions of bradykinin are mainly proinflamma-
tory, such as vasodilatation, increased vascular permeability,
pain production and so forth, so that the involvement of kinin
system in rheumatoid arthritis (RA) has been pointed out (Armstrong
et al., 1957, Goldfinger et al., 1964, Melmon et al., 1967, Jasani
et al., 1969, Eisen, 1970, Zeithin et al., 1976, Sharma et al.,
1976).

Evidence of the involvement of the system are not always easy to provide, since free kinin in plasma and body fluid are rapidly destroyed and active kallikrein is also easily inactivated by plasma inhibitors. Bradykinin is released preferentially from high molecular weight (HMW)-kininogen by plasma kallikrein, which becomes active from prekallikrein by active Hageman factor, so the assay of the residual HMW-kininogen is one of the way to prove the activation of plasma kallikrein-kinin system.

The present report descri es that 1) HMW-kininogen level was definitely reduced in synovial fluid of RA patients, particularly in the active phase, but not in that from osteoarthritis (OA) patients, 2) low molecular weight (LMW)-kininogen level in synovial fluid was not reduced in the patients with both diseases and 3) the levels of HMW-, LMW-, and total-kininogens in plasma of these patients were not different from those of healthy controls.

These results strongly indicate that plasma kallikrein-kinin system was activated only in local inflammatory site, synovial cavity, particularly when the disease became active.

MATERIALS AND METHODS

Patients. Synovial fluid and peripheral venous blood were obtained from patients with unilateral or bilateral knee joints effusion due to RA (11 females and 5 males) and OA (9 females and 3 males). Peripheral blood was also obtained from 12 females volunteers with average age of 38.9 years old (20-59 years old). These rheumatoid patients were classified as classical RA according to the criteria of the American Rheumatism Association (ARA), with average age 53.5 years old (24-72 years old). The average duration time of the disease was 10.3 years (2-16 years). The numbers of the patients in the functional class according to the ARA criteria were 1, 9 and 6 patients for class 1, 2 and 3 respectively. The numbers of the patients in the ARA anatomical stage were 5, 5 and 6 patients for stage II, III and IV. Blood sedimentation rate (BSR) of these rheumatoid patients was ranged from 20 mm/hr to 135 mm/hr and mean BSR (mm/hr) was 65 mm/hr. About 50% of these patients showed 3+ as C-reactive protein (CRP) value. The severity of the rheumatoid knee joint was evaluated in the following ways; the knee joint showing hydrops, pain and local heat as severe cases, hydrops and pain as moderate cases and only hydrops as mild cases. All patients received anti-inflammatory agents such as salicylates, indomethacin, phenylbutazone, gold, corticosteroids and others during the time of this study. For the study on the effect of withdrawal of indomethacin, 3 patients with classical RA were consented, showing severe inflammation in knee joints with high value of CRP (5+ - 6+) and BSR (72-100 mm/hr). These patients have received 75 mg to 100 mg/day of indomethacin. Synovial fluid and blood were

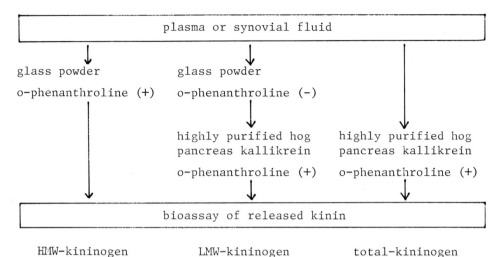

Fig. 1. A schematic diagram showing a differential assay method of high molecular weight (HMW)-, low molecular weight (LMW)-, and total-kininogens.

collected during drug administration and 71 hrs after the withdrawal.
    The OA patients affected by unilateral or bilateral knee joints showed characteristic radiological changes and no laboratory abnormalities, with average age of 71 years old (57-83 years old). No drug therapy have been received.

    Sample collection. Synovial fluid was removed from unilateral or bilateral knee joints and peripheral venous blood was collected from antecubital vein with plastic disposable syringe into plastic tube, containing heparin (2 units/ml, Sigma Co., St.Louis, Mo.). These sample were centrifuged at 3000 r.p.m. at room temperature for 15 min. Supernate or plasma were distributed into small plastic tubes and stored at -20°C untill use. All contact with glass or negatively charged surface were carefully avoided during whole procedure.

    Differential assay method of HMW-, LMW-, and total-kininogens. The sample was divided into three portions and assayed by the follwing different methods, as shown in Fig. 1. a) Total-kininogen. Plasma or supernate of synovial fluid (0.2 ml) was incubated with 0.1 ml of purified hog pancreas kallikrein (20 u/0.1 ml, a gift from DR. C. Kuzbach, Bayer, A. G., Germany) (1290 kallikrein units/ mg) in 0.2 M tris buffer (pH 7.4) in the presence of 0.2 ml of o-phenanthroline (2 mg/ml, Nippon Rikagaku Yakuhin Co. Ltd., Tokyo) for 30 min at 37°C (2 ml in total volume). The released kinin were separated and evaporated to dryness. The residue was dissolved by

saline and assayed on rat uterus. b) HMW-kininogen. Two tenths
ml of plasma or supernate of synovial fluid was incubated with 0.5
g of glass powder (Ballottini #14, 0.09-0.102 mm in diameter,
Jancons, England) in 0.2 M tris buffer (pH 7.4) in the presence of
0.2 ml of o-phenanthroline (2 mg/ml) for 30 min at 37°C (2 ml in
total volume). The released kinin was treated and assayed in the
same way as that for the total kininogen. c) LMW-kininogen. Half
ml of plasma or supernate of synovial fluid was incubated with 0.5
g of glass powder in 0.2 M tris buffer (pH 7.4) in absence of o-
phenanthroline for 30 min at 37°C (2 ml in total volume). An aliquot (0.8 ml) of this HMW-kininogen-depleted mixture was incubated
with 0.1 ml of purified hog pancreas kallikrein (20 u/0.1 ml) in
0.2 M tris buffer (pH 7.4) in the presence of 0.2 ml of o-phenanthroline (2 mg/ml) for 30 min at 37°C (2 ml in total volume). The
released kinin was treated and assayed in the same way as that for
total-kininogen.

Bioassay of bradykinin. Virgin rats weighting 150-250 g were
injected i.p. and s.c. with 5 mg of hexestrol (Hexron, Teikoku Zoki,
Tokyo). Contractions of the isolated rat uterus were recorded
using an isotonic transducer (ME Commercials Co. Ltd., Tokyo),
connected to a pen recorder (Rikadenki Kogyo Co. Ltd., Tokyo).
Synthetic bradykinin (Peptide Institute Inc., Osaka) was used as a
standard.

RESULTS

As shown in Table 1, the levels of HMW-, LMW-, and total-kininogen in plasma from OA patients as well as RA patients were not
significantly different from normal healthy subjects. Also HMW-,
LMW-, and total-kininogen levels in synovial fluid from OA patients
were not different from the levels in their own plasma, when the
levels are expressed as ng Bradykinin (BK) eq/mg protein.

On the contrary, only the level of HMW-kininogen in synovial
fluid from RA patients was significantly reduced, comparing with
that in plasma. LMW- and total-kininogen levels were not significantly different from those in plasma. This result strongly indicated that plasma kallikrein-kinin system was activated only in
synovial fluid of RA patients, but not in OA patients. So the reduction of HMW-kininogen was supposed to be the consumption.

The significant reduction of HMW-kininogen occurred particularly in the cases, in which inflammatory reactions of the patients
were very active, as shown by the fact that the value of C-reactive
protein (CRP) in plasma was more than 3+, and blood sedimentation
rate (BSR) was accelerated over 65 mm/hr, whereas the synovial
fluid from patients, who shows less than 3+ of the CRP value and
less than 65 mm/hr in BSR, did not show the significant reduction
of HMW-kininogen level (Table 2).

Table 1. Levels of high molecular weight (HMW)-, low molecular weight (LMW)-, and total-kininogen in plasma and synovial fluid from patients affected by rheumatoid arthritis (RA) or osteoarthritis (OA), compared with those in plasma from healthy control subjects.

		Kininogen (ng BK eq/mg protein) Mean ± SE		
		HMW	LMW	total
Healthy control	plasma (n=12)	9.98 ± 0.54	24.96 ± 1.06	36.99 ± 1.64
RA	plasma (n=14)	9.34 ± 0.84	23.39 ± 0.71	33.67 ± 0.99
	synovial fluid (n=20)	6.32 ± 0.55*	23.59 ± 1.61	31.49 ± 1.94
OA	plasma (n=9)	9.53 ± 1.02	24.73 ± 2.41	37.49 ± 3.43
	synovial fluid (n=13)	8.98 ± 1.27	32.11 ± 3.14	43.93 ± 4.29

* The HMW-kininogen level in synovial fluid from RA patients was significantly reduced from that in plasma (P < 0.005).

Table 2. Changes of kininogen levels in synovial fluid from RA patients, in relation to values of C-reactive protein (CRP) and blood sedimentation rate (BSR).

		Kininogen(ng BK eq/mg protein) Mean ± SE		
		HMW	LMW	total
cases CRP ≥ 3+ BSR ≥ 65 mm/hr	plasma (n=7)	10.83 ± 1.19	22.53 ± 1.03	33.82 ± 1.42
	synovial fluid (n=9)	7.02 ± 0.92*	25.81 ± 2.47	34.33 ± 3.12
cases CRP ≤ 3+ BSR < 65 mm/hr	plasma (n=3)	7.81 ± 1.30	23.77 ± 0.30	32.14 ± 0.38
	synovial fluid (n=6)	6.25 ± 0.94	22.61 ± 2.92	30.48 ± 2.88

* The HMW-kininogen level in synovial fluid from RA patients who showed high CRP values and high BSR, was significantly reduced from that in plasma (P=0.025).

The severity of the diseases certainly provides the difference in the consumption of HMW-kininogen. Patients with severe rheumatoid knee showed the significant reduction of HMW-kininogen in synovial fluid, but in the moderate and mild cases the HMW-kininogen level was not significantly reduced.

It was quite interesting to see the effect of the drug therapy on HMW-kininogen levels. When the levels of HMW-, LMW-, and total-kininogen in synovial fluid were compared before and after the withdrawal of indomethacin, the withdrawal caused the further reduction of the HMW-kininogen level in synovial fluid, whereas the total and LMW-kininogen levels were not significantly changed. The kininogen levels in plasma were certainly not changed before and after the withdrawal. The withdrawal of indomethacin induced clinical exacerbation, so that it could be concluded that plasma kallikrein-kinin system was activated and HMW-kininogen was further consumed after the withdrawal of indomethacin.

DISCUSSION

Differential assay method of the total-, HMW-, and LMW-kininogen, shown in Fig. 1, are fundamentally based on the established method in this laboratory (Uchida and Katori, 1978, in press). Only difference was that highly purified pancreas kallikrein was used to untreated plasma for conversion of kininogens to kinin. It was known that 20 units of the kallikrein induced the full conversion of kininogens to kinin (Uchida and Katori, 1978). Although the released kinin is kallidin, it is completely converted to bradykinin by the high levels of aminopeptidases in plasma and synovial fluid within 15 min. Thus, 30 min of incubation time in the present experiment was sufficient (Uchida and Katori, 1978). The levels of HMW-, LMW-, and total-kininogens were expressed as ng BK eq/mg protein, for comparison between those in plasma and synovial fluid, since protein contents in synovial fluid (2.7 ± 0.6 g/dl in OA and 4.0 ± 0.7 g/dl in RA) was lower than that in plasma of the same patients (7.6 ± 0.8 g/dl in OA, 7.7 ± 0.6 g/dl in RA and 7.4 ± 0.5 g/dl in control).

The total kininogen level in plasma of RA patients was not different from that of healthy subjects. This does not agree with the results of the papers (Sumita, 1974 and Sharma et al., 1976), in which the total-kininogen level in RA patients is approximately twice as much as that in healthy subjects. This discrepancy may be due to the assay methods, since Sumita used Diniz's method, which is known to produce bradykinin potentiator by trypsin (Aarsen, 1968 and Hamberg, et al., 1967), and Sharma et al. used other method (Brochlehurst and Zeitlin, 1967), comparing with the conversion of kininogen to kinin by purified pancreas kallikrein in the present study.

In the present experiments, the HMW-kininogen level was reduced in synovial fluid of RA patients, but the LMW-kininogen level
did not. This fact strongly suggests that plasma kallikrein-kinin
system was activated. In an inflammatory model of rat corrageenin
pleurisy (Katori et al., in press), and after intravenous injection
of Bromelain into rat (Oh-ishi et al., in press), the HMW-kininogen
in plasma was almost depleted in according with the marked reduction
of prekallikrein level. Thus, the reduction of HMW-kininogen level
could be interpreted as the consumption after activation of plasma
kallikrein-kinin system. The activation of plasma kallikrein-kinin
system occurred only in the synovial cavity, since the HMW-kininogen
level in synovial fluid was decreased, but that in plasma was not
changed. This, however, does not mean that the activation of the
system occurred by the migrated leucocytes, since the kallikrein-
kinin system was known to derive mainly from plasma (Jasani et al.,
1969).

It is interesting that the plasma kallikrein-kinin system was
not involved in OA, which is considered mainly as a degenerative
joint diseases. Conversely, it is not surprising that the kinin
system was much more involved in severe cases of RA. The fact that
HMW-kininogen was consumed more markedly in active phase, in which
the higher value of CRP ($\geq$ 3+) and the acceleration of BSR ($\geq$ 65
mm/hr) were shown, was very important.

Drug therapy is obviously effective in RA patients. The more
marked consumption of HMW-kininogen in synovial fluid after withdrawal of indomethacin clearly indicated that this drug prevented
the activation of plasma kallikrein-kinin system. As indomathacin
is known to inhibit prostaglandin biosynthesis with therapeutic
doses, the activation of plasma kallikrein-kinin system might occur
through the prostaglandin formation. The report that kininogen
levels in plasma was reduced by indomethacin (Sharma et al., 1976)
was not comfirmed by the present work.

ACNOWLEDGMENT

The authors would like to thank Dr. C. Kuzbach, Bayer A. G.,
Germany, for a generous gift of the highly purified hog pancreas
kallikrein and Miss K. Hayashi for skillful typing.

REFERENCES

Aarsen, P.N., 1968, Sensitization of guinea-pig ileum to the action
of bradykinin by trypsin hydrolysate of ox and rabbit plasma,
Br. J. Pharmacol. Chemother. 32, 453.

Armstrong, D., J.B.Jepson, C.A.Keele and J.W.Steward, 1957, Pain-
    producing substance in human inflammatory exudates and plasma,
    J. Physiol. (Lond.) 135, 350.

Brocklehurst, W.E. and I.J.Zeitlin, 1967, Depermination of plasma
    kinin and kininogen levels in man, J. Physiol. (Lond.) 191, 417.

Eisen, V., 1970, Plasma kinins in synovial exudates, Br. J. exp.
    Path. 51, 322.

Goldfinger, S., K.L.Melmon, M.E.Webster, A.Sjoerdsma and J.E.
    Seegmiller, 1964, The presence of a kinin-peptide in inflammato-
    ry synovial effusions, Arthr. and Rheum. 7, 311.

Hamberg, V., P.E.Elg and P.Stelwagen, 1969, Tryptic and plasmic
    peptide fragments increasing the effect of bradykinin on isolat-
    ed smooth muscle, Scand. J. Cli. Lab. Invest. 24, Suppl. 107, 21.

Jasani, M.K., M.Katori and G.P.Lewis, 1969, Instracellular enzymes
    and kinin enzymes in synovial fluid in joint diseases, Ann.
    rheum. Dis. 28, 497.

Katori, M., Y.Uchida, S. Oh-ishi, Y.Harada, A.Ueno and K.Tanaka,
    Involvement of plasma kallikrein-kinin system in rat carrageenin-
    induced pleurisy, Europ. J. Rheumatol. (in press).

Melmon, K.L., M.E.Webster, S.E.Goldfinger and J.E.Seegmiller, 1967,
    Presence of a kinin in inflammatory synovial effusion from arth-
    ritides of varying aetiologies, Arthr. and Rheum. 10, 13.

Oh-ishi, S., Y.Uchida, A.Ueno and M.Katori, Bromelain, a thiol-
    protease from pineapple stem, depletes high molecular weight
    kininogen through the activation of Hageman factor, Thromb. Res.
    (in press).

Sharma, J.N., I.J.Zeitlin, P.M.Brooks and W.C.Dick, 1976, A novel
    relationship between plasma kininogen and rheumatoid disease,
    Agents and Actions. 6, 148.

Sumita, A., 1974, Studies on the plasma kinin system in the plasmas
    of rheumatoid arthritis patients, J. Nagoya City Univ. Med. Assoc.
    24, 426.

Uchida, Y. and M.Katori, Differential assay method for high molecu-
    lar weight and low molecular weight kininogens, Thromb. Res.
    (in press).

Zeitlin, I.J., J.N.Sharma, P.M.Brooks and W.C.Dick, 1976, Raised
    plasma kininogen levels in rheumatoid patients-Response to
    therapy with nonsteroidal anti-inflammatory drugs, in Advances
    in Experimental Medicine and Biology (eds. F.Sicuteri, Nathan
    Back and G.L.Haberland) Vol. 70, p.335 Plenum Press, N.Y.

Kallikrein—Kinin Systems and
Cellular Function

THE ISOLATION OF LEUKOKININ-H AND LEUKOKININOGEN FROM HUMAN ASCITES FLUID; THEIR PROPERTIES AND ROLE

L. M. Greenbaum, G. Semente, P. Grebow, S. Roffman

College of Physicians and Surgeons, Columbia University

630 West 168th Street, New York, New York 10032

There is increasing emphasis on the role of kinins, both bradykinin and leukokinins, in the pathology of diseased states such as inflammatory reaction, ascites fluid accumulation, resulting from neoplastic disease (Greenbaum et al, 1977), as well as kidney disorders such as Bartter's syndrome (Vinci et al, 1978). In addition to these pharmacological and pathological actions of the kinins, there is now very good evidence that bradykinin can stimulate formation of prostaglandins from precursors of prostaglandins, as well as influence enzymes causing conversion of PGE into PGF_2 (Wong et al, 1977).

Our laboratory has been particularly concerned with the role of kinins in clinical aspects of disease. Thus over a period of years we have been studying the formation, structure and pharmacological properties of kinins, which are produced by acid proteases present in neoplastic and white cells. These kinins are known as leukokinins. More recently, through the expertise of Dr. Roffman, we have been able to study the precursor protein of leukokinins, leukokininogen, and finally with the aid of an acid protease inhibitor (pepstatin) we have been able to demonstrate that human and murine peritoneal ascites fluids are formed as a result of the action of an acid protease, cathepsin D (or cathepsin D-like enzyme), contained in neoplastic cells.

We were the first to demonstrate that acid proteases, such as cathepsin D (or cathepsin D-like enzymes), can catalyse the formation of kinins from a protein substrate at acid pH. These kinins were termed leukokinins to differentiate them from bradykinin and its analogues formed by the action of kallikrein. The name

TABLE 1.

Amino acid residues of leukokinins.

Amino Acid	PMN	M	A	H	BK
Alanine	1	2	1	1	0
Arginine	2	3	4	2	2
Aspartic acid	1	1	1	0	0
Cystine 1/2	0	0	0	0	0
Glutamic acid	1	2	1	2	0
Glycine	2	2	0	0	1
Histidine	1	1	1	0	0
Isoleucine	0	0	0	0	0
Leucine	1	1	1	3	0
Lysine	2	3	3	1	0
Methionine	0	0	0	0	0
Phenylalanine	1	1	1	1	2
Proline	3	3	3	2	3
Serine	2	2	1	2	1
Threonine	1	1	1	2	0
Tyrosine	2	1	1	2	0
Valine	1	2	1	4	0
Total A. A.	21	25	20	23	9

The abbreviations represent the source of enzyme
which catalyzed the formation of peptide. PMN-
polymorphonuclear leukocyte (rabbit), M-alveolar
macrophage (rabbit), A-ascites fluid, mastocytoma
(mouse), H-ascites fluid, ovarian carcinoma
(human). BK, bradykinin.

leukokinin originally was derived from the fact that the acid protease was first found in leukemic cells (L-1012 cells of mice)
(Greenbaum and Yamafuji, 1966), and in a variety of leukocytes
including rabbit PMN cells and rabbit macrophages (Freer et al,
1972; Chang et al, 1972). It was later demonstrated that similar
enzymes could be found in mouse fibroblasts (Li et al, 1977).

Properties of Leukokinins

Leukokinins are polypeptides with 21 and 25 amino acids

TABLE 2

Comparison of leukokinin activities with bradykinin[*]

	Lk-H	Lk-A	Lk-PMN	Lk-M
Permeability				
Rabbit	0.20	0.37	1.3	4.5
Guinea Pig	0.30	–	1.3	–
Blood Pressure				
Rat	0.09	–	10.0	–
Rabbit	0.05	0.22	3.5	1.0
Rat Uterus	0.03	0.15	0.80	0.26
Guinea pig ileum	0.001	0.08	0.08	0.08

*Bradykinin is equal to 1.0

(Table 1). Four leukokinins have so far been isolated. The letters following the term leukokinin indicate the source of enzyme which catalyzed their formation. Thus leukokinin-PMN refers to the leukokinin generated by rabbit PMN cells (Freer et al, 1972); "M" refers to rabbit macrophage generated leukokinin (Chang et al, 1972); "A" to leukokinin generated in ascites fluid of the mouse (Johnston and Greenbaum, 1973), and the first leuko-kinin isolated from human ascites fluid--leukokinin-H (Grebow et al, 1978).

There are two major differences when the leukokinins are com-pared to bradykinin. One is that the leukokinins are larger polypeptides (bradykinin has 9 amino acids). Second, the leuko-kinins have only one phenylalanine in their molecule while bradykinin has two. These differences no doubt account for the differences in the pharmacology of the leukokinins and bradykinin as shown in table 2.

In table 2, the pharmacology of each of the leukokinins are compared with one another as well as with bradykinin. The higher the numerical value, the greater the potency. It may be seen that all of the leukokinins are potent permeability agents having potencies of at least 20 per cent of bradykinin. Since the latter

is considered one of the most potent permeability mediators,
leukokinins would have high marks in this regard. Indeed,
leukokinins-M & PMN are more potent than bradykinin in terms of
increasing vascular permeability. In contrast to bradykinin, the
leukokinins have little or no activity on the guinea pig ileum
and less potency than bradykinin on the rat uterus although the
latter is used to bioassay leukokinin (Freer et al, 1972).

Isolation of Leukokinin-H

The first leukokinin so far isolated from human sources is
leukokinin-H, isolated by Grebow et al (1978), in our laboratory
from human ascites fluid. Purity studies including end group
analysis, high voltage paper electrophoresis, thin layer silica-
gel chromatography and polyacrylamide gel electrophoresis all
demonstrated a single component following the final purification
step.

Sequence of Leukokinin-H

The partial sequence of Leu-Ala-Tyr-Thr- has been found at
the amino terminal position of leukokinin-H, which has 23 amino
acids. This sequence is not known to be present in bovine or
human bradykininogens. This would indicate that leukokininogen,
the precursor of leukokinins, is a different protein than the
bradykininogens. Isolation of human leukokininogen in our
laboratory by Dr. Roffman from ascites fluid has confirmed that
leukokininogen and bradykininogen are distinctly different proteins (see below).

Leukokinin Detection by Bioassay and Fluorescamine
     Modification

The isolated rat uterus is a useful bioassay for leukokinins
(Freer et al, 1972). Nanogram quantities may be detected by this
procedure. A chemical procedure,which we have recently developed,
is extremely useful to identify leukokinin-H and to distinguish it
from bradykinin and bradykinin analogues. The procedure is to
modify the kinins with fluorescamine and electrophorese the
products on 12% polyacrylamide gels at pH 4.2 or 9.8 (Prakash et al
1978). 1-4 nanomoles of peptide are required. Using this procedure,
leukokinin-H is clearly distinguishable from bradykinin, lys-
bradykinin and met-lys-bradykinin. The technique also distinguishes
bradykinin from met-lys-bradykinin and from lys-bradykinin. The
procedure cannot distinguish lys-bradykinin from met-lys-
bradykinin. The use of this procedure in conjunction with scanning
techniques for fluorescamine-modified peptides (Soh et al, 1977)
makes for an elegant quantitative procedure.

TABLE 3.

Physicochemical Properties of Bradykininogens and Leukokininogen

Kininogen	Molecular Weight	Isoelectric pH
Leukokininogen (Human Ascites)	41,000	4.5-4.9
HMW Kininogen (Human)	200,000 70,000	4.5-4.7
LMW Kininogen (Human)	50-60,000	4.9
HMW Kininogen (Bovine)	76,000	4.5
LMW Kininogen (Bovine)	48,000	3.3

Leukokininogen

Human leukokininogen, the protein which releases leukokinin-H, has been isolated for the first time from a patient with ovarian carcinoma (Roffman and Greenbaum, 1978). Leukokininogen has a molecular weight of 41,000 daltons (table 3). Studies on the amino acid composition,as well as its immunological properties, demonstrate that leukokininogen is distinct from human and from bovine high and low molecular weight bradykininogen. Leukokininogen does not release bradykinin or related kinins when incubated with plasma kallikrein. It releases leukokinin, however, when incubated with the acid protease (cathepsin D-like enzyme) from neoplastic cells.

Leukokininogen is also present in calf and rat skin in material which sediments following extraction at 300,000 X g (Greenbaum and Houck, 1978). This is of particular interest in terms of inflammation of the skin since it may mean that acid proteases in white cells present in dermal areas can liberate leukokinins.

Leukokininogen does not circulate in the blood. It does appear in pathological fluids such as burn blister fluid (Greenbaum, 1972), and ascites fluid (Johnston and Greenbaum, 1973; Greenbaum, et al, 1975). The most plausible explanation for this

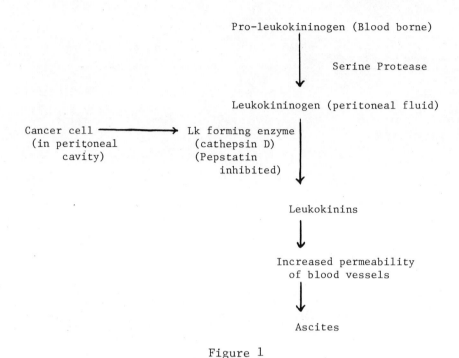

Pro-leukokininogen (Blood borne)

Serine Protease

Leukokininogen (peritoneal fluid)

Cancer cell ⟶ Lk forming enzyme
(in peritoneal   (cathepsin D)
cavity)   (Pepstatin
                        inhibited)

Leukokinins

Increased permeability
of blood vessels

Ascites

Figure 1

is that leukokininogen is a pathological protein which normally
circulates in precursor form as pro-leukokininogen. The latter
is converted to leukokininogen which then may be attacked by
Cathepsin D or cathepsin D-like enzymes liberated from cellular
sources such as neoplastic cells or white cells to liberate the
leukokinins (Figure 1). The conversion of pro-leukokininogen
into leukokininogen is blocked by aprotinin (Trayslol) thus indicating that a serine protease is probably mediating this conversion (Greenbaum, 1972). The cleavage of leukokininogen by cathepsin
D is blocked by pepstatin, a protease inhibitor isolated from
actinomycetes (Greenbaum et al, 1975). Pepstatin itself has become a useful tool to block leukokinin-mediated pathological
reactions.

Pepstatin (An Inhibitor of Leukokininogenases) and its
Action in Inhibiting Ascites Fluid Formation in Neoplastic
Disease:

Pepstatin has been used to demonstrate that leukokinins are
no doubt major mediators in the formation of ascites fluid resulting from neoplastic diseases in mouse models and in humans
with ovarian carcinoma. When pepstatin is adminstered in doses
of 80 mg/kg to mice previously inoculated with cancer cells,

TABLE 4.

In Vivo Tissue Cathepsin D Activity
Following Pepstatin Administration

Tissue	Specific Activity		% Inhibition
	Untreated	Treated	
Liver	25,356	6,998	72
Kidney	27,567	2,663	90
Lung	32,721	16,915	48
Skin	3,777	0	100
Spleen	33,346	28,143	16
Brain	18,207	10,119	44
Heart	42,943	22,042	37
Ascites Fluid	1,448	0	100

Treated mice received 80 mg/kg x 3 days s.c. before being
sacrificed.

there is a dramatic reduction in the rate of ascites formation.
This has been demonstrated in our laboratory (Greenbaum, et al,
1975; Greenbaum and Semente, 1977; Greenbaum et al, 1978) and
confirmed by collaborative effort with Drs. Esumi, Sato and
Sugimura at the National Cancer Center in Japan. These data are
the first to illustrate that ascites formation is not simply a
function of poor lymphatic drainage but is probably mediated in
good part by permeability agents such as the leukokinins (figure 1).

Of significance in human disease, is the finding of the
of the leukokinin-generating system (leukokininogen and cathepsin
D containing neoplastic cells) in ascites fluids of women with
ovarian carcinoma (Greenbaum et al, 1975; Greenbaum and Semente,
1977). The ascites formation occurs in the peritoneal cavity

following metastasis of the cells into the cavity from the primary
site in the ovaries. Our current thinking is that the neoplastic
cells liberate or secrete cathepsin D which catalyzes the formation of leukokinins from leukokininogen present in the peritoneal
cavity in a fluid medium. Just how leukokininogen is produced and
gets to the peritoneal cavity is an important question and may be
the key to the generation of leukokinins in neoplastic disease and
inflammatory reactions. It should be noted that the leukokinin
generation may be blocked by pepstatin, in human ascites fluid in
vitro just as it is blocked in vivo in the mouse. This means that
pepstatin may have significant potential as what may be termed an
"ascites retardant" in human neoplastic disease. At this writing
however, pepstatin has not been used in humans for such a purpose.

Cathepsin-D "Free" Animals Following Pepstatin Administration

We have postulated that the action of pepstatin to reduce
ascites fluid accumulation proceeds by reduction of cathepsin D
activity liberated into the fluid of the peritoneal cavity from
the neoplastic cells present. This hypothesis is strongly supported by experiments which demonstrate (table 4) that following pepstatin administration, the cathepsin D activity in vivo in the
fluid of the peritoneal cavity (indicated in the table as ascites
fluid) is eliminated. What is also very noteworthy is that the
specific activity of cathepsin D in many organs is also very significantly reduced particularly in liver, kidney, skin and lung.
The spleen seems resistant to the pepstatin effect.

Summary

The leukokinin-leukokininogen system is a pathological kinin
generating system which is catalyzed by acid proteases present in
neoplastic cells, white cells and even normal tissues. The components of the human system including leukokinin-H and leukokininogen
have now been isolated and characterized. Very specific protease
inhibitors of the system such as pepstatin have been found and are
now known to prevent "in vivo" the formation of pathological fluids
such as neoplastic ascites. Strong evidence has been previously
published and additional evidence has been presented here which
indicates that pepstatin's actions are related to the inhibition
of cathepsin-D in vivo and the inhibition of leukokinin formation.

Both leukokinins and leukokininogens have been clearly defined
and shown to differ from bradykinin and human bradykininogens.
This clearly demonstrates the presence in pathological systems of
a kinin-generating system which is separate and distinct from the
bradykinin generating system.

The importance of the leukokinin-leukokininogen system in disease would seem to be very great. The finding that pepstatin can inhibit the system in vivo opens the way for studies of pepstatin and related protease inhibitors as therapeutic agents in neoplastic disease and protease mediated inflammatory disorders.

This research is supported by a grant from the American Cancer Society and Grant No. CA24235 of the National Cancer Institutes, USPHS.

References

Chang, J., R. Freer, R. Stella and L. M. Greenbaum, 1972, Studies on leukokinins II, Biochem Pharmacol. 21, 3095.

Grebow, P., A. Prakash, and L. M. Greenbaum, 1978, Leukokinin-H generated from human ascites fluids, Agents and Actions--in press.

Greenbaum, L. M., 1972, Leukocyte kininogenases and leukokinin from normal and malignant cells, Am. J. Path. 68, 613.

Greenbaum, L. M., H. Esumi, S. Sato, and T. Sugimura, 1978, Further studies on the effect of pepstatin on ascites accumulation in tumor bearing mice--in preparation.

Greenbaum, L. M., P. Grebow, M. Johnston, A. Prakash, and G. Semente, 1975, Pepstatin, an inhibitor of leukokinin formation and ascitic fluid accumulation, Cancer Research 35, 706.

Greenbaum, L. M. and J. Houck, 1978, (Unpublished observations).

Greenbaum, L. M. and G. Semente, 1977, Pepstatin, an ascites retardant of L-1210 tumor bearing mice, J. Natl. Cancer Inst. 59, 259.

Greenbaum, L. M. and K. Yamafuji, 1966, The in vitro inactivation and formation of kinins by cathepsins, Br. J. Pharmacol. Chemother. 27, 230.

Li, H., W. F. McLimans and N. Back, 1977, Purification and Characterization of kinin-forming acid protease from mouse fibroblasts, Biochem. Pharmacol. 26, 1187.

Prakash, A., S. Roffman and L. M. Greenbaum. 1978, The differentiation of fluorescamine-modified kinins by gel electrophoresis, Analytical Biochem. 89, 257.

Roffman, S., and L. M. Greenbaum, 1978, The properties of leuko-
    kininogen isolated from human neoplastic ascites, Biochem.
    Pharmacol.--in press.

Soh, G. L., J. L. Pace, D. L. Kemper and W. L. Ragland, 1977,
    Fluorometric scanning of fluorescamine-labeled peptides in
    polyacrylamide gels, Analytical Letters 10, 111.

Vinci, J. M., and H. R. Keiser, 1976, The kallikrein-kinin system
    in Bartter's Syndrome, Abst. Clinical Research, 24, 414A.

Wong, P., D. A. Terragno, N. A. Terragno and J. C. McGiff, 1977,
    Dual effects of bradykinin on prostaglandin metabolism,
    Prostaglandins 13, 1113.

THE KININ-FORMING ACID PROTEASE SYSTEM IN MURINE FIBROBLASTS L-929

Hsin C. Li and Nathan Back

Department of Biochemical Pharmacology, State University

of New York at Buffalo, Buffalo, New York 14260

Kinin-forming protease systems have been identified recently
in malignant tissue and fluids. Both alkaline (1-3) and acid
proteases (4-7) capable of forming vasopeptide kinins have been
isolated from the rodent Murphy-Sturm lymphosarcoma (1,4), malignant cells and ascites tumor fluid (2,3,5,6), and rodent fibroblasts grown in stationary cell culture (7,8). This report will
summarize the studies on the purification and characterization of
the acid protease isolated from the fibroblast L-929 cell line
as well as the rat plasma kininogen substrate (8). In addition,
the isolation, purification, and partial chemical characterization
of the kinin peptides formed during incubation of the acid protease with the kininogen substrate will be described.

MATERIALS AND METHODS

Acid Protease Isolation and Purification

L-929 Fibroblast Cell Line Culture. Mouse L-929 fibroblast
cells (Grand Island Biological Co., Grand Island, N.Y.) were
cultured continuously in Minimum Essential Medium (Becton,
Dickinson & Co., Cockesville, Md.) containing 10% fetal calf serum
and 0.4% lactalbumin, under automatically controlled conditions
(9). Cell viability was 85-98% as determined by the trypan blue
exclusion test (10).

Isolation. 300-500 mg protein quantities of homogenized L-929
cells were centrifuged at 3000 rpm, sonicated for 1.5 min. 5 times,
centrifuged for 15 min at 10,000 rpm in a refrigerated centrifuge,
and the supernatant dialyzed for 48 hr against 0.01 M NaH_2PO_4:Na_2HPO_4

buffer, pH 6.8, in 0.1 M NaCl and 1.0 mM EDTA. The dialyzed supernatant had a protein concentration of 5.91 mg/ml. Protease activity
was measured initially on a denatured hemoglobin substrate. All
subsequent fractions were assayed for kinin-forming activity on the
isolated perfused rat uterus following incubation with rat plasma
kininogen substrate (7). Specific activity was calculated in terms
of ng kinin released per mg protein using synthetic bradykinin as
a reference standard.

Purification. A 9.0 ml volume of dialyzed homogenate supernatant 6.38 mg protein/ml first was applied onto a G-200 Sephadex
column, 2.5x90 cm. Active eluant fractions (17. ml) with a protein
concentration of 3.8 mg/ml then were applied onto a hydroxylapatite
column, 2x30 cm, equilibrated with 0.01 M phosphate buffer, pH 6.8.
Pooled active fractions with a protein concentration of 0.65 mg/ml
(14 ml) were activated by 18 hr dialysis against 0.1 M KH_2PO_4:K_2HPO_4
buffer, pH 6.8 in 0.1 M KCl containing 5 mM cysteine. This fraction,
0.73 mg protein/ml (11 ml) was applied onto a DEAE-A50 ion exchange
column, 1x20 cm, equilibrated with 0.01 M KH_2PO_4:K_2HPO_4 buffer,
pH 6.8 in 0.1 M KCl and 2.5 mM mercaptoethanol.

Rat Plasma Kininogen Purification.

Citrated rat plasma (25 ml) was dialyzed for 10 hr at 4°
against 0.01 M sodium phosphate buffer, pH 6.8, in 0.1 M NaCl and
1.0 mM EDTA. The dialysate was centrifuged at 3000 rpm for 30 min
and the supernatant (20 ml, 39 mg protein/ml) applied onto a DEAE-
A50 column, 2.5x30 cm, with appropriate buffers (8). Fractions
were assayed for kininogen by incubating aliquots for 18 hrs at
38° with purified acid protease and kinin formed assayed on the
rat uterus. Active peaks (I, 1.64 mg/ml; II, 7.75 mg/ml) were
applied onto a G-100 Sephadex column, 2.5x90 cm equilibrated with
a phosphate buffer in KCl and mercaptoethanol.

The pH profile for the kinin-forming activity of the purified
acid protease was determined over a pH range of 1.0-12.0 during a
15 hr incubation of 0.2 ml acid protease (0.6 mg/ml) with 0.2 ml
kininogen (1.2mg/ml) at 37°. Kinin release with respect to both
time and enzyme concentration also was determined. Both the
protease and kininogen were studied for extent of homogeneity by
disc gel electrophoretic technique (11), and molecular weight
determinations made on a Sephadex G-200 gel filtration column,
1x57 cm using the following markers of known molecular weight:
aldolase, ovalbumin, chymotrypsinogen, and ribonuclease.

Isolation and Purification of Fibroblast Kinins

Extractions of Kinins. A mixture of 20 ml of citrated rat
plasma was incubated at 37° for 92.5 hrs with 6.4 ml of homogenized
L-929 fibroblast cell supernatant (12,000 g fraction, 54.2 mg) in

30 ml of 0.50 M acetate buffer, pH 4.0 containing aprotinin (500,000 KIU) and 1,10 phenanthroline (10 mg). Boiling ethyl alcohol, 10 ml, containing 0.07 gm of p-toluene-sulfonic acid was added to the incubation mixture, the mixture centrifuged for 40 min at 12,000 g, the supernatant filtered under reduced pressure, and dried with a rotary evaporator. Citrated plasma without fibroblast incubated under similar conditions did not yield any spontaneous activity.

Purification. Four ml of the filtrate (representing 17 μg bradykinin equivalents), dissolved into 0.05 M ammonium formate, pH 3.75, was applied onto a G-25 Sephadex column (1x115 cm) equilibrated with ammonium formate. Kinin activity in each fraction was assayed and the pooled active fractions (9.6 mg bradykinin equivalents) lyophilized, redissolved in formate buffer and applied onto a CM-C50 Sephadex column (2.5x15 cm). Fractions appropriately eluted were assayed for kinin activity, and the two major peak fractions (I, II) were applied onto a Biogel P-4 column (1x110 cm) with a calculated total volume of 86.4 ml and void volume of 34 ml. The column also was calibrated with the following markers: glucagon, methionyl-lysyl-bradykinin(K_{11}), lysyl-bradykinin(K_{10}), and bradykinin (Kg). Kinin activity of each eluted fraction was assayed on the isolated rat uterus.

Thin Layer Chromatography. The following known kinins and fibroblast kinins were dansylated by mixing with 5 mg/ml dansyl chloride (15-30 μl) and 0.2 M sodium bicarbonate (15-30 μl) for 1 hr at 37-40°: bradykinin (25 μg), lysyl-bradykinin (5-7.5 μg) methionyl-lysyl-bradykinin (5-25 μg), fibroblast kinin I (0.4 μg), and fibroblast kinin II (0.3-0.48 μg). Approximately 10 μl of each incubation mixure was applied onto a silica gel thin layer chromatographic plate which then was developed with pyridine:acetic acid: butanol:water (40:14:68:25). The migration spots were examined under a longwave-length ultraviolet lamp. Two dimensional TLC also was carried out using chloroform:methanol:25% ammonia (2:2:1) in the first dimension and pyridine:glacial acetic acid:butanol: H_2O (40:14:68:25) in the second dimension.

Molecular weight estimation. Information on molecular weight was obtained from the Biogel P-4 column elution volume data plotted against log molecular weight.

Acid hydrolysis and amino acid composition of fibroblast kinin. The CM-50 Sephadex purified fibroblast kinins were purified further on a G-25 Sephadex column (1x115 cm). The two kinin peaks were lyophilized in hydrolysis vials to which was added 0.5 ml of 5.7 N HCl. The mixture was frozen with dry ice-acetone, and flushed with nitrogen. This procedure was repeated 3 times. The frozen hydrolysis vials then were evacuated to 50 micron mercury pressure, flame sealed, and hydrolyzed at 105° for 24 hours. The amino

acid compositon of each hydrolysate was determined with a Beckman
automatic amino acid analyzer.

RESULTS

Acid Protease Purification. The elution profiles of the fibroblast acid protease through G-200 Sephadex, hydroxylapatite, and
DEAE-A50 Sephadex are shown in Fig. 1, Fig. 2, and Fig. 3, respectively. Compared to the activity of the supernatant dialysate, the
final purification factor was almost 10-fold (Table 1).

Rat Plasma Kininogen Purification. Two kininogen substrate
peaks (PI, PII) were obtained when rat plasma was fractionated on
the DEAE-A50 ion exchange column, Fig. 4. Further fractionation
of PII fraction through a G-100 Sephadex column yielded a major
peak in fractions 14-20 and a smaller peak in fractions 21-23,
Fig. 5. A summary of the kininogens purification is noted in
Table 2.

pH Profile of Acid Protease. The acid protease formed kinin
within a relatively narrow pH range, Fig. 6. At pH 4.0, 137 ng
kinin/mg substrate/mg enzyme were formed after 15 hours of incubation at 37°.

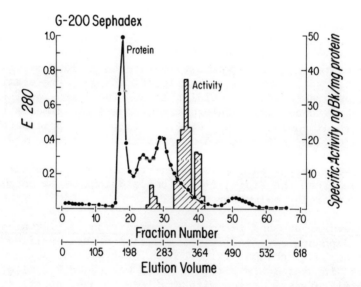

Figure 1. Elution profile of fibroblast L-929 cell homogenate
           dialysate on G-200 Sephadex column (2.5 x 90 cm).

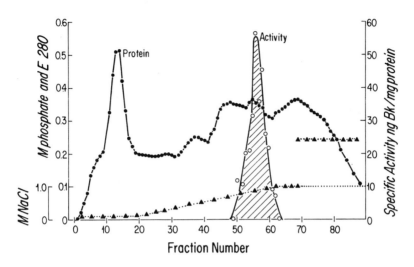

Figure 2.   Elution profile of G-200 Sephadex-purified acid
protease (17 ml, 3.8 mg/protein/ml) on hydroxylapatite
column (2 x 30 cm).

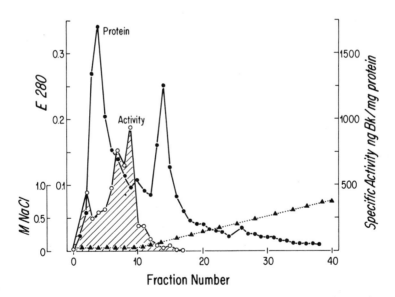

Figure 3.   Elution profile of hydroxylapatite-purified acid
protease (11.0 ml, 0.73 mg protein/ml) on DEAE-A50
ion exchange column (1 x 20 cm).

Table 1. Summary of purification of acid protease from L 929 fibroblast

Procedures	Vol (ml)	Protein (mg/ml)	Kinin-forming activity* (ngBK/ml)	Specific activity ngBK/mg protein	Yield (%)	Purification factor
L929 cell (10⁹) Supernatant dialysate	17.0	8.8	1940.0	220.5	100	1
G-200 Sephadex	17.0	3.8	1978.7	520.7	102	2.4
Hydroxylapatite (After dialysis vs cysteine)	13.0	0.73	727.0	1064.8	34.9	4.8
DEAE-A50 Sephadex	11.0	0.20	412.5	2062.5	13.8	9.4

*Activity in terms of kinin formed following 24 hr incubation of 0.5 ml fraction with 0.2 ml rat plasma

Table 2. Summary of purification of rat plasma kininogen

Procedures	Vol (ml)	Protein (mg/ml)	Activity ngBK/ml	Specific activity ngBK/mg Protein	Yield %	Purification factor
Rat Plasma	25.0	39.0	1124	28.8	100	1
DEAE Sephadex						
Peak I	8.0	1.64	37.6	22.9	1.06	0.8
Peak II	8.7	7.75	600.0	77.4	18.6	2.7
G-100 Sephadex	30	0.36	40.3	112.2	4.3	3.9

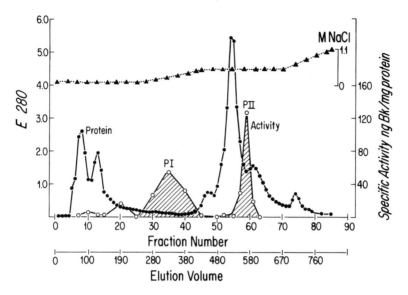

Figure 4.   Elution profile of rat plasma through DEAE–A50
            Sephadex column (2.5 x 30 cm) for initial isolation
            of rat plasma kininogen.

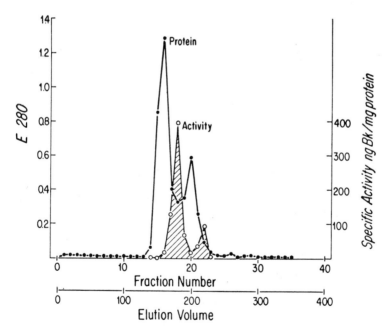

Figure 5.   Elution profile of DEAE–A50 Sephadex purified rat
            plasma kininogen through a G–100 Sephadex column
            (2.5 x 90 cm).

Time Course of Kinin Release. At a fixed substrate concentration, kinin release was directly proportional to enzyme concentration, Fig. 7. At higher enzyme concentrations, kinin formation
appeared to increase non-linearly.

Disc Gel Electrophoresis. Apparent homogenous acid protease
was obtained as indicated by a single band with protease activity
obtained by disc gel electrophoresis. With the rat plasma kininogen, disc gel electrophoretic patterns indicated a major kininogen
protein band and a major band of protein impurity.

Molecular Weight Determination. From the G-200 gel filtration
data, the molecular weight of the acid protease was estimated at
38,000-39,000, Fig. 8. The molecular weight of the peak II
kininogen was estimated to be 115,000.

Extraction of Fibroblast Kinins. After 92 hours of incubation,
the total fibroblast kinin activity generated was 41,100 ng bradykinin equivalents. The ethyl alcohol extraction step yielded
28,000 ng bradykinin equivalents whereas the rotary evaporation
step yielded 17,100 ng bradykinin equivalents of fibroblast kinin
activity. At the rotary evaporation step the yield was 41.6%.

Purification of Fibroblast Kinins. After 92 hours of incubation
the total fibroblast kinin activity generated was 41,100 ng bradykinin equivalents. The ethyl alcohol extraction step yielded
28,000 ng bradykinin equivalents whereas the rotary evaporation
step yielded 17,100 ng bradykinin equivalents of fibroblast kinin
activity. At the rotary evaporation step the yield was 41.6%.

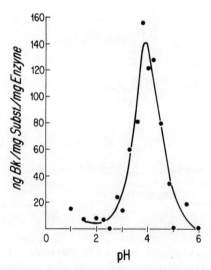

Figure 6.   pH profile of the kinin-forming activity of the acid
            protease on rat plasma kininogen.

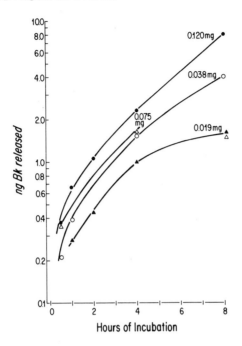

Figure 7.   Time course of kinin release at various amounts of
            DEAE-A50 Sephadex-purified acid protease incubated at
            37°, pH 4.0 with 0.075 ng DEAE-A50 Sephadex-purified
            rat plasma kininogen.

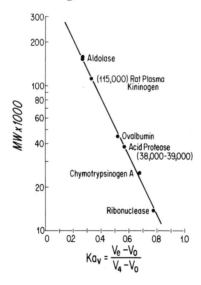

Figure 8.   Gel filtration of purified acid protease and
            kininogen through G-200 Sephadex column (1x57 cm)
            for estimation of molecular weight.

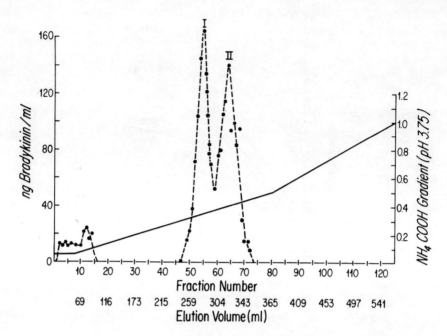

Figure 9. Elution profile of G-25 Sephadex-purified fibroblast
kinins on CM-C50 Sephadex column (2.5 x 15 cm).

Purification of Fibroblast Kinins. When the fibroblast kinin
preparation, 22 ml with an activity of 774 ng/ml bradykinin equivalents was passed through a G-25 Sephadex column, activity appeared
in fraction #7-14, amounting to a pool of 46 ml with a total kinin
activity of 370 ng bradykinin equivalents per ml. When passed
through a CM=C50 Sephadex column, two peaks with kinin activity
separated as seen in the exchange profile, Fig. 9. Fibroblast
kinin I peak appeared in fractions #49-57 and fibroblast kinin II
peak in fractions #61-72 with a yield of 12.8% and 14.9% respectively
and respective bradykinin equivalents/ml of 594 ng and 694 ng.
Elution volumes of the kinins and marker agents obtained from the
Biogel P-4 column chromatography, seen in Fig. 10, were as follows:
glucagon, 50.4 ml; K_{11}, 63.5 ml; K_{10}, 67.5 ml; K_9, 72.5 ml; fibroblast kinin I, 66.2 ml, and fibroblast kinin II, 72.5 ml. The
final yield for kinin I and kinin II was 17.2% and 12.9% respectively.

Thin Layer Chromatography. The results of the thin layer
chromatography fluorescene spot tracing are depicted in Fig. 11
and the R_f values for the various kinin peptides summarized on
Table 3. The R_f values of the fibroblast kinins are distinctly
different from those of the other kinins. Two dimensional TLC

showed the fibroblast kinins to be homogenous.

Molecular Weight Estimations.   Using least square analysis
of the elution volume data, the molecular weights of the fibroblast
kinin I and kinin II were estimated to be 1450 and 1000 respectively,
Fig. 12.

Amino Acid Composition of Fibroblast Kinins.   The amino acid
composition of the fibroblast kinins, expressed in molar ratio as
well as amino acid residues, is shown in Table 4.

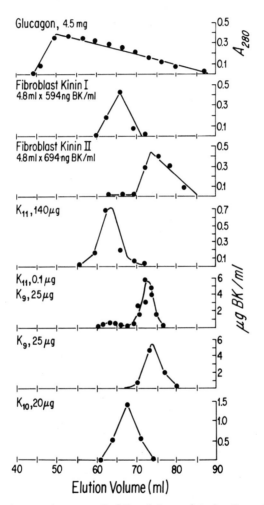

Figure 10.   Elution volumes of fibroblast kinin I and II,
            glucagon, bradykinin (K_9), lysyl-bradykinin (K_{10}),
            and methionyl-lysyl-bradykinin (K_{11}) on a Biogel
            P-4 column (1 x 110 cm).

TABLE 3. R_f values for various kinin peptides on silica
              gel thin layer chromatographic plate

Kinin peptides	R_f values *
Bradykinin (K_9)	0.890 (5)
Lysyl-bradykinin (K_{10})	0.708 (4)
Methionyl-lysyl-bradykinin (K_{11})	0.868 (4)
Fibroblast kinin I	0.451 (3)
Fibroblast kinin II	0.648 (3)

( ) = Number of measurements
 * = with respect to control

TABLE 4.   Amino acid composition of fibroblast kinins*

Fibroblast kinin	
I	II
.050 (1)	.048 (1)
.030 (0)	.032 (0)
.048 (1)	.063 (1)
.064 (1)	.083 (1)
.143 (2)	.075 (1)
.068 (1)	.055 (1)
.076 (1)	.073 (1)
.059 (1)	.033 (0)
.000 (0)	.000 (0)
.017 (0)	.010 (0)
.062 (1)	.038 (0)
.037 (0)	.074 (1)
.062 (1)	.031 (0)
.145 (2)	.186 (2)
.055 (1)	.052 (1)
.089 (1)	.150 (2)

 * = Amino acid-composition expressed as molar ratio
( )= Number of amino acid residues

DISCUSSION

Acid proteases capable of forming kinin-like peptides from appropriate substrates are present in a variety of normal and malignant cell types and tissues. An acid protease kinin-forming system was identified in the Murphy-Sturm lymphosarcoma (4). Both the protease and kininogen substrate were isolated and purified, and the molecular weight of the kininogen estimated to be 46,000 (12). Three kinin peptides isolated from incubated tumor tissue homogenates were purified and their molecular weights chromatographically estimated to be 1080, 1150, and 1170 respectively (12). This kinin-forming system as well as that in the fibroblasts bears a striking similarity to the leukokinin system described initially in polymorphonuclear leukocytes (13), leukemic (14) and neoplastic ascites cells (15). The fibroblast acid protease does differ with regard to the substrate requirements since leukokininogen is considered not to be present in normal plasma (16), and the fibroblast kinin amino acid compositions differ from those of the leukokinins (17).

The widespread distribution of fibroblasts in many rapidly proliferative tissues, as in tumors, suggest the possibility that this cell type may provide such factors as proteases and local chemical mediators essential in cell growth regulatory mechanisms. Evidence supporting the involvement of proteases in important

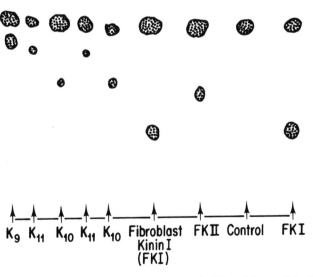

K_9 K_{11} K_{10} K_{11} K_{10} Fibroblast FKII Control FKI
                         Kinin I
                          (FKI)

Figure 11. Thin layer chromatography of fibroblast kinin I and II, bradykinin (K_9), lysyl-bradykinin (K_{10}), and methionyl-lysyl-bradykinin (K_{11}). Approximately 10 µl of each incubation was applied to the silica gel thin layer plate

cellular events is mounting (18). Fibroblast-associated protease
and kinin activities may affect the vascular permeability and
microcirculation of tumor tissue and possibly contribute chemotactic
and vasculogenesis actions in association with other proteases
systems and factors as schematically depicted in Fig. 13.

SUMMARY

Components of an acid protease kinin-forming enzyme system
were isolated and purified from the murine fibroblast L-929 cell
line grown in stationary cell culture. The enzyme, was purified
from the 10,000 g supernatant cell fraction by sequential passage
through G-200 Sephadex, hydroxylapatite, DEAE-A50 Sephadex and
affinity chromatography columns. The specific activity was determined on a rat plasma kininogen purified on DEAE and G-100 Sephadex
columns as assayed for kinin-forming activity on the isolated
perfused rat uterus. Both enzyme and substrate showed a single
band pattern by disc gel electrophoresis technique. Optimum
protease activity was obtained at pH 3.8, and kinin release was

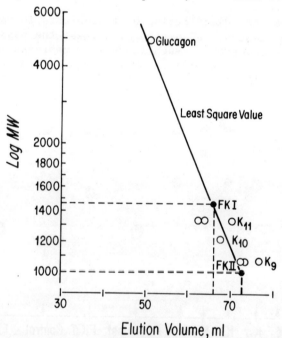

Figure 12. Plot of log molecular weights of glucagon, bradykinin (K_9), lysyl-bradykinin (K_{10}), and methionyl-
lysyl-bradykinin (K_{11}) against their respective
elution volumes obtained from elution volume data
from Biogel P-4 column (Fig. 10). Elution volumes
of the fibroblast kinins were fitted into the plot
for estimation of molecular weights.

both time- and enzyme-dependent at 37°. The molecular weight of
the protease and kininogen, estimated on a G-200 Sephadex column,
was 39,000 and 115,000 respectively. Two fibroblast kinins were
isolated from a mixture of 12,000 g fraction of fibroblast homogenate and rat plasma incubated at 37°, pH 4.0 for 92 hours. The
two fibroblast kinins (I, II) were separated and purified on G-25
Sephadex, CM-C50 Sephadex, and Biogel P-4 columns. The purity of
the kinins was ascertained by thin layer chromatography. The
molecular weight of fibroblast kinin I was estimated to be 1450 with
a 14-amino acid composition consisting of AspThrSerProGluGlyAlaVal-
LeuTyrPheLysHisArg. Fibroblast kinin II had an estimated molecular
weight of 1000 with a 12-amino acid composition that included Asp-
SerProGluGlyAlaLeuTyrLysHisArg. The kinins were relatively rich
in arginine and did not contain the bradykinin sequence.

ACKNOWLEDGEMENTS

This work was supported by USPHS grant #11492.

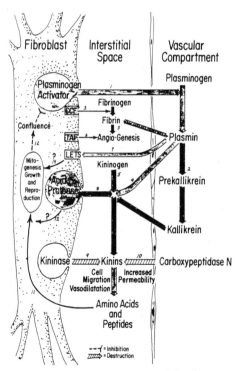

Figure 13.   Proposed scheme on relationship between fibroblast
             factors and the vasopeptide kinin and fibrinolysin
             systems.

BIBLIOGRAPHY FOR FIBROBLAST SCHEME.

1. Reich, E.: Plasminogen Activator: Secretion by Neoplastic Cells
    and Macrophages. In: Proteases and Biological Control (Eds.
    E. Reich, D.B. Rifkin, and E. Shaw) Cold Spring Harbor Conf.
    on Cell Proliferation. Cold Spring Harbor Laboratory. 1975.
    pp. 333.
    Holley, R.W.: Factors Controlling the Growth of 3T3 Cells and
    Transformed 3T3 Cells. In: Proteases and Biological Control
    (Eds. E. Reich, D.B. Rifkin, and E. Shaw). Cold Spring Harbor
    Conference on Cell Proliferation. Cold Spring Harbor Laboratory
    1975. pp. 777.
    Unkeless, J.C., Dano, K., Kellerman, G.M., and Reich, E.:
    Fibrinolysis Associated with Oncogenic Transformation: Partial
    Purification and Characterization of the Cell Factor - A Plas-
    minogen Activator. J. Biol. Chem. 249: 4295, 1973.
2. Webster, M. and Pierce, J.B.: Studies on Plasma Kallikrein and
    its Relationship to Plasmin. J. Pharmacol. Exp. Therap. 130:
    484, 1960.
3. O'Meara, R.A.Q. and Jackson, R.D.: Cytological Observations
    in Carcinoma. Irish J. Med. Sci. 391: 327, 1958.
    Thorns, R.D.: Fibrinogen and the Interstial Behavior of Cancer.
    In: Endogenous Factors Influencing Tumor-Host Balance. (Eds.
    R.W. Wissler, T.L. Dao, and S. Wood, Jr.) University of Chicago
    Press. 1967. pp. 255.
4. Back, N. and Steger, R.: Activation of Bovine Bradykininogen
    by Human Plasmin. Life Sci. 4: 153, 1965.
5. Habermann, E.: Kininogens. In: Handbook of Experimental Pharma-
    cology. Vol. 25. (Ed. E.G. Erdos). Springer-Verlag, Berlin,
    N.Y. 1970, pp. 250.
6. Klagsbrun, M., Knighton, D., and Folkman, J.: Tumor angiogenesis
    Activity in Cells Grown in Tissue Culture. Can. Res. 36: 110,
    1976.
7. Hynes, R.O. and Bye, J.M.: Density and Cell Cycle Dependence
    of Cell Proteins of Hamster Fibroblasts. Cell 3: 113, 1974.
    Hynes, R.O., Wyke, J.A., Bye, J.M., Humphryes, K.C., and Pearl-
    stein, E.S.: Are Proteases Involved in Altering Surface Proteins
    During Viral Transformation? In: Proteases and Biological
    Control (Eds. E. Reich, D.B. Rifkin, and E. Shaw). Cold Spring
    Harbor Conference on Cell Proliferation. Cold Spring Harbor
    Laboratory. 1975. pp. 931.
8. Back, N. and Steger, R.: Kinin-Forming Activity of Cultured
    Mouse Fibroblasts. Proc. Soc. Exper. Biol. Med. 143: 769,
    1973.
    Li, H.C., McLimans, W.F., and Back, N.: Purification and
    Characterization of Kinin-Forming Acid Protease from Mouse
    Fibroblasts L-929. Biochem. Pharmacol. 26: 1187, 1977.
9. Back, N. and Steger, R.: Kinin Destroying (Kininase) Activity
    of Rodent Fibroblasts L-929. Proc. Soc. Exp. Biol. & Med.
    153: 175, 1976.

10. Erdos, E.G.: Enzymes that Inactivate Polypeptides. In: Meta-
    bolic Factors Controlling Duration of Drug Actions. (Eds.
    B.B. Brodie and E.G. Erdos). Oxford Pergamon Press. 1962,
    pp. 159.
11. Holley, R.W.: (repeat under ref. #1).
12. Roblin, R., Chou, I.N., and Black, P.H.: Role of Fibrinolysin
    T Activity in Properties of 3T3 and SV3T3 Cells. In: Proteases
    and Biological Control (Eds. E. Reich, D.B. Rifkin, and E.
    Shaw). Cold Spring Harbor Conference on Cell Proliferation.
    Cold Spring Harbor Laboratory. 1975. pp. 869.
13. Bosmann, H.B., Lockwood, T., and Morgan, H.R.: Surface Bio-
    chemical Changes Accompanying Primary Infection with Rous
    Sarcoma Virus. Exp. Cell Res. 83: 25, 1974.

REFERENCES

1. N. Back and R. Steger In: Bradykinin and Related Peptides:
    Càrdiovascular, Biochemical and Neural Actions. (Eds. F.
    Sicuteri, M. Rocha e Silva, N. Back) Plenum Press, 1970.
    Characterization of pre-kallikrein activity in developing
    transplanted mammalian tumors. pp. 225-237.
2. T. Moriguchi and S. Okamoto In: Proc. 9th International Cancer
    Conf. Existence of kinin-forming system in ascitic tumor
    of animals. Springer-Verlag, 1966. pp. 164.
3. P.P. LeBlanc and N. Back, Proteases during the growth of Ehrlich
    ascites tumor II. The kallikrein system. J. Nat'l. Cancer
    Inst. 54: 1107, 1975.
4. N. Back and R. Steger In: Vasopeptides: Biochemistry, Pharma-
    cology and Pathophysiology. (Eds. N. Back, F. Sicuteri) Acid
    dependent kinin-forming system in mammalian malignant and
    normal tissue. Plenum Press, N.Y. 1972, pp. 417-434.
5. L.M. Greenbaum. Leukocyte kininogenases and leukokinins from
    normal and malignant cells. Am. J. Path. 68: 613, 1972.
6. L.M. Greenbaum, A. Prakash, G. Semente and M. Johnston. The
    leukokinin system: Its role in fluid accumulation in malig-
    nancy and inflammation. Agents & Actions 315: 332, 1973.
7. N. Back and R. Steger. Kinin-forming activity of cultured
    mouse fibroblast L-929. Proc. Soc. Exp. Biol. Med. 143: 769,
    1973.
8. Li, H.C., McLimans, W.F. and Back, N. Purification and charac-
    terization of kinin-forming acid protease from mouse fibro-
    blasts L-929. Biochem. Phcol. 26: 1187, 1977.
9. W.F. McLimans, E.V. Davis, F.L. Gover and G.W. Rake. The sub-
    merged culture of mammalian cells - the Spinner culture.
    J. Immunol. 79: 425, 1957.
10. Pappenheimer, A.M. J. exp. Med. 25: 633, 1917.
11. A.H. Gordon. In: Laboratory Techniques in Biochemistry and
    Molecular Biology.(Eds. T.S. Work, E. Work.)pp.1, 1969. The
    North Holland Publ. Co., Amsterdam, London.

12. N. Back, R. Steger, and H.J. Wilkens. Isolation and purification of kininogen and kinins from Murphy-Sturm lymphosarcoma solid tumor. Fed. Proc. 37: 602, 1978.

13. L.M. Greenbaum and K. Yamafuji. The role of cathepsins in the inactivation of plasma kinins. In: Hypotensive Peptides.(Eds. Erdos, E.G., Back, N. and Sicuteri, F.) Springer Verlag, New York, pp. 252, 1966.

14. L.M. Greenbaum, R. Freer, G. Chang, G. Semente and K. Yamafuji. PMN-kinin and kinin metabolizing enzymes in normal and malignant leukocytes. Brit. J. Pharmacol. 36: 623, 1969.

15. M.M. Johnston and L.M. Greenbaum. Leukokinin-forming system in ascites fluid of a murine mastocytoma. Biochem. P 22: 1386, 1973.

16. L.M. Greenbaum. In: Proteases and Biological Control.(Eds. E. Reich, D.B. Rifkin, and E. Shaw.) Cold Spring Harbor Laboratory. pp. 223, 1975.

17. J. Chang, R. Freer, R. Stella and L.M. Greenbaum. Studies on leukokinins. II. Studies on the formation, partial amino acid and PMN. Biochem. Pharmacol. 21: 3095, 1972.

18. E. Reich, D.B. Rifkin and E. Shaw. In: Proteases and Biological Control. Conference on Cell Proliferation. Cold Spring Harbor Laboratory, 1975.

BASOPHIL KALLIKREIN OF ANAPHYLAXIS (BK-A) - PURIFICATION AND

CHARACTERIZATION

Harold H. Newball, Ronald W. Berninger, Richard C. Talamo,
and Lawrence M. Lichtenstein

The Johns Hopkins University School of Medicine
Departments of Medicine and Pediatrics
O'Neill Research Laboratories, Baltimore, Maryland

ABSTRACT

These studies describe the IgE-mediated release of a basophil
kallikrein of anaphylaxis (BK-A) that has arginine esterase activity
and is inhibited by plasma, DFP, and Trasylol. The interaction of
BK-A active fractions from ion exchange (DEAE-Sephacel) and gel filtration (Sepharose 6B) chromatography, with human plasma kininogen
generates immunoreactive kinin. The BK-A and kinin-generating activities co-chromatograph on DEAE-Sephacel and Sepharose 6B columns,
and the quantity of kinin generated is, in general, proportional to
the BK-A activity of the column fractions, suggesting that these two
activities are subserved by the same protease. These data suggest
that kallikrein-like activity can be generated from human basophils
as a direct result of a primary IgE-mediated immune reaction, thus
providing a potential link between reactions of immediate hypersensitivity and the plasma and/or tissue kinin-generating systems.

INTRODUCTION

Kallikrein is a generic term used for the designation of serine
proteases capable of generating peptides called kinins from protein
substrates (27). These proteases have been found in plasma (plasma
kallikrein) (29), urine (urinary kallikrein) (13) as well as glandular tissues (glandular kallikrein) (13-14). Greenbaum et al. (6-7)
have reported kallikrein-like activity from the rabbit polymorphonuclear leukocyte (PMN) and human lymphocytes. In contrast to the
former several proteases, the kinin-generating enzyme reported by
Greenbaum et al. (6) is an acid protease. The above proteases
(plasma, urinary and glandular kallikreins) are variably inhibited

233

by plasma, SBTI, DFP and Trasylol (7-9).

There have been reports of the immune release of a kallikrein-like kinin-generating factor from perfused, sensitized guinea pig lung (3,9). This release process, however, was not calcium dependent, and more recent studies on this system suggest that the kinin-generating factor was not produced by the primary immune reaction, but, rather, as the result of a secondary event (30).

The present studies describe the IgE-mediated release of a kallikrein-like protease [basophil kallikrein of anaphylaxis (BK-A)] which is an arginine esterase (hydrolyses TAMe), and is inhibited by plasma, DFP, and Trasylol. A protease which is generated by IgE-mediated mechanisms and co-chromatographs with the BK-A, generates a kinin from human plasma kininogen. The data suggest that this kinin-generating protease and the BK-A TAMe esterase activity are subserved by the same enzyme. Thus, kallikrein-like activity can be generated from human basophils as a result of a primary IgE-mediated immune reaction, providing a potential link between reactions of immediate hypersensitivity and the kinin-generating systems.

METHODS

Materials. The ^{3}H – TAMe (210 mCi/mmol) was purchased from Biochemical and Nuclear Corp., Burbank, Calif. Tris buffers used in the release of histamine and the arginine esterase from basophils were made of 0.025 M pre-set Tris, pH 7.35 at 37° C (Sigma Chemical Co., St. Louis, Mo.), 0.12 M sodium chloride, 5 mM potassium chloride, and 0.03% HSA (Behring Werke, Marburg, Germany). The above constitutes Tris-A: Tris-ACM contains, in addition, calcium 0.6mM and magnesium 1.0 mM (11). The following were purchased from Schwarz-Mann, Orangeburg, N.Y.: acetyl-tyrosine methyl ester (ATMe); tosyl-arginine methyl ester (TAMe); and benzoyl-arginine methyl ester (BAMe). Soybean trypsin inhibitor (SBTI), acetyl-lysine methyl ester (LMe) and DTE were purchased from the Sigma Chemical Co., St. Louis, Mo.; L-alanyl-L-alanyl-L alanine methyl ester (AMe) from Vega-Fox Biochemicals, Tucson, Az.; and Sepharose 6B, pre swollen DEAE-Sephacel, Sephadex G-200 and Ficoll from Pharmacia Fine Chemicals, Inc., Piscataway, N.J. Antigen E was kindly provided by Dr. T.P. King of the Rockefeller University, New York, anti-IgE by Dr. K. Ishizaka, and the ionophore A23187 by Dr. R. Hamill, The Lilly Research Laboratories, Indianapolis, Indiana; and Trasylol (10000 KIU/ml) by Dr. M.E. Webster, NHLI, NIH, Bethesda, Md. (purchased from Farbenfabricken Bayer AG, Leverkusen, Germany).

Leukocyte preparations. Human leukocytes from donors allergic to ragweed or grass and from normal volunteers were separated from the other formed elements of blood by sedimentation for 60 to 90 minutes in a mixture of dextran-EDTA and dextrose. The cells were

washed twice in a Tris-A buffer, then resuspended in a serum-free
Tris-ACM buffer at a concentration of about 10^7 cells per ml, as
previously described (11). The immunologic reaction was initiated
by the addition of antigen or anti-IgE to the cell preparations and
the reaction allowed to proceed for 30 or 45 minutes in the dose-
response studies, or for periods of 90 minutes when generating large
quantities of BK-A. At the completion of the reaction, the cells
were centrifuged and the esterase released into the supernatant as
well as that present in an aliquot of untreated cells was determined
by the radiochemical technique of Beaven et al. (2), as previously
described (18).

Arginine esterase activity. Arginine esterase activity of the
supernatant was determined by a radiochemical technique employing
p-toluenesulfonyl-L-arginine ^{3}H -- methyl ester (^{3}H -- TAMe) (18)
which was devised by Beaven et al. (2) for the measurement of human
urinary kallikrein and modified for the determination of arginine
esterase activity in supernatants (28). The experimental tubes with
leukocytes were run in duplicate, while the determinations of arginine esterase activity were run in quadruplicate. The total cellular
arginine esterase activity was determined using sonicated aliquots
of untreated cells. Sonication studies with 1 ml aliquots of leukocyte preparations showed that when cells were sonicated for 30 second
periods, maximal arginine esterase activity was released with 2.5
minutes of sonication (Branson Sonic Power Co., Plainview, N.Y.).

Definition of TAMe unit. A TAMe unit is defined as that quantity of BK-A which hydrolyses one picomole (pmol) of the substrate
^{3}H- TAMe per minute. The activity of a sample is expressed as units
per ml of the sample, or pmol per minute per ml of sample. The specific activity of the ^{3}H-TAMe used in these studies is such that cpm
per 10 µl of sample reported in this manuscript may be converted to
units per ml by simply dividing cpm by 10,000.

Kinin-forming activity. The ability of BK-A purified by chromatography to generate immunoreactive kinin was tested using kininogen substrate prepared from normal human plasma by the method of
Diniz and Carvalho (5). The plasma was prepared by drawing venous
blood from normal donors into plastic tubes containing sodium citrate
(1 volume of 3.8% sodium citrate per 9 volumes of blood), and cen-
trifuging at 4° C for 20 minutes. Aliquots of 100 µl of Sepharose
6B or DEAE-Sephacel eluates, buffer, or trypsin (100 µg, Worthington
Biochemicals) were incubated in duplicate for 20 minutes at 25° C
in 200 µl of kininogen substrate in the presence of 3 mM 1, 10-phen-
anthrolene, and the reaction was terminated by addition of 20 µl of
20% trichloracetic acid. After addition of 1 ml of 0.1 N acetic
acid, the entire reaction mixture was applied to 3 cm columns (in
siliconized transfer pipets) of CG-50 gel (100-200 mesh) in 0.1 N
acetic acid. After washing with 10 ml of 0.1 N acetic acid, the

kinin bound to the columns was eluted with 5 ml of 50% acetic acid, concentrated by flash evaporation and quantitated by a kinin radio-immunoassay, as previously described (21).

RESULTS

Dose-response. Dose-response curves of arginine esterase re-lease have been studied with leukocyte preparations that were challenged with either the purified protein antigens from ragweed (AgE) (10) or grass (GP I) (12) or with highly specific anti-IgE (18). A typical arginine esterase dose-response curve is shown in Fig. 1. The precision of the arginine esterase assay for quadruplicate determinations is approximately 3% as is indicated by the standard deviations (Fig. 1).

Purification of the basophil arginine esterase. To generate large quantities of the basophil arginine esterase, leukocytes from 200 to 400 ml of blood were challenged with either anti-IgE or AgE. The supernatants from these preparations were concentrated 10-fold by vacuum dialysis at 4° C using Collodiun bags No. 100 and stored at -70° C until used for chromatographic studies. BK-A, obtained by challenge of leukocytes with anti-IgE was sequentially chromato-graphed on Sephadex G-200, DEAE-Sephacel and Sepharose 6B. The re-covery after chromatography on the three columns was variable, but averaged approximately 20%.

Sephadex G-200. A 2.6-X 40-cm column was packed with Sephadex G-200 to a height of 35 cm, and equilibrated with 0.02M PO_4 buffer, pH 6.8 at 4° C. Ten to fifteen ml of concentrated supernatant was applied to the column and the pattern developed by upward flow of 10 ml/hr using a peristaltic pump. Eighty 3-ml fractions were col-lected and we determined arginine esterase activity, and absorbance (280 nm). Only one major esterase-active area was observed when concentrated supernatant was applied to Sephadex G-200 (Fig. 2). This esterase-active area eluted with the first O.D. peak (the void volume). The esterase-active fractions from Sephadex G-200 were further purified by ion exchange chromatography (DEAE-Sephacel).

DEAE-Sephacel. A 1.6 X 20-cm column was packed with Sephacel to a height of 10 cm, and equilibrated with 0.02 M PO_4 buffer, pH 6.8 at 4° C. Forty to 60 ml of esterase-active eluate of the Sepha-dex G-200 were applied to the column and the pattern developed by downward flow of 30 ml/hr using a peristaltic pump. The column was washed with 200 ml of the equilibrating buffer and eluted with a linear salt gradient of 30 ml of equilibrating buffer and 30 ml of 0.02 M PO_4 buffer, pH 6.8 containing 0.50 M NaCl. A second-step salt gradient was developed with 30 ml of equilibrating buffer con-taining 0.50 M NaCl and 30 ml of 0.02 M PO_4, pH 6.8 containing 1 M NaCl. Thirty 2-ml fractions were collected from each salt gradient

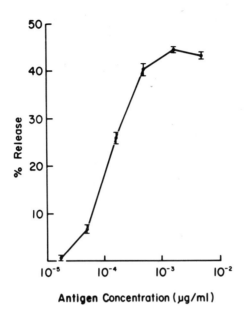

Figure 1.   IgE-mediated release of BK-A.

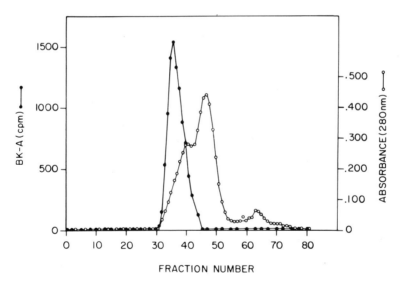

Figure 2.   Sephadex G-200 chromatography of preparations rich in
            BK-A.

and we determined arginine esterase activity, conductivity, and absorbance (280 nm). Only one esterase-active area was observed when Sephadex G-200 esterase-active fractions were applied to Sephacel. This esterase-active area eluted with the first NaCl gradient, and coincided with an O.D. peak. A second O.D. peak eluted with the second gradient, however, it had no esterase activity. The esterase-active fractions eluted with a conductivity of 10 mMhos, corresponding to a salt concentration of 0.1 M NaCl. The esterase-active fractions from DEAE-Sephacel were further purified by molecular sieve chromatography (Sepharose 6B).

Sepharose 6B. A 1.6-X 100-cm column of Sepharose 6B was equilibrated with 0.02 M PO_4 buffer, pH 6.8 at 4° C and calibrated with blue dextran, thyroglobulin, ferritin, catalase, and HSA (Mannheim-Boehringer). Six to 8 ml of concentrated esterase-active fractions from DEAE-Sephacel were applied to the column and the pattern developed by upward flow of 10 ml/hr using a peristaltic pump. One hundred 3-ml fractions were collected and we determined arginine esterase activity and absorbance (280nm). One major esterase-active area was observed (Fig. 3). This esterase-active area coincided with the first O.D. peak and eluted with an estimated molecular weight of 1.2 million. A second arginine esterase-active area is often present, and is quantitatively of smaller magnitude and of smaller molecular weight (approximately 400,000). A third arginine esterase-active area is variably present, and is quantitatively of smaller magnitude than the 1.2 million or the 400,000 forms. This third form also has the smallest molecular weight (approximately 80,000). The esterase-active fractions were used for further studies, including kinin generation and SDS-polyacrylamide disc gel electrophoresis.

Linear gradient polyacrylamide gel electrophoresis. BK-A from Sepharose 6B eluates with an estimated molecular weight of 1.2 million were inactivated with DFP (10mM final concentration) and subjected to a 2.5% to 27% linear gradient polyacrylamide gel (rods from Isolab, Inc.) electrophoresis using Tris-borate-EDTA buffer, pH 8.4, stained with 0.25% Coomassie Blue and destained by diffusion (1,25). BSA (68,000), HSA (69,000), bovine thyroglobulin (670,000), and human IgM 920,000 (Cappel Laboratories) were incubated as molecular weight markers. Fig. 4 compares the electrophoretic pattern of BK-A (gel 2 containing 50 µg in 50 µl) with human IgM (gel 1) and HSA (gel 3). The molecular weight of BK-A was estimated to be 950,000 ± 70,700 (mean ± SD) in four runs. Analyses of overloaded gels containing up to 200 µg of BK-A protein (in 200 µl) failed to reveal low mol. weight proteins.

SDS-polyacrylamide disc gel electrophoresis. SDS-polyacrylamide (3.3%) disc gel electrophoresis was performed according to the method of Weber et al. (25). Gels were cast in 5.5 mm (ID) X 12.5 cm siliconized tubes to a height of 10 cm. Urea was not added to

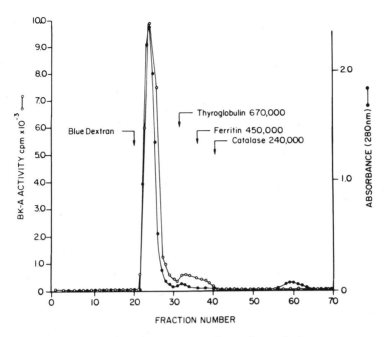

Figure 3. Sepharose 6B chromatography of arginine esterase active
fractions from DEAE-Sephacel.

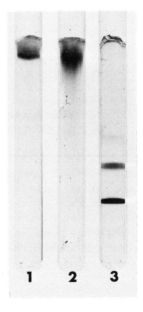

Figure 4. 2.5 to 27% linear gradient polyacrylamide gel electrophoresis of BK-A.

samples. BK-A from Sepharose 6B eluates with an estimated mol weight of 1.2 million were inactivated with DFP (10mM final concentration), and denatured with 2% SDS and 2% DTT (if reduced) at 100° C X 1 min or 37° C X 2 hr. Gels were stained with Coomassie Blue, destained by diffusion, and visually inspected. Each run contained the following standards: RNA polymerase (39,000; 155,000; 165,000), BSA (68,000), bovine thyroglobulin (670,000), human IgM (920,000) as well as concentrated buffer containing HSA (69,000). Studies showed that   both reduced (gel 1) and unreduced (gel 2) samples of DFP inactivated BK-A subjected to 100° C and 37° C denaturing conditions yielded bands with the following mol weight (mean ± SD, estimated relative intensity): 16,000 ± 0, dark; 30,500 ± 700, faint; 46,000 ± 1400, faint; 90,000 ± 700, dark. In addition to these bands, unreduced samples of BK-A (gel 2) exhibited a faint band with a mol. weight of 135,000. The reduced, concentrated buffer (in which the leukocytes were challenged) containing HSA is shown in gel 3. Analysis of BK-A samples which had not been inactivated with DFP usually resulted in a diffuse staining of the bottom two-thirds of the gel (low mol. weight proteins).

Attempts were made to correlate protein bands with esterolytic activity by staining one gel and slicing an identical unstained gel into 1.5 mm sections. These sections were crushed and the protein eluted by suspension in 300 μl of 0.01M sodium phosphate, pH 7.4 with and without 2% Triton X-100 or 6.0 M urea (24) at 37° C for 2 hours, followed by centrifugation. Unfortunately, the esterolytic activity of the BK-A was lost.

Kinin generation by the basophil arginine esterase. The interaction of the basophil arginine esterase with the plasma kinin-generating system was studied. In these experiments, the esterase-active chromatographic fractions from antigen or anti-IgE challenged cells, or buffer, were incubated with a crude kininogen preparation in duplicate and the kinin generated was assayed in quadruplicate by radio-immunoassay (21). Figure 5 shows that esterase-active fractions from Sepharose 6B generated kinin, and that the quantity of kinin generated is, in general, proportional to the esterase activity of the column fraction. Because the kinin radioimmunoassay is extremely time consuming, not all fractions were assayed; rather, we assayed those fractions with TAMe esterase activity. The data suggest that, for equivalent TAMe esterase activity, BK-A is about twice as active as human plasma kallikrein in the proteolytic cleavage of human plasma kininogen. Purified human plasma kallikrein (kindly provided by Drs. John Griffin and Charles Cochrane, Scripps Research Foundation, La Jolla, Calif.) and BK-A (sequentially purified on Sephadex G-200, DEAE-Sephacel and Sepharose 6B) were incubated with human plasma kininogen. For equivalent arginine esterase activity (0.4 TAMe units) plasma kallikrein generated 110 while BK-A generated 213 ng of kinin per ml of substrate. 100 μg of trypsin was used as a positive control and it generated 250 ng of kinin. Studies to determine the kinetics of kinin generation with purified high and low molecular weight kininogens (20) are currently ongoing.

Inhibitors of the arginine esterase. In the following experiments, we studied the inhibitory capacity of certain agents on the activity of BK-A. The pharmacological effects of the agents were determined by adding aliquots of a constant amount of BK-A to a series of test tubes containing variable concentrations of the agents. The percent inhibition resulting from each agent was determined from the equation: % Inhibition = $(C-E)/C \times 100$, where C and E represent the esterase activity of BK-A in the control (C) and experimental (E) tubes, respectively. The arginine esterase activity of the BK-A was minimally inhibited by SBTI (11% at 0.1 mM). Unlike its inhibition of plasma kallikrein (23), SBTI only poorly inhibits BK-A. With respect to its inhibition by SBTI, the basophil esterase is unlike the kallikreins of sweat glands, intestinal wall, brain, and carcinoid tumors; but similar to the kallikrein of urine which is unaffected by SBTI (23). Plasma diluted as much as 1:28 inhibits the basophil esterase activity. As with other kallikreins, C 1 esterase inhibitor may be the main plasma protein responsible for inhibition of the BK-A activity (23). Trasylol and DFP, likewise, inhibit the basophil arginine esterase activity (Figs. 6-7). As with other kallikreins, Trasylol does not completely inhibit the basophil esterase activity, even at concentrations of 1000 KIU per ml. This may be explained by the relatively high dissociation constant of the kallikrein-inhibitor complex (23).

Substrate specificity. The studies with substrates showed that the pattern of substrate specificity of the basophil esterase for synthetic amino acid ester substrates is generally similar to that reported for plasma kallikrein (26). In our studies, we looked at the competitive inhibition of "cold" TAMe, BAMe, LMe, ATMe and AMe on the hydrolysis of ^{3}H-TAMe by the basophil arginine esterase. The inhibition pattern was similar for TAMe, BAMe, and ATMe.

Temperature inactivation. Studies show that BK-A is totally inactivated when incubated at 61° C for 30 minutes. Incubation of BK-A for 30 minutes at 4° C and 25° C led to no loss of arginine esterase activity, while incubation for 30 minutes at 56° C and 61° C led to 85% and 98% inactivation, respectively.

pH optimum. Arginine esterase activity, reflecting the hydrolysis of ^{3}H-TAMe by BK-A, was optimum at pH 8.5. Non-enzymatic hydrolysis of the substrate ^{3}H-TAMe was increased above pH 8.0. The signal to noise ratio, that is, the enzymatic to non-enzymatic hydrolysis ratio, was optimal at pH 8.5. Hence, pH 8.5 is now being used for all assay procedures.

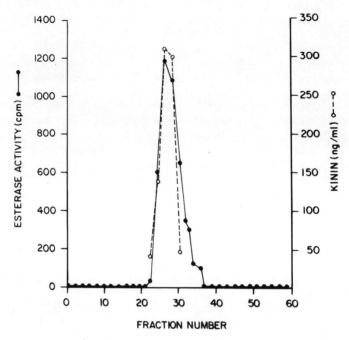

Figure 5.   Arginine esterase activity and kinin generation by BK-A.

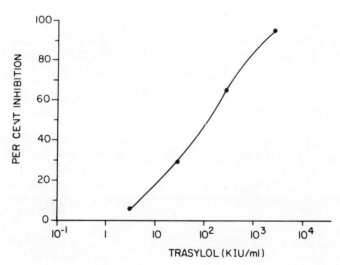

Figure 6.   Inhibition of arginine esterase activity of BK-A by
            Trasylol.

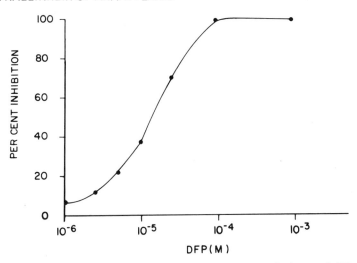

Figure 7. Inhibition of arginine esterase activity of BK-A
           by DFP.

DISCUSSION

        We earlier reported the IgE-mediated release of a TAMe esterase
(BK-A) from anti-IgE stimulated peripheral human leukocytes. The
supernatants from anti-IgE stimulated peripheral leukocytes also
had kinin-generating activity (26). The purpose of these studies
was to attempt to purify and characterize the BK-A and kinin-generating activities, and determine whether the two activities were subserved by the same protease. It is reasonable to assume that the
kinin-generating kallikrein and the basophil kallikrein-like arginine esterase activity (BK-A) might be subserved by the same protease,
since, like all known kallikreins (22-23), the basophil kallikrein-
like activity (BK-A) is an arginine esterase, and, like many kallikreins, it is variably inhibited by plasma, DFP, and Trasylol (Figs.
6-7). Moreover, the IgE-generated BK-A and kinin-generating activities co-chromatograph on both Sepharose 6B and DEAE-Sephacel (Fig.
5). Furthermore, the BK-A active fractions from Sepharose 6B and
DEAE-Sephacel generate kinin and the quantity of kinin generated is
proportional to the BK-A activity of the column fractions. The data
support the hypothesis that the basophil-derived arginine esterase
activity (BK-A) and the basophil-derived kinin-generating activity
are subserved by the same protease.

        To purify the BK-A, leukocytes from peripheral blood were chal-
lenged with anti-IgE and the supernatant was sequentially chromatographed on Sephadex G-200, DEAE-Sephacel and Sepharose 6B. Fig. 2
illustrates the elution profile of BK-A on Sephadex G-200. A major
arginine esterase active area is observed, which elutes in the void

volume. Chromatography on Sephadex G-200 accomplished two purposes:
a) the BK-A was desalted for subsequent chromatography on DEAE-Sephacel and b) the BK-A was partially purified since it eluted in the
void volume, thus allowing separation from smaller molecular weight
proteins. The arginine esterase active fractions from the void
volume of Sephadex G-200 were further purified on DEAE-Sephacel.
Only one BK-A esterase-active area is eluted from DEAE-Sephacel with
the first NaCl gradient. The second-step NaCl gradient eluted more
protein which had no esterase activity. The esterase-active fractions from DEAE-Sephacel were chromatographed on Sepharose 6B. The
major BK-A activity eluted with an estimated molecular weight of
1.2 million (Fig. 3). A second esterase-active area was often present, but quantitatively of smaller magnitude and molecular weight
(approximately 400,000). A third esterase-active area was variably
present, and had a molecular weight of less than 100,000. The relationship of one form of the enzyme to the other is not clearly
understood. The smaller molecular weight proteins seen on SDS-PAGE
suggest that the large form of BK-A might represent aggregated units,
or alternatively, BK-A has been digested, or fragmented by SDS.

The BK-A generates a kinin(s) from human plasma kininogen.
Plasma kininogen may not, however, be the natural substrate of BK-A.
There are more than one type of kininogen substrate, i.e. low and
high molecular weight kininogens (25). There may be another kininogen, i.e. a tissue kininogen that may be a better substrate for
BK-A. The data suggest, however, that BK-A is at least as active
as plasma kallikrein in the proteolytic cleavage of human plasma
kininogen. The continuous elaboration of BK-A over a prolonged IgE-
mediated event could conceivably lead to the generation of sufficient
quantities of kinins that would be important in the pathogenesis of
inflammation. Studies are in progress to determine the nature of
the kinin being generated. The antibody used in the kinin radioimmunoassay is able to detect all kinins containing the bradykinin
nonapeptide sequence, including lys-bradykinin, Met-lys-bradykinin
and the pachykinin Gly-Arg-Met-Lys-bradykinin (19).

Greenbaum et al. (6-7) have reported that kallikrein-like enzymes are found in leukocytes. These enzymes are acid proteases and
cleave leukokinins from a protein substrate known as leukokininogen.
Leukokinins are polypeptides having 20-25 amino acids, and are distinct from the nonapeptide bradykinin. Moreover, leukokinins do not
contain the bradykinin sequence in their molecule and would not be
detected by our radioimmunoassay. The substrate from which leukokinins are cleaved (leukokininogen) is not a normal constituent of
plasma (7).

Movat et al. (15) have described a neutral protease released
by polymorphonuclear leukocytes (PMN) after their interaction with
antigen-antibody complexes or IgG-coated latex particles. This protease has alanine esterase activity in contrast to the basophil pro-

tease (26)   and recent evidence suggests that the PMN protease
is an elastase (H. Movat, personal communication). Wintroub et al.
(31) have described a neutrophil-dependent pathway for the generation
of a neutral peptide which is cleaved from a plasma protein substrate
by an α-1-antitrypsin-inhibitable serine protease. This peptide is
distinguished from the kinin peptides by a neutral isoelectric point,
susceptibility to inactivation by trypsin, as well as chymotrypsin,
and activity on the isolated, atropinized, and antihistamine-treated
guinea pig ileum with relatively little action on the estrous rat
uterus.

A variety of immune complexes have been tested for their ability
to activate isolated human Hageman Factor (4). The data failed to
show interaction of Hageman Factor with the immune complexes, or
activation of Hageman Factor - the initial step in the cascade of
reactions which generate bradykinin in human plasma. This report
indicates that kallikrein-like activity (BK-A) can be generated from
human basophils as a result of a primary immune reaction. BK-A may
generate kinins directly by the proteolytic cleavage of human plasma
kininogen. BK-A may also generate kinins indirectly through the
activation of human Hageman Factor (31). Thus, this kinin-generating
activity (BK-A) which we have described appears to be unique, in
that it is the first recognized mechanism whereby IgE-mediated immune reactions may directly activate the kallikrein-kinin system.
Kinins are believed to mediate a variety of allergic and inflammatory conditions. The demonstration of the IgE-mediated release
of a basophil kallikrein of anaphylaxis (BK-A) allows us to begin
the study of the role of this system in the pathogenesis of allergic
and inflammatory processes.

ACKNOWLEDGEMENTS

This work was supported in part by Grants No. HL18526, HL14153,
AI07290, and AI07007 from the National Heart, Lung and Blood Institute and National Institute of Allergy and Infectious Diseases,
National Institutes of Health. The authors thank Ms. Judy Mason
for her technical assistance.

REFERENCES

1. Anderson, L.O., H. Borg, and M.M. Ikaelsson, 1972, Molecular
        weight estimations of proteins by electrophoresis in poly-
        acrylamide gels of graded porosity, FEBS Letters 20, 199.
2. Beaven, V.H., J.V. Pierce and J.J. Pisano, 1971, A sensitive
        isotopic procedure for the assay of esterase activity: Measure-
        ment of human urinary kallikrein, Clin. Chim. Acta. 32, 67.
3. Brocklehurst, W.E. and S.C. Lahiri, 1962, Formation and destruct-
        ion of bradykinin during anaphylaxis, J. Physiol. 165, 39.

4. Cochrane, C.G., et al., The structural characteristics and acti-
    vation of Hageman Factor, 1972, in: Inflammation: Mechanisms
    and Control, eds. I.H. Lepow and P.A. Ward, (Academic Press,
    New York) p. 119.
5. Diniz, C.R. and I.F. Carvalho, 1963, A micromethod for determin-
    ation of bradykininogen under several conditions, Ann. N.Y.
    Acad. Sci., 104, 77.
6. Engleman, E.G. and L. M. Greenbaum, 1971, Kinin-forming activity
    of human lymphocytes, Biochem. Pharmacol. 20, 922.
7. Greenbaum, L.M., et al., The leukokinin system; its role in fluid
    accumulation in malignancy and inflammation, 1973, in: Agents
    and Actions, (Birkhauser Verlag, Basel) p. 332.
8. Ishizaka, T., C.S. Sotta and K. Ishizaka, 1973, Mechanisms of
    passive sensitization III. Number of IgE molecules and their
    receptor sites on human basophil granulocytes, J. Immunol.,
    3, 500.
9. Jonasson, O. and E.L. Becker, 1966, Release of kallikrein from
    guinea pig lung during anaphylaxis, J. Exp. Med. 123, 509.
10. King, T.P., P.S. Norman, and J.T. Connell, 1964, Isolation and
    characterization of allergens from ragweed pollen, Biochem.
    3, 458.
11. Lichtenstein, L.M. and A.G. Osler, 1964, Studies on the mechan-
    isms of hypersensitivity phenomena, J. Exp. Med. 120, 507.
12. Marsh, D.G., F.H. Milner and P. Johnson, 1966, The allergenic
    activity and stability of purified allergens from the pollen
    of common rye grass (Lolium perenne), Int. Arch. Allergy 29,
    521.
13. Moriya, H., J.V. Pierce and M.E. Webster, 1963, Purification
    and some properties of three kallikreins, Ann. N.Y. Acad.
    Sci., 104, 172.
14. Moriya, H., et al., Human salivary kallikrein and liberation of
    colostrokinin, 1966, in: Hypotensive Peptides, eds.E.G. Erdos,
    N. Back and F. Sicuteri (Springer Verlag, N.Y.) p. 161.
15. Movat, H.Z., et al., 1973, Demonstration of kinin-generating
    enzyme in the lysosomes of human polymorphonuclear leukocytes,
    Lab. Invest., 29, 669.
16. Newball, H.H., R.C. Talamo and L.M. Lichtenstein, 1975, Release
    of leukocyte kallikrein mediated by IgE, Nature 254, 635.
17. Newball, H., et al., 1978, Cleavage of Hageman Factor (HF) by
    a basophil kallikrein of anaphylaxis (BK-A), Clin. Research,
    26, 519A.
18. Newball, H.H., et al., Activation of human Hageman Factor by a
    leukocytic protease, 1978, in: Proceedings of the International
    Symposium on Kinins, eds. T. Suzuki and H. Moriya, (Plenum
    Press, N.Y.).
19. Rocha E Silva, M., Bradykinin and bradykininogen - introductory
    remarks, 1974, in: Chemistry and Biology of the Kallikrein-
    Kinin System in Health and Disease, eds. J. Pisano and
    F. Austen, DHEW Publication No. (NIH) 76-791, 7.

20. Saito, H., 1977, Purification of high molecular weight kinin-
    ogen and the role of this agent in blood coagulation, J. Clin.
    Invest., 60, 584.
21. Talamo, R.C., E. Haber and K.F. Austen, 1969, A radioimmunoassay
    for bradykinin in plasma and synovial fluid, J. Lab. Clin.
    Med., 74, 816.
22. Trautschold, I., Assay methods in the kinin system, 1970, in:
    Handbook of Exper. Pharmacol., ed. E.G. Erdos, (Springer-
    Verlag, N.Y.) Vol. XXV, 52.
23. Vogel, R. and E. Werle, Kallikrein inhibitors, 1970, in: Hand-
    book of Exper. Pharmacol., ed. E.G. Erdos, (Springer-Verlag,
    N.Y.) 25, 213.
24. Weber, K. and D. J. Kuter, 1971, Reversible denaturation of
    enzymes by sodium dodecyl sulfate, J. Biol. Chem., 246, 4504.
25. Weber, K., J.R. Pringle and M. Osborn, Measurement of molecular
    weights by electrophoresis on SDS-acrylamide gel, 1972, in:
    Methods in Enzymology XXVI, 1.
26. Webster, M.E. and J.V. Pierce, 1961, Action of the kallikreins
    on synthetic ester substrates, Proceedings of the Society for
    Experimental Biology and Medicine, 107, 186.
27. Webster, M.E., 1970, in:Handbook of Exper. Pharmacol., ed.
    E.G. Erdos,(Springer-Verlag, N.Y.) Vol. XXV, 659.
28. Webster, M.E., et al., 1974, Release of histamine and arginine-
    esterase activity from passively sensitized human lung by
    ragweed antigen, Ciencia E Cultura, 26, 372.
29. Werle, E., 1936, Uber kallikrein aus Blut, Biochem. Z. 287,
    235.
30. Wintroub, B.U., et al., Characterization of and immunoassays
    for components of the kinin-generating system, 1973, in:
    Mechanisms in Allergy, eds. L. Goodfriend, H. Sehon and
    R.P. Orange, (Marcel Dekker, Inc., N.Y.) p. 495.
31. Wintroub, B.U., E.J. Goetzl and K.F. Austen, 1974, A neutrophil-
    dependent pathway for the generation of a neutral peptide
    mediator; partial characterization of components and control
    by α-1-antitrypsin, J. Exp. Med., 140, 812.

BIOLOGICAL AND PHYSIOLOGICAL CONSIDERATIONS ARISING FROM CELLULAR

LOCALIZATION AND OTHER RECENT OBSERVATIONS ON KALLIKREINS

M. Schachter

Department of Physiology
University of Alberta
Edmonton, Alberta, Canada

The application of immunocytochemical techniques to the localization of various kallikreins (E.C.3.4.21,8) in recent years has led to their localization, albeit incomplete, in several glandular tissues, viz., in salivary, pancreatic, and coagulating (sex) glands; also in sperm acrosome (acrosin). The significant conclusion is that these extremely similar enzymes differ so markedly in their cellular localizations that they must have different specific functions, and probably act on different substrates in each instance.

Thus, in the salivary glands of the mouse, rat, cat, guinea-pig and pig, kallikrein is located in duct cells, possibly in small secretory granules (Ekfors and Hopsu-Havu, 1971; Barton *et al.*, 1975; Brandtzaeg *et al.*, 1976; Hojima *et al.*, 1977; Dietl *et al.*, 1978; Schachter *et al.*, 1978). In the coagulating gland of the guinea-pig, in contrast, it is located in all the secretory cells of the gland, apparently in the cytosol rather than in secretory organelles (Barton *et al.*, 1973; Schachter *et al.*, 1978). In the pancreas, in contrast to the salivary glands, it occurs in the acinar secretory granules and appears to be absent from duct cells (Dietl *et al.*, 1978). In the pancreas, it is found in the acinar granules, together with the other similar serine proteases such as trypsin, chymotrypsin, and elastase. The latter lack the carbohydrate moiety which, in general, is a component of the kallikreins (see Stroud, 1974; Fiedler *et al.*, 1977; Fritz *et al.*, 1977).

The above immunocytochemical findings, which suggest diverse physiological roles of the kallikreins, are supplemented by other

observations which confirm the probable diversity of function of
these enzymes. *First*, there are the recent discoveries of new
biological or physiological effects of kallikreins or kinins such
as natriuretic and other possible transport effects, involvement
in blood coagulating "cascade" phenomena, in cell proliferation or
as a possible "wound hormone", in enhancing sperm motility, and
other actions (see Pisano and Austen, 1976; Hojima *et al*., 1977;
Nustad *et al*., 1978). *Second*, many widely distributed serine
proteases of diverse functions are so similar chemically to one
another, and to the kallikreins, that they are all considered to
have arisen from a single ancestral molecule. These include,
among others, trypsin, chymotrypsin, elastase, thrombin, plasmin,
"cocoonase", some lysosomal proteases, some bacterial trypsins (see
Stroud, 1974), and a number of tumour proteases (see Reich *et al*.,
1975). The widespread distribution in nature of inhibitors for
these serine proteases is also consistent with the evolution of
these enzymes from an ancestral molecule with increasing diversi-
fication of their functions accompanied by minor variations in
their structures (see Frey *et al*., 1968; Schachter, 1969; Wunderer
et al., 1976). Recently, Neurath and Walsh (1976) have also
suggested that the serine proteases are biological regulators with
diverse functions, and that they exert their actions by specific
and limited proteolysis. Thus, their known properties could
qualify them for functions not only in blood coagulation and in
digestion, where they now have known roles, but also possibly in
fertilization (via acrosin), in wound healing, repair and cell
growth; and also in embryonic development and differentiation, and
possibly in producing some of the properties of tumour cells. The
serine proteases are well known for activating proenzymes to
active enzymes, e.g., trypsinogen, chymotrypsinogen, proelastase,
etc. There is also recent evidence that human urinary kallikrein
converts inactive plasma renin to the active enzyme (Sealey *et al*.,
1978). The possibility also exists that kallikrein-like serine
proteases, with their remarkable substrate specificities, also
play a part in the conversion of some prohormones to hormones (e.g.
proinsulin, proglucagon, etc.). There is, in fact, recent
evidence that the γ subunit of NGF is a specific protease (an
arginyl-esteropeptidase) which may be the activator of pro-NGF
(Bergen and Shooter, 1977). It is therefore of interest that
kallikrein-, trypsin- and chymotrypsin-like proteases, and NGF,
are all located in the duct cells of the submandibular gland (see
Schwab *et al*., 1976; Maranda *et al*., 1978; Schachter *et al*., 1978).
Perhaps of relevant interest is that of the activation of the
highly toxic promellitin in bee venom by a specific protease of
the bee (Kreil, 1978).

There is little doubt that the recent developments in the
chemistry of the kallikreins and of the related serine proteases
and their inhibitors, together with the new knowledge of their

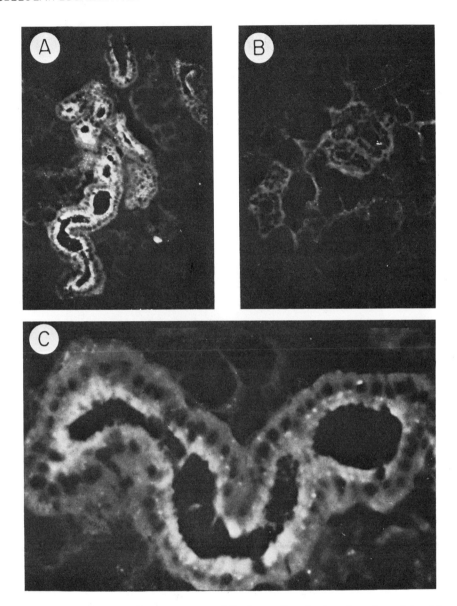

Fig. 1. Sections of cat submandibular gland showing localization
of kallikrein by immunofluorescence microscopy. A, after reaction
with antibody to kallikrein. Note intense fluorescence in apical
region (bordering lumen) of striated duct cells. Fluorescence in
acinar and demilune cells as well as in surrounding tissue. x200.
B, control section prepared as A but without addition of antibody
to kallikrein shows only mild and diffuse nonspecific fluorescence.
C, part of area of specific fluorescence in duct cells shown in A
but at higher magnification. x500. (From Hojima *et al*., 1977)

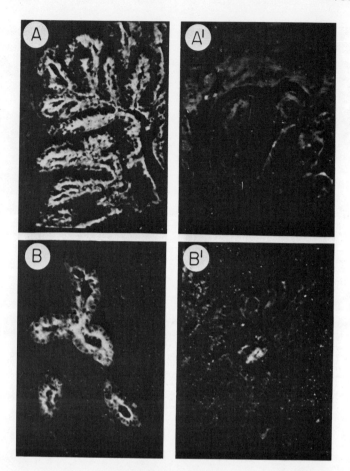

Fig. 2. Localization of kallikrein in guinea-pig coagulating and
submandibular glands by immunofluorescence microscopy. x200. The
antibody in both instances was raised in rabbits injected with
guinea-pig coagulating gland kallikrein (CGK).
Upper panels: coagulating gland. A, after reaction of tissue with
antibody to kallikrein. Note the diffuse yellow-green specific
fluorescence in all the secretory cells surrounding the crypts and
lumen; only the nuclei, located in the basal portions of these
cells, are nonreactive. The surrounding connective tissue shows
no specific fluorescence. A^1, control tissue section without
addition of antibody to kallikrein. There is only a slight and
nonspecific fluorescence throughout.
Lower panels: submandibular gland. B, after reaction of tissue
with antibody to kallikrein. Note specific yellow-green fluorescence that is concentrated near the luminal border of striated
duct cells. The surrounding acinar and interstitial tissue is
nonreactive. B^1, control tissue section.
(From Schachter, Maranda and Moriwaki, 1978).

cellular localizations and physiological actions, will provide new
and interesting insights into their biological significance.

ACKNOWLEDGEMENTS

    Support for research by the Medical Research Council of
Canada and the Alberta Heart Foundation is acknowledged.

REFERENCES

Barton, S., E.J. Sanders, M. Schachter and M. Uddin, 1975, Auto-
    nomic nerve stimulation, kallikrein content and acinar cell
    granules of the cat's submandibular gland, J. Physiol. (Lond.)
    251, 363.
Barton, S., J. Wimalasema and M. Schachter, 1973, Subcellular
    location of the kininogenase in the coagulating gland of the
    guinea-pig, Biochem. Pharmacol. 22, 1121.
Berger, E.A. and E.M. Shooter, 1977, Evidence for pro-B-nerve
    growth factor, a biosynthetic precursor to β-nerve growth
    factor, Proc. Natl. Acad. Sci. 74, 3647.
Brandtzaeg, P., K.M. Gautvik, K. Nustad and J.V. Pierce, 1976, Rat
    submandibular gland kallikreins: purification and cellular
    localization, Brit. J. Pharmacol. 56, 155.
Dietl, T., J. Kruck and H. Fritz, 1978, Localization of kallikrein
    in porcine pancreas and submandibular gland as revealed by
    the indirect fluorescence technique, Hoppe-Seyler's Z. Physiol.
    Chem. 359, 499.
Ekfors, T.O. and V.K. Hopsu-Havu, 1971, Immunofluorescent locali-
    zation of trypsin-like esteropeptidases from the mouse sub-
    mandibular gland, Biochem. Pharmac. 3, 415.
Fiedler, F., W. Ehret, G. Godec, C. Hirschauer, G. Schmidt-Kastner
    and H. Tschesche, The primary structure of pig pancreatic
    kallikrein B, 1977, in: Kininogenases 4, Int. Symp. Acad. Sci.
    Lit., Mainz, eds. G.L. Haberland, J.W. Rohen and T. Suzuki
    (Schattauer, New York-Stuttgart) p. 7-14.
Frey, G.K., H. Kraut and E. Werle, 1968, Das Kallikrein-Kinin
    System und Seine Inhibitoren (Ferdinand Enke, Stuttgart).
Fritz, H., F. Fiedler, T. Dietl, E. Warwas, H. Truscheit, J. Kolb,
    G. Mair and E. Tschesche, On the relationships between por-
    cine, pancreatic, submandibular and urinary kallikreins, 1977,
    in: Kininogenases 4, Int. Symp. Acad. Sci. Lit., Mainz, eds.
    G.L. Haberland, J.W. Rohen and T. Suzuki (Schattauer, New
    York-Stuttgart) p. 15-28.
Hojima, Y., B. Maranda, C. Moriwaki and M. Schachter, 1977, Direct
    evidence for the location of kallikrein in the striated ducts
    of the cat's submandibular gland by the use of specific anti-
    body, J. Physiol. (Lond.) 268, 793.
Kreil, G., 1978, Biochemical surprise of a bee sting, New Scientist
    Aug. 31, 618-620.

Neurath, H. and K.A. Walsh, 1976, Role of proteolytic enzymes in biological regulation, Proc. Natl. Acad. Sci. U.S.A. 73, 3825.

Nustad, K., T.B. Ørstavik, K.M. Gautvik and J.W. Pierce, 1978, Glandular kallikreins, Gen. Pharmacol. 9, 1.

Pisano, J.J. and K.F. Austen, eds., Symposium, Chemistry and Biology of the Kallikrein-Kinin System in Health and Disease, 1976, Fogarty International Center Proceedings, U.S. Govt. Printing Office, Washington, D.C.

Reich, E., D.B. Rifkin and E. Shaw, eds., Symposium, Proteases and Biological Control, 1975, Cold Spring Harbor Conferences on Cell Proliferation, Vol. 2.

Schachter, M., 1969, Kallikreins and kinins, Physiol. Rev. 49, 509.

Schachter, M., B. Maranda and C. Moriwaki, 1978, Localization of kallikrein in the coagulating and submandibular glands of the guinea-pig, J. Histochem. Cytochem. 26, 318.

Schwab, M.E., K. Stockel and H. Thoenen, 1976, Immunocytochemical localization of Nerve Growth Factor (NGF) in the submandibular gland of adult mice by light and electron microscopy. Cell Tissue Res. 169, 289.

Sealey, J.E., S.A. Atlas, J.H. Laragh, N.B. Oza and J.W. Ryan, 1978, Human urinary kallikrein converts inactive to active renin and is a possible physiological activator of renin, Nature (Lond.) 275, 144.

Stroud, R.M., 1974, A family of protein-cutting proteins, Sci. Am. 231, 74.

Wunderer, G., L. Beress, W. Macleidt and H. Fritz, Broad specificity protease inhibitors from sea anemones, 1976, in: Protides of the Biological Fluids, 23rd Colloquium, ed. H. Peeters (Pergamon, Oxford-New York).

IMMUNOGENICITY OF GUINEA-PIG SUBMANDIBULAR AND COAGULATING GLAND KININOGENASES

Kanti D. Bhoola, Jean Higginson[†], Marius J.C. Lemon, Robin W. Matthews[*] and John T. Whicher[†]

Departments of Pharmacology, Dental Medicine[*] and Chemical Pathology[†], University of Bristol, Bristol BS8 1TD, England

ABSTRACT

The antigenic relationship between submandibular and coagulating gland kininogenases of the guinea-pig has been examined using Ouchterlony double diffusion, crossed and rocket immunoelectrophoresis and immunofluorescent techniques. The evidence suggests a partial immunological identity between submandibular and coagulating gland kininogenases of the guinea-pig. In this respect these enzymes seem to differ from the glandular kallikreins of other species (porcine, human and rat) which apparently share a complete immunological identity.

INTRODUCTION

Immunological studies indicate that the glandular kallikreins share a common antigenic identity. Such a relationship has been demonstrated for porcine submandibular, pancreatic and urinary kallikreins by immunodiffusion and immunoelectrophoresis (Fritz, Fiedler, Dietl, Warwas, Truscheit, Kolb, Mair and Tschesche, 1977). Antibodies raised to human urinary kallikrein cross reacted with human saliva and pancreatic juice (Mann and Geiger, 1977). Similarly, antibodies produced against rat urinary kallikrein specifically precipitated rat submandibular kallikrein (Bradtzaeg, Gautvik, Nustad and Pierce, 1976). Because the glandular kallikreins of some of these species appeared to possess complete immunological identity, it was of importance to determine whether such an antigenic relationship existed between the guinea-pig submandibular and coagulating gland kininogenases; particularly since in immunofluorescent studies the submandibular enzyme was localized in both

acini and ducts whereas antibodies raised with coagulating gland
kininogenase only reacted with antigens in the apical region of the
duct cells.

METHODS

Kininogenases: Pooled guinea-pig submandibular glands were
homogenized in ice-cold acetic acid (100 mM), neutralized and the
supernatant mixed with DEAE-cellulose slurry. Subsequent purification was by gel filtration on Sephadex G-100 and chromatography on
DEAE-Sephadex A-50 column. The purified enzyme (SGK_O) was used to
raise antibodies in rabbits. On further purification, SGK_O was
separated into two protein components, one with low (SGK_1) and the
other with high (SGK_2) benzoyl-arginine esterase activity.
Antibodies were raised to both SGK_1 and SGK_2. The coagulating
gland kininogenase (CGK) was purified by Professor C. Moriwaki and
very kindly donated by Professor M. Schachter. The purified CGK
preparation was used to raise antibodies in rabbits.

Unpurified preparations of glandular kininogenases were also
used in the immunoelectrophoretic experiments. The various glands
considered to contain kininogenase activity were homogenised in
ice-cold Tris-HCl buffer (4^oC, 50 mM, pH 7.0).

Immunological techniques: In all gel experiments barbitone
(0.02 m, pH 8.6) buffer was used. The support medium was 1% Litex
HSA agarose. For the crossed immunoelectrophoresis studies samples
containing 1 mg/ml antigen were diluted ten fold with 0.15 M sodium
chloride. 5 µl of the diluted antigen was applied to the first
dimension gel which was carried out at 10 V/cm for 30 min (4^oC).
The second dimension separation was performed at 8 V/cm for 4 hr
(4^oC) in a gel containing 2% antibody. In experiments involving
rocket immunoelectrophoresis samples of purified antigens and gland
homogenates were diluted varyingly between 1 in 2 and 1 in 100 with
0.15 M sodium chloride. 5 µl samples were applied to antibody (2%)
containing gels which were run at 10 V/cm for 2 hr (4^oC).
Ouchterlony double diffusion was performed using 5 µl samples and
a 7 mm spacing between wells. Precipitation of the antigen by the
antibody was allowed to proceed over a period of 24 to 48 hr. On
completion of each experiment, the gels were prepared for staining,
washed and the precipitates visualised with Coomassie Brilliant blue.

Immunofluorescent studies: Freshly removed tissue was frozen
in isopentane chilled in liquid nitrogen. The tissue was freeze
dried, fixed by diethylpyrocarbonate vapour for 3 hr at 60^oC and
embedded in paraffin wax. Fluorescent staining was performed on
dewaxed sections according to Coon's "sandwich" technique.
Specificity of the fluorescence was verified by non-immune serum
and by blocking the antibody with the appropriate antigen. The

fluorescence was visualised on a Leitz Ortholux II microscope.

RESULTS

Ouchterlony double diffusion gels showed a partial fusion of the CGK precipitation line with that of SGK_2 (Fig. 1). This finding suggested that a partial antigenic identity may exist between the coagulating and submandibular gland kininogenases. Immuno-electrophoresis, however, revealed no precipitating antibodies to preparations of submandibular kininogenase (SGK_0, SGK_1 and SGK_2) in the CGK-immune serum and similarly the coagulating gland kinino-genase (CGK) did not react with antisera raised against SGK_0, SGK_1 SGK_2. Two dimensional immunoelectrophoresis of CGK and SGK_0 through a mixture of Anti-CGK and Anti-SGK_0 sera also produced separate and distinct precipitin lines with no evidence of identity. These findings were supported by rocket immunoelectrophoresis experiments. CGK was run through Anti-SGK_2 serum and SGK_2 passed through Anti-CGK without reaction (Fig. 2); each antigen precipitating only antibodies in its own antiserum.

Because CGK reacted immunofluorescently with submandibular gland tissue, the question arose whether its antigenicity could be demonstrated using tissue extracts. Homogenates of mixed coagulating and prostate glands (CG-PG), kidney, pancreas, parotid, sublingual and submandibular glands were electrophoresed through Anti-CGK, Anti-SGK_0, Anti-SGK_1 and Anti-SGK_2 sera. Antibodies in the Anti-CGK serum were precipitated by CG-PG, kidney and pancreas but not by the salivary gland homogenates. Alternatively, precipitation in Anti-SGK_0, Anti-SGK_1 and Anti-SGK_2 sera was observed with the sublingual and submandibular extracts, a trace reaction with pancreas but none with CG-PG.

The Ouchterlony immunodiffusion finding of a partial antigenic identity between CGK and SGK was supported by some of the immunofluorescent studies. Premixing of CGK (1 mg/ml) with Anti-SGK (0.02%) did not block the duct cell localization whereas the reactivity of SGK_2 (but not SGK_0; 1 mg/ml) was reduced by premixing with Anti-CGK (0.02%).

DISCUSSION

The immunodiffusion (Ouchterlony double diffusion) experiments indicate a partial identity between submandibular and coagulating gland kininogenases. However, both cross and rocket immunoelectro-phoresis failed to detect any immunological identity between CGK and SGK_0, SGK_1 or SGK_2. One possible explanation may be that these methods are not sufficiently sensitive to detect partial antigenicity,

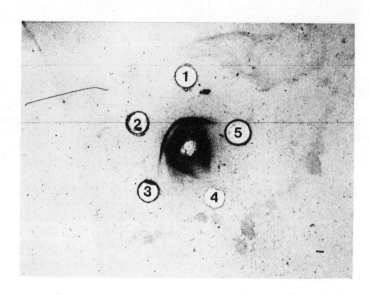

Fig. 1. Immunodiffusion of submandibular and coagulating gland
kininogenases against SGK_2- and CGK- specific rabbit antisera.
C = Centre well containing 5 µl Anti-SGK_2 and 5 µl Anti-CGK. 5 µl
of each antigen (1 mg/ml) was added to the outer wells, 1 = SGK_2
2 = SGK_1, 3 = CGK, 4 = blank, 5 = CGK

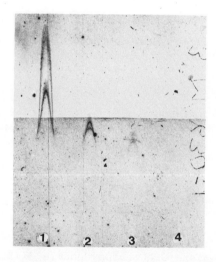

Fig. 2. Rocket immunoelectrophoresis of submandibular gland
kininogenase (SGK_2) through CGK- and SGK_2- specific rabbit antisera.
A = gel containing antiserum to SGK_2 (2%), B = gel containing
antiserum to CGK (2%). 5 µl of different dilutions of SGK_2 was
applied to wells, 1 = 1 mg/ml, 2 = 0.1 mg/ml, 3 = 0.02 mg/ml,
4 = blank.

and probably signify that SGK$_2$ and SGK$_1$ contain some antigenic
determinants that are not present on the CGK molecule.

The finding of a partial identity between the two kininogenases
may explain the common immunofluorescent localization of these
enzymes in the duct cells of the submandibular gland. So far we
have failed to clarify whether the submandibular gland acinar cell
localization of SGK (Bhoola, Matthews and Lemon, 1977) was due to
a granule protein contaminant, precursor molecule of the kininogenase or a low affinity arginine esterase. The submandibular and
coagulating gland kininogenases appear to only share a partial
immunological identity and seem to be different from the glandular
kallikreins of other species which show complete identity.

Acknowledgements: We thank the Wellcome Trust and Royal Society
for financial support. M.J.C. Lemon is a Wellcome Research Fellow.
The Leitz Ortholux II was obtained with a Royal Society Equipment
Grant.

RERERENCES

Bhoola, K.D., M.J.C. Lemon and R.W. Matthews, 1977, Immunofluorescent
    localization of kallikrein in guinea-pig submandibular gland,
    J. Physiol. (Lond.) 272, 28.
Brandtzaeg, P., K.M. Gautvik, K. Nustad and J.V. Pierce, 1976, Rat
    submandibular gland kallikreins: purification and cellular
    localization, Br. J. Pharmac. 56, 155.
Fritz, H., F. Fiedler, T. Dietl, M. Warwas, E. Truscheit, H.J. Kolb,
    G. Mair and H. Tschesche, On the relationships between porcine
    pancreatic, submandibular and urinary kallikreins, 1977, in:
    Kininogenases 4, eds., G.L. Haberland, J.W. Rohen and T. Suzuki
    (F.K. Schattauerverlag, Stuttgart-New York) p.15.
Mann, K. and R. Geiger, Radioimmunoassay of human urinary kallikrein,
    1977, in: Kininogenases 4, eds. G.L. Haberland, J.W. Rohen and
    T. Suzuki (F.K. Schattauerverlag, Stuttgart-New York) p. 55.

STUDIES ON THE BIOLOGICAL FUNCTION OF GLANDULAR KALLIKREIN

E. Fink*, T. Dietl**, J. Seifert***, and H. Fritz*

*Abteilung fur Klinische Chemie und Klinische Biochemie
in der Chirurgischen Klinik der Universitat Munchen,
Nussbaumstr. 20, D-8000 Munchen 2, Germany
**Anatomisches Institut der Universitat Erlangen,
Krakenhausstr. 9, D-8520 Erlangen, Germany
***Institut fur Chirurgische Forschung an der Chirurgischen
Klinik der Universitat Munchen, Nussbaumstr. 20, D-8000
Munchen 2, Germany

INTRODUCTION

The physiological role of glandular kallikrein is still a
matter of speculation. The same holds true for the mechanism of
action by which administered kallikrein produces the many biological effects which have been observed (Haberland et al., 1977).
Investigations which might contribute to the clarification of
these problems include the cellular localization of glandular
kallikrein, the measuring of physiological concentrations in
tissues and body fluids and the tracing of administered kallikrein
within the organism by sensitive and specific assay methods. In
our studies on the physiological role of endogenous glandular
kallikrein and the fate of administered kallikrein we applied
immunofluorescent methods for the cellular localization and the
radioimmunoassay technique for the sensitive and highly specific
measurement of kallikrein in biological samples.

MATERIALS AND METHODS

Materials

Pig pancreatic kallikrein used in cellular localization
studies and in the radioimmunoassay was a highly purified, neura-
minidase treated preparation (Fiedler, 1976) kindly provided by

Dr. F. Fiedler, Munich, guinea pig coagulation gland kallikrein
was a gift of Dr. C. Moriwaki, Tokyo, guinea pig submandibular
gland and pig submandibular gland kallikreins (Lemon et al., 1976)
and pig urinary kallikrein (Tschesche et al. 1976) were kindly
provided by Dr. M. Lemon, Bristol and Dr. G. Mair, Munich. Pig
pancreatic kallikrein used in experiments on intestinal absorption
(1 180 KU/mg) and antisera and immunoglobulin G directed against
pig pancreatic kallikrein were gifts of Bayer AG, Wuppertal.

Radioimmunoassay

The radioimmunoassay for pig pancreatic kallikrein is described
elsewhere (Fink and Guttel, 1978).

Gel Filtration

For gel filtration experiments Sephacryl S 200, Pharmacia,
was used. Column size: 0.9 x 95 cm, elution buffer: 0.015 mol/1
NaH_2PO_4, 0.15 mol/1 NaCl, 0.01 mol/1 EDTA, 200 mg/1 NaN_3, pH 7.4,
flow rate: 3-4 ml/h.

Cellular Localization

Production of kallikrein antibodies, tissue preparation and
indirect immunofluorescent technique are described elsewhere
(Dietl et al., 1978).

RESULTS AND DISCUSSION

Radioimmunoassay

The determination of kallikrein is generally achieved by
measuring the rate of hydrolysis either of synthetic substrates or
of the natural substrate kininogen. These assays are not specific
for kallikrein, since the substrates are hydrolyzed also by other
proteases. For physiological studies, which include the measurement of kallikrein in tissues and body fluids where other proteases
may be present, a more specific assay is required. This requirement is met by the radioimmunoassay technique.

With the radioimmunoassay developed in our laboratory (Fink
and Guttel, 1978) the lower detection limit for pig pancreatic
kallikrein is 40 - 300 pg, corresponding to concentrations of 0.2
- 1.5 ng/ml. The assay is highly specific for pig glandular kallikreins. Pig urinary and pig submandibular kallikreins show an
immunological reactivity indistinguishable from that of pig pancreatic kallikrein under radioimmunoassay conditions as indicated
by the parallel dose-response curves (Fig. 1). No cross-reactivity
was detected with porcine trypsin, bovine trypsin and chymotrypsin

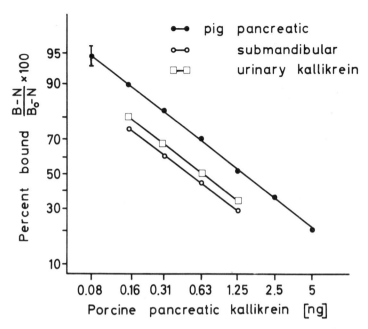

Fig. 1. Dose-response curves of pig glandular kallikrein.

and kallikreins of guinea pig submandibular glands and guinea pig coagulation glands.

Intestinal Absorption

The radioimmunoassay was employed to investigate whether kallikrein can be absorbed in the intestinal tract using the rat as a model (Fink et al., 1978; Fink et al., in press). The experiments were done both with rats which had fasted for 24 hr and with unfasted rats. 10 mg hog pancreatic kallikrein dissolved in 1 ml 0.9% saline were injected into the lumen of the duodenum of anesthetized rats. Lymphatic fluid, collected from the thoracic duct, and blood samples, drawn from the tail vein, were measured by radioimmunoassay. Kallikrein was detected in the samples in concentrations up to 200 ng/ml within 4 hr after injection, demonstrating that intestinal absorption had taken place. However, the absorption kinetics were highly variable within series of identical experiments, both with fasted and unfasted rats, in some experiments even no absorption at all was observed. Figure 2 gives an example of two completely different absorption kinetics, the two experiments were done under identical conditions with fasted rats.

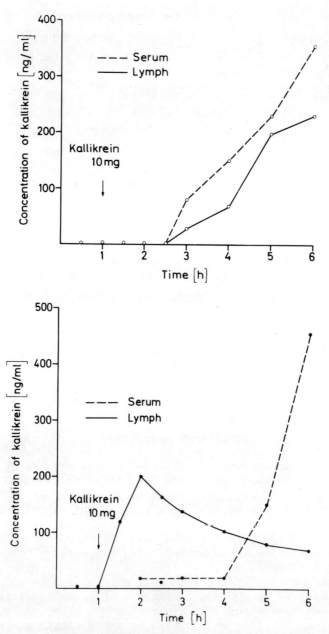

Fig. 2. Kinetics of intestinal absorption of pig pancreatic
         kallikrein into serum and lymph of rats after intra-
         duodenal administration.

In Table 1 those two rats of the fasted and unfasted group
are compared which showed the highest absorption within each group.
The data suggest that fasting has a stimulating effect on the
intestinal absorption of kallikrein.

Table 1.

INTESTINAL ABSORPTION OF PIG PANCREATIC
KALLIKREIN IN THE RAT

	Rat A (without fasting)	Rat B (24 hr fasting)
Dose administered	10 mg	10 mg
Total amount of kallikrein in lymphatic fluid	300 ng (30 ppm)	15,000 ng (1,500 ppm)
Maximal concentration in lymphatic fluid	800 ng/ml	33,000 ng/ml
Maximal concentration in serum	700 ng/ml	4,700 ng/ml

In order to clarify, whether or not the radioimmunoassayable
material consisted of low molecular weight degradation products,
samples of lymphatic fluid were subjected to gel filtration and
the eluate was tested by radioimmunoassay (Fig. 3). Two main
peaks of immunochemically reactive material were found, the smaller
one in an elution position corresponding to the molecular weight
of about 80,000, indicating that most of the absorbed kallikrein
was bound to a plasma protein, probably α_1-antitrypsin. Immunochemically reactive material could not be found in the low
molecular weight region where degradation products are to be
expected.

In spite of the high variability discussed above our results
demonstrate that glandular kallikrein can be absorbed by the intestine without detectable degradation. The partial binding to -
presumably - α_1-antitrypsin suggests that a large part of the absorbed kallikrein is enzymatically active. Furthermore, the
results indicate a significant role of the lymphatics in the
intestinal absorption of pancreatic kallikrein, in addition to the
absorption via mesenteric vein routes. Absorption via mesenteric
vein route was demonstrated also by Moriwaki et al. (1973) using
a mesenteric perfusion system.

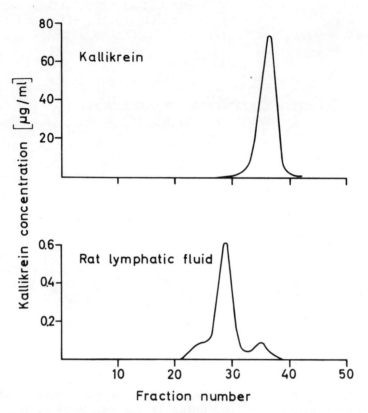

Fig. 3.   Gel filtration of pig pancreatic kallikrein and rat
          lymph (from experiments on intestinal absorption) on
          Sephacryl S 200. The fractions were assayed for pig
          pancreatic kallikrein by radioimmunoassay.

Glandular Kallikrein in Blood

The radioimmunoassay was further applied to investigate
whether endogenous glandular kallikrein is present in the blood.
We found glandular kallikrein in pig serum in concentrations of
10 - 20 ng/ml (Fink et al. 1978; Fink et al., in press). In order
to ascertain that the radioimmunoassayable substance was not a low
molecular weight degradation product, serum samples were subjected
to gel filtration and the fractions tested by radioimmunoassay.
Generally two peaks were found, one in the elution position of
kallikrein, the other one in a position which would correspond to
the complex with α_1-antitrypsin (Fig. 4). In similar experiments
with boar seminal plasma mainly one peak was detected corresponding

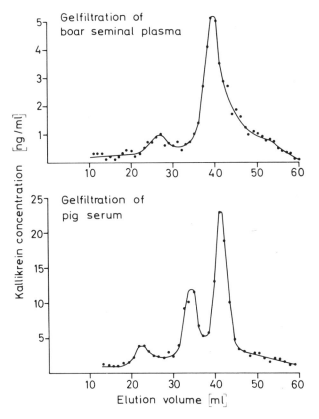

Fig. 4. Gel filtration of boar seminal plasma and pig serum
         on Sephacryl S 200. The fractions were assayed by a
         radioimmunoassay for pig pancreatic kallikrein.

to free kallikrein. Comparable results were found both for human
blood (Fink et al. 1978; Geiger et al., this volume) and for rat
blood (Nustad et al. 1978). Hence, the occurrence of glandular
kallikreins in the blood is established now for three species.
The exact origin of the glandular kallikrein in blood is unknown.
The discrimination by radioimmunoassay is impossible because of
the immunological cross-reactivity of the various glandular kallikreins (Fig. 1). The findings of other authors and our observations
suggest that glandular kallikreins have access to the circulation
via intestinal absorption and/or via release into the local
glandular circulation.

Renal Excretion of Glandular Kallikrein

The presence of glandular kallikrein in blood leads us to the assumption that renal excretion might contribute to some extent to the amount of kallikrein present in urine. Some recent experiments on the renal excretion of pig pancreatic kallikrein after intravenous infusion into dogs corroborate this assumption.

0.5 mg pig pancreatic kallikrein, dissolved in 250 ml saline, were infused over a period of 2 hr into the femoral vein of anesthetized dogs. Blood samples were drawn every 15 or 30 min from the femoral artery. Urine was collected from the two catheterized ureters. The results of one experiment are summarized in Figure 5.

The plasma level of pig pancreatic kallikrein during the infusion (about 45 ng/ml) was comparable to the physiological concentration in porcine blood (10-20 ng). The fact that the kallikrein concentration in the urine samples was twice to three times higher than in plasma, demonstrates that the kallikrein found in urine was excreted by the kidney, and did not originate from the small amount of blood by which the urine samples were contaminated. The lower panel in Figure 5 shows the amounts of kallikrein excreted during each urine collection period. The total excreted kallikrein amounted to 2% of the administered dose.

These results demonstrate that glandular kallikrein can be excreted by the kidney. This is not surprising considering that glomerular filtration of proteins with molecular weights up to 70,000 is possible, and that the molecular weight of pig pancreatic kallikrein is only about 30,000 (for other glandular kallikreins, values of 25,000 - 45,000 are reported). Taking into account that glandular kallikrein is physiologically present in the blood, as demonstrated by radioimmunoassays for man, pig and rat, it seems very likely to us that urinary kallikrein is not pure kidney kallikrein but contains also other glandular kallikrein(s).

Cellular Localization

For cellular localization studies we employed the indirect immunofluorescence technique on cryosections of pig submandibular gland, kidney and pancreas (Dietl et al. 1978).

Submandibular gland. Strong and specific fluorescence indicates location of kallikrein in striated and also collecting ducts of the submandibular gland (Fig. 6). Kallikrein is present there in the apical portion of the duct cells, where the zymogen granules are located. Our results are in agreement with the

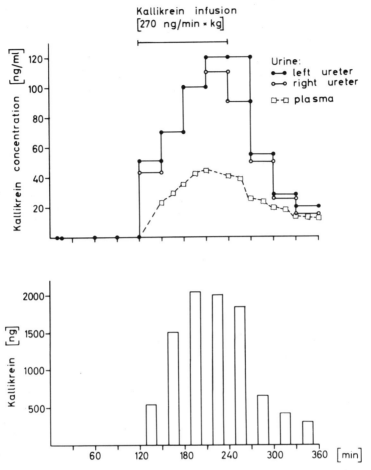

Fig. 5.   Renal excretion of pig pancreatic kallikrein infused
          into the femoral artery of a dog. The samples were
          assayed for pig pancreatic kallikrein by radioimmunoassay.

location of kallikrein in submandibular glands of rat and cat as
described by other groups (Berg Ørstavik et al. 1975; Brandtzaeg
et al. 1976; Hojima et al. 1977). Only in guinea pigs additional
fluorescence was found in acinar cells (Bhoola et al. 1977).

   Pancreas. In the pancreas strong and specific fluorescence
could be observed in the acinar cells, mainly in the apical regions
(Figure 7a and b). In contrast to the submandibular gland, we
observed no specific fluorescence in the interlobular ducts of
the pancreas. The islets of Langerhans were also unstained. This

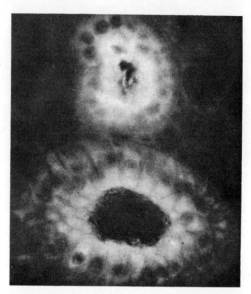

Fig. 6.   Localization of kallikrein in porcine submandibular
          gland as revealed by immunofluorescence (x 400)(Dietl
          et al. 1978).

indicates that pancreatic kallikrein is, like other proteases,
located in the exocrine cells. We suppose, therefore, that the
zymogen granules in the apical region of the acinar cells contain
the kallikrein.

    Kidney. Differing from the results in the rat kidney, where
kallikrein was found in the distal tubular cells (Ørstavik et al.
1976) by direct fluorescence-antibody technique, no proper localization of kallikrein was achieved by us in the porcine kidney:
Specific fluorescence could not be observed by employing the same
technique as for porcine pancreas and submandibular glands. This
might be due to the much lower amount of kallikrein present in the
kidney compared to pancreas and submandibular gland or to a special
mode of binding of kallikrein to kidney organelles so that its
antigenic sites are inaccessible to the antibody.

    Immunological crossreactivity. In immunodiffusion experiments
precipitation patterns of identity were obtained for porcine
kallikreins from pancreas, submandibular gland and urine with
antibodies directed against each of the kallikreins. When we
applied the three antibodies in the localization studies, each of
them yielded the same immunofluorescence pattern in the submandi-

bular gland and in the pancreas, respectively. This finding demonstrates that the tissue-bound kallikreins, probably prekallikreins,
also crossreact with antibodies produced against the three active
enzymes.

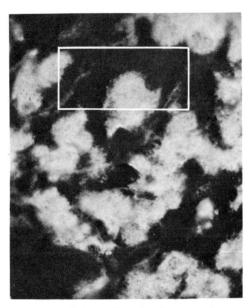

Fig. 7a. Localization of kallikrein in porcine pancreas as
          revealed by immunofluorescence (x 400) (Dietl et al.
          1978).

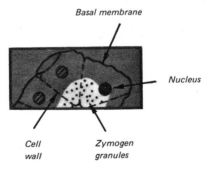

Fig. 7b. Schematic drawing of acinar cells. Nucleus and basal
          membranes, but not cell walls, are visible in Fig. 7a.
          Zymogen granules are located in the region of fluores-
          cence (Dietl et al. 1978).

ACKNOWLEDGEMENTS

This work was generously supported by grants of the Deutsche Forschungsgemeinschaft (Fi 204/3,4 and Sonderforschungsbereich 51, Munchen). We are very grateful to Prof. C. Scriba for the kind permission to use the facilities of his laboratory for radioactive work. The excellent technical assistance of Mrs. C. Guttel, Mrs. E. Kraus and Mrs. H. Kruck is greatly appreciated. We are also indebted to Dr. M. Warwas (scholarship holder of the Alexander von Humboldt-Stiftung) for immunizations of rabbits and for isolation of antikallikrein IgG fractions.

REFERENCES

Bhoola, K.D., M.J.C. Lemon and R.W. Matthews (1977). Immunofluorescent localization of kallikrein in the guinea pig submandibular gland. J. Physiol. 272, 28P.

Bollmann, J.L., J. Cain and J.H. Grindlay (1948). Techniques for the collection of lymph from the liver, small intestine, or thoracic duct of the rat. J. Lab. Clin. Med. 33, 1349-1352.

Brandtzaeg, P., K. Gautvik, K. Nustad and J. Pierce (1976). Rat submandibular gland kallikreins: purification and cellular localization. Brit. J. Pharmacol. 56, 155-167.

Dietl, T., J. Kruck and H. Fritz (1978). Localization of kallikrein in porcine pancreas and submandibular gland as revealed by the indirect immunofluorescence technique. Hoppe-Seylers Z. Physiol. Chem. 359, 499-505.

Fiedler, F.(1976). Pig pancreatic kallikreins A and B. In: L. Lorand (Ed.), Methods in Enzymology, Vol. 45, Academic Press, New York, pp. 289-303.

Fink, E. and C. Guttel (1978). Development of a radioimmunoassay for pig pancreatic kallikrein. J. Clin. Chem. Clin. Biochem. 16, 381-385.

Fink, E., J. Seifert and C. Guttel (1978). Development of a radioimmunoassay for pig pancreatic kallikrein and its application in physiological studies. Fresenius Z. Anal. Chem. 290, 183.

Fink, E., J. Seifert, R. Geiger and C. Guttel (in press). Studies on the physiological function of glandular kallikrein by radioimmunoassay. In: Current Concepts in Kinin Research, G. L. Haberland and U. Hamberg (Eds.), Pergamon Press, Oxford

Geiger, R., E. Fink, K. Mann, U. Stuckstedte and B. Forg-Brey (this volume). Human urinary kallikrein-Biochemical and physiological aspects.

Haberland, G.L., J.W. Rohen and T. Suzuki (1977). Kininogenases IV. Kallikrein, F.K. Schattauer Verlag, Stuttgart - New York.

Hojima, Y., B. Maranda, C. Moriwaki and M. Schachter (1977). Direct evidence for the location of kallikrein in the striated ducts of the cat's submandibular gland by the use of specific antibody. J. Physiol. 268, 793-801.

Lemon, M., B. Forg-Brey, and H. Fritz (1976). Isolation of por-
     cine submaxillary kallikrein. In: F. Sicuteri, N. Back and
     G.L. Haberland (Eds.), Kinins. Pharmacodynamics and Biological
     Roles. Plenum Press, New York and London, pp. 209-216.
Moriwaki, C., H. Moriya, K. Yamaguchi, K. Kizuki and H. Fujimori
     (1973). Intestinal absorption of pancreatic kallikrein and
     some aspects of its physiological role. In: G.L. Haberland
     and J.W. Rohen (Eds.), Kininogenases I. Kallikrein, F.K.
     Schattauer Verlag, Stuttgart - New York, pp. 57-66.
Nustad, K., B. Østavik, K.M. Gautvik and J.V. Pierce (1978).
     Glandular kallikreins. Gen. Pharmac. 9, 1-9.
Ørstavik, B., P. Brandtzaeg, K. Nustad and K. Halvorsen (1975).
     Cellular localization of kallikreins in rat submandibular
     and sublingual salivary glands. Immunofluorescence tracing
     related to histological characteristics. Acta histochem. 54,
     183-192.
Ørstavik, T.B., K. Nustad, P. Brandtzaeg and J.V. Pierce (1976).
     Cellular origin of urinary kallikreins. J. Histochem. Cyto-
     chem. 24, 1037-1039.
Seifert, J. (1976). Enterale Resorption grossmolekularer Proteine
     bei Tieren und Menschen. Z. f. Ernahrungswissenschaft, Suppl.
     18.
Tschesche, H., G. Mair, B. Forg-Brey and H. Fritz (1976). Isolation
     of porcine urinary kallikrein. In: F. Sicuteri, N. Back and
     G.L. Haberland (Eds.), Kinins. Pharmacodynamics and Biological
     Roles, Plenum Press, New York and London, pp. 119-122.

ENDOTHELIAL CELLS AND COMPONENTS OF THE KALLIKREIN-KININ SYSTEM

Una S. Ryan, James W. Ryan, Douglas L. Habliston, and
Guillermo A. Pena

Department of Medicine, University of Miami School of
Medicine, Miami, Florida 33101, USA

ABSTRACT

Endothelial cells are a major source of kininase enzymes
including kininase II. Kininase II is situated along the plasma
membrane, not as an ecto-enzyme but as an enzyme synthesized by
the endothelial cells themselves. However, it is likely that
endothelial cells do more than degrade kinins. These cells are
contractile and may possess kinin receptors; a possibility supported by the fact that kinins stimulate endothelial cells to form
and release prostaglandin-related substances. In addition, we
have found that endothelial cells in culture are reactive with
antibodies to α_2-macroglobulin. Endothelial cells can hydrolyze
$[^3H]$Pro-Phe-Arg-anilide, a kallikrein substrate, but the reaction
is not inhibited by soya bean trypsin inhibitor (SBTI) or Trasylol.
Possibly kallikrein or a related trypsin-like enzyme is bound to
α_2-macroglobulin and is not free to react with the inhibitors.
Thus, endothelial cells can bind and inhibit kallikrein-like
enzymes, degrade kinins and respond to kinin stimulation.

INTRODUCTION

As is well known, endothelial cells, especially those of the
lungs, possess enzymes capable of inactivating kinins (Ryan and
Smith, 1973; Ryan and Ryan, 1975; Ryan et al., 1975, 1976a,b,c).
Thus, only a small fraction of kinins arriving in central venous
blood survive passage into the systemic arterial circulation (cf.
Ferreira and Vane, 1967). Kininase II is perhaps the best known
of these enzymes, but a number of other enzymes also participate
(Ryan et al., 1968, 1970a).

Much of the present understanding of the disposition of
kininase enzymes on pulmonary endothelial cells has come from
studies in which the cells were maintained in culture (cf. Ryan
and Smith, 1973; Chiu et al., 1975; Ryan et al., 1976b, 1978a).
Through our examination of endothelial cells in culture, it has
become evident that endothelial cells possess other components
which may affect the overall functioning of the kallikrein-kinin
system and the renin-angiotensin system. The cells possess
plasminogen activator (Loskotoff and Dieter, 1978), a kallikrein-
like enzyme, and α_2-macroglobulin antigen. Further, their
responses to kinins in terms of prostaglandin release may imply
the existence of receptors (see also Ryan, U.S., et al., this
volume).

MATERIALS AND METHODS

Isolation and Culture of Endothelial Cells

Cells of bovine main-stem pulmonary artery and of guinea pig
pulmonary vascular bed were isolated and maintained in culture
using methods described previously (Ryan et al., 1976b, 1978a;
Habliston et al., in press). The kininase II inhibitor, BPP_{9a},
was synthesized in this laboratory. SQ 14,225 was the kind gift
of Dr. Z. Horovitz, Squibb Institute for Medical Research).

Assays

Unless noted otherwise, angiotensin converting enzyme was
assayed using [^{3}H]benzoyl-Phe-Ala-Pro as described by Ryan et al.
(1978b). Kallikrein-like activity was measured using the radioassay described elsewhere in this volume (Chung et al.). Protein
was measured by the Folin-Lowry method or by the use of the Bio-Rad
reagents for microanalysis of protein. Intrinsically labelled
kinins and α-L-Asp-[^{3}H]benzylamide were provided by Alfred Chung.
Studies of α_2-macroglobulin were performed using reagents from
Behring Diagnostics (Calbiochem). ^{14}C-Arachidonic acid was
obtained from Amersham Corp. and ^{14}C- and ^{3}H-ADP were obtained from
New England Nuclear Corp.

RESULTS AND DISCUSSION

Synthesis of Kininase II

Previously we have shown that the kininase II activity of
endothelial cells is not lost during culture. Endothelial cells in
their 59th passage show no diminution of kininase II activity.
However, as a routine, our cells are carried in medium containing
fetal calf serum, itself a source of kininase II. Thus, further to

clarify the origins of kininase II, we cultured bovine pulmonary artery endothelial cells using heat-inactivated fetal calf serum (cf. Das and Soffer, 1976). Kininase II does not survive heating at 56°C.

The primary cultures were propagated through 4 passages. The average number of progeny in the 4th passage was 6,400 with respect to each cell in the original isolate. The cells were assayed using [^{3}H]benzoyl-Phe-Ala-Pro (Ryan et al., 1978b) as substrate. The specificity of the assay was tested by using SQ 14,225 (10^{-5} M), a specific inhibitor of angiotensin converting enzyme (Ondetti et al., 1977). The results are summarized in the Table.

Table 1

SYNTHESIS OF ANGIOTENSIN CONVERTING ENZYME
BY PULMONARY ENDOTHELIAL CELLS

Endothelial cells of 14 pulmonary arteries (calf) were seeded into five 25 cm^2 flasks at a density of approx. 10^5 cells/flask. The cells were grown to confluency (~5 days). Three flasks were used for assays and two were transferred (trypsinization) to five new flasks. Every five days the process was repeated until the fourth passage was obtained at confluency. The fetal calf serum used in these experiments was heated at 56°C for 30 min.

Passage	Cells/flask	Progeny/ orig. cell	ACE/cell* (μ units)
1	10^6	10	0.533
2	10^6	100	0.647
3	8.5×10^5	850	0.471
4	7.6×10^5	6,400	1.035

Overall increase of ACE per original cell:

12,428-fold

*ACE = angiotensin converting enzyme. Enzyme activity was measured as described in the text (cf. Ryan et al., 1978b).

(Reproduced with permission of the publishers from Ryan, U.S., E. Clements, D. Habliston and J.W. Ryan, Tissue & Cell, 10, 535, 1978)

Inhibition of Kininase II

As we have reported at previous kinin symposia (Ryan and Ryan, 1976; Ryan et al., 1976c), kininase II is situated along the luminal surface of endothelial cells. However, there are a number of other enzymes capable of inactivating bradykinin, and their cellular and subcellular dispositions are less clearly defined. As a practical matter, it would appear to be important to obtain clearer characterization of the other enzymes in both cellular and molecular terms. If current clinical trials using SQ 14,225 continue to be successful, it is likely that as many as 10 million patients in the U.S.A, and far more worldwide, will be under treatment with drugs that inhibit angiotensin converting enzyme (kininase II). This means that a large number of people will have to find means of living without kininase II.

We have found that even relatively large concentrations of SQ 14,225 do not prevent endothelial cells in culture from inactivating bradykinin. Two flasks of guinea pig lung endothelial cells (each flask with approx. 10^6 endothelial cells) were incubated at 37°C with $[^3H]Phe^5$-bradykinin (7 Ci/mmole; 10 ng/ml in 5 ml of medium 199), with or without SQ 14,225 at 10^{-7} M. At timed intervals (5-30 min), samples were collected, heated in a boiling water bath for 5 min, and then applied to a Bio-Gel P-2 column (1.1 by 100 cm). A blank incubation mixture (medium 199 and $[^3H]$-Phe^5-bradykinin, but without cells) was examined in parallel. In the absence of cells, bradykinin was not degraded. However, the cells rapidly degraded bradykinin. Only the pattern of degradation was changed by SQ 14,225. In the absence of SQ 14,225, $[^3H]Phe^5$-bradykinin was metabolized to yield four radioactive metabolites: Phe-Ser (53%) and three larger peptides, which are not yet identified. In the presence of SQ 14,225, two radioactive metabolites were formed: des-Arg^1-bradykinin and the C-terminal pentapeptide, Phe^5---Arg^9. We were unable to find evidence of the participation of a carboxypeptidase B-like enzyme. Nonetheless, even at the shortest time interval, using a relatively small number of cells, SQ 14,225 did not preserve bradykinin. It would appear that there are important alternative means by which bradykinin can be eliminated.

Kallikrein-like Enzymes

Other members of our laboratory (Chung et al., this volume) have developed a sensitive, apparently highly selective radioassay for kallikrein. The assay uses Pro-Phe-Arg-$[^3H]$benzylamide as substrate, and enzyme is measured in terms of formation of $[^3H]$-benzylamide.

The substrate is hydrolyzed briskly by endothelial cells in monolayer culture, in suspension, or as a homogenate, all at pH 8.0 or pH 9.5. At pH 8.0, substrate (400 nM) was hydrolyzed at a rate of $1\%/min/10^6$ cells. However, the reaction is not inhibited by soya bean trypsin inhibitor (10 µg/ml), and is inhibited only weakly (~15%) with Trasylol (10 µg/ml). If, in fact, the relevant enzyme is a kallikrein-like enzyme, its response to inhibitors is reminiscent of results obtained when kallikrein is bound to a α_2-macroglobulin (cf. Vogt and Dugal, 1977). Clearly, further characterization is required, yet it should be emphasized (see below) that bovine pulmonary artery endothelial cells are reactive with antibodies to human α_2-macroglobulin.

Plasmin is unlikely to explain our result, as it shows little reactivity with Pro-Phe-Arg-[^{3}H]benzylamide. Similarly, cathepsin B would not be expected to have much activity at relatively high pH. If the activity of angiokinase or plasminogen activator parallels that of urokinase, the substrate would not be hydrolyzed. Urokinase does not hydrolyze Pro-Phe-Arg-[^{3}H]benzylamide at pH 8.0 or 9.5 (Chung et al., this volume).

Kallikrein Inhibitors

As mentioned above, bovine pulmonary endothelial cells are reactive with antibodies to α_2-macroglobulin (cf. Ryan et al., 1978a; see also Becker and Harpel, 1976). However, this may not show that endothelial cells are capable of inhibiting kallikrein via α_2-macroglobulin.

Both Harpel (1976) and Vogt and Dugal (1977) have shown that the inhibitor-enzyme complex loses its reactivity to antibodies against plasmin or kallikrein, but retains its reactivity with antibodies to α_2-macroglobulin. It has not been ruled out that endothelial cells, like macrophages, possess receptors for inhibitor-enzyme complex. However, either possibility is worth pursuing: Free α_2-macroglobulin associated with endothelial cells might provide a means of limiting the action of plasmin or kallikrein within the vascular space. On the other hand, receptors for inhibitor-enzyme complex would have implications for elimination of the complex.

As a point of technical interest, free inhibitor might help explain why relatively large amounts of trypsin are required to lift endothelial monolayers from their culture flasks.

Converting Enzymes

The occurrence of angiotensin converting enzyme on endothelial cells has been discussed previously. However, it appears likely that other converting enzymes also occur. Johnson and Erdös (1977)

have reported evidence of an aminopeptidase A-like enzyme
associated with human umbilical vein endothelial cells, and we have
found an enzyme capable of hydrolyzing α-L-Asp-[^{3}H]benzylamide,
using bovine pulmonary artery endothelial cells in monolayer
culture. The enzyme is inhibited completely by penicillamine at
10^{-4} M and by EDTA at 10^{-3} M. The use of monolayers is important
in our view, as enzymic activities demonstrable with cells in
monolayer culture imply that at least a portion of the enzyme has
access to exterior substrates. Whether the substrate remains in
the extracellular space has bearing on the disposition of the
active site of the enzyme. We have found that Asp-[^{3}H]benzylamide
is hydrolyzed, but is not taken up by endothelial cells in monolayer culture.

Whether our data can be interpreted in terms of the mechanisms
by which angiotensin II is converted into angiotensin III remains
to be seen. However, in our early studies on the conversion of
angiotensin I into angiotensin II by isolated lungs, we found that
a major metabolite of [^{14}C]Leu^{10}-angiotensin I is a ^{14}C-labelled
metabolite not distinguished from des-Asp^1-angiotensin I (Ryan et
al., 1970b).

Contractility

Majno and colleagues have adduced indirect data in support of
the concept that endothelial cells are capable of contraction
(Majno, 1965). Further, we and others have shown that endothelial
cells, especially those of pulmonary artery (Smith et al., 1971;
Smith and Ryan, 1973) and cells of the bronchial circulation
(Pietra et al., 1971), contain actin-like filaments. The actin-
like filaments are clearly visible in endothelial cells in culture
(Ryan et al., 1978a). Becker and Murphy (1969) have shown endothelial cells to be reactive with antibodies to actinomyosin of
uterine smooth muscle. Bovine endothelial cells removed from
pulmonary arteries by collagenase digestion are detached as sheets
linked by junctions as in situ. The cuboidal shape of the isolated
cells is much like the shape endothelium assumes in constricted
arterioles (Fig. 1).

Fig. 1. Electron micrograph of freshly isolated endothelial cells
obtained from calf pulmonary artery by washing with 0.25% collagenase. The endothelial cells detach as sheets and are centrifuged
to obtain a pellet. Sections of the pellet indicate that the
isolated cells retain their polarity, the original luminal surface
having smoother contours, while the abluminal surface shows many
anchoring processes and traces of basement membrane (*). The cells
are linked by junctions (arrows) as in situ. The cuboidal shape of
the cells and irregular nuclear outlines suggest that the cells are
capable of contracting even after removal from adjoining smooth
muscle layers.   x   5,000

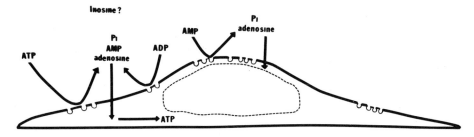

Fig. 3. Metabolism of adenine nucleotides by pulmonary endothelial cells.

Kinins and Prostaglandin Synthesis

Endothelial cells incubated with $1-^{14}C$-arachidonate rapidly remove arachidonate from the culture medium and then release ^{14}C-metabolites (Ryan et al., 1978c). In our experience PGE_2 is the major product, but a substance which is not distinguished from 6-keto-prostaglandin $F_{1\alpha}$, a breakdown product of PGI_2, is released in highly variable quantities. A difference chromatogram obtained in one such experiment is shown in figure 2.

Once labelled with $1-^{14}C$-arachidonic acid, pulmonary endothelial cells in culture respond to bradykinin (0.1 - 1 mg/ml) by releasing precisely the same pattern of metabolites. Under these latter conditions, arachidonic acid itself does not appear to be released into the culture medium. Possibly all of the arachidonate presumed to be mobilized by kinin-stimulated phospholipase is processed intracellularly.

CONCLUDING REMARKS

Although it has been evident for some time that pulmonary endothelial cells do more than provide a barrier between blood and air (cf. Heinemann and Fishman, 1969; Smith and Ryan, 1973), it seems likely that we are only approaching the threshold of understanding of how these cells participate in hemostasis and in the overall functioning of the kallikrein-kinin system and renin-angiotensin system. However, it would be a mistake to limit considerations only to these three areas.

We have shown that pulmonary endothelial cells metabolize the adenine nucleotides, AMP and ATP (Smith and Ryan, 1970a; Ryan and Smith, 1971). More recently Crutchley et al. (1978) have shown that ADP is cleared during passage through isolated, blood-free lungs, and we have found that a vigorous ADPase enzyme occurs on the surface of pulmonary endothelial cells in culture (Habliston et al., 1978; Ryan et al., in preparation). As a by-product of the latter study, it became evident that lung cells like those of the aorta (Pearson et al., 1978; Alain Junod, personal communication) rapidly take up adenosine, the second product formed on metabolism of ADP, and reincorporate it into intracellular ATP (see Fig. 3). Clearly there is much more to be learned about the metabolic properties of cells in general and pulmonary endothelial cells in particular.

REFERENCES

Becker, C.G. and P.C. Harpel, 1976. α_2-Macroglobulin on human vascular endothelium. J. Exp. Med., 144: 1.

Becker, C.G. and G.E. Murphy, 1969. Demonstration of contractile protein in endothelium and cells of the heart valves, endocardium, intima, arteriosclerotic plaques, and Aschoff bodies of rheumatic heart disease. Am. J. Pathol., 55: 1.

Chiu, A.T., J.W. Ryan, U.S. Ryan and F.E. Dorer, 1975. A sensitive radiochemical assay for angiotensin converting enzyme (kininase II). Biochem. J., 149: 297.

Chung, A.C., J.W. Ryan, G.A. Pena and N.B. Oza. (this volume). A simple radioassay for human urinary kallikrein.

Crutchley, D.J., T.E. Eling and M.W. Anderson, 1978. ADPase activity of isolated perfused rat lung. Life Sciences. 22: 1413.

Das, M. and R.L. Soffer, 1976. Pulmonary angiotensin converting enzyme antienzyme antibody. Biochemistry, 15: 5088.

Ferreira, S.H. and J.R. Vane, 1967. The disappearance of bradykinin and eledoisin in the circulation and vascular beds of the cat. Br. J. Pharmac., 30: 417.

Habliston, D.L., C. Whitaker, M.A. Hart, U.S. Ryan and J.W. Ryan, (in press). Isolation and culture of endothelial cells from the lungs of small animals. Amer. Rev. Resp. Dis.

Harpel, P.C., Circulating inhibitors of human plasma kallikrein, 1976. In: Chemistry and Biology of the Kallikrein-Kinin System in Health and Disease, eds. J.J. Pisano and K.F. Auster, (U.S. Government Printing Office, Washington, D.C.), p. 169.

Heinemann, H.O. and A.P. Fishman, 1969. Nonrespiratory functions of mammalian lung. Physiol. Rev., 49: 1.

Johnson, A.R. and E.G. Erdos, 1977. Metabolism of vasoactive peptides by human endothelial cells in culture, J. Clin. Invest. 59: 684.

Loskutoff, D.J. and P. Dieter, 1978. Intracellular plasminogen activator activity in growing and quiescent cells. J. Cell Physiol., 97: 9.

Majno, G., Ultrastructure of the vascular membrane, 1965. In: Handbook of Physiology, (Am. Physiol. Soc.), p. 2293.

Ondetti, M.A., B. Rubin and D.W. Cushman, 1977. Design of specific
    inhibitors of angiotensin converting enzyme: New class of
    orally active antihypertensive agents. Science. 196: 441.
Pearson, J.D., J.S. Carleton, A. Hutchings and J.L. Gordon, 1978.
    Uptake and metabolism of adenosine by pig aortic endothelial
    and smooth-muscle cells in culture. Biochem. J., 170: 265.
Pietra, G.G., J.P. Szidon, M.M. Leventhal and A.P. Fishman, 1971.
    Histamine and interstitial pulmonary edema in the dog. Circ.
    Res., 29: 323.
Ryan, J.W., A. Chung, L.C. Martin and U.S. Ryan, 1978b. New sub-
    strates for the radioassay of angiotensin converting enzyme
    of endothelial cells in culture. Tissue & Cell, 10: 555.
Ryan, J.W., A.R. Day, U.S. Ryan, A. Chung, D.I. Marlborough and
    F.E. Dorer, 1976. Localization of angiotensin converting
    enzyme (kininase II), Tissue & Cell, 8: 111.
Ryan, J.W., J. Roblero and J.M. Stewart, 1968. Inactivation of
    bradykinin in the pulmonary circulation. Biochem. J. 110: 795.
Ryan, J.W., J. Roblero and J.M. Stewart, 1970a. Inactivation of
    bradykinin in rat lung. Adv. Exp. Med. Biol., 8: 263.
Ryan, J.W. and U.S. Ryan. Biochemical and morphological aspects of
    the actions and metabolism of kinins, 1976. In: Chemistry
    and Biology of the Kallikrein-Kinin System in Health and
    Disease, eds. J.J. Pisano and K.F. Austen, (U.S. Government
    Printing Office, Washington, D.C.), p. 315.
Ryan, J.W. and U.S. Ryan. Metabolic activities of plasma membrane
    and caveolae of pulmonary endothelial cells, with a note on
    pulmonary prostaglandin synthetase, 1975. In: Lung Metabolism,
    eds. A.F. Junod and R. de Haller, (Academic Press, New York),
    p. 399.
Ryan, J.W., U.S. Ryan, D.H. Habliston and L. C. Martin. 1978a. (in
    press). Synthesis of prostaglandins by pulmonary endothelial
    cells. Trans. Assoc. Amer. Phys.
Ryan, J.W., U.S. Ryan, D.R. Schultz, C. Whitaker, A. Chung and
    F.E. Dorer, 1975. Subcellular localization of pulmonary angio-
    tensin converting enzyme (kininase II). Biochem. J., 146: 497.
Ryan, J.W., J.M. Stewart, W.P. Leary and J.G. Ledingham, 1970b.
    Metabolism of angiotensin I in pulmonary circulation, Biochem.
    J., 120: 221.
Ryan, J.W. and U. Smith, 1971. Metabolism of adenosine-5'-mono-
    phosphate during circulation through the lungs. Trans. Assoc.
    Am. Phys., 84: 297.
Ryan, J.W. and U. Smith, The metabolism of angiotensin I by endo-
    thelial cells, 1973. In: Protides of the Biological Fluids,
    Vol. 20, ed. H. Peeters, (Pergamon Press, Oxford, England),
    p. 379.
Ryan, U.S., E. Clements, D. Habliston and J.W. Ryan, 1978a.
    Isolation and culture of pulmonary artery endothelial cells.
    Tissue & Cell, 10: 535.

Ryan, U.S., J.W. Ryan and A. Chiu, 1976c. Kininase II (angiotensin converting enzyme) and endothelial cells in culture. Adv. Exp. Med. Biol., 70: 217.

Ryan, U.S., J.W. Ryan and C. Whitaker, (this volume). How do kinins affect vascular tone?

Ryan, U.S., J.W. Ryan, C. Whitaker and A. Chiu, 1976b. Localization of angiotensin converting enzyme (kininase II). Tissue & Cell, 8: 125.

Smith, U. and J.W. Ryan, 1970. An electron microscopic study of the vascular endothelium as a site for bradykinin and ATP inactivation in rat lung. Adv. Exp. Med. Biol., 8: 249.

Smith, U. and J.W. Ryan, 1971. Pinocytotic vesicles of the pulmonary endothelial cell. Chest, 59: 12S.

Smith, U. and J.W. Ryan, 1973. Electron microscopy of endothelial and epithelial components of the lungs: Correlations of structure and function. Fed. Proc., 32: 1957.

Smith, U., J.W. Ryan, D.D. Michie and D.S. Smithm 1971. Endothelial projections: As revealed by scanning electron microscopy, Science, 173: 925.

Vogt, M. and B. Dugal, 1976. Generation of an esterolytic and kinin-forming kallikrein-α_2-macroglobulin complex in human serum by treatment with acetone. Arch. Pharmac., 294: 75.

ANGIOTENSIN I CONVERTING ENZYME (KININASE II) IN HUMAN ENDOTHELIAL

CELLS IN CULTURE

A.R. Johnson and E.G. Erdos

Departments of Pharmacology and Internal Medicine

University of Texas Health Science Center at Dallas, Tx.

The vascular endothelium provides an extensive surface where vasoactive peptides can be metabolized. The lung is a major site for the metabolism of bradykinin and angiotensin (Van, 1969) since peptidyl dipeptidase (E.C. 3.4.15.1; kininase II, or angiotensin I converting enzyme) is associated with pulmonary endothelium (Caldwell et al., 1976; Ryan et al., 1976). Peripheral vascular endothelium (Kreye and Gross, 1971; Collier and Robinson, 1974) also metabolizes angiotensin I to angiotensin II, and the enzyme is associated with endothelial cells isolated from pig arterial vessels (Ody and Junod, 1977) and endothelial cells cultured from human umbilical cord vessels (Johnson and Erdos, 1977).

The dual activity of peptidyl dipeptidase (Yang et al., 1970; 1971) places it in a key position to control blood flow and pressure in specific vascular beds. Recent studies on inhibition of the enzyme by hypoxia (Leunberger et al., 1978) and by albumin fragments (Klauser et al., 1979) indicate that its activity may be controlled by physiologic mechanisms.

Human endothelial cells in culture provide a convenient tool for the study of peptidyl dipeptidase. The enzyme on the plasma membrane of the cells is retained through a number of passages in culture (Johnson and Erdos 1977). This study describes the influence of inhibitors and growth factors on the activity of peptidyl dipeptidase in cells cultured from various human vessels.

METHODS

Endothelial cells were cultured from human umbilical cord

287

vessels and described previously (Johnson and Erdos, 1977). Cells were cultured from human aorta and pulmonary vessels by similar techniques (Johnson, 1979). All endothelial cells were grown in monolayers in medium 199 supplemented with 20% fetal calf serum and 10% human serum. The cultures were maintained in a 37° incubator supplied with 5% CO_2.

Experiments with epidermal growth factor (EGF) were performed as described in detail elsewhere (Johnson et al., 1979). Briefly, the influence of EGF was determined in subconfluent cultures by measuring the uptake of ^{3}H-thymidine into DNA and increases in protein and cell number. The number of cells was determined by counting in a Coulter counter and by measurement of DNA (Burton, 1968). Protein was measured by the method of Lowry et al., (1951).

The activity of peptidyl dipeptidase was assayed with two substrates: bradykinin (2 μM) and ^{3}H-hippuryl glycylglycine (Hip-Gly-Gly; 3 mM). When bradykinin was the substrate, inactivation of the peptide was measured by bioassay on the rat uterus. When ^{3}H-Hip-Gly-Gly was the substrate (Ryan et al., 1977), ^{3}H-hippuric acid was extracted and measured in a liquid scintillation counter. SQ 20881 (0.1 mM) was used to establish the specificty of the assay for peptidyl dipeptidase. Inhibitors were added to the cells 15 min before addition of the substrate.

RESULTS

Human endothelial cells in culture, whether from umbilical or pulmonary vessels, had peptidyl dipeptidase activity as shown by the inactivation of bradykinin and the hydrolysis of ^{3}H-Hip-Gly-Gly. The enzymatic activity was inhibited completely in cells that were incubated with SQ 20881 (0.1 mM). Peptidyl dipeptidase activity was retained by cultured endothelial cells for at least 6 passages in culture, and was found in cells that were tested as late as 10 passages. Cells from aorta, pulmonary artery or umbilical artery had approximately 3-5 times more activity than cells from pulmonary or umbilical veins. This pattern was observed when either bradykinin or ^{3}H-Hip-Gly-Gly was the substrate.

Kininase activity of cultured endothelial cells was inhibited when intact cells were incubated with a goat antibody to human lung peptidyl dipeptidase. In 5 experiments with cells from umbilical veins the enzyme was inhibited 45% (range 30-66%) by 30 μg/ml of the immunoglobulin fraction of goat antiserum. In 3 experiments with pulmonary arterial endothelial cells peptidyl dipeptidase was inhibited 47% (range 35-53%) by the antibody (Table 1). Non-immune serum globulin did not inhibit the enzyme activity. Similarly, concanavalin A partially inhibited the activity of peptidyl dipeptidase on endothelial cells from both umbilical veins and

Table 1

Effect of Inhibitors on Peptidyl Dipeptidase Activity in
Endothelial Cells

Cell Source	Treatment	Activity (nmol/hr/10^6 Cells)	% Inhib.
Umbilical Vein	None	12.2 ± 1.0	---
	Antibody (30 µg/ml)	6.7 ± 0.7	45
	Concanavalin A (1 mg/ml)	7.1, 8.8	35
Pulmonary Artery	None	36.3 ± 4.4	---
	Antibody (30 µg/ml)	19.1 ± 3.9	47
	Concanavalin A (1 mg/ml)	25.4 ± 3.8	30

Endothelial cells were treated with inhibitors 15 min prior to
addition of bradykinin (2 uM).

Table 2

Influence of Cortisol on Peptidyl Dipeptidase Activity

Cell Source	Treatment	Activity (nmol/hr/10^6 Cells)
Umbilical Vein	None	2.8 ± 0.2
	Cortisol	2.0 ± 0.8
Pulmonary Artery	None	10.5 ± 1.8
	Cortisol	10.0 ± 2.0
Pulmonary Vein	None	3.5 , 1.6
	Cortisol	2.8 , 2.2

The cells were treated with 15 µM cortisol 72 hr prior to measurement of enzymatic activity with ^{3}H-Hip-Gly-Gly as substrate.

pulmonary arteries. The inhibition was approximately 30% in 2
experiments with cells from vein and 3 experiments with cells
from artery (Table 1).

Because corticosteroids have been reported to induce the activity of peptidyl dipeptidase in other cultured cells (Friedland
et al., 1977; 1978) we added cortisol to endothelial cultures for
periods of 48-72 hrs. Addition of 15 µM cortisol to the cultures
72 hr prior to measurement of enzymatic activity did not affect
the enzymatic activity of endothelial cells. Although cells from
three different vessels were tested (umbilical vein, pulmonary
vein and pulmonary artery) cortisol did not enhance the peptidyl
dipeptidase activity in any of them (Table 2).

Cell growth and replication was stimulated in 7 cultures from
umbilical veins when EGF (50 ng/ml) was added to the culture medium.
In 72 hr after application of the growth factor there was a significant (p < .01) increase in both the total protein in the dishes
and the amount of ^{3}H-thymidine taken up into the cells. In contrast,
cells from the pulmonary artery did not respond to EGF, and in 4
experiments the changes in protein and ^{3}H-thymidine uptake were
not different from control (untreated) cells (Table 3).

The activity of peptidyl dipeptidase did not increase in parallel with the cell growth in cells from umbilical veins. In 3
experiments there was a small but significant (p < .01) decrease
in enzymatic activity of cells that were treated with EFG. In two
separate experiments with pulmonary arterial endothelial cells,
the enzyme activity did not change when the cultures were treated
with EFG (Table 3).

                              DISCUSSION

We found that the characteristics and behavior of human endothelial cells in culture depends upon their vascular origin. Cells
from arteries consistently had more peptidyl dipeptidase than did
cells from veins. The enzyme in all of the cultured cells was
inhibited by SQ 20881, a specific inhibitor of peptidyl dipeptidase
(Ondetti et al., 1971).

Others found that the activity of peptidyl dipeptidase can be
blocked by specific antibody. Oshima et al. (1974) reported that
rabbit antibody to hog kidney enzyme inhibited the enzyme from
hog kidney, hog lung and hog plasma to approximately the same
extent, ranging between 42 and 48%. We found that peptidyl dipeptidase of human endothelial cells was similarly inhibited. The
enzyme from umbilical vein cells was inhibited by 45% and that
from pulmonary artery cells by 47%.

Lanzillo and Fanburg (1976) investigated the inhibition of
peptidyl dipeptidase from guinea pig lung and serum. They found
that concanavalin A (0.4 mM) inhibited the enzyme from either
source by 35%. Our findings with human endothelial cell enzyme

Table 3

Influence of Growth Factors on Peptidyl Dipeptidase Activity
and Replication in Endothelial Cells

Cell Source	Treatment	Uptake of ^{3}H-Thymidine (CPM/Dish)	Protein (μg/Dish)	Enzyme Activity (nmol/hr/10^6 Cells)
Umbilical Vein	None	10,040 ± 1,500	190 ± 15	5.3 ± 0.2
	EGF	22,525 ± 1,220*	341 ± 16*	3.4 ± 0.3*
Pulmonary Artery	None	35,420 ± 1,514	340 ± 77	55.1 , 74.9
	EGF	34,345 ± 2,830	362 ± 71	50.0 , 63.5

EGF (50 ng/ml) was added to cultures 72 hr before measurements were made.
^{3}H-thymidine (0.1 uCi/ml) was added at the same time. The enzymatic activity was measured with 3H-Hip-Gly-Gly in parallel cultures treated with EGF
but not with ^{3}H-thymidine.

* Significantly different from control (untreated) cells, p ≤ .01.

are similar to theirs. Since the enzyme from either venous or
arterial endothelial cells was similarly inhibited by SQ 20881,
specific antibody to human lung peptidyl dipeptidase and concanavalin A, the enzyme in different vessels presumably has the same
antigenic and glycoprotein components.

    We also investigated the effects of cortisone and EGF on pep-
tidyl dipeptidase activity in endothelial cells. Others reported
that glucocorticoids affect morphologic and biochemical characteristics of endothelial cells. Maca et al. (1978) found that treatment of the cultures with hydrocortisone, dexamethasone or predni-
sone for 24-48 hr increased the surface area of the cells and
increased protein synthesis without affecting DNA synthesis or
cell replication. These authors did not measure specific proteins,
however.

    Friedland et al. (1977; 1978) measured the activity of pep-
tidyl dipeptidase in cultures of alveolar macrophages from rabbits
and monocytes from humans. They found significant enhancement of
enzyme activity when the cells were cultured with steroids for
24-72 hr in the presence of 10% fetal calf serum. We did not find
this phenomenon in endothelial cell cultures. Although the cells
grew readily in medium that contained cortisol (15 μM), there
was no increase in enzymatic activity. Since cortisol has the
same effect as dexamethasone on protein synthesis in cultured endothelial cells (Maca et al., 1978), it should have the same effect
as dexamethasone on peptidyl dipeptidase activity. Probably other
factors, such as the presence of 20% fetal calf serum and 10% human
serum in our culture medium affect the response to steroids. It
is known that endothelial cells from hog aorta that are grown in
serum-free medium have enhanced activity and release peptidyl
dipeptidase into the medium (Hayes et al., 1978). Thus, the synthesis of the enzyme in cultured cells may be regulated by serum
factors.

    We reported that endothelial cells from umbilical cord vessels
respond to polypeptide growth factors with an increase in DNA and
protein synthesis and enhanced cell replication (Johnson et al.,
1978; 1979). The present study compares the influence of EGF on
cells from different vessels and on the activity of peptidyl dipeptidase. Only cells from umbilical vessels responded to the growth
factor with increased cell replication. Cells from pulmonary
arteries showed neither increased protein synthesis nor increased
labeling of DNA after treatment with EGF. Other investigators
noted a difference in the sensitivity of cells from bovine aorta
and human umbilical cord to growth factors. Gospodarowicz et al
(1978) suggested that the human cells require thrombin as a co-
mitogen. Our data suggest that pulmonary endothelial cells may be
more sensitive to suppressor regulatory mechanisms, or possibly

that they lack receptors for EGF.

Endothelial cells that were stimulated by EGF had decreased activity of peptidyl dipeptidase relative to control cells. This decrease in enzymatic activity in rapidly replicating cells may be due to an increase turnover of cell surface protein, since the enzyme is localized on the surface of these cells (Johnson and Erdos, 1977).

We conclude that peptidyl dipeptidase is associated with human endothelial cells derived from aorta, umbilical and pulmonary vessels. The inhibition of the enzyme by SQ 20881, antibody and concanavalin A is similar in cells from different vessels. Thus, there is no remarkable qualitative difference in the enzyme from these different vessels. Enzymatic activity was not induced by cortisol in any of the cells, and it decreased rather than increased with enhanced cell replication. The failure of pulmonary endothelial cells to respond to EGF suggests that factors such as age, lack of receptors or the presence of serum inhibitors can influence endothelial cell replication.

ACKNOWLEDGEMENTS

We are grateful for the assistance of Mrs. Shashi Rattan and Mrs. Lavinia Nogueira with the culture of endothelial cells and biochemical assays. The goat antibody to peptidyl dipeptidase was kindly provided by Mrs. Katy Hammon.

These studies were supported by NIH USPHS HL 18826, and HL 14187.

REFERENCES

Burton, K.: Determination of DNA concentration with diphenylamine. Methods Enzymol. 12(Part B): 163-166, 1968.

Caldwell, P.R.B., Seegal, B.C. and Hsu, K.C.: Angiotensin-converting enzyme: vascular endothelial localization. Science 191: 1050-1051, 1976

Collier, J.G. and Robinson, B.F.: Comparison of effects of locally infused angiotensin I and II on hand veins and forearm arteries in man: evidence for converting enzyme activity in limb vessels. Clin. Sci. Molec. Med. 47: 189-192, 1974.

Friedland, J., Setton, C. and Silverstein, E.: Angiotensin converting enzyme: induction by steroids in rabbit alveolar macrophages in culture. Science 197: 64-65, 1977.

Friedland, J., Setton, C. and Silverstein, E.: Induction of angiotensin converting enzyme in human monocytes in culture. Biochem. Biophys. Res. Comm. 83: 843-849, 1978.

Gospodarowicz, D., Brown, K.D., Birdwell, C.R. and Zetter, B.R.:
    Control of proliferation of human vascular endothelial cells.
    Characterization of the response of human umbilical vein endo-
    thelial cells to fibroblast growth factor, epidermal growth
    factor and thrombin. J. Cell Biol. 77: 774-788, 1978.

Hayes, L.W., Goguen, C.A., Ching, S.-F. and Slakey, L.L.: Angio-
    tensin-converting enzyme: Accumulation in medium from cultured
    endothelial cells. Biochem. Biophys. Res. Comm. 82: 1147-1153,
    1978.

Johnson, A.R.: The culture of human pulmonary endothelial cells.
    Comparison of enzymatic activities in cells from arteries and
    cells from veins. Submitted for publication, 1979.

Johnson, A.R. and Erdos, E.G.: Metabolism of vasoactive peptides
    by human endothelial cells in culture. Angiotensin I converting
    enzyme (kininase II) and angiotensinase. J. Clin. Invest. 59:
    684-695, 1977.

Johnson, A.R., Boyden, N.T. and Wilson, C.M.: Stimulation of growth
    in cultured endothelial cells. Fed. Proc. 37: 474, 1978.

Johnson, A.R., Boyden, N.T. and Wilson, C.M.: Growth-promoting
    actions of extracts from mouse submaxillary glands on human
    endothelial cells in culture. Submitted for publication, 1979.

Klauser, R.J., Robinson, C.J.G. and Erdos, E.G.: Inhibition of
    kininase II (angiotensin I converting enzyme) by human serum
    albumin and its fragments. In: Kinin '78 Tokyo, Eds. H. Moriya
    and T. Suzuki, Plenum Press, New York, 1979.

Kreye, V.A.W. and Gross, F.: Conversion of angiotensin I to angio-
    tensin II in peripheral vascular beds of the rat. Am. J.
    Physiol. 220: 1294-1296, 1971.

Lanzillo, J.J. and Fanburg, B.L.: Angiotensin I-converting enzyme
    from guinea pig lung and serum. A comparison of some kinetic
    and inhibition properties. Biochim. Biophys. Acta 445: 161-
    168, 1976.

Leunberger, P.J., Stalcup, S.A., Mellins, R.B., Greenbaum, L.M.
    and Turino, G.M.: Decrease in angiotensin I conversion by
    acute hypoxia in dogs. Proc. Soc. Exp. Biol. Med. 158: 586-
    589, 1978.

Lowry, O.H., Rosenbrough, N.J., Farr, A.L. and Randall, R.J.: Pro-
    tein measurement with the Folin phenol reagent. J. Biol. Chem.
    193: 265-275, 1951.

Maca, R.D., Fry, G.L. and Hoak, J.C.: The effects of glucocorticoids
    on cultured human endothelial cells. Brit. J. Haem. 38: 501-
    509, 1978.

Ody, C. and Junod, A.F.: Converting enzyme activity in endothelial
    cells isolated from pig pulmonary artery and aorta. Am. J.
    Physiol. 232: C95-C98, 1977.

Ondetti, M.A., Williams, N.J., Sabo, E.F., Pluscec, J., Weaver, E.
    R. and Kocy, O.: Angiotensin-converting enzyme inhibitors from
    the venom of Bothrops jararaca. Isolation, elucidation of
    structure, and synthesis. Biochemistry 10: 4033-4039, 1971.

Oshima, G., Gecse, A. and Erdos, E.: Angiotensin I-converting enzyme
     of the kidney cortex. Biochim. Biophys. Acta 350: 26-37, 1974.
Ryan, J.W., Chung, A., Ammons, C. and Carlton, M.L.: A simple radio-
     assay for angiotensin-converting enzyme. Biochem. J. 167:
     501-504, 1977.
Ryan, U.S., Ryan, J.W., Whitaker, C. and Chiu, A.: Localization of
     angiotensin converting enzyme (kininase II). II. Immunocyto-
     chemistry and immunofluorescence. Tissue and Cell 8: 125-145,
     1976.
Vane, J.R.: The release and fate of vaso-active hormones in the
     circulation. Br. J. Pharmacol. 35: 209-242, 1969.
Yang, H.Y.T., Erdos, E.G. and Levine, Y.: A dipeptidyl carboxy-
     peptidase that converts angiotensin I and inactivates brady-
     kinin. Biochim. Biophys. Acta 214: 374-376, 1970.
Yang, H.Y.T., Erdos, E.G. and Levine, Y.: Characterization of a
     dipeptide hydrolase (kininase II; angiotensin I converting
     enzyme). J. Pharmacol. Exptl. Therap. 117: 291-300, 1971.

THE EFFECT OF HUMAN GRANULOCYTE PROTEINASES ON KININOGENS

B. Dittman*, R. Wimmer*, R. Mindermann*, and K. Ohlsson**

*Abteilung fur Klinishce Chemie und Klinische Biochemie
der Chirurgischen Klinik der Universitat Munchen, NuB-
baumstr. 20, D-8000 Munchen, 2, Germany
** Department of Clinical Chemistry and Surgery, Univ.
of Lund, Malmo General Hospital, Malmo, Sweden

INTRODUCTION

Substances such as endotoxin, antigen-antibody complexes and
complement components induce loss of lysosomal enzymes from PMN-
leukocytes into the surrounding medium. The main contributors of
the powerful enzyme capacity thus released are the neutral proteinases elastase, cathepsin G, collagenase and the acid proteinases
cathepsin B and D. Besides their biological function - e.g.
digestion of invading microorganisms after phagocytosis, local
fibrinolysis of fibrin deposits and vascular thrombi - they are
involved in destructive processes under pathological conditions.
The granulocytic enzymes are capable of degrading connective tissue
proteins such as collagen, microfibrillar elastin, basement membranes and cartilage proteoglycans. It is evident, therefore, that
these enzymes participate in circumscribed inflammatory injuries,
for example, in local hemorrhagic Shwartzman and Arthus reactions,
glomerulonephritis, arthritic diseases, pulmonary emphysema and
so on. Severe bleeding tendency may occur in patients suffering
from acute myeloblastic or myelomonocytic leukemia and septicemia
indicating that degranulation of inflammatory cells leads also to
a systemic degradation and cleavage of circulating proteins in
the blood, especially of clotting factors, complement components
and immunoglobulins. It is worth mentioning, that inactivation
of these factors occurs in spite of an exceeding plasmatic inhibitory potential directed against the leukocytic proteinases, as
clearly stated by Egbring and Haveman (1978). The in vitro and
in vivo experiments of these authors showed that the decrease of
clotting factor levels was not due to a triggering of blood coagulation and subsequent activation of fibrinolysis. The granulo-

cytic proteinases broke down the factors by direct unspecific proteolysis, this is no consumption caused by increased turnover of
clotting factors, but resulting in prolonged clotting times as
well.

Conscious of the above cited aspects the question arises whether
kininogens are also attacked unspecifically by granulocytic enzymes
resulting in partial or total elimination from their biological
function. In addition, we were eager to know whether potent naturally
occuring inhibitors of these enzymes are capable of inhibiting the
unspecific degradation thus perhaps also interrupting a patholo-
gically increased turnover. Their therapeutical application might
then be possible in the future to decline the inflammatory response.

Our main interest was focused on the degradation of human HMW-
kininogen, because it is not merely a central component of the
kallikrein-kinin system. This substance is connected by complicated
interplays with other regulatory systems. Best investigated is its
participation in the solid-phase activation of the intrinsic pathway of coagulation (Kato et al., 1977). Destruction of the clotting
promoting activity of HMW-kininogen might also be responsible for
severe bleeding tendency during septicemia or acute leukemia.

MATERIALS AND METHODS

The substrates we used for the degradation studies were:
(1) Bovine HMW-kininogen, isolated according to the method of
Komya, et al. (1974). (2) Human HMW-kininogen, isolated recently
in our laboratory to electrophoretic homogeneity. Determination
of N-terminal amino acids revealed no contaminating proteins. The
electrophoretic mobility was slightly faster than that of the
bovine material. The molecular weight (estimated by SDS-electro-
phoresis) was 120,000. The specific activity was estimated to 13.5
bradykinin equivalents per unit of absorbancy at 280 nm. The
isolation procedure consisting of three steps (chromatography on
DEAE Sephadex A50, CM Sephadex C50 and Sephacryl S200) will be
published in detail elsewhere. (3) Human LMW-kininogen, partially
purified recently in our laboratory (R. Mindermann, Diplomarbeit
1977, Technical University of Munich).

The neutral proteinases from human polymorphonuclear granulocytes elastase, cathepsin G and collagenase were isolated by K.
Ohlsson, Malmo. Elastase and cathepsin G purification was achieved
by affinity chromatography on Trasylol-Sepharose followed by ion
exchange chromatography on CM cellulose as described by Travis
et al., (1978). For the isolation of collagenase affinity chromatography on collagen-Sepharose 4B was used (Ohlsson 1978).

The mixture of the acid proteinases cathepsin B and D was

isolated in our laboratory by H. Schiessler and M. Arnhold according
to the method described by Barrett (1973).

The inhibitors we used were preferably the eglins and the Bowman-Birk inhibitor from soybeans. Eglins from the leech Hirudo
medicinalis were isolated and characterized by Seemuller et al.
(1977) in our laboratory. The eglins are strong inhibitors of
chymotrypsin, subtilisin and the PMN-granulocytic proteinases
elastase and cathepsin G. In this respect their inhibition specificity is very similar to that of the inhibitors from human plasma
α_1-antitrypsin and α_2-macroglobulin and mucous secretions (the
antileukoprotease HUSI-I) (Schiessler 1976). The molecular weight
of the eglins is remarkably low (~7,000) and, a structural pecularity,
they contain no disulfide bridge. The trypsin-chymotrypsin inhibitor from soybeans (Bowman-Birk type), Mr~8,000, was isolated by the
team of H. Schiessler in our laboratory according to the methods
of Birk (1974) and Smirnoff et al. (1976).

RESULTS AND DISCUSSION

Unspecific Degradation of Kininogens by Granulocytic Proteinases

For the degradation studies we incubated bovine and human HMW-
kininogen with each of the following enzymes: the neutral proteinases
elastase, cathepsin G and collagenase and with a mixture of the
acid proteinases cathepsin B and D. To reduce the reaction time,
the experiments were performed applying equimolar amounts of substrate and enzyme. Polyacrylamide gel electrophoresis of the degradation products, performed at pH 8.3, showed a characteristic
protein band pattern for each enzyme, cf. Figure 1 and 2.

The neutral proteinase elastase turned out to be most effective
in kininogen digestion as estimated by the rate of disappearance
of the native kininogen band in the electrophoretic protein band
pattern. The effectiveness of this enzyme in the degradation of
clotting factors was demonstrated recently by Egbring and Haveman
(1978). On the other hand, complete removal of the native kininogen
band by collagenase was achieved only within the reaction time (45
min) if a hundred fold higher amount of this enzyme was applied.

The mixture of the acid proteinases cathepsin B and D was also
capable of breaking down the HMW-kininogens. The electrophoretical
protein band patterns obtained were clearly different from those
produced by the other enzymes. The mixture of the cathepsins B
and D was nearly as effective at pH 5.5 as elastase. At neutral
pH, however, degradation by these enzymes was clearly delayed.
This latter finding is in accordance with results reported recently
by Baggiolini (1978).

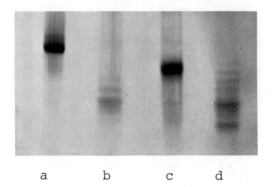

Figure 1.   Polyacrylamide gel electrophoresis (7% gel, pH 8.3)
of bovine HMW-kininogen before (a) and after degradation
with elastase (b), collagenase (c) and cathepsin G (d).

Equimolar amounts of enzyme and substrate were incubated
in 0.1 M Tris-HCl, pH 7.5 at 37°C for 45 min.

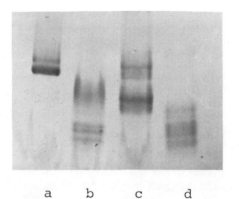

Figure 2.   Polyacrylamide gel electrophoresis (7% gel, pH 8.3)
of human HMW-kininogen before (a) and after degradation with elastase (b), collagenase (c) and
cathepsin G (d).

Equimolar amounts of enzyme and substrate were
incubated in 0.1 M Tris-HCl, pH 7.5 at 37°C
for 45 min.

When the degradation products formed by each of the neutral proteinases were reacted with human plasma kallikrein (isolated by R. Geiger in our laboratory; cf. Heber et al. 1978) in a further step, only about 9-15% of the amount of kinin released from native kininogens was detectable with the bioassay on the oestrogeneous rat uterus. Incubation with trypsin led to the liberation of the original amount of kinin, except from the cathepsin G digest yielding clearly lower kinin activity. This observation indicates that the kinin moiety was not cleaved by alastase and collagenase, with cathepsin G, however, cleavage seems to occur; cf. below.

Due to loss of the native conformation of the kinin moiety containing peptides, the latters are, on the other hand, not or only very slowly susceptible to hydrolysis by plasma kallikrein. The remaining clotting activity of the degradation products of the HMW-kininogen digests was not examined up to now.

The degradation patterns of bovine and human HMW-kininogen produced by the granulocytic enzymes are not identical (cf. Fig. 1 and 2) indicating differences in the primary structure of both kininogens. The existence of such differences was stated earlier by Nagasawa (1978) and discussed also by others during this meeting.

Preliminary experiments performed with human LMW-kininogen as substrate indicate that this molecule is not so easily susceptible to degradation by granulocytic neutral proteinases as HMW-kininogen, only one protein band with changed electrophoretic mobility could be found in the digests.

Digestion of HMW-kininogen by elastase and cathepsin G could be prevented by preincubating these enzymes with eglins or inhibitor AA from soybeans. The action of collagenase on HMW-kininogen could be inhibited by α_2-macroglobulin but not by EDTA. This is in accordance with the inhibitory spectrum of this enzyme being characterized as collagenolytic enzyme but not as true collagenase. Degradation of HMW-kininogen by the mixture of acid proteinases cathepsin B and D was prevented by the eglins but not by more specific inhibitors of these enzymes such as antipain and/or pepstatin. It is not unlikely, therefore, that the enzyme preparation applied contained an additional proteinase not yet characterized. This finding needs further investigation.

Failure to Detect Kininogenase Activity in Granulocytic Proteins

Movat et al. (1976) reported recently that a granulocytic enzyme resembling elastase exhibits kininogenase activity. There is strong evidence, however, that pure elastase is not able to release kinins from kininogens as shown in our laboratory, cf. Fritz (1978). In contrast, degradation of kininogens is unspecific,

cf. above. Similar results were obtained with the other neutral
and acidic proteinases applied, that means, in no case liberation
of kinin activity was detectable with the bioassay on oestrogeneous
rat uterus.

Kininase Activity of Granulocytic Proteinases

Movat and coworkers (Wasi et al. 1978) found two kininases
in neutrophils, one in the cytosol fraction and the other in the
lysosomal granules. The lysosomal enzyme was tentatively called
"catheptic carboxypeptidase" because of its carboxypeptidase-like
substrate specificity.

We found potent kininase activity in fractions obtained by
M. Baggiolini from azurophil granules of human PMN-leukocytes by
zonal sedimentation of subcellular components. These fractions
contained cathepsin B as shown by cleavage of the synthetic substrate carbobenzoxy-ala-arg-arg-4-methoxy-β-naphtylamide. Isolation
of cathepsin B from PMN-leukocyte granules according to the procedure
published by Barrett (1973) resulted so far in a cathepsin B preparation exhibiting also potent kininase activity. Inhibition of
both, cleavage of the synthetic substrate and the kininase activity
by antipain but not by phenanthrolin and EDTA is in favor to the
assumption that the observed kininase activity is an intrinsic
property of cathepsin B.

On the other hand, the failure to find the total amount of
kinin present in native kininogen after treatment of the cathepsin
G digest with trypsin indicates, that either this chymotrypsin-
like enzyme exhibits also kininase activity or there is still
another not yet identified kininase present in our purified
cathepsin G preparation.

SUMMARY

From the results obtained in preliminary in vitro experiments
we may conclude that the unspecific breakdown of kininogens by
neutral and acidic granulocytic proteinases may occur also in the
organism during pathological conditions. Inhibitor application
may serve as a valuable tool to prevent unspecific proteolytic
degradation and thus elimination of kininogens and other clotting
or complement factors from their biological function. Furthermore,
specific cleavage products of the kininogens produced by granulocytic enzymes may be useful in the diagnosis of a beginning septicemia as well as in elucidation of the primary structure of the
human kininogens.

ACKNOWLEDGEMENTS

This work was supported by grant B/3 of the Deutsche Forschungsgemeinschaft, Sonderforschungsbereich 51, Munchen. We are indebted
to A. Steger, Munich, for samples of human HMW-kininogen. We are
very grateful to A. Henschen-Edman, Max-Planck-Institut fur Biochemie, Martinsried bei Munchen, for determinating N-terminal amino
acids. The excellent technical assistance of Mrs. R. Hell is gratefully appreciated. We would also like to thank Prof. H. Fritz
for the initiation of this work and for his stimulating comments.

REFERENCES

Baggiolini, M. 1978. Lysosomal enzymes and neutral proteinases
as mediators of inflammation. International Congress of Inflammation. Bologna.

Barrett, A.J. 1973. Human Cathepsin B1, Purification and Some
Properties of the Enzyme. Biochem. J. 131: 809-822.

Birk, Y. 1974. In: Bayer Sympos. V, Proteinase Inhibitors. Eds.
Fritz, H., Tschesche, H., Greene, L.J. and E. Truscheit.
pp. 355-361, Springer Verlag, Berlin.

Egbring, R. and K. Havemann. 1978. Possible Role of Polymorpho-
nuclear Granulocyte Proteases in Blood Coagulation. In: Neutral
Proteases of Human Polymorphonuclear Leukocytes. Eds.
Havemann, K and A. Janoff.

Fritz, H. 1978. Necessity of a critical consideration of the homo-
geneity of PMN-proteases applied to biological assay systems:
Failure to detect intrinsic kininogenase activity in PMN
elastase. In: Neutral Proteases of Human Polymorphonuclear
Leukocytes. Eds. Havemann, K. and A. Janoff. Urban und
Schwarzenberg Verlag

Heber, H., R. Geiger and N. Heimburger. 1978. Human Plasma Kallikrein: Purification, Enzyme Characterization and Quantitative
Determination in Plasma. Hoppe-Seylers Z. Physiol. Cheml 359:
659-669.

Kato, H., J.N. Han, S. Iwanaga, N. Hashimoto, T. Sugo, S. Fuji,
T. Suzuki. 1977. Mammalian Plasma Kininogens: Their Structures
and Functions. In: Kininogenases - Kallikrein IV. Eds. Haberland, G.L., J. W. Rohen and T. Suzuki., F.K. Schattauer Verlag,
Stuttgart

Komiya, M., H. Kato, T. Suzuki. 1974. Bovine plasma kininogens I.
Further purification of HMW-kininogen and its physiochemical
properties. J. Biochem. 76: 811-822.

Movat, H., F.M. Habal and D.R.L. MacMorine. 1976. Neutral Proteases
of Human PMN-Leukocytes with Kininogenase Activity. Int.
Archs. Allergy appl. Immun. 50: 257-281.

Nagasawa, S., T. Nakayasu. 1978. Enzymatic and chemical cleavages
of human kininogens. Conference Abstracts Vol. 16, #5, p.791.

Ohlsson, K. 1978.   Purification and properties of granulocyte colla-
     genase and elastase. In: Neutral Proteases of Human Polymorpho-
     nuclear Leukocytes. Eds. Havemann, and A. Janoff., Urban and
     Schwarzenberg Verlag.

Schiessler, H., M. Arnhold, K. Ohlsson, and H. Fritz. 1976.
     Inhibitors of Acrosin and Granulocyte Proteinases from Human
     Genital Tract Secretions. Hoppe Seylers Z. Physiol. Chem.
     357: 1251-1260.

Seemuller, U., M. Meier, K. Ohlsson, H.P. Muller and H. Fritz. 1977.
     Isolation and Characterization of a Low Molecular Weight Inhi-
     bitor (of Chymotrypsin and Human Granulocytic Elastase and
     Cathepsin G) from Leeches. Hoppe Seylers Z. Physiol. Chem.
     358: 1105-1117.

Travis, J., R. Baugh, P.J. Giles, D. Johnson, J. Bowes and C.F.
     Reilly. 1978. Human leukocyte elastase and cathepsin G:
     isolation, characterization and interaction with plasma pro-
     teinase inhibitors. In: Neutral Proteases of Human Polymorpho-
     nuclear Leukocytes. Eds. Havemann, K. and A. Janoff. Urban
     und Schwarzenberg Verlag

Wasi, S., H. Movat, E. Pass and J.Y.C. Chan. 1978.   Production,
     Conversion and Destruction of Kinins by Human Neutrophil
     Leukocyte Proteases. In: Neutral Proteases of Human Poly-
     morphonuclear Leukocytes. Eds. Havemann, K. and A. Janoff.
     Urban und Schwarzenberg Verlag.

EFFECT OF PANCREATIC KALLIKREIN, SPERM ACROSIN AND HIGH MOLECULAR
WEIGHT (HMW) KININOGEN ON CERVICAL MUCUS PENETRATION ABILITY OF
SEMINAL PLASMA-FREE HUMAN SPERMATOZOA

W.-B. Schill, G. Preissler, B. Dittmann and W.P. Muller

Andrology Units of the Dept. of Dermatology and Dept.
of Clinical Chemistry and Clinical Biochemistry. The
Ludwig-Maximilians University School of Medicine,
Munich, FRB.

INTRODUCTION

In vitro-stimulation of sperm motility by components of the
kallikrein-kinin system was first demonstrated by Schill and coworkers (Schill et al., 1974; 1976). Involvement of the kinin
system in reproductive functions by affecting sperm motility is
supported by the fact that all components of the kinin system are
present in the male and female genital secretions (Palm and Fritz,
1975).

Hog pancreatic kallikrein yields the following effects in
hypokinetic ejaculated human spermatozoa (Leidl et al., 1975;
Wallner et al., 1975; Schill et al., 1976; Schill and Preissler,
1977; Steiner et al., 1977).

a)   Increase of the percentage of motile spermatozoa
b)   Shift of the number of spermatozoa with poor motility
     to those with very good forward progression.
c)   Increase of mean velocity.
d)   Slight improvement of sperm viability.
e)   Stimulation of sperm metabolism.
f)   Improvement of cervical mucus sperm penetration.

Palm and Fritz (1975) showed that the acrosomal penetration
enzyme acrosin is a potent kinin-liberating proteinase. Therefore,
acrosin may play a significant role in the female genital tract by
enhancing sperm migration within the uterus. It is suggested that
the release of acrosin in the presence of kininogen will lead to a
self-stimulation of uterine spermatozoa facilitating sperm-egg
contact in order to achieve fertilization.

The following investigation was undertaken to study whether acrosin is able to stimulate sperm migration within the uterine secretions determined by cervical mucus penetration tests with seminal plasma-free human spermatozoa. The result of this study should help to clarify the suggested role of acrosin as sperm stimulating agent within the female genital tract.

MATERIAL AND METHODS

Spermatozoa: Seminal plasma-free human spermatozoa (SPFS) from oligozoospermic men, 2 x washed (600 xg, 5 min, 22°C) in Lindholmer solution without albumin (Schill and Preissler, 1977), resuspension in the same buffer medium (22°C).

Substances: Highly purified hog pancreatic kallikrein (EC 3.4.21.8), specific activity: 1190 KU/mg (Bayer Co., Germany), final concentration: 0.7 KU/ml.

Highly purified boar acrosin (EC 3.4.21.10), specific activity: 13.2 U/mg, final concentration: 55 mill/ml.

Highly purified HMW bovine kininogen (1 mg kininogen released 0.6 ug bradykinin equivalents within the bioassay after 30 min of incubation with 10 mg trypsin), final concentration: 0.17 µg/ml.

Methods: Cervical mucus penetration ability of washed human spermatozoa was studied in vitro using the capillary tube test according to Kremer (see Schill and Preissler, 1977). Capillary tubes: 7 cm length, 0.6 mm outer diameter.

Experimental procedure: 0.2 ml sperm suspension + 0.05 ml buffer medium containing test substances. All penetration tests were performed in duplicate.

The following parameters were determined: (a) penetration depth after 20 min of migration at 22°C (linear penetration); (b) penetration density 20, 60 and 120 min after mucus-semen contact by calculating the number of spermatozoa at various migration points.

RESULTS

Figure 1 shows the effect of bradykinin on sperm migration.

Figures 2, 3, and 4 show the effect of kallikrein and HMW kininogen on sperm migration.

Figures 5 and 6 show the effect of acrosin on sperm migration compared to kallikrein in the presence of HMW kininogen.

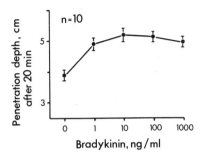

Figure 1.   Effect of different concentrations of bradykinin on
            linear penetration of SPFS in cervical mucus (Mean ±
            SEM of 10 experiments).

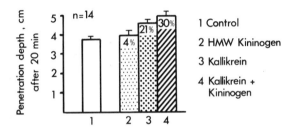

Figure 2.   Linear penetration of SPFS in cervical mucus after 20
            min of incubation (Mean ± SEM of 14 experiments).

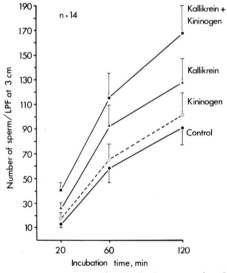

Figure 3.   Penetration density of SPFS in cervical mucus
            determined after 20, 60, and 120 min of incubation
            at 22°C.

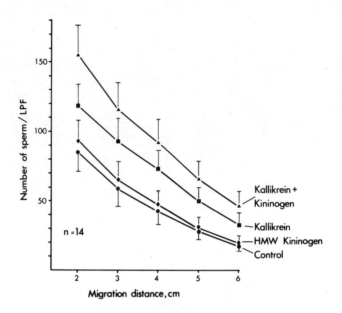

Figure 4.   Penetration density of SPFS determined at various
             migration points after 60 min of incubation at
             22°C.

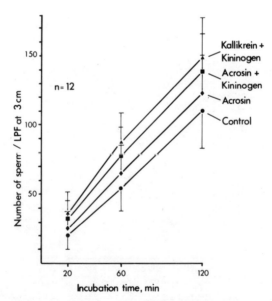

Figure 5.   Penetration density of SPFS determined after 20, 60 and
             120 min of incubation at 22°C (Mean ± SEM of 12 experiments

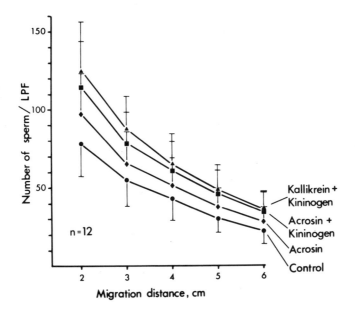

Figure 6.   Penetration density of SPFS determined at various migration points after 60 min of incubation at 22°C.

CONCLUSIONS

Bradykinin is able to stimulate sperm migration of SPFS; HMW kininogen does not effect sperm migration of SPFS; Kallikrein and acrosin induce small stimulation of sperm migration of SPFS indicating traces of kininogen attached to the sperm surface enabling liberation of kinins; In the presence of kininogen, kallikrein and acrosin significantly improve cervical mucus penetration of SPFS; Lastly, from the presented studies there is experimental evidence that acrosin is involved in stimulation of sperm migration within the female genital tract due to liberation of kinins from kininogen (see Figure 7.).

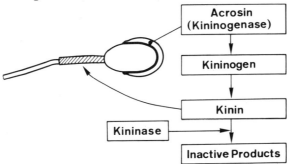

Figure 7.

ACKNOWLEDGEMENTS

Supported by Deutsche Forschungsgemeinschaft Schi 86/5 and SFB 51 (B/3) and World Health Organization, Geneva, Grant No. 76357 and 75080.

REFERENCES

Leidl, W., R. Prinzen, W.-B. Schill and H. Fritz, 1975. The effect of kallikrein on motility and metabolism of spermatozoa in vitro, In: Haberland, G.L., J.W. Rohen, C. Schirren and P. Huber (eds.), Kininogenases. Kallikrein 2. Schattauer, Stuttgart-New York, pp. 33-40.

Palm, S. and H. Fritz, 1975. Components of the kallikrein-kinin system in human midcycle cervical mucus and seminal plasma, In: Haberland, G.L., J.W. Rohen, C. Schirren and P: Huber (eds), Kininogenases. Kallikrein 2, Schattauer, Stuttgart-New York, pp. 17-21.

Schill, W.-B. and G. Preissler, 1977. Improvement of cervical mucus spermatozoal penetration by kinins - a possible therapeutical approach in the treatment of male subfertility, In: Insler, V. and G. Bettendorf (eds)., The Uterine Cervix in Reproduction. Thieme, Stuttgart, pp. 134-146.

Schill, W.-B., O. Braun-Falco and G.L. Haberland, 1974. The possible role of kinins in sperm motility. Int. J. Fertil. 19: 163-167.

Schill, W.-B., O. Wallner, S. Palm and H. Fritz, 1976. Kinin stimulation of spermatozoa motility and migration in cervical mucus. In: Hafez, E.S.E. (ed.), Human Semen and Fertility Regulation in Man. Mosby Company, St. Louis, Miss. pp.442-451.

Steiner, R., N. Hofmann, R. Kaufmann and R. Hartman, 1977. The influence of kallikrein on the velocity of human spermatozoa measured by Laser-Doppler-spectroscopy, In: Haberland, G.L., J.W. Rohen and T. Suzuki (eds.) Kininogenases. Kallikrein 4. Schattauer, Stuttgart-New York, pp. 229-235.

Wallner, O., W.-B. Schill, A. Grosser and H. Fritz, 1975. Participation of the kallikrein-kinin system in sperm penetration through cervical mucus - in vitro studies. In: Haberland, G.L., J.W. Rohen, C. Schirren and P. Huber (eds). Kininogenases. Kallikrein 2. Schattauer, Stuttgart-New York, pp. 63-70.

THE EFFECT OF THE KALLIKREIN-KININ SYSTEM AND PROSTAGLANDINS E ON THE MOTILITY OF HUMAN SPERMATOZOA MEASURED BY THE LASER-DOPPLER METHOD

R. Hartmann, R. Steiner, N. Hofmann and R. Kaufmann

Lehrstuhl für Klinische Physiologie und Andrologische Abteilung, Universität Düsseldorf und Med.Einrichtungen Universitätsstrasse 1, D-4000 Düsseldorf, FRG

Laser-Doppler Spectroscopy has proved to be a powerful tool in observing pharmacological effects on human spermatozoa by allowing for continuous measurement of mean velocity (1,3). The earlier instrumental setup has been improved by a multiple sample holder which provides for simultaneous computer-controlled data evaluation of 10 different samples.

We have studied the dose- and time-dependence of the effects produced by substances such as Kallikrein, bradykinin, and prostaglandins E1, E2, F1α. In earlier studies (1) we have already reported that Kallikrein exerts a stimulating effect on the mean velocity of human spermatozoa. Maximum stimulation could be achieved with a concentration of 4 KE/ml. These results are consistent with those previously reported by Schill (2) and Schill and Haberland (4). These authors used conventional microscopic observation. The mechanism which Kallikrein stimulates the motility of sperms is not well understood. The present in vitro experiments may contribute to the understanding of the mechanism involved. In this investigations we mainly used washed human spermatozoa resuspended in an isotonic salt solution. Washing procedure followed the method of Peterson and Freund (5), however, washing- and resuspension-media have been improved. Aliquots of human blood serum have been added as source for kininogen.

RESULTS

PGE2 when added in concentrations between 0.03 and 3 µg/ml was found to increase mean sperm velocity. The stimulating effect of PGE2 had its maximum at a concentration of 300 ng/ml (fig. 1).

311

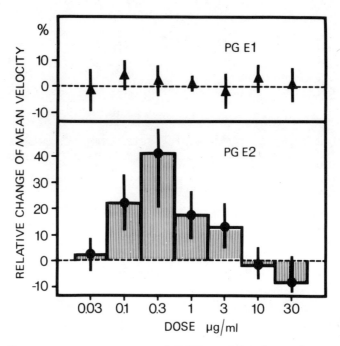

Figure 1: Dose-response curves of PGE1 and PGE2 on the mean velocity of human sperms.

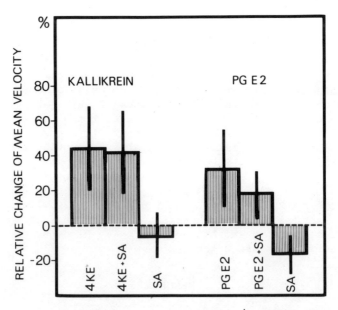

Figure 2: Stimulating effects of Kallikrein and PGE2 (100 ng/ml) on human sperm motility with and without salicylic acid (SA, 0.3 mg/ml).

PGE1 added in the same concentration range was absolutely ineffective. Experiments with PGF1α, which are not shown, gave identical
results as PGE1.

A comparison of the stimulating effects produced by either Kallikrein or prostaglandin E2 is shown in figure 2. The addition of
either acetylsalicylic acid (ASA) or salicylic acid (SA) did not
produce different effects. The Kallikrein effect was not influenced
by salicylic acid. SA itself sometimes slightly decreases sperm motility usually by a nonsignificant amount. However, an enhanced
motility caused by the addition of PGE2 could be reduced by SA.

Bradykinin as one of the substances which are liberated by Kallikrein has also been tested for its stimulating effect on human
sperm motility (Synthetic Bradykinin, Sandoz, Switzerland). The
results are summarized in figure 3. When bradykinin was added to
native semen in doses from 100 ng/ml to 3 μg/ml, a small but significant increase in the mean velocity of sperms (40 experimental
points) could be observed. With washed spermatozoa, however, this
effect did not appear. To ascertain the pharmacological activity
of the bradykinin used, samples were tested on isolated cat uterus
smooth muscle and were found to produce its well known normal
actions.

In figure 4 mean sperm velocity was continuously measured over a
period of about 9 hours for PGE1, PGE2, Kallikrein and a control
specimen. Maximum stimulating effects on velocity were reached at
the 2nd hour, thereafter motility steadily decreased, but tended
to level off at still higher levels in comparison to the control
specimen. These curves are one of the examples demonstrating the
benefits of the computerized and automatically evaluated motility
measurements.

DISCUSSION

The way of action of Kallikrein has already been discussed by other
authors. Palm et al. suggested that Kallikrein acts somehow via a
prostaglandin dependent mechanism (7). Alternatively one has also
suggested a direct influence of Kallikrein induced liberation of
kinins.

However, in our experiments salicylic acid did not depress
the Kallikrein induced increase of sperm motility. That means that
the first of the above mentioned mechanisms is rather unlikely to
occur. With other words, one may conclude that the action of Kallikrein on sperm motility is independent on the prostaglandin synthesis. However, there is a stimulating effect of PGE2 which is clearly
dose-dependent. With prostaglandin synthesis inhibited by salicylic
acid only exogeneous PGE2 can be active in stimulating sperm moti-

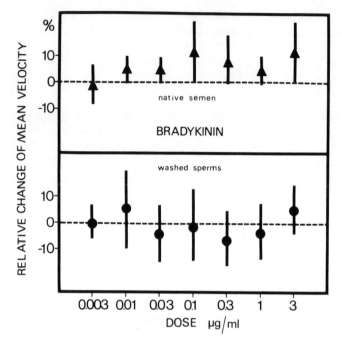

Figure 3: Dose-response curves of bradykinin on the mean velocity
          of human sperms.

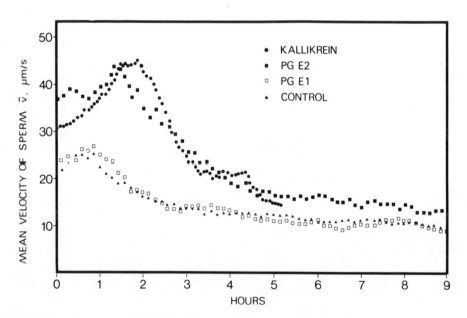

Figure 4: Mean sperm velocity continuously measured for about
          9 hours. Maximum stimulating effects occur at the 2nd
          hour.

lity. This effect is supposed to be smaller than under conditions
where prostaglandin synthesis is unimpaired. This indicates that
SA may exert some unspecific effect or that other prostaglandins
are involved. The latter appears to be rather unlikely since we
did not find other prostaglandins, such as PGE1 or PGF1α to be
active motility stimulators.

Prostaglandin synthesis is most active during epididymical sperm
maturation. It is therefore possible that in ejaculates the pro-
staglandinsynthetase activity may vary with the degree of maturation (9). A clinical observation supports our results that SA reduces sperm motility slightly. When patients with chronical unspecific infections of the genital tract are treated with indomethacin the motility of sperms is reduced (this substance acts
like salicylic acid as an inhibitor of the prostaglandinsynthe-
tase (6)).

To compare the possible unspecific effects of SA to the
action of drugs known to be specific inhibitors of prostaglandin-
synthetase, arachidonic acid (5,8,11,14-eicosatetraenoic acid) as
well as linoleic acid (cis-9-cis-12-octadecadienoic acid) in concentrations of 3.6 mM have been applied (6). (Both compounds were supplied by Sigma Chemical Company, USA). Astonishingly enough, these
substances showed a deleterious effect on human sperm motility
which was completely abolished within 5 minutes.

Also the direct influence of kinin on sperm motility has been
tested, but with bradykinin only. The increase in mean velocity
of sperms in native semen induced by the addition of bradykinin
is less than observed by Schill and Haberland (8). It is not possible so far to explain why, in washed spermatozoa, bradykinin is
ineffective.

ACKNOWLEDGEMENTS

We are grateful to Bayropharm, Köln, for supply with highly purified Kallikrein, and Upjohn GmbH, Heppenheim, for supply with PGE1
(U-10136), and PGE2 (U-12062).

This work has been supported by the Ministry for Science and
Technology, NRW, Germany.

REFERENCES

(1) R. Steiner, N. Hofmann, R. Hartmann, R. Kaufmann: The influence of Kallikrein on the velocity of human spermatozoa measured by laser-doppler-spectroscopy.
In: G.L. Haberland, J.W. Rohen, T. Suzuki (eds.): Kininogenases 4. Schattauer-Verlag, Stuttgart-New York (1977)
(2) Schill, W.B.: Influence of the Kallikrein-kinin system on human sperm motility in vitro.
In: Haberland, G.L., J.W. Rohen, C. Schirren, P. Huber (eds.):
Kininogenases 2. Schattauer-Verlag, Stuttgart-New York (1975)
(3) R. Steiner, N. Hofmann, R. Hartmann, T. Baumeister, R. Kaufmann: Laser-doppler spectroscopy, a useful technique for objective measurements of sperm motility parameters.
In: Proceedings of the Vth European Congress on Sterility and
Fertility, Venice, October 2.-6. 1978
(4) Schill, W.B., G.L. Haberland: In vitro stimulation of human
sperm motility by Kallikrein.
In: Exerpta Medica International Congress Series No. 394,
VIIIth World Congress of Fertility and Sterility, Buenos Aires,
November 3.-9. 1974, Exerpta Medica, Amsterdam
(5) Peterson, R.N. and M. Freund: Reversible inhibition of the
motility of human spermatozoa by tetraphenylboron.
J. Reprod. Fert. 47, 33-38 (1976)
(6) E.W. Horton: Prostaglandins.
Springer-Verlag, Berlin-Heidelberg-New York (1972)
(7) Palm, S., Schill, W.B., Wallner, O., Prinzen, R., Fritz, H.:
Occurence of components of the Kallikrein-kinin system in human genital tract secretions and their possible function in
stimulation of sperm motility and migration.
In: Kinins: Pharmacodynamics and Biological Roles (eds.): Sicuteri, F., Back, N., Haberland, G.L., Plenum Publishing Corporation, New York (1976)
(8) W.B. Schill, G.L. Haberland: Wirkungen von verschiedenen Kom-
ponenten des Kallikrein-Kinin-Systems auf die Spermatozoen-
Motilität in vitro.
Klin. Wschr. 53, 73-79 (1975)
(9) J.M. Johnson and L.C. Ellis: The histochemical localization of
prostaglandin synthetase activity in reproductive tract of the
male rat.
J. Reprod. Fert. 51, 17-22 (1977)

Kallikrein Inhibitor Therapy

RECENT ADVANCES IN MICROBIAL SECONDARY METABOLITES: INHIBITORS OF HYDROLYTIC ENZYMES

Hamao Umezawa

Institute of Microbial Chemistry

14-23 Kamiosaki 3-Chome, Shinagawa-ku, Tokyo

Since 1944, the author has been engaged in the study of antibiotics and other bioactive microbial products. In 1965, the author initiated the study of enzyme inhibitors produced by microorganisms and found nearly 50 small molecular inhibitors (Umezawa, 1976). Among them, protease inhibitors have been used for the identification of enzymes and in the analysis of a role of a protease in biological functions and disease processes. They are used to prevent the proteolysis of bioactive tissue proteins during the extraction. They may be useful in the study of kinin system and inflammation. Inhibitors of enzymes on the cellular surface enhance or suppress immune response.

It is often said that microorganisms in nature compete with each other and produce antibiotics which suppress the growth of others. Most enzyme inhibitors produced by microorganisms do not have a significant antimicrobial activity. Microbial products which have no obvious function in the growth of microbial cells are called microbial secondary metabolites. The findings of various antibiotics and various enzyme inhibitors indicate that microorganisms in nature have aquired the ability to produce numerous secondary metabolites which have various chemical structures.

In this paper, the author will review his studies on the genetic control in the biosynthesis of microbial secondary metabolites and on small molecular inhibitors of hydrolytic enzymes and their actions.

GENETIC CONTROL IN THE BIOSYNTHESIS OF MICROBIAL
SECONDARY METABOLITES

There are many groups of antibiotics each of which contains
a same characteristic structural part. If kanamycin found by the
author is taken as an example, a kanamycin-producing strain produces not only kanamycins A, B and C but also other four similar
compounds (Murase et al., 1970). They all contain 2-deoxystrep-
tamine. Moreover, about a hundred 2-deoxystreptamine-containing
compounds have been found in culture filtrates of streptomyces,
micromonospora, nocardia and bacteria. This indicates that a gene
set for the biosynthesis of 2-deoxystreptamine has been distributed
among various strains of actinomycetes and bacteria. In fact, we
have confirmed that the ability to produce kanamycin is eliminated
by acriflavine treatment and many kanamycin-nonproducing mutants
thus obtained produce kanamycin in media to which 2-deoxystrepta-
mine was added. It can be proposed that a gene involved in the
biosynthesis of a characteristic structural part of a secondary
metabolite has been generated and the product like 2-deoxystrepta-
mine thus produced is transformed or modified by enzymes which are
produced by following the control of other genes and the products
thus formed are released extracellularly. In the natural environment, changes should have further occurred in chromosomes and the
product like 2-deoxystreptamine is further differently modified.
If a gene involved in the biosynthesis of the characteristic structural part was transferred to a plasmid, then it was possible that
this plasmid was transferred into other cells of the same or the
different species where the product like 2-deoxystreptamine was
further differently modified. The secondary metabolites do not
have a function in the growth of microbial cells and it is possible
that numerous genes or gene sets involved in the biosynthesis of
secondary metabolites have been generated in microorganisms and
many or some of them have been transferred into other cells.

The author first noticed the possible involvement of a plasmid
in the biosynthesis of an antibiotic. In the screening of an
inhibitor of plasmin and trypsin, we found leupeptin which was
acetyl or propionylleucylleucylargininal in culture filtrates of
many strains belonging to more than 18 species of streptomyces
(Aoyagi et al., 1969; Umezawa, 1976). Since leupeptin was produced
by strains belonging to so many species, a gene set involved in
its biosynthesis was suggested to lie on a plasmid. We succeeded
in the extraction of a multienzyme which catalyzed the biosynthesis of leupeptin acid, acetyl or propionylleucylleucylarginine
from acetate (or propionate), leucine, arginine in the presence
of ATP (Hori et al., 1978). On this multienzyme, leupeptin acid
is synthesized starting from the synthesis of acetyl leucine.
The ability to produce this multienzyme was transferred from a
methione-requring leupeptin-producing mutant to an arginine-
requiring leupeptin-nonproducing mutant (Umezawa et al., 1978).

It indicates that a gene set involved in the biosynthesis of leupeptin acid, an intermediate peptide to leupeptin, lies on a plasmid.

INHIBITORS OF SERINE AND THIOL PROTEASES

As described above, microorganisms have aquired the ability to produce numerous secondary metabolites which have various chemical structures. Therefore, it is rational to search for microbial products with useful bioactivities. We found inhibitors of various serine and thiol proteases (Umezawa, 1976).

Leupeptin inhibits trypsin, plasmin, papain and cathepsin B. PMR indicates that most leupeptin in the aqueous solution exists mainly in its hydrated and hydroxypiperidine forms as shown in Fig. 1.

The racemization of the asymmetric center in the argininal moiety of leupeptin easily occurs: after 4 days in pH 8.0 aqueous solution at room temperature, this asymmetric center is completely racemized and the activity is reduced to 50%. The L-argininal moiety is the absolute structure requirement for the activity. If it is oxidized to acid or reduced to alcohol, the activity almost disappears. L-argininal and N^α-acetylargininal do not show any activity. Acetyl-L-leucyl-L-argininal shows the almost same activity as leupeptin (Maeda et al., 1971).

Leupeptin prolongs the blood coagulation time of rabbit and human. This inhibition of blood coagulation by leupeptin is temporary and is recovered after 30 to 60 minutes. This inhibition of blood coagulation is not seen in the blood of mice, rats

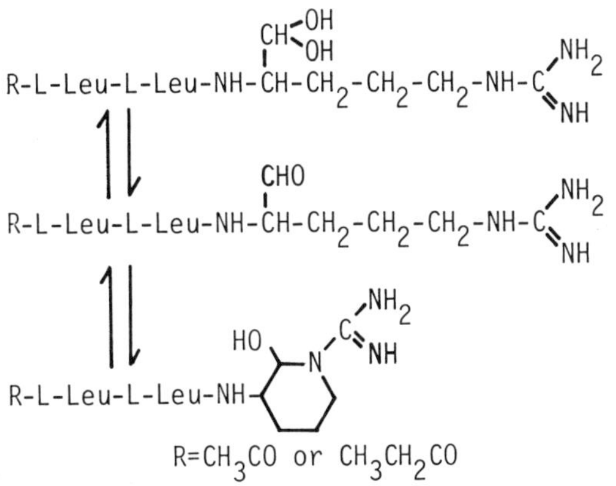

Figure 1. Structures of Leupeptin in its Aqueous Solution

and dogs.   LD$_{50}$ value by intravenous injection to rabbits is
smaller compared with those to mice and rats as follows:
      Mice: I.V.   118 mg/kg; S.C.   1450 mg/kg; Oral >1550 mg/kg
      Rats: I.V.   125 mg/kg; S.C. >4000 mg/kg; Oral >4000 mg/kg
      Rabbits: I.V.   35 mg/kg; S.C. >4000 mg/kg; Oral >1550 mg/kg

The smaller LD$_{50}$ value by intravenous injection to rabbits
may be related to the inhibition of blood coagulation.   Oral 500
mg/kg daily administration for 180 days causes no toxicity in
rabbits.

Leupeptin inhibits carrageenin edema.   Leupeptin ointment (1%)
applied immediately after a burn suppresses pain and blister formation and has been used in the authors' laboratories.

Leupeptin has been reported to inhibit chemical carcinogenesis and the metastasis in experimental animal models (Hozumi et
al., 1972; Matsushima et al., 1977; Kakizoe et al., 1977a and
1977b).

The other peptide, antipain, which also contains argininal
has also been found in culture filtrates of actinomycetes (Umezawa,
1976).

Antipain (Fig. 2) inhibits papain, trypsin, cathepsins A and
B.   The action on plasmin is very much weaker than that of leupeptin.   It shows inhibition of carrageenin edema and prolongs the
blood coagulation time of human and rabbit.   As well as leupeptin,
antipain has been reported to inhibit a chemical carcinogenesis.

Antipain also has a low toxicity.   Absorption of antipain by
rabbits has been studied comparatively with leupeptin.   Blood level
of antipain after oral administration to rabbits is lower than
leupeptin and the amount extracted in urine is less than that for
leupeptin.   In a rabbit liver homogenate, the activity of antipain
decreased rapidly.

As described above, both leupeptin and antipain contain L-
argininal and inhibit trypsin which hydrolyzes the carboxyl side
of arginine and lysine in peptides.   Chymostatin (Fig. 2) and elastatinal (Fig. 2) found by screening the activity of culture filtrates to inhibit chymotrypsin or pancreas elastase also contain
L-phenylalaninal or L-alaninal (Umezawa, 1976).   These aldehyde
structures for inhibition of serine and thiol proteases were first
found in these inhibitors produced by streptomyces.

Chymostatin inhibits all chymotrypsins but not trypsin.   It
inhibits also papain, but this action is much weaker than that
against chymotrypsins.   Chymotrypsin is known to inhibit carrageenin edema.   Intraperitoneal injection of chymostatin also in-

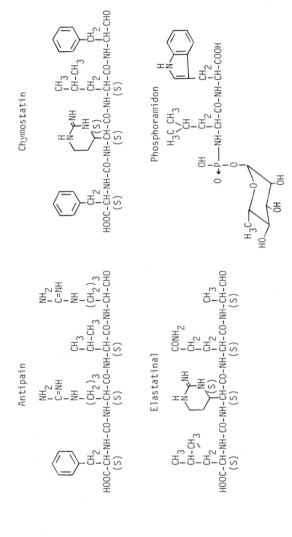

Figure 2. Structures of Antipain, Chymostatin, Elastatinal and Phosphoramidon

hibits this edema. Elastatinal inhibits elastase but not the
other proteases and its inhibition is competitive with the substrate. Ki observed was 2.4 x 10^{-7}M with acetyl-alanyl-alanyl-
alanine p-nitroanilide and 2.1 x 10^{-7}M with acetyl-alanyl-alanyl-
alanine methyl ester. Chymostatin and elastatinal have a low
toxicity. The intravenous injection of 250 mg/kg causes no toxicity in mice. Elastatinal also inhibits carrageenin edema. It is
noticeable that elastatinal inhibits chemical mutagenesis shown
by Ames method and also a malignant transformation (Umezawa, K.
et al., 1977).

On the basis of the activities to inhibit serine and thiol
proteases, various effects on biological functions and disease
processes have been studied as summarized in Table 1. It has been
suggested that human leucocyte proteases may play a primary role
in the inflammatory process and may be involved in causing pulmonary emphysema and certain types of joint diseases. Chymostatin
was reported by Janoff et al. to be a powerful inhibitor of a
chymotrypsin-like protease of human leucocytes. Elastatinal was
reported by the same authors to show only a weak inhibition of
human leucocyte elastase. Stracher et al. reported a therapeutic
effect of leupeptin on hereditory chicken muscle dystrophy. Leupeptin decreases the rate of protein break down in rat skeletal
and cardiac muscles and in denervated rat muscles. Inhibitors of
proteases may be useful in the study of muscle dystrophy and some
of them, for instance, chymostatin and leupeptin, may exhibit
therapeutic effect on some types of muscle dystrophy. Stracher
et al. also observed an effect of pepstatin on chicken muscle dystrophy. According to Rao, chymostatin shows a therapeutic effect
on pancreatitis of his animal model. It may be necessary to study
the effect of protease inhibitors on pancreatitis more in detail.

An inhibitor of thiol proteases (papain and cathepsin B) has
been found in aspergillus japonicus by Hanada et al. This inhibitor designated as E-64 was determined to be N-[N-(L-trans-
carboxyoxiran-2-carboxyl-L-leucyl]-agmatine. This trans-
epoxysuccinic acid moiety was essential for the action (Hanada et
al., 1978a, 1978b and 1978c).

INHIBITION OF CARBOXYL PROTEASES

In the study of inhibitors of pepsin, we found pepstatins in
culture filtrates of various species of actinomycetes. As shown
by the structure formula, various pepstatins are different from
one another in the fatty acid moiety, and the pepstatin containing
an isovaleryl group has been most widely used for biological and
biochemical studies. This pepstatin and the other containing a
n-caproyl group are the main components of the active agents produced by a strain belonging to Streptomyces testaceus. As minor
components, other pepstatins, pepstanones and hydroxypepstatins

TABLE 1.   BIOLOGICAL EFFECTS OF LEUPEPTIN (LP), ANTIPAIN (AP),
               CHYMOSTATIN (CS) AND ELASTATINAL (ES)

Inhibition of carrageenin edema and low toxicity ....LP, AP, CS, ES

Prevention of pain and blister in burn ....LP, (AP)

Inhibition of chemical carcinogenesis in skin, colon,
            esophagus and mammary gland of rats ....LP, AP

Suppression of chemical mutagenesis of bacteria ....ES

Inhibition of polyoma-transformed baby hamster cells ....LP

Inhibition of Vascular metastasis of hepatoma to lung in rats ......LP

Inhibition of emphysema ....CS, (ES)

Inhibition of chicken muscle dystrophy ....LP, CS

Possible therapeutic effect on pancreatitis ....CS

Inhibition of protozoa growth in reticulocytes ....LP, AP, CS

Inhibition of fertilization of sea urchin ....CS, LP, AP

TABLE 2.   BIOLOGICAL EFFECT OF PEPSTATIN

Inhibition of leukokinin formation from leukokininogen and
     inhibition of ascites formation

Inhibition of focus formation of YH-7 mouse cells by murine
     sarcoma virus

Inhibition of carrageenin edema

Inhibition of growth of protozoa in reticulocytes

Inhibition of metamorphosis of tadopole

Possible therapeutic effect on stomach and duodenal ulcer

Possible therapeutic effect on cerebral damage

Possible therapeutic effect on arthritis (rheumatism)

Possible therapeutic effect on renal hypertension

Pepstatins:

RCO-L-Val-L-Val-AHMHA-L-Ala-AHMHA

$$\text{AHMHA} = \begin{array}{c} H_3C \\ H_3C \end{array}\!\!>\!\!CH-CH_2-\overset{\overset{NH_2}{|}}{\underset{H}{C}}-\overset{\overset{OH}{|}}{\underset{H}{C}}-CH_2-COOH$$

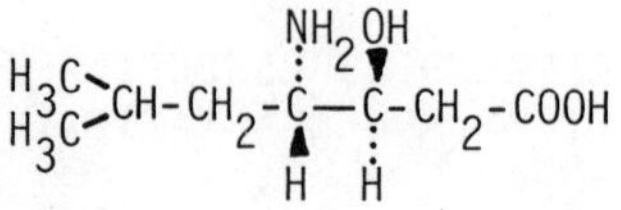

$R=CH_3(CH_2)_n-$, n=0-20; $(CH_3)_2CH(CH_2)_n-$, n=1-17

Pepstanones:

RCO-L-Val-L-Val-AHMHA-L-Ala-AMHN

$$\text{AMHN} = \begin{array}{c} H_3C \\ H_3C \end{array}\!\!>\!\!CH-CH_2-\overset{\overset{NH_2}{|}}{\underset{H}{C}}-\overset{\overset{O}{||}}{C}-CH_3$$

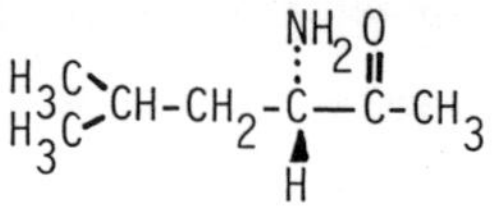

$R=CH_3(CH_2)_n-$, n=0-20; $(CH_3)_2CH(CH_2)_n-$, n=1-17

Hydroxypepstatins:

RCO-L-Val-L-Val-AHMHA-L-Ser-AHMHA

$R=CH_3(CH_2)_n-$, n=0-20; $(CH_3)_2CH(CH_2)_n-$, n=1-17

Figure 3.   Structures of Pepstatins, Pepstanones and
Hydroxypepstatins

are produced in the culture filtrates of the same strain (Fig. 3)
(Umezawa, 1976).

Pepstatins containing acetyl, propionyl or butyryl groups
are produced by strains belonging to other species such as Streptomyces parvisporogenes. A pepstatin containing an isobutyryl
group is also produced by a streptomyces.

As already described for leupeptin, peptide antibiotics are
biosynthesized on multienzyme systems specific for each of them,
but not on the ribosome system. Pepstatin also seems to be biosynthesized by similar means. ^{14}C-labeled AHMHA is not incorporated into pepstatin during fermentation, but ^{14}C-leucine and [14]C-
acetate are incorporated into this amino acid moiety in pepstatin
(Morishima et al., 1974). The formation of pepstanone can be
understood to be due to the decarboxylation of the terminal leucyl
acetate of a biosynthetic intermediate. The ability to produce
pepstatin is eliminated by treatment of its producing strain with

acriflavine and the presence of a gene set is suggested for the biosynthesis of a multienzyme.

As shown by the structure of pepstanone, the terminal carboxyl group is not involved in the activity. Esters and amide of pepstatin, pepstatinal and pepstatinol in which the carboxyl is reduced to aldehyde or alcohol shows a similar activity as pepstatin against pepsin. The inner 4-amino-3-hydroxy-6-methylheptanoic acid moiety is necessary for the activity. (3S,4S)-4-Amino-3-hydroxy-6-methylheptanoic acid (AHMHA) or its N-acyl derivative has no activity. The N-acetylvalyl derivative shows activity and the addition of another valine between the acetyl and valyl groups does not increase its activity. Addition of L-alanine to the C-terminal group increases the activity about 100 times. It suggests that the acyl-valyl-AHMHA-L-alanine moiety may be involved in binding with pepsin and cathepsin D (Aoyagi et al., 1972). Kinoshita et al. (1973) have synthesized acetyl-L-valyl-L-valyl-[(3S, 4R)-4-amino-3-hydroxy-6-methyl]heptanoic acid. It shows no activity. It suggests that the 4S-configuration of AHMHA is the requirement for the activity.

Pepstatins, pepstanones and hydroxypepstatins are active against pepsin and cathepsin D, but pepstatins are more active against renin than pepstanones and hydroxypepstatins. It has also been reported pepstatin inactivates bovine renin (Chang et al., 1973). Activity of pepstatin against rennin increases with an increase in the number of carbon atoms in the fatty acid moiety (Aoyagi et al., 1972). An enzyme which hydrolyzes pepstatins to the fatty acid, L-valine and the residual tetrapeptide has been found in Bacillus sphaericus (Tone et al., 1975a and 1975b). From this tetrapeptide, water-soluble pepstatin analogs (benzoyl or lactoyl-L-valyl-AHMHA-L-alanyl-AHMHA etc.) have been synthesized. They show a similar activity as pepstatin to inhibit pepsin and cathepsin D (Matsushita et al., 1975). Therefore, it is possible to prepare water-soluble pepstatin analogs exhibiting strong inhibition against pepsin and cathepsin D. But these water soluble derivatives have very low activity against renin. Recently, Corval found that pepstanoyl L-aspartic acid is soluble in water and shows the same activity as pepstatin in inhibiting renin. This water-soluble pepstatin showed hypotensive effect (Corval, 1978).

Pepstatin has contributed to the study of the function and chemistry of renin. It became possible to purify renin by using pepstatin affinity chromatography (Corval et al., 1973; Devaux et al., 1976; McKnown et al., 1974; Murakami et al., 1973 and 1975; Orth et al., 1974).

As shown by the extremely small Ki value, that is, 10^{-10}M, the tight binding with pepsin and cathepsin D is strong enough to use pepstatin for titration of these enzymes. The equimolar pepsin-pepstatin complex can be shown by Sephadex chromatography. Pepstatin affinity chromatography has been used also for purification of cathepsin D (Kregar et al., 1975). However, the binding of pepstatin to pepsin and cathepsin D may be too strong and its less active derivatives such as its O-acyl derivatives may be more useful for this purpose (Yago et al., 1975).

Pepstatin shows a strong inhibition of cathepsin D of various sources: swine liver, rabbit liver, human liver, beef lung, rabbit lung, rabbit alveolar macrophages, oil induced rabbit peritoneal macrophage, human cartilage, pig brain and mouse leukemia L-1210. Based on the inhibition of cathepsin D, possible therapeutic effects on cerebral cleavage and arthritis have been suggested. Greenbaum et al. (1975) reported the inhibition of leukokinin formation from leukokininogen and a possible use of pepstatin to inhibit ascites formation in cancer patients has been suggested. As summarized in Table 2, various biological effects of pepstatin have been reported.

Pepstatin has very low toxicity: LD_{50} by intravenous injection; 1,000 mg/kg to mice, 820 mg/kg to rabbits, 450 mg/kg to dogs; LD_{50} by oral administration larger than 2,000 mg/kg. Daily oral administration of 200 mg/kg and 1,000 mg/kg for 180 days caused no toxicity in rats. Daily oral administration of 1,000 mg/kg to monkeys also caused no toxicity. Pepstatin orally given is not practically absorbed.

AN INHIBITOR OF METALLO-ENDOPEPTIDASES

After inhibitors of serine, thiol and carboxyl proteases had been found, our study was extended to find inhibitors of all other proteases. Thermolysin is a zinc enzyme, and its inhibitor has been found in streptomyces. The structure of this inhibitor was elucidated to be N-(α-L-rhamnopyranosyloxyhydroxyphosphinyl)-L-leucyl-L-tryptophan (Fig. 2) and named phosphoramidon (Umezawa, 1976). It inhibits thermolysin (Ki = 2.8 x 10^{-9}M) and related enzymes. It inhibits a thermolysin type enzyme which is called an elastase of Pseudomonas aeruginosa, causing pneumonia in minks. The partially hydrolyzed product, phosphoryl-L-leucyl-L-tryptophan exhibits a 10 times higher activity to inhibit thermolysin (Ki = 2.0 x 10^{-9}M). Thermolysin hydrolyzes the amino side of the hydrophobic aminoacyl group in the peptides. It suggests that the N-phosphate of a hydrophobic amino acid would be the active structure (Komiyama et al., 1975). N-(α-L-rhamnopyranosyloxyhydroxyphosphinyl)-L-leucyl methyl ester shows almost no activity and N-(α-L-rhamnopyranosyloxyhydroxyphosphinyl)-L-leucyl-L-histidine shows a lower activity than phosphoramidon. It indicates that addition of tryptophan or another amino acid to C-terminal group of phosphoryl-L-leucine is necessary for the activity. Phosphoramidon has a low toxicity and the LD_{50} is higher than 1.0 g/kg in mice by intravenous injection.

INHIBITORS OF HYDROLYTIC ENZYMES ENHANCING
OR SUPPRESSING IMMUNE RESPONSES

As already described, enzyme inhibitors can be used in the
treatment of diseases where an enzyme activity is raised abnormally.
In this case, a concentration of an inhibitor high enough to
suppress the raised enzyme activity should be maintained in the
body. However, in case of a sequential change which occurs as the
result of the inhibition of an enzyme continues for a long period,
the intermittent administration of an inhibitor can produce its
effect.

Coriolin group antibiotics (Fig. 4) found by the author, that
is, sesquiterpene antibiotics produced by a cultured mushroom
(Coriolus consor), inhibit Na–K–ATPase (Kunimoto et al., 1973).
Very low doses of coriolins and diketocoriolin B such as 0.01–10
μg/mouse increased the number of mouse spleen cells producing
antibody against sheep red blood cells (Ishizuka et al., 1972).
This effect can be observed also in mouse spleen cells cultured
in vitro. In the experiment shown in Table 3, spleen cells were
cultured with sheep red blood cells for 24 hours under rocking;
cell clusters were dispersed with a syringe and cultured for 2
hours without rocking; the non-adherent cells were transferred to
a fresh dish and the number of antibody-forming cells/10^6 non-
adherent cells was counted. The addition of 0.1 ng of diketocoriolin B at the start or 24 hours of the culture increased the
number of B cells forming antibody against sheep red blood cells.
In this experimental condition, adherent cells, that is, macrophages, were removed. This action of diketocoriolin B occurs even
in the experimental condition where T cells were destroyed by
addition of anti-θ serum and complement. Therefore, diketocoriolin
B should act on B lymphocytes and cause their blastogenesis.

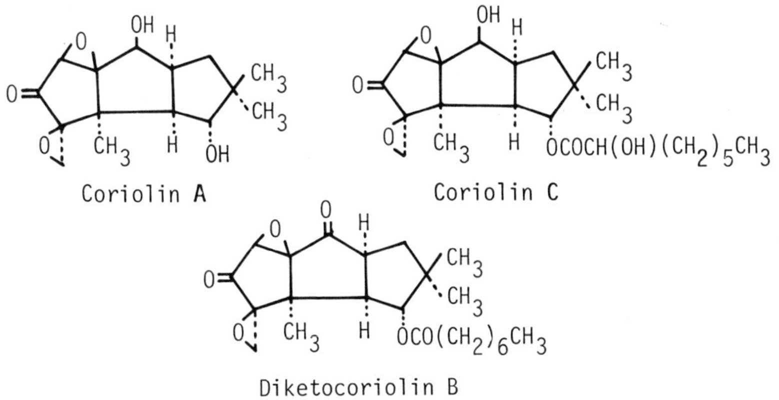

Figure 4. Structures of Coriolins

Glycopeptides such as lectins bind to the surface of immune cells, cause mitogenesis and enhance immune response. The action of coriolin and diketocoriolin B to increase the number of antibody-forming cells may be due to their binding to Na-K-ATPase on the surface of B cells. Therefore, the author thought that small molecular compounds which bound to the surface of immune cells might enhance immune response. The author searched for inhibitors of enzymes on the surface of animal cells. Aminopeptidases which hydrolyzed N-terminal peptide bonds were located not only in cells but also on the cell surface of all kinds of animal cells but not released extracellularly (Aoyagi et al., 1976). That is, intact cells hydrolyzes N-terminal peptide bonds but the enzyme can not be found in the culture medium. Alkaline phosphatase and esterase are also located on the cellular surface. The author et al. (1976a) found bestatin (Fig. 5) which inhibited aminopeptidase B and leucine aminopeptidase. Bestatin is a strong inhibitor of these enzymes and Ki values are 6.0×10^{-8}M against aminopeptidase B and 2.0×10^{-8}M against leucine aminopeptidase. The type of inhibition is competitive with substrates such as arginine β-naphthylamide and leucine β-naphthylamide. Bestatin inhibits the hydrolysis of arginine β-naphthylamide by rat macrophages, lymphocytes and mouse spleen cells. It indicates the binding of bestatin to these cells. The binding of bestatin to these cells has also been shown by experiments using ^{3}H-bestatin. Bestatin enhances activation of small lymphocytes by concanavalin A.

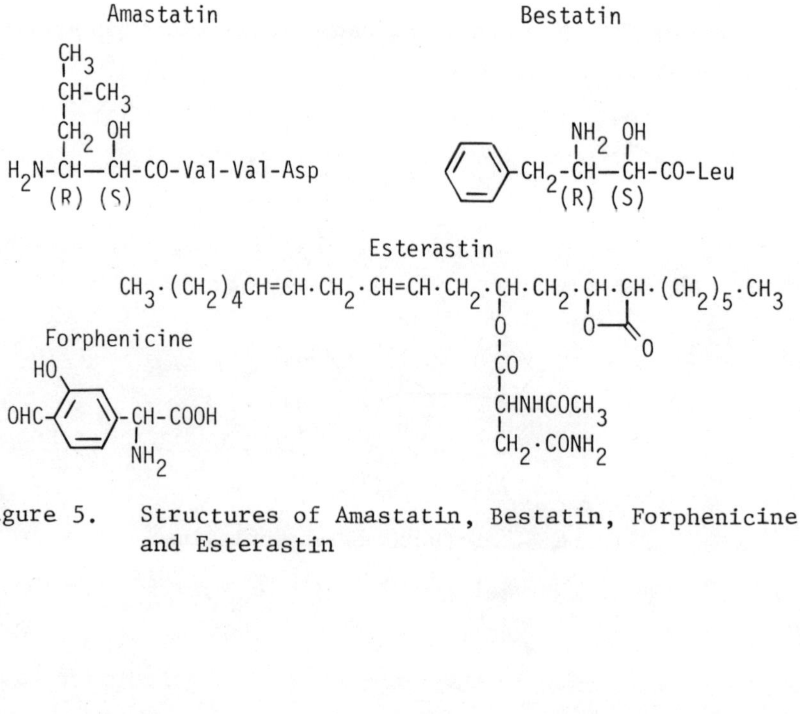

Amastatin

$$CH_3$$
$$|$$
$$CH-CH_3$$
$$|$$
$$CH_2 \quad OH$$
$$| \quad |$$
$$H_2N-CH—CH-CO-Val-Val-Asp$$
$$(R) \quad (S)$$

Bestatin

$$NH_2 \quad OH$$
$$| \quad |$$
⟨benzene⟩$-CH_2-CH—CH-CO-Leu$
$$(R) \quad (S)$$

Esterastin

$$CH_3 \cdot (CH_2)_4 CH=CH \cdot CH_2 \cdot CH=CH \cdot CH_2 \cdot \underset{\underset{CO}{\overset{|}{|}}}{CH} \cdot CH_2 \cdot \underset{\underset{O}{|}}{CH} \cdot CH \cdot (CH_2)_5 \cdot CH_3$$
$$O$$
$$|$$
$$CO$$
$$|$$
$$CHNHCOCH_3$$
$$|$$
$$CH_2 \cdot CONH_2$$

Forphenicine

$$HO$$
$$OHC-⟨benzene⟩-CH-COOH$$
$$|$$
$$NH_2$$

Figure 5.   Structures of Amastatin, Bestatin, Forphenicine and Esterastin

Bestatin enhanced delayed-type hypersensitivity shown by mouse footpad test (Umezawa et al., 1976b). In order to test the activity to enhance delayed-type hypersensitivity, it is necessary to test the activity against aged mice, because the immune response is reduced parallel to the age. Bestatin enhances delayed-type hypersensitivity of mice older than 8 weeks after the birth. If mice are sensitized to sheep red blood cells and the reaction is elicited by human red blood cells, or vice versa, bestatin shows no effect.

Oral, intraperitoneal or intravenous administration of bestatin at the time of sensitization enhances delayed-type hypersensitivity but the administration at the time of the elicitation of the reaction does not. A large dose such as 1,000 µg/mouse of bestatin increases the number of antibody forming cells but does not enhance delayed-type hypersensitivity significantly. Oral, intravenous and intraperitoneal administration of bestatin shows the same action but subcutaneous injection does not always produce the effect.

TABLE 3.   EFFECT OF DKC ON ELIMINATION OF ADHERENT CELLS FROM SPLEEN CELL CULTURE FOR ANTIBODY FORMATION IN VITRO

	whole cells	without adherent cells*
	PFC/10^6 nucleated cells on day 4	
SRBC	395.0	543.3
" + DKC (0)**	653.8	784.9
" + DKC (24)**	856.2	1308.7**

DKC 0.1 ng/culture

*Mouse spleen cells were cultured for 24 hr under rocking; cell clusters were dispersed with syringe and the dispersed cultures were kept for 2 hr without rocking. The non-adherent cells with the cultured fluid were transferred to fresh dishes. 4 days after the culture, the number of plaques forming the antibody against sheep red blood cells was counted.

**DKC was added 0 or 24 hr after the removal of the adherent cells.

TABLE 4.   EFFECT OF BESTATIN ON IMC-CARCONOMA

Bestatin µg/mouse/day	Treatment days and % inhibition mean (range)			
	-7 - -1	1 - 5	8 - 12	14 - 18
1	—	43.1 (52 - 27)	48.7 (89 - 0)	55.0 (76 - 3)
10	—	41.7 (75 - 26)	82.0 (89 - 76)	71.0 (84 - 58)
100	42.3 (91 - 0)	36.3 (63 - 0)	71.6 (82 - 61)	71.3 (81 - 62)

Bestatin (Fig. 5) has three asymmetric carbon atoms and all stereoisomers were synthesized. Then, the configuration of the α-carbon atom of 3-amino-2-hydroxy-4-phenylbutanoyl moiety was shown to be the absolute requirement for inhibition of amino-peptidase B and leucine aminopeptidase (Suda et al., 1976). All isomers containing R configuration of this carbon atom shows much weaker inhibition of these enzymes than the others containing S-configuration. The isomers which inhibit aminopeptidase B strongly enhance delayed-type hypersensitivity in almost the same degree as bestatin. It suggests that the enhancement of delayed-type hyper-sensitivity is due to the binding of bestatin to cells involved in immune response.

If 10, 100 or 1,000 µg/mouse of bestatin is administered and 24 hours thereafter mouse spleen cells are cultured for 48 hours and the ^{3}H-thymidine incorporation is tested, the incorporation into DNA is increased by 50-100%. Bestatin (1 µg/ml) added to mouse spleen cells cultured in vitro increases ^{3}H-thymidine in-corporation into DNA by 50-100%, but if macrophages are removed or T cells are destroyed by addition of anti-θ serum and complement, the effect of bestatin increasing ^{3}H-thymidine incorporation is not observed. It suggests that the mitogenesis of T lymphocytes might occur following the action of bestatin on macrophages.

Bestatin shows therapeutic effect on experimental animal solid tumors which grow slowly and on which the growth can be examined for more than 30 days. In this condition, it inhibits the growth of Gardner lymphosarcoma: when 0.5 or 5 mg/kg of bestatin was orally given for 5 days during day 1 to day 5 of the inoculation of 10^5 cells and the size of the tumor was measured on day 31 of the inoculation, 59-77% inhibition was observed. The effect on IMC carcinoma which appeared spontaneously in CDF$_1$ mice in the author's laboratory is shown in Table 4. If 0.05, 0.5 or 5.0 mg/kg of bestatin is given daily orally for 5 days, the treatment during 8-12 or 14-18 days after the inoculation of tumor cells exhibits a stronger therapeutic effect than the treatment started 1 day after the inoculation.   Daily oral administration of 10 or 100 μg/mouse shows a suppressive effect on induction of squamous cell carcinoma in mouse skin by methylcholanthrene.

Bestatin has low toxicity and clinical studies have been started two years ago. Daily administration of 5 or 30 mg per person has been continued for more than a half year. Daily administration of 300 mg/person for 4 weeks does not show any toxic sign.

The gas chromatographic method of determining bestatin in blood or urine has been developed by Miyazaki et al., Nihon Kayaku Co. Institute. About 80% of bestatin orally administered is excreted into urine. About 1 hour after the oral administration of 30 mg of bestatin, the blood level reaches 1-2 μg/ml. The mass spectroscopic analysis of bestatin in urine indicates that most of bestatin administered is excreted as itself, and 3-10% of bestatin administered is oxidized to p-hydroxybestatin.

Derivatives and analogs of bestatin have been synthesized. Modification of the benzene ring gives more active compounds than bestatin in inhibiting aminopeptidase B and leucine aminopeptidase. p-Hydroxybestatin is one of the derivatives which have a stronger action to inhibit aminopeptidase B than bestatin. It enhances delayed-type hypersensitivity as well as bestatin. Low doses of hydroxybestatin not only enhances delayed-type hypersensitivity but also increases the number of antibody-forming cells. The administration at the time of the elicitation of the reaction also enhances delayed-type hypersensitivity.

On the basis of the experimental data, it has been examined, whether the treatment with 5 or 30 mg of bestatin orally daily or two or three times a week might increase T cells in human patients. Increase of the number of T cells in peripheral blood and increase of T cell percent have been observed in cancer patients. The increase of the number of total lymphocytes was also observed frequently. Thus, the results indicate that bestatin can exhibit the same effect on human immune system as on a mouse immune system. The clinical studies have suggested a favourable effect of bestatin on various tumors. Adverse effect has never been observed in bestatin treatment.

In the last 10 years, cancer immunotherapy using BCG, dead streptococci or high molecular compounds have been studied in detail. The principal difference between high molecular and small molecular immune-enhancing agents is their positive or negative antigenicity. In the case of macromolecular agents, it is possible

that immune response against themselves is enhanced together with
that against tumors. In the case of small molecular immune-
enhancing agents like bestatin, they are not antigenic and immune
response against themselves should not occur.

In preliminary experiments, when the oral bestatin treatment
of IMC carcinoma was started from 8 days after the inoculation of
tumor cells, the simultaneous daily intraperitoneal administration
of a protein (bovine γ-globulin) decreased the therapeutic effect
of bestatin. It suggests that in some cases of the reduced immune
stage of cancer-bearing animals or patients the administration of
antigenic materials might reduce the therapeutic action of immune-
enhancing agents. Moreover, it suggests that small molecular
immune-affecting agents would be useful in analysis of the
immune-response process.

Since we established a method to find immune-enhancing agents,
it is possible to find active agents in natural products. As
already described, aminopeptidase A which hydrolyzes the N-terminal
glutamyl and aspartyl bonds appears on the surface of animal cells
but not released extracellularly. In the screening of this
inhibitor, we found a tetrapeptide which we named amastatin (Fig.
5) (Aoyagi et al., 1978a). It contains (2S,3R)-3-amino-2-hydroxy-
5-methylhexanoic acid. It inhibits aminopeptidase A and leucine
aminopeptidase. IC_{50} against these enzymes was about 0.5 µg/ml.
It does not inhibit aminopeptidase B and endopeptidases. Amastatin
inhibits the hydrolysis of glutamic acid β-naphthylamide and
leucine β-naphthylamide by human thymocytes and rat thymocytes.
It also inhibits aminopeptidase B activity of human thymocytes but
not of rat thymocytes. Bestatin inhibits aminopeptidase B of these
thymocytes but aminopeptidase A only weakly. Amastatin also inhibits not only the action of aminopeptidase A and leucine aminopeptidase of lymphocyte B cell lines but also inhibits the aminopeptidase B of these cell lines. These results indicate that
amastatin can bind to immune cells. Intraperitoneal injection of
10 or 100 µg of amastatin at the time of immunization increased
the number of sheep red blood cell antibody-forming cells 2.5-3.5
times.

As shown in Table 5, amastatin, bestatin and hydroxybestatin
inhibit the activities of aminopeptidases A and B, and leucine
aminopeptidases of all cancer cells cultured: FM3A, mouse mammary
carcinoma cells; AH66 and AH66F, rat hepatoma cells, Ehrlich carcinoma cells. These inhibitors all inhibit the hydrolysis of
glycylprolylleucine or glycylhistidyllysine β-naphthylamide by
these cells. Glycylhistidyllysine has been reported to promote
the growth of human hepatoma cells (Schlessinger et al., 1977).

As already described, alkaline phosphatase appears on the
surface of cells. In the screening of inhibitors against chicken

TABLE 5.   INHIBITORY ACTIVITIES OF AMASTATIN, BESTATIN AND
           HYDROXYBESTATIN AGAINST AMINOPEPTIDASES OF TUMOR CELL

| | Aminopeptidase | IC_{50} (μg/ml) | | | |
		FM3A	AH66	AH66F	Ehrlich
Amastatin	A	0.01	0.03	0.05	0.01
	B	0.08	0.4	0.1	0.01
	Leu	0.1	0.8	0.3	0.4
	Gly-Pro-Leu	10	0.3	1	0.2
	Gly-His-Lys	0.05	0.1	0.5	0.1
Bestatin	A	1	0.2	0.2	0.05
	B	0.2	0.2	0.2	0.3
	Leu	1	5	5	8.5
	Gly-Pro-Leu	46	1.6	4.2	3
	Gly-His-Lys	1	0.8	2	2
Hydroxy-bestatin	A	0.2	0.1	0.1	0.05
	B	0.2	0.1	0.1	0.4
	Leu	2	5	5	13
	Gly-Pro-Leu	28	2	5	3.5
	Gly-His-Lys	1	1	2	2.5

The homogenates of cells were prepared by Dounce homogenizer.

intestine alkaline phosphatase, we found a new amino acid which
was named forphenicine (Fig. 5) (Aoyagi et al., 1978b). It inhibits
chicken intestine alkaline phosphatase very strongly.   But it
inhibits only very weakly alkaline phosphatases from other sources.
The type of inhibition is very interesting and uncompetitive with
the substrate (p-nitrophenyl phosphate).   The binding of forphenicine to animal cells including lymphocytes can be shown by
using its labeled analog.   Intraperitoneal administration of
1-1,000 μg/mouse of forphenicine at the time of the immunization
enhanced delayed-type hypersensitivity to sheep red blood cells
and intraperitoneal administration of 10-1,000 μg/mouse increased
the number of antibody-forming cells.   Intraperitoneal injection
at the time of the elicitation of the reaction also enhanced
delayed-type hypersensitivity shown by mouse footpad test.

The action to increase the number of antibody-forming cells
can also be shown by its effect on cultured mouse spleen cells.
If macrophages are pretreated with forphenicine, then the number
of antibody-forming cells is increased.   It indicates that forphenicine acts on macrophages.   The intraperitoneal administration
of 10 or 100 μg/mouse showed the same inhibitory action against
Gardner lymphosarcoma and IMC carcinoma as bestatin.

An inhibitor of esterase which we named esterastin (Fig. 5)

was also found in streptomyces (Umezawa et al., 1978). As shown
by its Ki value it is a very strong inhibitor. The type of the
inhibition was competitive with the substrate (p-nitrophenyl
acetate). Intraperitoneal injection of not less than 62 µg/mouse
suppressed both delayed-type hypersensitivity and antibody-
formation.

In Table 6, there are shown Ki values of bestatin against
aminopeptidase B (rat liver) and leucine aminopeptidase (hog
kidney), amastatin against aminopeptidase A (rat kidney) and leucine aminopeptidase, forphenicine against chicken intestine alkaline phosphatase and esterastin against esterase (hog pancreas).
Ki value of esterastin is in the order of 10^{-10}M and extremely
small compared with Ki values of others. It is not yet certain
whether the enhancement or the suppression of immune response is
due to the binding strength or to the kinds of receptors for the
binding.

As described above, inhibitors of enzymes which appear on
the surface of macrophages and lymphocytes enhance or suppress
immune response. We are continuing the study of enzymes on immune
cells and their inhibitors. Some of them will become useful in
treatment of cancer. If we have various inhibitors which affect
immune response, they will be useful for analysis of immune reaction process. They also affect inflammation and may be useful
in the analysis of inflammatory processes.

TABLE 6.   KINETIC CONSTANTS OF INHIBITORS AGAINST ENZYMES

Inhibitors	Enzymes	Substrates	$Km(\times 10^{-4}M)$	$Ki(\times 10^{-8}M)$	Type of inhibition
Amastatin	AP-A[1]	L-Glutamic acid NA[2]	1.0	15	Competitive
	Leu-AP	L-Leucine NA	37	160	Competitive
Bestatin	AP-B	L-Arginine NA	1.0	6.0	Competitive
	Leu-AP	L-Leucine NA	5.8	2.0	Competitive
Forphenicine	Alkaline phosphatase	PNPP[3]	4.6	16.4	Uncompetitive
Esterastin	Esterase	PNPA[4]	4.0	0.016	Competitive

1) Aminopeptidase A   2) L-Glutamic acid β-naphthylamide
3) p-Nitrophenyl phosphate   4) p-Nitrophenyl acetate

CONCLUSION

We initiated the study of small molecular enzyme inhibitors produced by microorganisms and found about 50 new compounds. In this paper, the author reviewed our studies on inhibitors of various proteases and enzymes on the surface of animal cells. Small molecular inhibitors of cellular surface enzymes enhanced or suppressed immune response. Studies on kinin and its related areas are rapidly progressing as shown by papers presented in this symposium. Parallel to the progress in these areas, it will become possible to establish new screening methods and to find new compounds useful in the study of kinin and its related systems.

REFERENCES

Aoyagi, T., S. Miyata, M. Nanbo, F. Kojima, M. Matsuzaki, M. Ishizuka, T. Takeuchi and H. Umezawa, 1969. Biological activities of leupeptins, J. Antibiotics 22: 558.

Aoyagi, T., H. Morishima, R. Nishizawa, S. Kunimoto, T. Takeuchi, H. Umezawa and H. Ikezawa, 1972. Biological activity of pepstatins, pepstanone A and partial peptides on pepsin, cathepsin D and renin. J. Antibiotics, 25: 689.

Aooyagi, T., H. Suda, M. Nagai, K. Ogawa, J. Suzuki, T. Takeuchi and H. Umezawa, 1976. Aminopeptidase activities on the surface of mammalian cells. Biochim. Biophys. Acta 452: 131.

Aoyagi, T., H. Tobe, F. Kojima, M. Hamada, T. Takeuchi, and H. Umezawa, 1978a. Amastatin, an inhibitor of aminopeptidase A, produced by actinomycetes. J. Antibiotics 31: 636.

Aoyagi, T., T. Yamamoto, K. Kojiri, F. Kojima, M. Hamada, T. Takeuchi and H. Umezawa, 1978b. Forphenicine, an inhibitor of alkaline phosphatase produced by actinomycetes, J. Antibiotics 31: 244.

Chang, W. and K. Takahashi, 1973. The structure and function of acid proteases. II. Inactivation of bovine renin by acid protease-specific inhibitors, J. Biochem. 74: 231.

Corval, P., 1978. (National Institute of Health and Medical Research, Paris), An active water soluble pepstatin derivative (pepstanoylaspartic acid) against renin. Personal communication.

Corval, P., C. Devaux and J. Menard, 1973. Pepstatin, an inhibitor for renin purification by affinity chromatography, FEBS Letters 34: 189.

Devaux, C., J. Menard, P. Sicard and P. Corval, 1976. Partial characterization of hog renin purified by affinity chromatography, Eur. J. Biochem. 64: 621.

Greenbaum, L.M., P. Grebow, M. Gohnston, A. Prekash and G. Semente, 1975. Pepstatin, an inhibitor of leukokinin formation and ascitic fluid accumulation, Cancer Res. 35: 706.

Hanada, K., M. Tamai, S. Morimoto, T. Adachi, S. Ohmura, J. Sawada
    and I. Tanaka, 1978a. Inhibitory activities of E-64 derivatives
    on papain, Agric. Biol. Chem. 42: 537.
Hanada, K., M. Tamai, S. Ohmura, J. Sawada, T. Seki and T. Tanaka,
    1978b. Structure and synthesis of E-64, a new thiol protease
    inhibitor, Agric. Biol. Chem. 42: 529.
Hanada, K., M. Tamai, M. Yamagishi, S. Ohmura, J. Sawada and I.
    Tanaka, 1978c. Isolation and characterization of E-64, a new
    thiol protease inhibitor, Agric. Biol. Chem. 42: 523.
Hori, M., H. Hemmi, K. Suzukake, H. Hayashi, Y. Uehara, T. Takeuchi
    and H. Umezawa, 1978. Biosynthesis of leupeptin. J. Antibiotics,
    31: 95.
Hozumi, M., M. Ogawa, T. Sugimura, T. Takeuchi and H. Umezawa, 1972.
    Inhibition of tumorigenesis in mouse skin by leupeptin, a
    protease inhibitor from Actinomycetes, Cancer Res. 32: 1725.
Ishizuka, M., H. Iinuma, T. Takeuchi and H. Umezawa, 1972. Effect
    of diketocoriolin B on antibody formation. J. Antibiotics 25:
    320.
Kakizoe, T., H. Esumi, K. Kawachi, T. Sugimura, T. Takeuchi and
    H. Umezawa, 1977a. Further studies on the effect of leupeptin,
    a protease inhibitor, on induction of bladder tumors in rats
    by N-butyl-4-(4-hydroxybutyl)nitrosamine, J. Natl. Cancer Inst.
    59: 1503.
Kakizoe, T., T. Sano, T. Kawachi, T. Sugimura, T. Takeuchi and H.
    Umezawa, 1977b. Effect of leupeptin on induction of lympho-
    blastic leukemia in mice by N-nitrosobutylurea, Gann 68: 281.
Kinoshita, M., S. Aburaki, A. Hagiwara and J. Imai, 1973. Absolute
    configuration of 4-amino-3-hydroxy-6-methylheptanoic acid
    present in pepstatin A and stereospecific synthesis of all four
    isomers. J. Antibiotics 26: 249.
Komiyama, T., H. Suda, T. Aoyagi, T. Takeuchi, H. Umezawa, K. Fuji-
    moto and S. Umezawa, 1975. Studies on inhibitory effect of
    phosphoramidon and its analogs on thermolysin, Arch. Biochem.
    Biophys. 171: 727.
Kregar, I., I. Urh, H. Umezawa and V. Turk, Isolation of cathepsin
    D by affinity chromatography on immobilized pepstatin, 1975.
    In: Intracellular protein catabolism II, eds. V. Turk, N. Marks,
    A.J. Barrett and J.F. Woessner (Plenum Press, New York) p. 250.
Kunimoto, T. and H. Umezawa, 1973. Kinetic studies on the inhibition
    of Na^+-K^+-ATPase by diketocoriolin B, Biochim. Biophys. Acta
    318: 78.
Maeda, K., K. Kawamura, S. Kondo, T. Aoyagi, T. Takeuchi and H.
    Umezawa, 1971. The structure and activity of leupeptins and
    related analogs. J. Antibiotics 24: 402.
Matsushima, T., T. Kakizoe, T. Kawachi, K. Hara, T. Sugimura, T.
    Takeuchi and H. Umezawa,Effects of protease inhibitors of
    microbial origin on experimental carcinogenesis, 1977, In:
    Fundamentals in Cancer Prevention, eds. P.N. Magee et al.,
    (University of Tokyo Press and University Park Press, Tokyo)
    p. 57.

Matsushita, Y., H. Tone, S. Hori, Y. Yagi, A. Takamatsu, H. Morishima, T. Aoyagi, T. Takeuchi and H. Umezawa, 1975. N-Acylated derivatives of a peptide obtained by enzymatic degradation of pepstatin, J. Antibiotics 28: 1016.

McKnown, M.M., R.J. Workman and R.I. Gregerman, 1974. Pepstatin inhibition of human renin. Kinetic studies and estimation of enzyme purity. J. Biol. Chem. 249: 7770.

Morishima, H., T. Sawa, T. Takita, T. Aoyagi, T. Takeuchi and H. Umezawa, 1974. Biosynthetic studies on pepstatin. Biosynthesis of (3S,4S)-4-amino-3-hydroxy-6-methylheptanoic acid moiety, J. Antibiotics 27: 267.

Murakami, K. and T. Inagami, 1975. Isolation of pure and stable renin from hog kidney. Biochem. Biophys. Res. Commun. 62: 757.

Murakami, K., T. Inagamin, A. Michelakis and S. Cohen, 1973. An affinity column for renin, Biochem. Biophys. Res. Commun. 54: 482.

Murase, M., T. Ito, S. Fukatsu and H. Umezawa, Studies on kanamycin related compounds produced during fermentation by mutants of streptomyces kanamyceticus. Isolation and Properties, 1970. In: Progress in Antimicrobial and anticancer chemotherapy (Proceedings of the 6th International Congress of Chemotherapy) (University of Tokyo Press, Tokyo) p. 1098.

Orth, H., E. Hackenthal, J. Lazar, U. Miksche and F. Gross, 1974. Kinetics of the inhibitory effect of pepstatin on the reaction of hog renin with rat plasma substrate. Circulation Res. 35: 52.

Schlessinger, D.H., L. Pickart and M. M. Thaler, 1977. Growth-modulating serum tripeptide is glycyl-histidyl-lysine, Experimentia 33: 324.

Suda, H., T. Aoyagi, T. Takeuchi, and H. Umezawa, 1976. Inhibition of aminopeptidase B and leucine aminopeptidase by bestatin and its stereoisomers. Arch. Biochem. Biophys. 177: 196.

Tone, H., Y. Matsuchita, Y. Yagi, A. Takamatsu, T. Aoyagi, T. Takeuchi and H. Umezawa, 1975a. Purification and properties of pepstatin hydrolase from Bacillus sphaericus, J. Antibiotics 28: 1012.

Tone, H., N. Shibamoto, Y. Matsushita, T. Inui, A. Takamatsu, T. Aoyagi, T. Takeuchi and H. Umezawa, 1975b. Enzymatic degradation of pepstatin A to a new tetrapeptide, J. Antibiotics 28: 1009.

Umezawa, H., Structures and activities of protease inhibitors of microbial origin, 1976. In: Methods in Enzymology 45, Part B, eds. L. Lorand (Academic Press, New York) p. 678.

Umezawa, H., T. Aoyagi, T. Hazato, K. Uotani, F. Kojima, M. Hamada and T. Takeuchi, 1978. Esterastin, an inhibitor of esterase, produced by actinomycetes. J. Antibiotics 31: 639.

Umezawa, H., T. Aoyagi, H. Suda, M. Hamada and T. Takeuchi, 1976a. Bestatin, an inhibitor of aminopeptidase B, produced by actinomycetes, J. Antibiotics 29: 97.

Umezawa, H., M. Ishizuka, T. Aoyagi and T. Takeuchi, 1976b. Enhancement of delayed-type hypersensitivity by bestatin, an inhibitor
of aminopeptidase B and leucine aminopeptidase. J. Antibiotics
29: 857.

Umezawa, K., T. Matsushima and T. Sugimura, 1977. Antimutagenic
effect of elastatinal, a protease inhibitor from actinomycetes,
Proc. Japan. Acad. 53: Ser. B, 30.

Yago, N. and W.E. Bowers, 1975. Unique cathepsin D-type proteases
in rat thoracic duct lymphocytes and in rat lymphoid tissues.
J. Biol., Chem. 250: 4749.

KALLIKREIN INHIBITOR (APROTININ): PLASMA TURNOVER

AND EFFECTS ON COAGULATION IN RHESUS MONKEYS

Moacir De Sa Pereira

U. S. Army Medical Research Institute
of Infectious Diseases
Frederick, Maryland 21701 U.S.A.

Aprotinin (Trasylol^R = 10,000 KIU/ml) is a protease inhibitor obtained from bovine lung, and is known to inhibit kallikrein, trypsin and plasmin (1). In vitro, it has been shown to inhibit early reactions of blood coagulation and to prolong clotting time (2,3). In view of these properties, aprotinin has been proposed as therapy for disseminated intravascular coagulation (DIC) (2,4). Results of in vivo studies were contradictory as to the effects of aprotinin in human coagulation (2,5) but in preliminary clinical trials the net effect was found to be beneficial (4).

We studied the use of aprotinin in coagulation in the rhesus monkey model for DIC described by Wing et al (6). Initial efforts were directed toward the study of the pharmacology of the inhibitor in monkeys: one milliliter samples of aprotinin were iodinated by microdiffusion as described by Gruber and Wright (7).

The labeled product maintained the inhibitory properties of stock aprotinin as demonstrated by successful inhibition of the esterase activity of kallikrein on the substrates benzoyl arginine ethyl ester and tosyl-L-arginine methyl ester.

Eight monkeys were injected (via the saphenous vein) with 1 ml of ^{125}I-aprotinin and 40,000 KIU/kg of "cold" aprotinin. Two minutes after injection the 0 time sample was drawn from the contralateral femoral vein. Subsequent sampling was done at sequential intervals after infusion.

The radioactive content of these plasma samples was measured in a gamma counter. The values obtained were plotted on a logarithmic scale against time (Fig. 1). In each case, the disappearance curve of the injected label was fitted to a triple exponential equation.

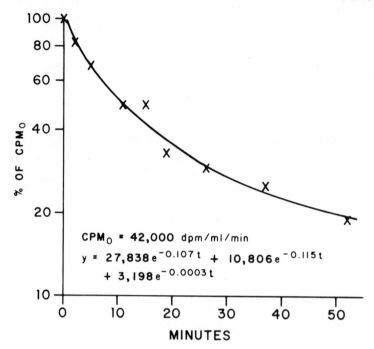

Fig. 1.   Plasma turnover of ^{125}I-aprotinin in a rhesus monkey. The points are results of a representative experiment (last 6 values not shown).   The equation that best fits the data is depicted.

In the equation (Table 1), y represents counts per minute, t represents time, λ_1, λ_2, λ_3, are the time constants with σ_1, σ_2, σ_3, the constants of the exponentials.   The equation that best fits the data for each test was obtained by linear regression analysis (8).

The calculated half-lives are represented in Table 1; since they were so short, it was decided that the only effective route of administration of aprotinin was continuous intravenous infusion. The fast turnover confirms the results of Werle and Trautschold in dogs and humans (9).   It also explains the results of Amris and Hilden (2) showing aprotinin effect on coagulation in early samples.   The negative results of Gormsen and Josephsen (5) are explained by the later sampling done by these authors.

The next step was to study the in vivo effect of an injection of aprotinin.   Thirteen monkeys were injected with 40,000 KIU/kg of aprotinin; blood samples were obtained at sequential time intervals after the end of the injection.   The activated partial thromboplastin time (APTT) peaked at 4.6 $\pm$ 1.0 min after the injection with an increase of 47.3 $\pm$ 5.0% without any significant

Table 1. Turnover of ^{125}I-aprotinin in plasma of rhesus monkeys.

$$y = \sigma_1 e^{-\lambda_1 t} + \sigma_2 e^{-\lambda_2 t} + \sigma_3 e^{-\lambda_3 t}$$

Monkey No.	Half-life (T-1/2 = $\frac{\ln 2}{\lambda}$)		
	λ_1 (min)	λ_2 (min)	λ_3 (h)
1	6.5	60	41
2	6.0	67	68
3	3.2	34	33
4	3.8	36	102
5	5.0	53	68
6	3.2	25	48
7	3.5	34	44
8	2.4	23	53
Mean $\pm$ SD	4.2 $\pm$ 1.4	41 $\pm$ 16	57 $\pm$ 22

Table 2. Effect of aprotinin 40,000 KIU/kg, on activated partial thromboplastin time of rhesus monkeys after i.v. injection

	Mean $\pm$ SD	
Min after end of injection	% Increase in APTT
2.2 $\pm$ 0.6	36.5 $\pm$ 15.0
6.4 $\pm$ 1.0	38.9 $\pm$ 19.6
12.3 $\pm$ 0.6	31.2 $\pm$ 18.2
15.8 $\pm$ 4.0	26.9 $\pm$ 18.2
26.3 $\pm$ 1.4	20.3 $\pm$ 16.3
33.1 $\pm$ 2.4	15.9 $\pm$ 16.5
46.6 $\pm$ 2.2	17.8 $\pm$ 16.6
61.2 $\pm$ 4.1	11.0 $\pm$ 14.1
125.3 $\pm$ 6.1	9.3 $\pm$ 23.6

change in prothrombin time. This effect was short-lived and by 1 hr the APTT values had returned to normal (Table 2).

The downward slopes in the first 20 min after the injection were similar when both experiments were done simultaneously in four monkeys, as shown by the correlation (Fig. 2) of the values for counts per minute in the pharmacokinetic studies and the increase in the APTT after injection.

In summary, these data indicate that aprotinin has a very short half-life in the plasma of rhesus monkeys and when circulating at high levels it can inhibit the initial phase of intravascular coagulation, as has been described in human plasma (2,4).

We have used aprotinin for therapy in Salmonella typhimurium-infected rhesus monkeys following the protocol (Fig. 3).

Preliminary data have failed to demonstrate any significant difference in the parameters measured between saline and aprotinin-treated monkeys. In platelet counts, for example (Fig. 4), all infected animals had significantly fewer circulating platelets than controls, independent of therapy.

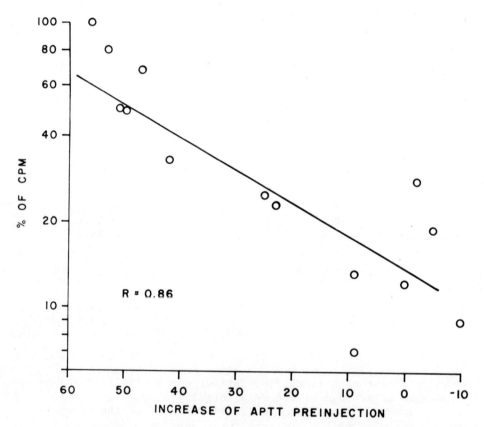

Fig. 2. Correlation between plasma level of ^{125}I-aprotinin and prolongation of APTT. The points are results of a representative experiment (same as Fig. 1).

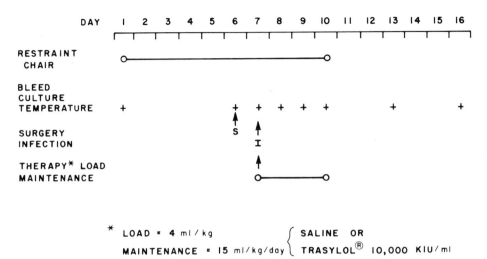

Fig. 3. Protocol for study of effects of aprotinin infusion in S. typhimurium-infected and appropriate control monkeys.

ACKNOWLEDGMENTS

The author thanks Drs. Tadataka Yamada and David Wing for their advice, comments and encouragement, Mrs. Phebe W. Summers for her editorial assistance and Mr. Glen Higbee for the computer analysis of the data. The technical skills of C. Paul Abshire, Charles Ambrose, Carol Heavner, Cathleen Schmidt and David Shapiro are gratefully acknowledged.

In conducting the research described in this report, the investigator adhered to the "Guide for the Care and Use of Laboratory Animals," as promulgated by the Committee on the Revision of the Guide for Laboratory Animal Facilities and Care of the Institute of Laboratory Animal Resources, National Research Council. The facilities are fully accredited by the American Association for Accreditation of Laboratory Animal Care.

The views of the author do not purport to reflect the positions of the Department of the Army or the Department of Defense.

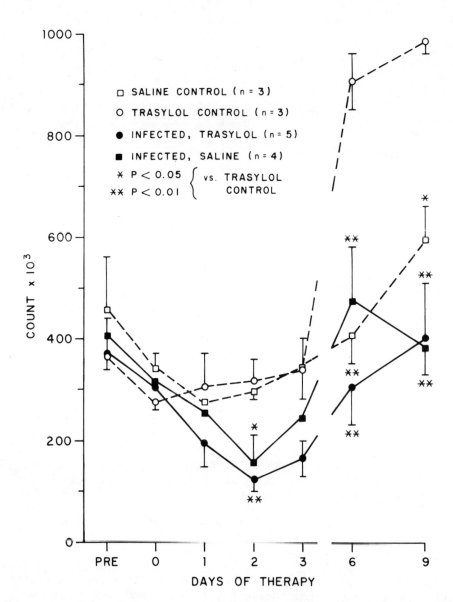

Fig. 4. Effect of aprotinin on platelet count in S. typhimurium-infected rhesus monkeys. The Pre value is the average of 2 samples obtained prior to infection. Bars are SEM. Significance was calculated by analysis of variance using the least significant difference between groups.

REFERENCES

1. Trautschold, I., E. Werle and G. Zickgraf-Rudel, 1966, Uber
    den Kallikrein-Trypsin-Inhibitor, Arzneim-Forsch. 16, 1507.

2. Amris, C. J. and M. Hilden, 1968, Anticoagulant effects of
    Trasylol^R: in vitro and in vivo studies. Ann. N.Y. Acad. Sci.
    146, 612.

3. Prentice, C. R. M., G. P. McNicol and A. S. Douglas, 1970,
    Studies on the anticoagulant action of aprotinin ("Trasylol").
    Thromb. Diath. Haemorrh. 24, 265.

4. Ambrus, J. L., C. M. Ambrus, L. Stutzman, G. Schimert, K. R.
    Niswander, M. W. Woodruff and I. V. Magoss, 1968, Treatment
    of fibrinolytic hemorrhage with proteinase inhibitors: a pre-
    liminary report. Ann. N.Y. Acad. Sci. 146, 625.

5. Gormsen, J. and P. Josephsen, 1967, The effect of Trasylol on
    blood coagulation after intravenous injection. Thromb. Diath.
    Haemorrh. 17, 51.

6. Wing, D. A., T. Yamada, H. B. Hawley and G. W. Pettit, 1978,
    Model for disseminated intravascular coagulation: bacterial
    sepsis in rhesus monkeys. J. Lab. Clin. Med. 92, 239.

7. Gruber, J. and G. G. Wright, 1967, Iodine-131 labeling of
    purified microbial antigens by microdiffusion. Proc. Soc.
    Exptl. Biol. Med. 126, 282.

8. Berman, M. and M. F. Weiss, 1967, SAAM Manual (U. S. Public
    Health Service Publ. No. 1703, U.S. Government Printing
    Office, Washington, D.C.).

9. Werle, E. and I. Trautschold, 1961, Bestimmung des Kallikrein-
    Inaktivators "Trasylol^R" im Blut und im Organen und seine
    Verteilung nach Injektionen. Munch. Med. Wschr. 103, 773.

THE EFFECT OF PROPHYLACTIC PROTEINASE INHIBITOR THERAPY ON

POST-TRAUMATIC PULMONARY INSUFFICIENCY AND PLATELET COUNTS

David S. Rosengarten, J.C. McMichan, E. Philipp

Department of Surgery, Monash Medical School
Alfred Hospital
Melbourne, Australia

ABSTRACT

In a prospective double blind clinical study of 70 patients with bony trauma and shock, 35 patients were allocated into each group receiving either a placebo or Aprotinin.

In both groups there was a high incidence of pulmonary insufficiency and thrombocytopaenia.

In the placebo group there was a higher incidence of pulmonary insufficiency, but not its severity, with greater volumes of blood transfusion and the most severe form occurred only after decompensated shock.

Thrombocytopaenia showed a similar pattern in all patients from both groups falling to a mean minimum on the 2nd day and rising thereafter. In the placebo group counts were lower in those with decompensated shock, and the fall was more profound, rapid and earlier in patients developing severe pulmonary insufficiency. Counts of less than 100,000 on the first day were associated with a high probability of severe pulmonary insufficiency subsequently occurring and this finding was not associated with greater volumes of blood transfusion.

In those patients receiving Aprotinin, the subsequent incidence of severity of pulmonary insufficiency was less and not associated with increased volumes of blood transfusion. The platelet counts were not lower in decompensated shock and there was a more rapid rise from the minimum level.

349

INTRODUCTION

Pulmonary insufficiency is a well recognized complication of
traumatic shock and often is the cause of death. Among the many
factors implicated in its aetiology, microvascular damage and
especially pulmonary microembolic occlusion either by fat (Parker et
al. 1972), fibrin deposition following disseminated intravascular
coagulation (McKay 1965, Bergentz et al. 1971, Hardaway 1966),
macroaggregates from infused stored blood (McNamara et al. 1972,
Davidson et al. 1975), and platelet aggregates (Blaisdell et al.
1970, 1973, 1974) have been considered important. Several animal
studies (Heideman et al. 1972, Peer et al. 1975) have provided
evidence to support the view of pulmonary trapping of platelet
aggregates being a major aetiological factor.

Following clinical reports (Zimmerman et al. 1972, Gurd 1972,
Haberland et al. 1970) of the beneficial effects of Aprotinin
(TRASYLOL) on this condition plus animal experimental findings of
a reduction in platelet trapping after traumatic shock in the
presence of this drug (Heideman et al. 1972), a prospective double
blind clinical study was designed to assess the relationship between
platelet counts and post-traumatic pulmonary insufficiency plus the
effect of Aprotinin on this relationship.

Aprotinin is a basic polypeptide which is a potent proteinase
inhibitor and inactivator of the Kallikrein - Kinin system, both of
which are known to be activated in shock states.

METHODOLOGY

Patients included were those with a combination of hypovolaemic
shock plus major fractures of the pelvis, femur and tibia.

Patients excluded from the study were those admitted more than
12 hours after injury and those with major head or chest injuries so
that local trauma would not confuse the clinical diagnosis of
pulmonary insufficiency.

After admission, the patients were allocated at random into
those to receive either placebo or Aprotinin intravenously in
unlabelled coded ampoules, the codes not being broken until the
conclusion of the study. These were added to a regimen designed to
intensively treat hypovolaemia. Microfilters were not used on any
patient in this study and the attending clinicians administered
oxygen on their own judgement; our research team had no role in any
clinical decision making.

Patients were assessed on admission, after any operative
procedure, and, thereafter, daily for 5 days, by taking paired venous

and arterial blood samples for serial platelet counts and arterial blood gases as well as inspired oxygen concentration (Fi 02) using a Beckman analyser.

The Aprotinin dosage was 500,000 K.I.U. intravenously with a maintenance dosage of 300,000 K.I.U. intravenously for 96 hours.

Shock was defined as compensated if vasoconstriction was present with a systolic blood pressure greater than 110mm. Hg. and decompensated if the systolic blood pressure was less than this level.

Pulmonary insufficiency (P.I.) was defined by the criterion of the P/F ratio $(\frac{Pa\ 02}{Fi\ 02\%})$.
If this was less than 300, significant pulmonary insufficiency was present (Horovitz et al. 1974). The use of this ratio has the advantages of simplicity and has an excellent correlation with the pulmonary shunt fraction and the alveolar arterial oxygen gradient, and is able to give an assessment of pulmonary function in a patient on oxygen supplementation.

As the P/F ratio is purely a qualitative criterion, an arbitrary quantitation of the severity of pulmonary insufficiency was made (Table 1). Discrimination between stages 1 and 2 was difficult as changes in pulse and respiratory rates were somewhat non specific.

RESULTS

Of the 70 patients studied, 35 were allocated to each group and these were comparable for all the parameters shown (Table 2).

TABLE 1.   QUANTITATION OF PULMONARY INSUFFICIENCY (P/F < 300)

		P/F	CLINICAL	
0	ABSENT	> 300	-	
1	↓	< 300	-	
2		< 300	R > 20	P > 100
3	SEVERE	< 300	CEREBRAL DYSFUNCTION	

TABLE 2. PATIENT DATA

	PLACEBO (35)	APROTININ (35)
MALE	22	27
FEMALE	13	8
AGE MEAN (YEARS)	30.6	30.9
SHOCK		
COMPENSATED	9	11
DECOMPENSATED	26(2.4HRS)	24(2.2HRS)
MEAN VOLUME BLOOD		
TRANSFUSED (LITRES)	1.6	1.2
BLOOD TRANSFUSION		
< 1 LITRE	16	22
> 1 LITRE	19	13
CRYSTALLOID INFUSION		
(LITRES) RESUSC.	3.3	3.5
DAY 1	2.2	2.3
TIME LAPSE (HRS)	3	2.9
OPERATION	33 (2HRS)	33 (1.6HRS)
HYPOXAEMIA ON ADMISSION	18	18

Pulmonary Insufficiency

The incidence of lesser degrees of pulmonary insufficiency (stages 1 and 2) was no different between the treatment groups. However there was a significantly lesser incidence of severe pulmonary insufficiency with cerebral symptoms in those patients receiving Aprotinin (Table 3).

Of the patients who did not have pulmonary insufficiency on admission, a significantly lesser incidence of pulmonary insufficiency subsequently occurred in those patients receiving Aprotinin (Table 4).

An analysis of respiratory support (Table 5) showed that those patients receiving Aprotinin needed less oxygen supplementation, both throughout the whole period of study and also from day 1 onwards. This was entirely due to those patients with decompensated shock. Overall all patients in both groups with decompensated shock required more oxygen supplementation than those with compensated shock. Only 5 patients in the whole study required ventilatory support and these all received the placebo.

TABLE 3. PULMONARY INSUFFICIENCY

STAGE	PLACEBO	APROTININ	
0	8	16	
1	9	10	
2	9	8	
3	9	1	P = 0.016
	35	35	

TABLE 4.

	PLACEBO	APROTININ
NO PI ADMISSION	20	31
↓		
PI DAY 1	11	7

$p < 0.02$

TABLE 5. RESPIRATORY SUPPORT

	PLACEBO(35)	APROTININ(35)	P
O$_2$ SUPPLEMENT			
WHOLE PERIOD	24	14	< 0.025
DAYS 1 - 5	23	10	< 0.005
SHOCK			
COMPENSATED	2	3	N.S.
DECOMPENSATED	22	11	< 0.01
MECHANICAL VENTILATION	5	0	0.026

Platelet Counts

The relative fall of platelet counts is shown in Figure 1. The platelet counts were corrected for the admission level in individual patients and the means plotted to give an assessment of the rate of change of the platelet counts (B.M.D. Program P2D University of California).

An overall pattern of platelet counts occurred in all patients irrespective of the presence of absence or severity of pulmonary insufficiency and regardless of the treatment given. This pattern was a fall from admission to a mean minimum on the second day which subsequently rose thereafter to approximate the admission level by the 5th day.

An analysis of covariance (B.M.D. Program P2V University of California) showed that:-
1. All patients showed this pattern (p < 0.0001).
2. There was no significant difference in either the fall or rise between groups 0, 1 and 2 in the placebo group.
3. There was no significant difference in the fall or rise between groups 0, 1 and 2 in the Aprotinin group.
4. Those patients developing severe pulmonary insufficiency in the placebo group had an earlier, more profound, and rapid fall than those of lesser degrees of pulmonary insufficiency
5. Those patients receiving Aprotinin had a significantly lesser fall and a more rapid rise in the placebo group.

The means of the absolute platelet counts in the placebo group (Figure 2) were lower in those who developed severe pulmonary insufficiency and this became significant (p < 0.02) at the 100,000 level.

On this basis, and to assess the effects of blood transfusion on thrombocytopaenia and the development of pulmonary insufficiency between the treatment groups, a multivariate analysis was performed (Table 6)

In the placebo group there was a significant increase in the incidence of pulmonary insufficiency if more than 1,000ml of blood transfusion was given. This was related entirely to the presence of pulmonary insufficiency but not to its severity (p < 0.006). This relationship was not present in those receiving Aprotinin. There was a strong association between platelet counts below 100,000 at any time in the study and the incidence of severe pulmonary insufficiency in the placebo group (p < 0.02). This relationship was even stronger if counts fell to this level or below on the 1st day after admission (p < 0.005). There was no association between increased volume of blood transfusion greater than 1,000ml. and

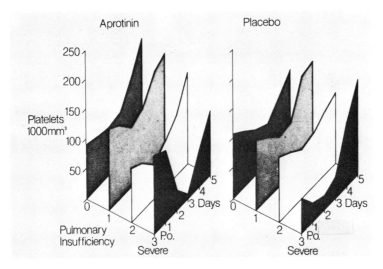

Figure 1. Relative fall of platelet counts. Estimated means corrected for prevalue covariance analysis BMD program P2V. University of
California. (p.o.= postoperative).

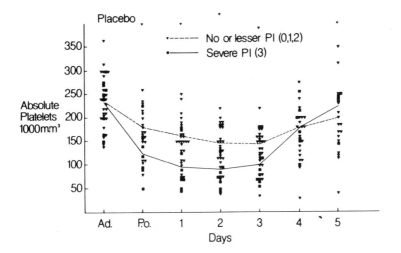

Figure 2. (p.o. = postoperative)

TABLE 6.   MULTIVARIATE ANALYSIS (BMD Program P3F University
                                              of California)

PLATELET COUNT	BLOOD TRANSFUSION	P.I.	TREATMENT
≳ 100,000	≳ 1000ML	YES	PLACEBO
		NO	APROTININ

PLACEBO	P	APROTININ
TRANSFUSION > 1000ML : PI ALL	< 0.03	N.S.
: PI 1 ONLY	< 0.006	N.S.
PLATELETS < 100,000 ANY DAY:SEVERE PI	< 0.02	N.S.
1ST DAY	< 0.005	N.S.
TRANSFUSION : PLATELETS	N.S.	N.S.
TRANSFUSION : PLATELETS : PI	N.S.	N.S.

platelet counts falling below 100,000. There was also no association
between a combination of blood transfusion requirements, platelet
counts, and pulmonary insufficiency.

The absolute platelet counts in those patients in the placebo
group with decompensated shock were lower than those with compensated
shock. This was not found to be so in those receiving Aprotinin
(Figure 3).

DISCUSSION

In this study it was found that there was a high incidence of
both pulmonary insufficiency and thrombocytopaenia.

The high incidence of pulmonary insufficiency, often clinically
undetectable, has confirmed that found by other workers (Ross 1970).

The predictable pattern of thrombocytopaenia seen in all
patients regardless of absence, presence, or severity of pulmonary
insufficiency appears to be a normal response to traumatic shock,
possibly due to a combination of local consumption at the site of
trauma and a minor degree of pulmonary platelet trapping.

Pulmonary platelet trapping would explain the modification of
this pattern found in the placebo group in those who sustained

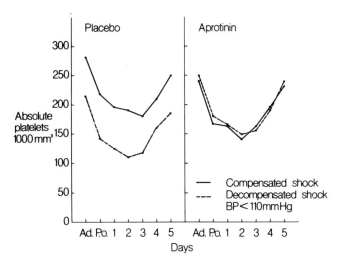

Figure 3. (p.o. = postoperative)

decompensated shock. Platelet aggregation is known to occur after
severe trauma and these aggregates would then be more easily trapped
in the pulmonary circulation.

As increasing volumes of bank blood transfusion, containing
macroaggregates, is not associated with the even more profound,
rapid, and earlier fall in platelet counts in those developing severe
pulmonary insufficiency, another factor must be implicated. This
could be an indicant of the degree of platelet aggregation or
trapping, due to the severity of trauma or duration of shock, or may
possibly involve other multifactorial local pulmonary mechanical or
chemical mechanisms such as fat deposition and break down, fibrin
deposition, the release of vasoactive amines, and over transfusion,
thus setting up a series of local pulmonary events which, in the
efflux of time, produces pulmonary damage and would explain the so
called "latent period" between trauma and clinical detection of
severe pulmonary dysfunction. The profound thrombocytopaenia
preceding severe hypoxia implies that the platelet trapping is a
primary causal factor rather than a secondary event.

The strong association of platelet counts falling to levels of
less than 100,000 on the 1st day prior to clinical detection of
severe pulmonary insufficiency could well be used as a clinical
predictor by which patients could be selected from a high background
incidence of pulmonary insufficiency who may be more likely to
develop severe pulmonary dysfunction and thus merit closer monitoring.
It is appreciated that the level of 100,000 is arbitrary and chosen
because statistical significance became apparent at this level. It
is possible that the rate of fall is of more importance.

The less profound fall of platelet counts in the presence of Aprotinin in conjunction with a lesser incidence of severe pulmonary insufficiency could also be explained on the basis of prevention of pulmonary platelet aggregation and trapping and would confirm controlled animal experimentation in this regard (Heideman et al. 1972). It is possible that Aprotinin also may produce deaggregation of platelets to explain the more rapid rise of the platelet counts.

To explain the increased incidence but not severity of pulmonary insufficiency with increasing blood transfusion greater than 1 litre the relationship of which is not present in those receiving Aprotinin, it is possible to hypothesize that Aprotinin may modify the macroaggregates present in stored bank blood to prevent their mechanical or chemical effects or to inhibit any proteinase activity present.

This study has found several associations explained only by hypotheses. It is difficult to ignore the importance of pulmonary platelet trapping as a causal factor in the development of severe pulmonary dysfunction which is probably superimposed on many other factors.

The exact mechanisms by which Aprotinin has its effects are unclear. However the facts presented show that, all other facts being equal, the presence of Aprotinin has a concomitant effect on both the pattern of thrombocytopaenia and a reduction in subsequent severity of pulmonary insufficiency, and also abolishes any association of pulmonary insufficiency with greater volumes of blood transfusion.

CONCLUSION

1. After major bony trauma and shock there is a high incidence of both pulmonary insufficiency and thrombocytopaenia.

2. Pulmonary insufficiency
    a. Is often subclinical.
    b. Its presence, but not severity,is associated in the placebo group with the transfusion of bank blood greater than 1,000mls.
    c. Its most severe form occurred only after decompensated shock.

3. Thrombocytopaenia
    a. Occurs as a normal response to major trauma and shock falling from admission to a minimum on the 2nd day and thereafter rising to approximate admission levels by 5th day.
    b. This pattern is affected in patients developing severe pulmonary insufficiency with cerebral symptoms in that it becomes

more profound and rapid and occurs earlier, often preceding the
clinical detection of this event. This occurred only with
decompensated shock and the levels in patients with decompensated
were significantly lower than those with compensated shock.

    c. A fall of the platelet counts to less than 100,000 on the 1st
day is a very strong predictor of the subsequent onset of severe
pulmonary insufficiency.

    d. This profound fall was not associated with increased volumes
of blood transfusion and leads to the possibility of pulmonary
platelet trapping occurring.

  4. The addition of aprotinin to hypovolaemic therapy reduced:-
    a. The degree of thrombocytopaenia and enhanced its rise.
    b. The incidence of severity of pulmonary insufficiency.
    c. The requirement of oxygen supplementation and ventilatory
support in patients with decompensated shock.
    d. The incidence of pulmonary insufficiency associated with
blood transfusions greater than 1 litre.

ACKNOWLEDGEMENTS

We wish to express our gratitude to Professor J. Clarke McNeur
for his encouragement and support, the surgical staff at the Alfred
Hospital for allowing us to study their patients, to Dr. K. Boehme
of the Biometrical Department of Bayer, Ag Wuppertal, Germany for
her assistance with the statistical analysis, and to Miss Kay Krygger
fo her patient secretarial help.

This study was financially supported by Bayer Germany and the
Alfred Hospital Research Fund.

REFERENCES

Bergentz, S-E., Leandoer, L., 1971 : Disseminated Intravascular
    Coagulation in Shock. Annls Chir. Gynaec. Fenn., 60:175-179
Blaisdell, F.W., Lim, R.C., Stallone, R.J., 1970 : The Mechanism of
    Pulmonary Damage following Traumatic Shock. Surgery Gynec.
    Obstet., 130:15-22
Blaisdell, F.W., Schlobohm, R.N., 1973 : The Respiratory Distress
    Syndrome: A Review. Surgery, 74:251-262.
Blaisdell, F.W., 1974 : Pathophysiology of Respiratory Distress
    Syndrome. Archs Surg., 108:44-49
Davidson, I., Barret, J.A., Miller, E., et al., 1975 : Pulmonary
    Microembolism Associated with Massive Transfusion: 1.
    Physiologic Effects and Comparison in vivo of Standard and
    Dacron Wool (Swank) Blood Transfusion Filters in its Prevention.
    Ann. Surg., 181:51-57.

Gurd, A.R., 1972 : Treatment of the Fat Embolism Syndrome. New
    Aspects of Trasylol Therapy, 5:137-140.
Haberland, G.L., P. Matis, 1970 : Trasylol, a proteinase inhibitor
    in surgical and internal indications. Med. Welt 18 (New Series):
    1367-1376
Hardaway, R.M., 1966 : Syndromes of Disseminated Intravascular
    Coagulation. Thomas, Springfield, Illinois.
Heideman, M., Bergentz S-E., Lewis, D.H., et al., 1972 : The Effect
    of Trasylol on the platelet Reaction after Trauma. New Aspects
    of Trasylol Therapy, 5:193-198.
Horovitz, J.H., Carrico, C.H., Shires, J.t., 1974 : Pulmonary
    Response to Major Injury. Archs Surg;, 108:349-355.
McKay, D.G., 1965 : Disseminated Intravascular Coagulation.
    New York, Harper Medical.
McNamara, J.J., Burran, E.L., Larson, E., et al. : Effect of
    Debris in Stored Blood on Pulmonary Microvasculature.
    Ann. thorac. Surg., 14:133-139.
Parker, F.b., Wax, S.D., Kusajima, K., et al., 1974 : Hemodynamic
    and Pathological Findings in Experimental Fat Embolism. Archs
    Surg., 108:70-74.
Peer, R.M., Schwartz, S.I., 1975 : Development and Treatment of
    Post-Traumatic Pulmonary Platelet Trapping.
    Ann. Surg., 181:447-451.
Ross, A.P.J., 1970 : The Fat Embolism Syndrome : With Special
    Reference to the Importance of Hypoxia in the Syndrome.
    Ann. Surg., 46:159-171.
Zimmermann, W.E., Vogel, W., Mittermayter, Ch., et al., 1972 : Gas
    Exchange and Metabolic Disorders in Traumatic-Hemorrhagic Shock
    and Septic Shock and their Treatment. New Aspects of Trasylol
    Therapy, 5:141-163.

EFFECT OF INTRAPERITONEAL APROTININ TREATMENT IN ACUTE AND CHRONIC PERITONITIS

P. Eckert*, M. Pfeiffer**, and H.P. Eichfuss**

* Hospital of Saarbruecken City-Department of General Surgery
** University Hospital of Hamburg-Department of General Surgery

The main complications of septic shock in peritonitis are: cardiovascular depression, pulmonary and renal insufficiency [1].

The mortality associated with peritonitis is high, the values stated in international literature range between 30% and 80% [2]. Septic shock can occur after bacteriaemia and toxinaemia. The peritoneum is the largest cavity with active surface in human. Soluble and non soluble substances can be resolved. The peritoneum uses its cellular digestion and exudation for the direct defence of bacteria and toxins.

Studies have shown that after the free perforation of hollow organs in the digestive tract, the high defensive power of the peritoneum is due to the three previously mentioned mechanisms, namely: translymphatic transportation, -pinocytosis, phagocytosis. The contents of the peritoneal ascites are fibrine, mucus and different enzymes (lysosomale enzymes). Statistically significant higher survival rates have been found by clinical application of TRASYLOL[R] in septic shock, when it is given early in a disease [3]. The pharmacological explanations for the enzyme inhibitors are multiple. Earlier works of MÖRL [4], NAGEL et al. [5] reported on less adhesions between the intestinal organs and statistically less pulmonal emboles after intraperitoneal injection.

These correlations between TRASYLOL[R] and pathogenesis are still unclear and hypothetic.

METHODS

The investigation was made with 60 wistar rats with an average
bodyweight of 250 gramms.

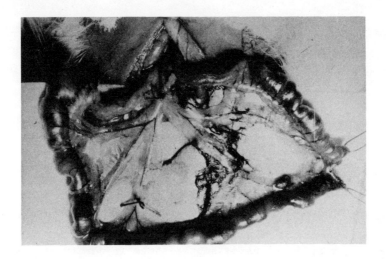

Fig. 1

Rats were laparotomized and an upper segment of the jejunum
was devascularised and opened by semicircular incision in ether
narkosis. [Group 1]. Immediately afterwards 10 rats were given
TRASYLOL^R (20,000 KIU/ 1 ml) into the peritoneal cavity. 10 rats
received likewise 10 ml of saline.

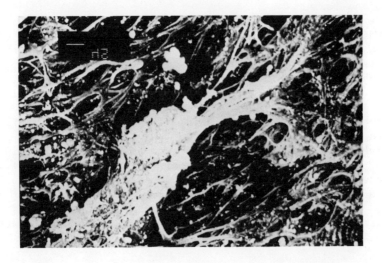

Fig. 2

20 animals, by intraperitoneal injection of a 5% talcum (SiO_2 and $CaHCO_3$) suspension on four consecutive days an irritation of the peritoneum was produced which is comparable to chronic peritonitis. 10 rats were treated in addition with TRASYLOL[R] (20,000 KIU/ 1 ml).

[Group 3]
Healthy animals received on four days either 1 ml of saline or TRASYLOL[R] (20,000 KIU/ 1 ml). -Three days after the operation or last injection, respectively, all animals were given an aminoglycoside antibiotic (TOBRAMYCIN[R] 1 mcg/ g bodyweight) intraperitonealy and this dose was repeated 12 hours later. 30 minutes afterwards the animals were laparatomized in NEMBUTAL[R] anaesthesia and blood was collected from the vena cava inferior. The concentration of aminoglycoside antibiotic in the sampled blood was determined by a microbiological assay (test germ : bact.esch.coli).

RESULTS

[Group 1]

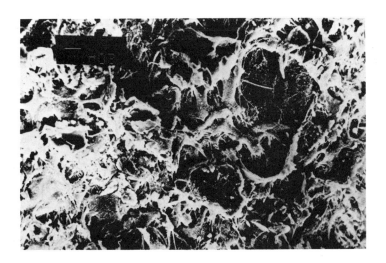

Fig. 3

The animals subjected to jejunal incision developed severe acute septic peritonitis. The scanning electron microscopical picture of peritoneum shows many dedrites of cells and unstructured fibrin without free cells.

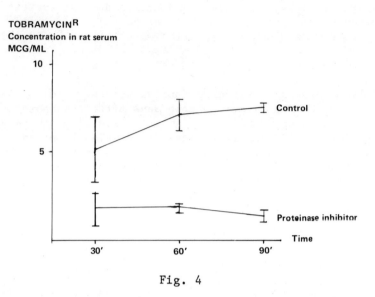

Fig. 4

Serum concentration 1 ss of the aminoglycoside antibiotic were significantly lower (p < 0.001) in rats treated with TRASYLOL[R] in comparison with those who were only given saline.

[Group 2]

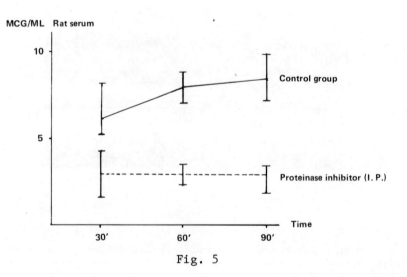

Fig. 5

The animals with intraperitoneal instillation of talcum showed inflammation of the peritoneum and fibrinous agglutination of the bowel (Fig. 2). In this group also the difference in serum concentrations of the aminoglycoside antibiotic was statistically highly significant in relation to TRASYLOL[R] or saline administration.

[Group 3]

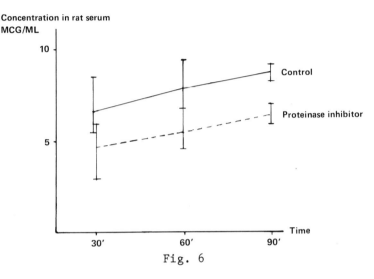

Fig. 6

This group served as a control. There was no difference in serum concentrations of the antibiotic in normal or healthy animals.

CONCLUSIONS

Our results demonstrate that peritoneal absorption even of large amounts of fluid is not restricted in either acute or chronic peritonitis. According to investigations reported elsewhere, antibiotics administered intraperitonealy can be found quantitatively in the serum, if peritoneal absorption is not impaired.

The retardation effect of proteinase inhibitor TRASYLOL[R] on peritoneal absorption in peritonitis may indicate that proteolytic processes are necessary to break up the proteinbinding of antibiotics which only then are able to permeate the peritoneal wall. This may also pertain to other substances of pharmacologic activity, like toxins -lipoproteins, lipopolysaccharides- and medicaments.

With respect to the clinical relevance of this effect it should be regarded as beneficial. Alternatively, the role of kallikrein/

kinin-system for transmembranous absorption of proteins and protein
split products has to be considered.

REFERENCES

Eckert,P., H.P.Eichfuss
    Peritonitis.
    G.Thieme Verlag, Stuttgart (1978)
Eckert,P., H.P.Eichfuss, H.W.Schreiber
    Frührelaparotomie
    Chirurg: 49, 33-36 (1978)
Eckert,P., K.Riesner, M.Doehn
    Indikationen zur Therapie mit Proteinasenhemmern in der
    Chirurgie.
    Med.Welt 25, 2154-2157 (1974)
Mörl,F.K.
    Die Peritonitis. In: Neue Aspekte der Trasylol-Therapie Bd. II,
    hrsg. R.Marx, H.Imdahl, G.L.Haberland
    F.K.Schattauer, Stuttgart, 138 (1967)
Nagel,M., W.Karl-Schuch, R.Ramanzadeh
    Untersuchungen zur zusätzlichen Proteaseninhibitor-Therapie bei
    der septischen Peritonitis. In: Neue Aspekte der Trasyslol
    Therapie. Bd.II, hrsg. R.Marx,H.Imdahl, G.L. Haberland
    F.K.Schattauer, Stuttgart, 129 (1967)

COMPARATIVE CLINICAL STUDY OF FOY AND TRASYLOL IN ACUTE PANCREATITIS

Norio Tanaka[1], Ryoichi Tsuchiya[2] and Kaneo Ishii[2]

1) Department of Surgery, Nagasaki University, School
   of Medicine, Sakamoto-cho, Nagasaki, Japan
2) Department of Internal Medicine, Asahikawa Medical
   College, Kagura-cho, Asahikawa, Japan

SUMMARY

In order to evaluate the efficacy and safety of FOY injectable ([ethyl-4-(6-guanidinohexanoyloxy) benzoate] methane sulfonate) on acute pancreatitis, a comparative clinical study was carried out using Trasylol as the control at 38 hospitals in Japan. Favourable results were obtained in 60 (71%) out of 84 patients in the FOY group and 29 (44%) out of 66 patients in the Trasylol group. The results showed that these both drugs were effective and the statistical analysis revealed considerable difference (χ^2 = 10.464, $p < 0.005$) between the two groups in this condition of clinical trial.

In addition, a double blind trial was carried out at 4 hospitals using FOY-305 ([n.n-dimethylcarbamoylmethy 4-(4-guanidinobenzoyloxy)-phenylacetate] methane sulfonate) oral capsule and inactive placebo. Favourable results were obtained in 18 (69%) out of 26 patients in the FOY-305 group and 8 (32%) out of 25 patients in the inactive placebo group, indicating a significant difference between the two groups (χ^2 = 8.930, $p < 0.01$). The results of the present study suggest that synthetic protease inhibitor, FOY or FOY-305, is beneficial in the treatment of acute pancreatitis.

INTRODUCTION

It is well known that a variety of proteolytic and lipolytic enzymes such as trypsin, kallikrein, elastase, lipase and phospolipase A play an important role in acute pancreatitis as aetiological factors. In particular, trypsin causes the autodigestion of the organ and the subsequent activation of some hydrolytic enzymes. Trapnell (1974) reported that Trasylol, trypsin and kallikrein inhibitor, was significantly beneficial in the treatment of acute pancreatitis as compared with inactive placebo. Similarly to Trasylol, FOY also has inhibitory activities on trypsin and kallikrein as described by Muramatsu and Fujii (1971, 1972). Fujii (1973, 1976) and Okegawa et al. (1974) reported that FOY suppressed the elevation of blood lipase and sugar levels, and reduced the mortality rate of dogs in which pancreatitis was experimentally produced by Elliott's method (1957). In our preliminary clinical study which was carried out at 54 hospitals, favourable results were obtained in 197 patients (77%) out of 257 patients with acute, relapsing and post-operative pancreatitis.

In addition, Fujii (1977) and Tamura et al. (1977) reported that a new analog of FOY, FOY-305 had more potent inhibitory effects than FOY on proteolytic enzymes. In particular, FOY-305 which was administered either by oral or intravenous route reduced the mortality rate of animals suffering from experimental pancreatitis and inhibited fibrinolytic system in rats and rabbits. In our preliminary clinical study, FOY-305 administered orally was effective in 68 (53%) out of 129 patients with acute, chronic or post-operative pancreatitis. Heartburn, as the side effect, was observed in two patients at the beginning of administration, but disappeared soon without reducing the dose.

In order to further evaluate the efficacy and safety of FOY injectable and FOY-305 oral capsule, a comparative controlled trial using Trasylol as the control and a small scale double blind trial using inactive placebo as the control were carried out, respectively.

METHODS & MATERIALS

Comparative Controlled Trial with FOY and Trasylol

The present study has been carried out at 38 hospitals in Japan. The patients with acute, relapsing or post-operative pancreatitis were subjected to the trial. The degree of severity was graded according to the Forell's criteria (1959). For random drug allocation, patients were allotted in alternative order to the treatment with FOY or Trasylol, that is, if the first patient

ETHYL-4-(6-GUANIDINOHEXANOYLOXY) BENZOATE

• METHANE SULFONATE

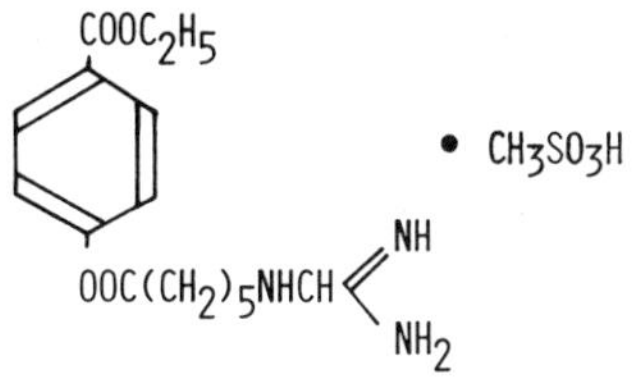

COOC$_2$H$_5$

• CH$_3$SO$_3$H

OOC(CH$_2$)$_5$NHCH

NH

NH$_2$

M.W. 417.78

Figure 1   Chemical structure of FOY

was assigned to the FOY treatment group, the second patient was assigned to the Trasylol treatment group.

FOY injectable, 100 mg/vial in lyophilized form, was supplied by Ono Pharmaceutical Co., Ltd. (Figure 1). FOY was used by dissolving one vial in 250 to 500 ml of intravenous fluid and infused by i.v. drip in one to two hours. The daily dose was adjusted according to the clinical course of the patients within a range from one to six vials.

Commercially available Trasylol (Bayer Co., Ltd.), 25,000 KIE/vial, was obtained and distributed to all participants. For it is difficult to standardize the administration method and dose of Trasylol, each physician was allowed to administer it according to his own method.

Each patient was carefully observed for subjective, objective and laboratory findings. When the treatment was completed, each physician assessed the efficacy of the drug based on the degree of improvement in these findings on the 3rd to 4th, 7th, 14th and 21st days after the start of administration (Figure 2). Separately, The Evaluation Committee which consisted of selected members assessed the efficacy of the drug under blind conditions. For convenience, the efficacy of the drug was expressed by the four categories as follows, "excellent", "good", "fair" and "poor". In addition, assessments of "excellent" and "good" categories were regarded as "effective" in order to summarize the results.

Double Blind Trial with FOY-305 and Inactive Placebo

The present study has been carried out at 4 hospitals. The patients with acute, chronic and post-operative pancreatitis were

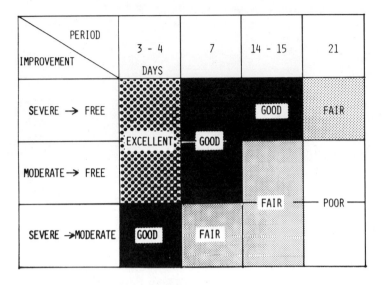

Figure 2   Criteria for efficacy judgement

subjected to the trial, but the patients with severe pancreatitis
were excluded from the trial because these patients were unable to
take a meal orally.   Six active or inactive capsules (Ono
Pharmaceutical Co., Ltd.) were administered daily in three divided
doses after each meal for 6 weeks.   An active capsule contained
100 mg of FOY-305.   The efficacy of the drug was assessed based on
the degree of the improvement of subjective, objective and
laboratory findings under attendance of all physicians.

RESULTS

Comparative Controlled Trial with FOY and Trasylol

One hundred fifty patients, 84 patients of the FOY group and
66 patients of the trasylol group, were subjected to the trial.
Since the drug allotted in alternative order was changed in some
patients because of positive reaction in the sensitivity test
against Trasylol, the number of patients treated with FOY became
greater than those with trasylol.   The age of the patients in the
FOY group ranged from 16 to 80 years old, with a mean of 47.
In the Trasylol group, the age ranged from 16 to 72 years old,
with a mean of 45.   Since there were no serious biases of drug
allocation with regard to the background factor, age, sex, and
type of disease (Table 1), further analyses were carried out.

Table 1   Background features

| | TOTAL CASES | SEX | | AGE (MEAN) | DIAGNOSIS | | |
		MALE	FEMALE		ACUTE	RELAPS-ING	POST-OPERATIVE
FOY	84	49	35	47.2	43	29	12
TRASYLOL	66	44	22	45.0	31	26	9

Table 2   Dose and administration period

	DOSE/DAY	PERIOD	TOTAL DOSE
FOY	239.3 (MG)	16.3 (DAYS)	3627.4 (MG)
TRASYLOL	123,000 (KIE)	16.5 (DAYS)	1767,000 (DIE)

The doses ranged from 100 to 600 mg/day, with a mean of 239.3 mg/day, in the FOY group, and from 25,000 to 700,000 KIE/day with a mean of 123,000 KIE/day, in the Trasylol group. Two hundred mg/day of FOY or 100,000 KIE/day of Trasylol was administered in the majority of patients.

The medication period ranged from 1 to 83 days, with a mean of 16.3 days, in the FOY group, and from 1 to 160 days, with a mean of 16.5 days, in the Trasylol group. The mean total dose in each group was 3,627.4 mg and 1,767,000 KIE, respectively.

There were 4 deaths, 1 in the FOY group and 3 in the Trasylol group. All of these patients were suffering from acute pancreatitis. Favourable results, judged by the Evaluation Committee as well as by attending physicians as "excellent" or "good" effect, were obtained in 60 cases (71%) of the FOY group and in 29 cases (44%) of the Trasylol group. (Figure 3)

The results of the trial clearly show that FOY is considerably effective as compared with Trasylol. When the efficacy of the drug was judged by the Evaluation Committee based on the type of disease,

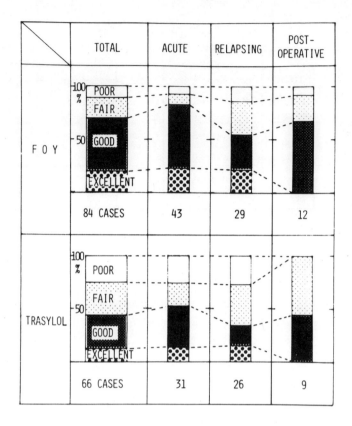

Figure 3   Efficacy of the drugs

it was noted that the efficacy rates of the FOY group were 84% in
the cases with acute pancreatitis, 55% in the cases with relapsing
pancreatitis and 67% in the cases with post-operative pancreatitis,
while those of the Trasylol group were 52%, 35% and 44%,
respectively.   As compared with the Trasylol group, the FOY group
showed over 20% higher efficacy rate for every type of disease.

     The degree of improvement in subjective findings was compared
between the two groups.   The patients without symptoms throughout
the medication period were excluded from the analysis.   The
improvement rate was always higher in the FOY group than in the
Trasylol group.   Especially, there was a considerable difference
between the two groups at one week after the start of administration
in abdominal pain and at 3 weeks in abdominal distention.
(Figure 4)

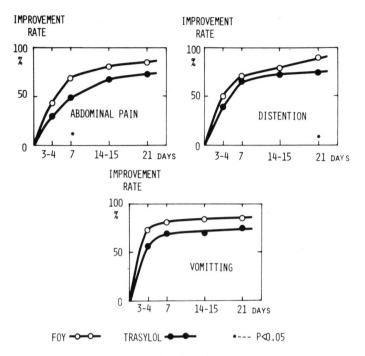

Figure 4   Improvement of subjective findings

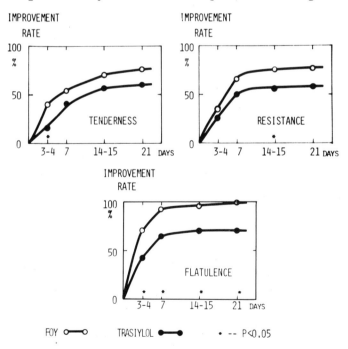

Figure 5   Improvement of objective findings

   We also analyzed the degree of improvement in objective
findings. The improvement of shock was observed in 4 of 7 cases
in the FOY group and 5 of 9 cases in the Trasylol group.

   Regarding other objective findings, the improvement rate was
rather higher in the FOY group. Especially, there was a
considerable difference between the two groups at 3 - 4 days after
the start of administration in tenderness, at 2 weeks in resistance
and at every occasion in flatulence. (Figure 5)

   In laboratory findings, similar results were obtained. The
improvement rate was rather higher in the FOY group, and there was
a considerable difference between the two groups at 1 week in serum
amylase level and at 2 and 3 weeks in urine amylase level.
(Figure 6)

   Side effects were observed in 7 out of 84 patients treated
with FOY, and in 4 out of 66 treated with Trasylol. In the FOY
group, any of the following side effects was observed in one case
each: elevation of BUN and GOT, hypotension, sternalgia, blurred
vision, and vasalgia and redness at the injection site. The degree
of elevation of BUN and GOT were so minimal that the administration
could be continued, and their levels were normalized in 2 weeks to
20 days. In the Trasylol group, any of the following side effects

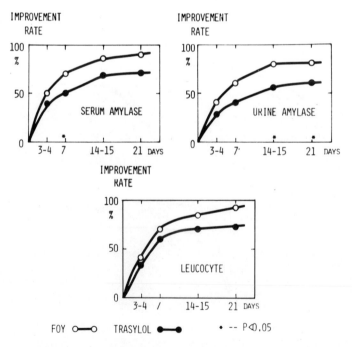

Figure 6   Improvement of laboratory findings

was observed in one case each: elevation of GOT, urticaria, eruption and erythema. The number of cases in which administration was discontinued due to side effects was one case of hypotension in the FOY group and 2 cases each of erythema and eruption in the Trasylol group. Although the elevation of BUN and the abnormality of hepatic function were observed in some cases, it is well recognized that these symptoms often appear in association with pancreatitis.

Double Blind Trial with FOY-305 and Inactive placebo

Fifty one patients, 26 patients of the active group and 25 patients of the inactive group, were subjected to the trial. The majority of patients were chronic pancreatitis with acute episodes. There were no serious biases of drug allocation with regard to the background factor, age, sex, type of disease and severity. (Table 3)

Favourable results were obtained in 18 cases, 69% of the active group. On the other hand, 8 cases, 32% of the inactive group, received favourable assessment. A significant difference was noted between the two groups. As to side effect, constipation was observed in one patient of the active group. (Figure 7)

The degree of improvement in abdominal pain and tenderness and in urinary amylase levels were compared between the two groups. The improvement rate of the active group was higher than that of the inactive group in each finding at 4 to 6 weeks after the start of administration. Especially, there were significant differences between the two groups at 6 weeks after the start of administration in each finding. (Figure 8)

DISCUSSION

Acute pancreatitis is a grave disease with a high mortality. Therefore, we judged it is difficult to conduct a double blind test with an inactive placebo, and tried to design a double blind test with Trasylol. However, a contradiction between the two

Table 3 Background features

| | NO.OF CASES | SEX | | AGE (MEAN) | DIAGNOSIS | | SEVERITY | |
		MALE	FEMALE		CHRONIC	ACUTE	MOD-ERATE	MILD
ACTIVE	26	16	12	39.6	21	5	19	7
INACTIVE	25	13	12	43.8	23	2	1	9

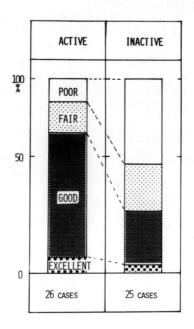

Figure 7　Efficacy of drugs

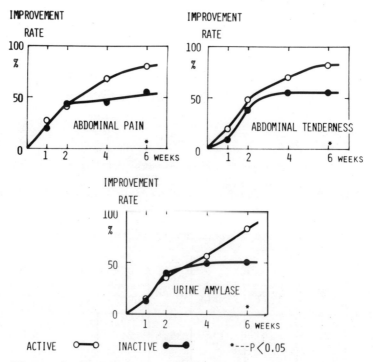

Figure 8　Improvement of abdominal pain, tenderness
and urine amylase levels

drugs arose in respect of dosage and administration method. The
recommended route of FOY is constant drip infusion, whereas Trasylol
is recommended to give by one shot i.v. injection of a large dose
at the initial stage. The opinions of attending physicians did
not come to an agreement regarding the initial large dosing and
one shot i.v. injection of Trasylol. In addition, in case that
Trasylol was given blindly, it would become impossible to prevent
anaphylactic reaction opportunely. Therefore we had to give up
the double blind test with Trasylol. Finally, a comparative
clinical study with FOY and Trasylol was conducted. The results
of the present study indicated that FOY was more effective than
Trasylol in the treatment of pancreatitis. However, the doses of
Trasylol widely varied from 25,000 to 700,000 KIE/day and its
efficacy appeared to depend upon the doses. Especially between
the patients whose initial doses were more than 100,000 KIE and
those less than 100,000 KIE, statistically significant difference
in the efficacy of the drug was observed.

Side effects were observed in 7 out of 84 patients in the
FOY group and in 4 out of 66 patients in the Trasylol group. The
elevation of BUN or the abnormality of hepatic function were
observed in 2 patients given FOY and one given Trasylol. It is
well known that the elevation of BUN and the abnormality of hepatic
function often appear as the symptoms of pancreatitis, and so it
seems rather appropriate to judge that the drug was not effective
than to regard the symptoms as side effects. In the FOY
group, vasalgia and redness at the injection site were observed
in one patient each, which seemed due to the drug's irritant
action. Besides, hypotension, sternalgia and blurred vision,
which seemed to be caused by the dilatation of vascular beds, were
observed in one patient each. On the other hand, in the Trasylol
group, allergic reaction appeared in 3 patients.

Now, we are conducting a multi-center double blind study with
FOY-305 at 24 hospitals to further evaluate the efficacy and
safety of this drug.

ACKNOWLEDGEMENT

We are indebted to many physicians who participated in
the trial: M. Namiki, T. Takebe (Asahikawa Medical College),
S. Nozaki (Sapporo Medical College), A. Hirayama (Tonan Hospital),
Y. Tamazawa (Iwate Medical College), Y. Saito (Tohoku University),
S. Tashiro (Niigata University), M. Oda (Shinshu University),
S. Naito (Juntendo University), M. Uchimura (Hamamatsu Medical
Center), Y. Toda (Nagoya University), I. Miyazaki (Kanazawa
University), I. Murata (Toyama Prefectural Hospital), S. Hosoda
(Shiga Medical College), K. Mori (Kyoto City Hospital),

Y. Tsukiyama (Ikeda City Hospital), T. Masujima, H. Sakashita
(Hiroshima University), M. Abe (Kyushu National Cancer Center),
H. Wakasugi (Kyushu University), M. Shimada (Kagoshima University),
Y. Murashima (Kosei Hospital), and H. Kizuno (National Rail-way
Hospital).

REFERENCES

Elliott, D. W., et al., 1957, Alterations in the pancreatic
resistance to bile in the pathogenesis of acute pancreatitis.
Annals Surg., 146, 669.

Forell, M. M., Dobovicnik, W., 1959, Über möglichkeiten und
Grezen der Erkrankung akuter und Chronischer Pankreaserkrankungen
auf Grund von Diastase-, Lipase-, und Trypsin-bestimmungen,
Klin. Wschr., 19, 1018.

Fujii, S., 1973, Enzymatic therapy of pancreatitis,
Jap. J. Clin. Exp. Med., 50(3), 682.

Fujii, S., 1976, Kinins: Pharmacodynamics and Biological Roles.
75, Edited by F. Sicuteri, Nathan Back and G. L. Haberland.

Fujii, S., 1977, Synthetic Protease Inhibitor. Metabolism and
Disease, Japan 14 (6), 1087.

Muramatsu, M. and Fujii, S., 1971, Inhibitory effects of ω-amino
acid esters on trypsin, plasmin, plasma kallikrein and thrombin.
Biochim. Biophys. Acta., 242, 203.

Muramatsu, M. and Fujii, S., 1972, Inhibitory effects of ω-guanidino
acid esters on trypsin, plasmin, plasma kallikrein and thrombin.
Biochim. Biophys. Acta., 268, 221.

Okegawa, T., 1974, Effect of FOY on experimental acute pancreatitis.
Gendai Iryo (Current Medicine), Japan. 6 (8), 1001.

Tamura, Y., Hirado, M., Okamura, K., Minato, Y. and Fujii, S., 1977,
Synthetic inhibitors of trypsin, plasmin, kallikrein, thrombin, C_1r
and C_1-esterase. Biochim. Biophys. Acta., 484, 417.

Trapnell, J. E., 1974, A controlled trial of Trasylol in the
treatment of acute pancreatitis. Br. J. Surg., 61 (3), 177.

TESTS TO LOCALIZE FREE PROTEOLITIC ENZYMES IN VIVO BY ^{14}C-CYSTEINE-APROTININ

F. Amenta, C. Cavallotti, M. Di Jorio, F. Porcelli, and G. Porcelli

Ist.Anatomia Umana University of Rome,
Ist.di Chimica, Fac.Med.,Università Cattolica S.Cuore
and Centro Chimica Recettori C.N.R., Rome, Italy

ABSTRACT

Aprotinin, a polyvalent protease inhibitor from bovine organs, has been labelled with ^{14}C-cysteine in 6 M urea to produce a radioactive conjugate, without effect on the inhibitor activity. 138×10^3 dpm of radioactive product, containing 5 mg of protein (20.000 kal. inhibitor units) in 5 ml of Locke's solution were perfused in anesthetized rabbits via ascending aorta. Then the anesthetized rabbit was killed and specimens of some organs were admitted to autoradiographic analysis. Small intestine, ischiatic nerve and testis have been the most rich radiolabelled organs (+++). In kidney, stomach, large intestine, liver and eye the radiolabelled aprotinin was found in fair amounts (++); while in pancreas, spleen, spinal cord, brain, cava vein and aorta of rabbit the ^{14}C-cysteine-Aprotinin was practically undetectable by autoradiography.

INTRODUCTION

The aprotinin is a polypeptide that inhibits proteolytic enzymes such as trypsin, chynotrypsin, some kallikrein and some proteases from plants (for ref. see Vogel et al., 1970; Kiernan and Stoddart, 1973). The aprotinin conjugated with fluorescein isothiocyanate was used for the specific staining of acidic mucosubstances (Kiernan and Sroddart, 1973). In this paper the aprotinin was labelled with ^{14}C-cysteine in 4-6 M urea. This ^{14}C-cysteine aprotinin compound was used to localize, in vivo, free proteolytic enzymes.

MATERIAL AND METHODS

Aprotinin (4,000 KIU/mg protein) was purchased from Bayer (Germany) and labelled with (U -14C)-cysteine HCl (19,7 m Ci/mM - Radiochemical Ctr. - Amersham - England) in 4 - 6 M urea according to the method previously described (Porcelli et al., 1978). The ^{14}C-cysteine-aprotinin was dissolved in a Locke's solution ($138x40^3$ dpm/mg of Aprotinin / ml). A number of 6 male albino rabbits were used in these experiments. The animals were anesthetized with ketamine HCl (Ketala-Parke Davis, 15 mg/kg i.m.). A cannula was introduced into the ascending aorta and animals were superfused with ^{14}C-cysteine-aprotinin at a rate of 5 ml/h during 60 min. The rabbits were killed with an overdose of Ketalar 5 min. after the onset of superfusion. Specimens of stomach, small and large intestine, liver, pancreas, spleen, kidney, testis, aorta, vena cava, spinal cord, brain, ischiatic nerve, and eye were rapidly removed and fixed in 10% neutralized buffered formalin. The specimens were then cut by a cryostat (sections of 5-15 um in thickness), placed on glass slides and coated by dipping with Ilford K5 emulsion diluted 1:1. After 8-20 days of exposure these autoradiographies were developed in D 19 b Kodak, stained in H.E., or P.AS or talnidine blue and examined in the light microscope.

RESULTS AND DISCUSSION

After superfusion with ^{14}C-cysteine-aprotinin a very weak and diffuse autoradiographic reaction was observed. The pattern of the distribution of silver grains is different in various organs studied. Small and large intestine, testis and ischiatic nerve are richest in silver grains. In the intestine the globet cells and surface mucin bind intensely by ^{14}C-cysteine-aprotinin; in the testis the radioactivity is well localized in the semini ferous tubules. In the kidney, stomach, liver and eye the radiolabeled aprotinin was found in fair amounts. In the kidney the silver grains are localized in the basement membranes of glomeruli, of Bowman's capsule and of the tubular epithelium. In the stomach the radiolabeled aprotinin is localized in the surface epithelium. In the liver the radioactivity is localized in correspondence of hepatocytes and in the basement membranes of blood veins and biliary ducts. In the eye the labeled aprotinin is localized in the retina and in correspondence of ocular muscles. In other organs studied the radioactivity is practically undetectable. The present results have demonstrated "in vivo" the localization of aprotinin. The inhibitor and binding properties of the ^{14}C-labeled aprotinin are unchanged, indicating that the biological activity of ^{14}C-aprotinin is not altered.

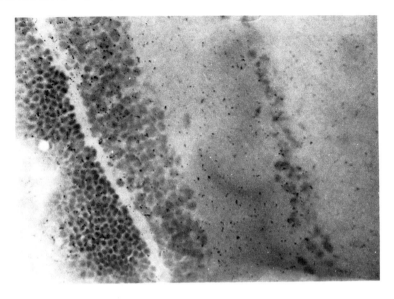

Fig. 1 Rabbit's retina
        Silver grains are localized in all organs of the retina

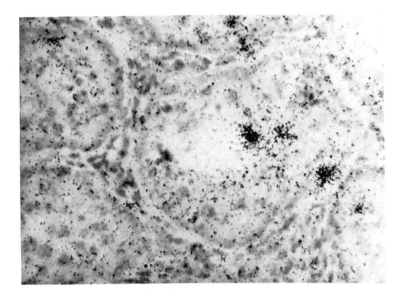

Fig. 2 Rabbit's testis
        Deposition of silver grains in correspondence of the
        tubules

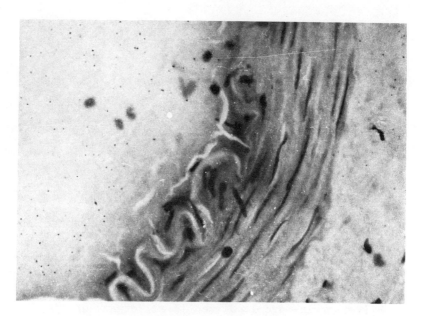

Fig. 3 Rabbit's vena cava
Note the negativity of the autoradiography

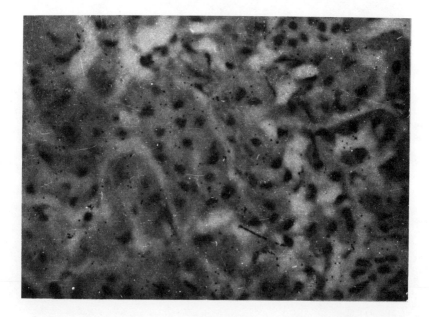

Fig. 4 Rabbit's kidney
The silver grains are localized in correspondence of proximal and distant tubules.

REFERNCES

1) Porcelli G., Di Jorio M., Ranieri M., Marini-Bettòlo G.B.,
   (1978), Preparation of ^{14}C-aprotinin, Il Farmaco, 33, 720
2) Stoddart R.W., Kiernan J.A., (1973),
   Aprotinin: a carbohydrate-binding protein, Histochemic., 34, 77
3) Vogel R. and Werle E., (1970),
   Kallikrein inhibitors, in Hdb. of Exp.Pharmacol., Vol. XXV, P.212

INHIBITORY EFFECTS OF GABEXATE MESILATE (FOY) ON EXPERIMENTAL DIC

Junichi Isobe

Department of Laboratory Medicine, Tokushima University

2-50, Kuramoto-cho, Tokushima 770, Japan

ABSTRACT

The inhibitory effects of a newly synthesized protease inhibitor, Gabexate mesilate (FOY), on experimental disseminated intravascular coagulation were studied as compared with those of aprotinin or heparin. Thrombin, tissue thromboplastin, and endotoxin were used as DIC trigger substances. As parameters on DIC, platelet counts, white blood cell counts, neutrophilic leukocyte counts, fibrinogen, fibrin degradation products, platelet retention, platelet aggregation, prothrombin time, partial thromboplastin time were served. The drug efficacy in each parameter were expressed by the score system and analyzed statistically. The results were summarized as follows; (1) In thrombin-induced DIC, FOY was apparently superior to the other drugs (p<0.05). (2) In thromboplastin-induced DIC, heparin was slightly more effective than FOY or aprotinin. (3) In endotoxin infusion, there were no significant differences among them.

In conclusion, the results of the present study suggest that FOY was more effective than heparin or aprotinin on experimental DIC.

INTRODUCTION

Extensive studies have been done on the diagnosis and/or therapy in disseminated intravascular coagulation (DIC)(Minna, et al., 1974). However, unknown things concerning the pathological findings are not a few, and it is necessary that we devise the treatment of DIC case by case. In general, heparin is used

clinically as a drug with antithrombin and antithromboplastin
effects (Lusch and Heene, 1974). Aprotinin, having such a combined
antitrypsin and antiplasmin action, has also been employed recently
(Sakuragawa, 1975). In Japan, Gabexate mesilate (FOY) has been
synthesized as a new therapeutic agent for pancreatitis (Fujii and
Muramatsu, 1972). It has been known that this protease inhibitor
acts on trypsin, kallikrein, plasmin, thrombin, and C_1-esterase.
In this paper, the inhibitory effects of FOY on experimental DIC
were investigated in comparison with those of aprotinin or heparin.

MATERIALS

36 rabbits (matured male, body weight from 2.5 kg to 3.0 kg)
were used as experimental animals and were divided into three
groups. Blood collections were done by disposable syringes from
a marginal ear vein in rabbits. Blood samples were partially
provided as citrated blood containing sodium citrate in a final
concentration of 0.38%. Platelet rich plasma, when necessary,
was obtained from the citrated blood by centrifugation at 1000 rpm
for 10 minutes, platelet poor plasma was separated by further
centrifugation at 3000 rpm for 20 minutes.

METHODS

A. Parameters and Their Determination Methods

Platelet counts were enumerated by Brecher-Cronkite's method.
White blood cells (WBC) and neutrophilic leukocytes (Neutro) were
determined by manual method. Fibrinogen levels were measured by
thrombin time method. Measurements of platelet retention were
done by Hellem II modified method, ADP-induced platelet aggregation
was investigated by turbidimetric method with a platelet aggregometer
(Bio/Data, Type PAP-III). Fibrin degradation products (FDP) were
examined by Ristocetin precipitation method (Watanabe and Tullis,
1977). The results were semiquantitatively expressed by five
degrees - (-1), (+), (+), (++), (+++) - according to the mass of
precipitates. Measurements of prothrombin time (PT) and partial
thromboplastin time (PTT) were done by one step method using
Simplastin (Warner-Lambert) or Platelin (Warner-Lambert) as reagents.
Preparations of rabbits with DIC, and the administration methods
of drugs are mentioned below. The number of animals in each group
was two for control and three for each drug group, and the results
obtained were expressed by mean values.

B. Preparations of Rabbits with DIC

1) <u>Thrombin- induced DIC</u>. Each parameter was determined
before, immediately after, and at 15, 30 and 60 minutes after the

infusion of 40 units/kg of thrombin (Parke-Davis) diluted with
20 ml of physiological saline (PS) for 30 minutes.

2) Tissue thromboplastin-induced DIC. Infusion of 8 ml/kg
of 10% tissue thromboplastin suspension (Simplastin, as 100% for
PT measurement) diluted with PS was done, for 30 minutes and each
parameter was checked at the same time intervals as mentioned above.

3) Endotoxin-induced DIC. Infusion of 40 μg/kg of endotoxin
(Lipopolysaccharides, Sigma, No. L-3129) diluted with 20 ml of PS
for 30 minutes, and each parameter was investigated before,
immediately after, and at 1, 3, 5 and 48 hours after.

C. Administration Methods of Drugs

20 mg/kg of FOY (Ono Pharmac. Co., Ltd., 100 mg/V), 10,000
KIE/kg of aprotinin (Teikokuzoki Corp., antikrein, 50,000 KIE/A)
or 400 units/kg of heparin (Kodama Corp., 5,000 units/A) were
infused with each 50 ml of PS for 30 minutes immediately after the
infusion of each DIC trigger substance. Control groups were given
the infusion of only 50 ml of PS for 30 minutes.

D. Score in Parameters

Table 1 indicates the criteria for drug efficacy in each
parameter.

The changes in each parameter, as compared with those of
intact animals were graded into five steps with scores from 1 to 5.
It means that as the total score becomes smaller, the inhibitory
effect of the drug on DIC becomes stronger.

RESULTS

A. Changes of Parameters in Thrombin-induced DIC

Control group. Figure 1 summarizes the changes in parameters.
Platelet counts, WBC and Neutro were rapidly reduced immediately
after thrombin infusion reaching the minimum at 15 minutes. Then,
WBC returned nearly to the initial level, but platelets remained
at low level even after 60 minutes. Fibrinogen was diminished
following the infusion and remained low till 15 minutes, but it
showed a sharp increase thereafter overshooting the initial level
at 30 minutes. The change of FDP was recognized in mirror image
relation with that of fibrinogen. The time course of the changes
in both retention and aggregation of platelets showed decrease.
PT and PTT were fairly prolonged in 15 or 30 minutes after infusion,
and then tended to show some recovery at 60 minutes.

TABLE 1.   SCORE IN PARAMETERS

Platelet	Score	WBC	Score	Neutrophils	Score
0 - 10	1	0 - 1	1	0 - 0.5	1
10 - 20	2	1 - 2	2	0.5 - 1.0	2
20 - 30	3	2 - 3	3	1.0 - 1.5	3
30 - 40	4	3 - 4	4	1.5 - 2.0	4
40 -	5	4 -	5	2.0 -	5

Fibrinogen	Score	PT	Score	PTT	Score
0 - 50	1	0 - 1	1	0 - 5	1
50 - 100	2	1 - 2	2	5 - 10	2
100 - 150	3	2 - 3	3	10 - 15	3
150 - 200	4	3 - 4	4	15 - 20	4
200 -	5	4 -	5	20 -	5

Retention	Score	Aggregation	Score	FDP	Score
0 - 10	1	0 - 10	1	(-)	1
10 - 20	2	10 - 20	2	(±)	2
20 - 30	3	20 - 30	3	(+)	3
30 - 40	4	30 - 40	4	(++)	4
40 -	5	40 -	5	(+++)	5

Platelet	$\times 10^4/\mu l$	Fibrinogen	mg/dl	Retention	%
W B C	$\times 10^3/\mu l$	P T	sec	Aggregation	%
Neutrophils	$\times 10^3/\mu l$	P T T	sec		

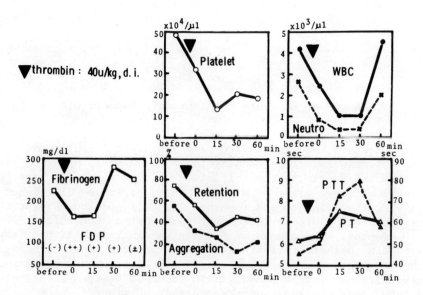

▼thrombin : 40u/kg, d. i.

Figure 1.   Thrombin-induced DIC

FOY group.   As shown in Figure 2, no apparent changes in all
parameters were seen.

Aprotinin group.   The changes in parameters were slight in
contrast to control, but platelet retention and FDP were fairly
changed.

Heparin group.   Degrees of the changes in parameters were
between those shown in FOY and aprotinin groups, and WBC and PTT
were considerably changed.

B.   Changes of Parameters in Tissue Thromboplastin (TP)-
     induced DIC

Control group.   At 15 minutes following the infusion of TP,
platelets were reduced from 32 x 10^4/µl to 10.5 x 10^4/µl and
neutrophils from 6000/µl to 1300/µl.   The apparent decrease in
fibrinogen, platelet retention and platelet aggregation and the
prolongation of PT and PTT were observed.   FDP was remarkably
elevated (++) at 30 minutes.   All parameters, except fibrinogen
overshooting the initial level, did not return to the initial
level in 60 minutes.

FOY group.   Figure 3 shows the time course of changes in
parameters, indicating the inhibitory effects of FOY on platelets,
fibrinogen, FDP, platelet function and PT.   Most of the parameters
recovered their initial levels at 60 minutes.

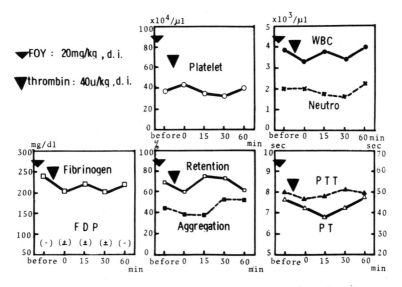

Figure 2.   Effect of FOY on Thrombin-induced DIC

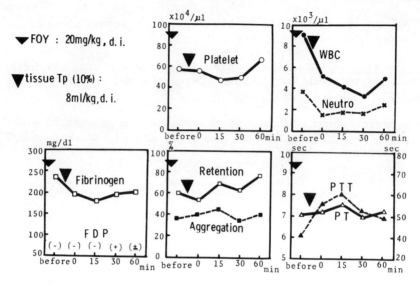

Figure 3.   Effect of FOY on Tissue-thromboplastin-induced DIC

Aprotinin group.   Fibrinogen was gradually decreased in course
of time, but the change in FDP tended to be slight.

Heparin group.   The changes in this group, in general, were
slight, though fibrinogen and PTT varied.

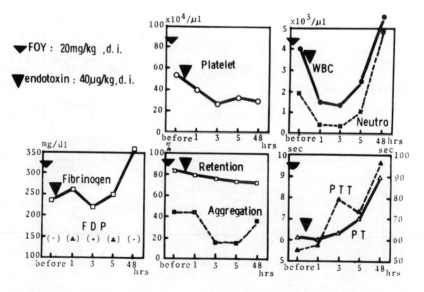

Figure 4.   Effect of FOY on Endotoxin-induced DIC

C.   Changes of Parameters in Endotoxin-induced DIC

Control group.   The changes in parameters were more remarkable than those in the above mentioned control groups.   Namely, specific patterns in this group were shown with rapid reduction or pro-longation, and with a long period of the inhibitory action.

FOY group.   Parameters, except PT and PTT, varied not so greatly.   FDP remained only slightly (+) at 3 hours (Figure 4).

Aprotinin group.   The potency of the inhibitory effects in this group was in the middle of those of FOY and heparin.

Heparin group.   Platelets, WBC, Neutro, platelet aggregation and PTT were fairly changed.

D.   Comparison of the Effects among Drugs

The total score of each group in thrombin-induced DIC was as shown in Table 2.   Scores in drug-pretreated groups were signifi-cantly smaller than those in control groups ($p < 0.05$).   In particular the score in FOY group was superior to those in the other drug groups statistically ($p < 0.05$).   In TP-induced DIC, scores were 35, 26, 24 and 20, in groups of control, FOY, aprotinin, and heparin, respectively, with no significant differences among the drug groups.

Scores in endotoxin-induced DIC were 39, 28, 29, and 31 in groups of control, FOY, aprotinin and heparin, respectively, showing no significant difference.

TABLE 2.   THROMBIN - INDUCED DIC

	Control	FOY	Aprotinin	Heparin
Platelet	5	1	1	1
WBC	4	1	3	4
Neutrophils	5	1	4	3
Fibrinogen	2	1	1	1
P T	1	1	1	1
P T T	3	1	3	5
Retention	3	1	2	1
Aggregation	4	1	5	3
FDP	4	2	4	2
Total score	31	10	24	21
N	2	3	2	3

DISCUSSION

It is acceptable that combined use of heparin and complementary therapy in the rule of DIC treatment (Matsuoka and Yamanaka, 1978). However, in some cases of DIC with thrombocytopenia and/or hypo-fibrinogenemia, we cannot use heparin becuase of the increase in haemorrhage (Merskey, 1972; Ingram, 1965). The heparin effects are not expected in cases with low levels of anti-thrombin III which is a heparin co-factor. Sakuragawa (1978) showed that the thrombin III decreased to less than 50% of normal level, and the author (1978) suggested that the affection of platelet factor 4 released by platelet destruction in DIC should not be neglected.

On the other hand, it has been known that aprotinin possesses antifibrinolytic and antithromboplastic activities (Amris and Hilden, 1968). Moreover, there are some reports that aprotinin is available instead of heparin (Sakuragawa, 1975). Nevertheless, the author regards the production of the antibody as dangerous when it is used repeatedly.

FOY, which was synthesized by Fujii et al., (1972), possesses the chemical structure as shown in Figure 5. It has been demonstrated to have the inhibitory effects on several enzyme systems, as illustrated in Figure 6, and is expected to work effectively for prevention of DIC. A recent paper on the effects of FOY in vitro reported that FOY showed the most potent inhibition on the factor Xa activity and that it was more potent in antithromboplastic activity and nearly equipotent in antifibrinolytic activity as compared to aprotinin (Yamada et al., 1978). It is the advantage of FOY that no antibody will be produced because of low molecular weight.

Depending on these details, the author examined these effects on experimental DIC of FOY, aprotinin and heparin comparatively, with the results that these drugs were significantly effective in comparison with controls, though differing from each other in the potency of activity. Especially, FOY was superior to the other drugs with significant differences ($p < 0.05$) in thrombin-induced DIC. This finding is very interesting, and it is suggested that

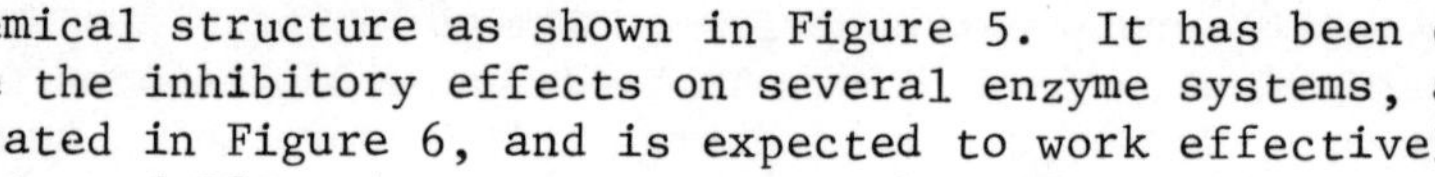

$$HN \diagdown / C \, NHCH_2CH_2 \, CH_2 \, CH_2 \, CH_2 \, COO - \langle \bigcirc \rangle - COOC_2H_5 \cdot CH_3 \, SO_3H$$

$N_3O_4 \cdot CH_3SO_3H$ M·W· 417·48

P—(6—guanidinohexanoyloxy)benzoate]

1esulfonate

Figure 5

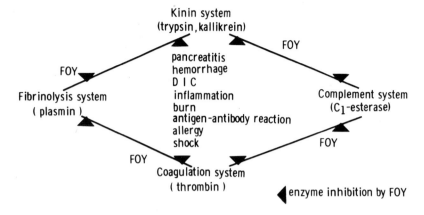

Figure 6

the results are regarded as the combined antitrypsin and anti-plasmin activities through α_1-antitrypsin, besides the antithrombin activity.

On the other hand, there were no such apparent differences among these drugs in thromboplastin-, or endotoxin-induced DIC as shown in thrombin-induced DIC. In particular, however, the antishock action of FOY must be noticed because the changes of WBC or neutrophils were minimal at the infusion of endotoxin.

In the future, the collections of clinical evidence in FOY trials will be expected.

REFERENCES

Amris, C.J. and Hilden, M. 1968. Anticoagulant effects of Trasylol in vitro and in vivo studies. Ann. N.Y. Acad. Sci., 146: 612.
Fujii, S. and Muramatsu, M. 1972. Inhibitory effects of ε-guanidino acid esters on trypsin, plasmin, plasmin kallikrein and thrombin. Biochem. Biophys. Acta. 268: 221.
Ingram, G.I.C. and Richardson, J. 1965."Anticoagulant Prophylaxis and Treatment", pp. 199. Charles C. Thomas, Springfield.
Isobe, J. 1978. Around the DIC syndrome. The 40th Congr. Japan Haemat. Soc., Symp. on DIC (in press).
Lasch, H.G. and Heene, D.H. 1974. Heparin therapy of diffuse intravascular coagulation (DIC). Thrombo. Diath. Haemorrh., 33: 105.
Matsuoka, M. and Yamanaka, M. 1978. Around the DIC syndrome. The 40th Congr. Japan Haemat. Soc., Symp. on DIC. (in press).
Merskey, C. Defibrination syndrome. "Human Blood Coagulation. Maemostasis and Thrombosis", ed. by Biggs R. Ist ed., 1972. pp. 444, Blackwell, Oxford.

Minna, J.D., Robboy, S.I. and Coleman R.W. 1974. "Disseminated
    Intravascular Coagulation in Man". Charles C. Thomas,
    Springfield.
Sakuragawa, N. 1975. Coagulation and fibrinolysis. J. Japan Soc.
    Int. Med., 64: 3 (in Japanese).
Sakuragawa, N. 1978. Around the DIC syndrome. The 40th Congr.
    Japan Haemat. Soc., Symp. on DIC. (in press).
Watanabe, K. and Tullis, J.L. 1977. Ristocetin precipitation test
    - a new method for determination of fibrin monomer and fibrin
    degradation products. Japan. J. Haemat., 18: 46 (in Japanese).
Yamada, S., et al. 1978. Inhibitory effects of gabexate mesilate
    (FOY) on coagulation and fibrinolysis in vitro. Acta Haemat.
    Jap. (Abstract), 41: 379 (in Japanese).

EXPERIMENTAL STUDIES ON THE EFFECT OF PROPHYLACTIC PROTEINASE

INHIBITOR THERAPY ON ENDOTOXIN SHOCK

Sajio Sumida

Department of Surgery, National Fukuoka Central

Hospital, Jonai 2-2, Fukuoka, 810, Japan

Sudden and simultaneous activations in the blood coagulation fibrinolysis, complement and kinin systems have been increasingly recognized as complications of septic shock due to a variety of gram-negative bacteria. Catecholamines stimulate all the three essential plasma cascades by the sequence of: microcirculation spasm, hypoxia, acidosis, sludging, lysosomal degradation, and then the proteinase activation. Severe hypotension and respiratory distress in the course of septic shock were believed to be due partly to the liberation of vasoactive substances including kinins into the circulation. This paper is concerned with the changes of plasma kinin level in endotoxin shock and the influence of the kallikrein-trypsin inhibitors.

METHODS

Endotoxin shock was produced in rats by the intravenous injection of Escherichia coli endotoxin. Rats ranging in weight from 450 to 500 g anesthetized lightly with intraperitoneal administration of 50 mg sodium pentothal , were placed on their backs on the operating table. A polyethylene tube (21 gauge) was inserted into the right atrium through the right jugular vein of each rat. Endotoxin (Difco B4 1 mg in a saline) and test drugs were administered through this tube. Test drugs were given several minutes before the administration of endotoxin. Shock occured at 50 to 60 minutes after injection of endotoxin as mentioned elsewhere (Sumida 1972). Sixty (60) minutes after the injection of endotoxin, 5 ml of blood was drawn without anticoagulant into a polyethylene test tube through the canula placed in the right jugular vein with a polyethylene syringe. Blood sample to estimate the normal value of plasma kinin was collected from other rats anesthetized without the administration of endotoxin. The blood was immediately inactivated within 10 sec by forcibly ejecting it through the needle into 15 ml of chilled 80% (v/v) ethanol in a stoppered polyethylene centrifuge tube, which was then shaken to give adequate dispersion to extract kinin in whole blood according to the method reported by Brocklehurst and Zeitlin (1967).

One horn of the isolated rat uterus was used for determination of free kinin. In our hands, the method of Brocklehurst and Zeitlin worked with a 71% yield. The contraction of the uterus was recorded using a force-displacement transducer (Nihon Koden Kogyo Co., Ltd Japan). Synthetic bradykinin (Nakarai Chemical Ltd. Japan) was used as the standard. The contraction of plasma kinin levels in venous blood was expressed in ng Bradykinin equivalent/ml plasma.

In order to observe the mortality, unanesthetized rats were used, endotoxin and test drugs were administered into the tail vein, and the mortality of 24 hour period was determined. Control rats received saline for test drugs.

Rats of 24 hour period or just before death were sacrificed by decapitation, and the histological examinations by the stain of hematoxylin eosin and pressure-volume curve determinations of resected lungs were performed.

RESULTS

Effect of Proteinase Inhibitors on Endotoxin Lethality in Rats.

The control rats without pretreatment of proteinase inhibitor possessed a significantly higher mortality than either the hydrocortisone, Trasylol (aprotinin), FOY (gebaxate mesilate), FOY + hydrocortisone or FOY + hydrocortisone + heparin rats receiving the same dose of endotoxin (Table 1). The protective effect of the single use of proteinase inhibitor on endotoxin shock in rats is still controversial.

Pressure-Volume Curve of the Resected Lung.

The resected lungs of control rats showed a remarkable decrease in lung compliance. They were easily collapsed when the intrapulmonary pressure was deflated (Figure 1). Inflation did not result in a change in appearance. The lungs of control rats were dark red, appeared hemorrhagic, and grossly resembled liver. The lungs of experimental rats with pretreatment of test drugs resulted in clearing much of the hemorrhagic appearance by inflation.

Table 1.   Endotoxin Lethality of Rats

Controls	96% (50/52)
Hydrocortisone	34% (5/22)
Trasylol	69% (11/16)
FOY	67% (12/18)
FOY+Hydrocortisone	31% (4/13)
FOY+Hydrocortisone+Heparin	27% (4/15)

(Hydrocortisone: 1 mg/100g body weight intravenous, Trasylol: 10^3 U/ 100g body weight, Heparin 0.1 mg/100g body weight, FOY: 0.5 mg/100g body weight intravenous)

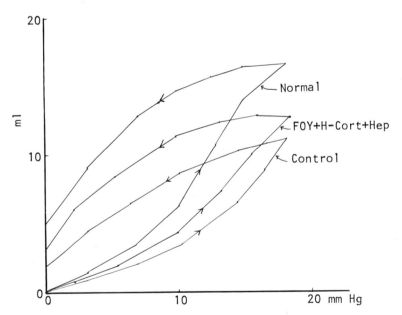

Figure 1. Pressure-Volume Curve of the Resected Lungs of Rats in Endotoxin Shock. Each curve consists of mathematical mean. H-Cort.: Hydrocortisone, Hep: Heparin.

Microscopic Changes of the Resected Lung.

In the control rats by 24 hours, severe congestion, interstitial hemorrhage, and edema are apparent (Figure 2-b) in contrast
to the normal lung. In severe cases, intra-alveolar edema and
hemorrhage were combined. Collapse of many alveoli and dense con-
solidation of segments and lobes were also seen. The lungs of
experimental rats, pretreated with proteinase inhibitor, especially
with FOY, had slight microscopic changes in the lung. The effect
of heparin on pulmonary changes were not distinct.

Plasma Kinin Levels in Venous Blood in Normal Conditions and in
Endotoxin Shock.

The normal level of free kinin in rat plasma was 5.1 Bk.eq/ml
(S.D.= 2.8). The release of plasma kinin in the state of shock and
the effect of test drugs on the inhibition of kinin formation is
shown in Table 2. The level of free kinin was found to increase
significantly in endotoxin shock, however, the release of kinin was
markedly prevented when the test drugs including kallikrein-trypsin
inhibitor, corticosteroid, and heparin were prophylactically and
intravenously administered. The combined uses of FOY + hydrocortisone
or FOY + hydrocortisone + heparin were more effective than the
single use of proteinase inhibitor (Table 2).

DISCUSSION

Plasma kinins produce vasodilation, edema, pain and hypotension.
Clinical importance of plasma kinins was first recognized in septic
shock, but now their role in all kinds of shock has been acknowledged.
In 1971 an International Symposium on Proteinase Inhibition in Shock
Therapy was held in Wiesbaden, and recently several interesting
works have appeared from the clinical fields (Berry et al., 1970;
Diniz et al., 1963; Seidel et al., 1972; Nagaoka et al., 1975;
Deklerk, 1977). However, only Trasylol (aprotinin) has been used
to suppress the activation of kallikrein-trypsin system and to treat
the state of shock. FOY is a new proteinase inhibitor having the
same inhibitory effects on fibrinolytic activity (Aichita et al.,

Table 2.   Free Plasma Kinin as Bradykinin (ng/ml plasma)
            in the Blood of Endotoxin Shock Rats

Controls (5)	34.5 ± 18.3
Hydrocortisone (3)	16.5 ± 11.6
Trasylol (3)	21.3 ± 8.8
FOY (7)	18.4 ± 9.4
FOY+Hydrocortisone (3)	14.9 ± 8.3
FOY+Hydrocortisone+Heparin (3)	11.0 ± 7.0

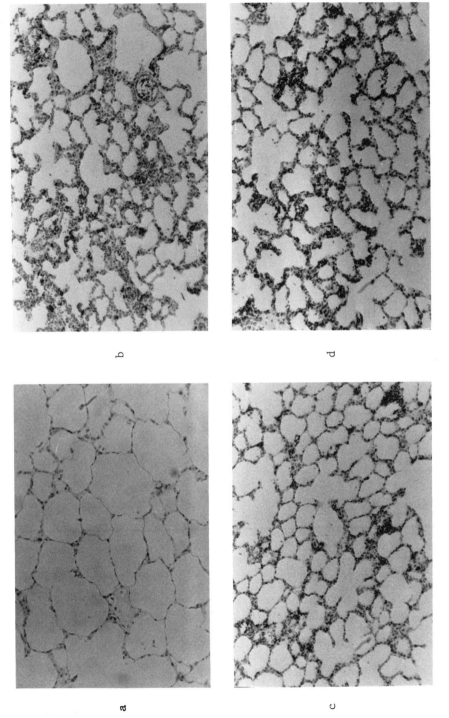

Figure 2. Microscopic Changes of the Endotoxin Shock Lung.
a = Normal Lung, b = Control, c = FOY, and d = Hydrocortisone.

1975). The molecular weight of FOY is 417, which is smaller than 6500-13900 of Trasylol (Bogel et al., 1966). And, FOY has no antigenicity in contrast to Trasylol. Toxicity of FOY is still in controversy, however, FOY is widely used to treat pancreatitis and peritoneal infection without any side effects (Hirayama et al., 1973; Tsukiyama et al., 1973; Namiki et al., 1972).

In this study, FOY was prophylactically effective to minimize the mortality and pulmonary complications for the treatment of shock and shock lung. As the plasma kinin level in endotoxin shock was suppressed by the proteinase inhibitors combined with other drugs as shown in Table 2, we can consider that FOY will be used without any hesitation for the purpose of prophylactic protein ase inhibitor therapy in any type of shock.

CONCLUSION

Prophylactic proteinase inhibitor therapy with Trasylol or FOY had significant effect on endotoxin lethality in rats. Corticosteroids for the same purpose was more effective than the single use of proteinase inhibitors. No significant difference of the effect on the endotoxin lethality between Trasylol and FOY was found. The combined therapy of FOY corticosteroids and heparin resulted in a decrease of the lethality in contrast with their single uses.

Fall in lung compliance was seen in the rats in endotoxin shock, which was slight when pretreatments had been performed. Those lungs were more difficult to inflate and easier to deflate than the normal lungs. It was also confirmed by the morphologic changes observed in those lungs: interstitial edema, vascular congestion and alveolar collapse. Alveolar edema was also seen in severe cases.

Liberation of plasma kinin in endotoxin shock was suppressed by the prophylactic protease inhibitor therapy. The combined use of FOY with corticosteroids and heparin suppressed intensively the liberation of plasma kinin in contrast to the single use of each one of them.

The data indicate these agents, especially the combined uses, do exert their prophylactic effect on the treatment of endotoxin shock, not only experimentally but clinically.

REFERENCES

Aishita, H., Okegawa, T., Akimoto, A., et al., 1975. Effects of methanesulfonate (FOY) on kinin formation and fibrinolytic activity. Folia pharmacol. japan. 71: 89-99.

Berry, H.E., Collier, J.G., and Vane, J.R., 1970. The generation of kinin in the blood of dogs during hypotension due to hemorrhage. Clinical Science 39: 349-365.

Bertelli, A., and Back, N. 1970. Shock. Biochemical, Pharmacological, and Clinical Aspects. Advances in Experimental Medicine and Biology. Vol. 9.

Brocklehurst, W.E., and Zeitlin, I.J. 1967. Determination of plasma kinin and kininogen levels in man. J. Physiol. 191: 417-426.

Deklerk, J., Benzer, H., Haider, Q., Pauser, G., und Stellwag, F. 1977. Beeinflussung des Kininogen-Kininsystems durch einen Kallikreinhemmer bei Operationen am offenen Herzen in extra-corporaler Zirkulation. Anaesthesist 26: 639-643.

Diniz, C.R. and Carvalho, I.F. 1963. A micromethod for determination of bradykininogen under several conditions. Ann. N.Y. Academy Sciences 104: 77-89.

Hirayama, S., Uehara, S., Itagaki, H. et al. 1973. Clinical effect of FOY on Pancreatitis. Gendai-Iryo 6: 741-744.

Nagaoka, H., and Katori, M. 1975. Inhibition of kinin formation by a kallikrein inhibitor during extracorporeal circulation in open-heart surgery. Circulation 52: 325-332.

Namiki, M. 1972. Clinical effect of FOY on pancreatitis. Gendai-Iryo 4: 421-426.

Seidel, G., Meyer-Burgdorff, C., and Habel, E. 1972. Liberation of kinin during extracorporeal circuation. Experientia 28(10): 1193-1194.

Sumida, S. 1972. Effect of proteinase inhibitor on renal blood flow and CVP in septic shock. In: New Aspects of Trasylol Therapy No. 5. F.K. Schattauer Verlag, Stuttgart-N.Y. pp.233.

Tsukiyama, Y. 1973. Clinical experiences on the use of FOY for the treatment of pancreatitis. Rinsho-to-Kenkyu 50(12): 271-274.

Vogel, R., Trautschold, I., und Werle, E. 1966. Natuerliche Proteinasesn-Inhibitoren. Georg Thieme Verlag, Stuttgart.

CHANGES IN BLOOD LEVEL OF KININOGEN, PROSTAGLANDIN E AND
HEMODYNAMICS DURING EXPERIMENTAL ACUTE MYOCARDIAL ISCHEMIA
WITH AND WITHOUT FOY-007

Keiichi Hashimoto, Hiroshi Mitamura, Yuichiro Honda,
Shigeru Kawasumi, Teruo Takano, Eiichi Kimura and Michio
Tsunoo*

Department of Internal Medicine and Department of Pharmacology*, Nippon Medical School, Tokyo, Japan

ABSTRACT

Changes in kininogen, prostaglandin E and hemodynamics were
studied during 2 hours after left anterior descending artery ligation in 19 anesthetized dogs with and without FOY-007, an inhibitor of kinin forming enzyme.

Significant decrease in kininogen in aorta and great cardiac
vein (aorta > great cardiac vein) and increase in prostaglandin E
in great cardiac vein were observed after ligation, indicating
release of kinin and prostaglandin E from ischemic area. Both
kininogen and prostaglandin E changes were inhibited by FOY-007
but further decrease in cardiac output and increase in systemic
vascular resistance were observed. In summary, myocardial release
of both kinin and prostaglandin E was inhibited by FOY-007, with
increase of afterload of the heart.

INTRODUCTION

Bradykinin and prostaglandins have a potent pain producing
and a vasodilating action, and have been suggested as one of the
causes of chest pain and hypotension in acute myocardial ischemia
(4,11,12,13). Although the release of bradykinin and prostaglandins
during myocardial ischemia has been previously reported by us (6,7,
8,9,11) and others (1,2,3,5,13,14), the role of and the interrelationships between bradykinin and prostaglandins in such pathological
conditions have not yet been elucidated. Thus, we studied the influences of FOY-007 (an inhibitor of kinin forming enzyme, Ono
Pharmaceutical Co., Japan) on changes in blood levels of prosta-

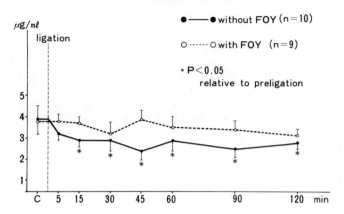

Fig. 1. Changes in kininogen levels in aorta after coronary artery
ligation in two groups with and without FOY treatment.

glandin E (PGE) and kininogen (KGN), a precursor of kinin, and
hemodynamics in acute coronary occlusion in dogs.

MATERIALS AND METHODS

Nineteen dogs, weighing between 20 and 30 kg, were divided
into two groups; 10 dogs were served as non-treated group and 9
dogs as FOY treated group. Dogs were anesthetized with 30mg/kg of
pentobarbital sodium given intravenously. The heart was exposed
through a left thoracotomy under artificial respiration and suspended in a pericardial cradle. The catheters were inserted into
left ventricle, aorta and great cardiac vein via carotid and femoral
artery and jugular vein, respectively. The electromagnetic flow
probes were placed around the root of aorta and the left circumflex
coronary artery, and the strain gauge arches were sutured in the
epicardium of the ischemic and non-ischemic zone. The epicardial
unipolar electrocardiograms were also obtained from ischemic and
non-ischemic zone.

Left anterior descending artery was completely ligated, and
blood was drawn from aorta and great cardiac vein before and 5, 15,
30, 45, 60, 90 and 120 minutes after ligation, and assayed for PGE
and KGN following the methods of Jaffe et al (10) and Wilkens and
coworkers (15), respectively. Simultaneously with blood sampling,
such hemodynamic parameters as heart rate, aortic and left ventricular pressure, left ventricular max dp/dt, cardiac output, coronary
flow, myocardial contractility, systemic vascular resistance, stroke
work index and ECG ST segment elevation in ischemic and non-ischemic

zone were obtained. In the FOY treated group, FOY-007 was continuously administered via femoral vein at the dose of 0.3 mg/kg/minute.
All values described in the text and figures are means ± SEM. Significance of all results was determined using Student's t-test.

RESULTS

Figure 1 shows the changes in KGN in aorta after coronary artery
ligation. Solid line indicates the changes in KGN in the group
without FOY and broken line represents the group with FOY treatment.
Significant decrease in KGN after ligation was observed in the group
without FOY, while no significant change occurred in the group with
FOY treatment.

Changes in KGN in great cardiac vein are illustrated in figure
2. Marked decrease in KGN was observed after coronary ligation in
the group without FOY, while no significant change occurred in the
group with FOY. This indicates that the activation of kallikrein-
kinin system during acute myocardial ischemia was blocked by FOY,
an inhibitor of kinin forming enzyme.

The transmyocardial KGN changes, calculated by KGN in aorta
minus GCV, are shown in figure 3. In the group without FOY, it
tended to increase until 30 minutes after ligation, but no significant change was observed in the group with FOY treatment. This
suggests that the myocardial ischemic area is the site of activation
of kallikrein-kinin system in the early phase of myocardial infarction.

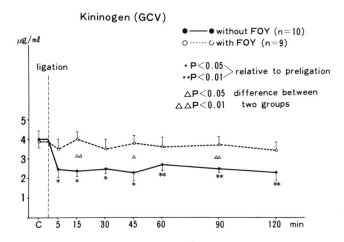

Fig. 2. Changes in kininogen levels in great cardiac vein (GCV)
after coronary artery ligation in two groups with and without FOY
treatment.

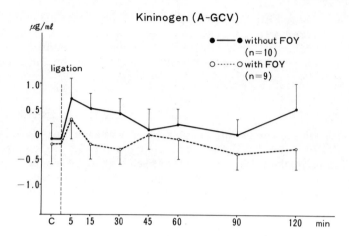

Fig. 3.   Changes in A-GCV differences of kininogen after coronary
artery ligation in two groups with and without FOY treatment.

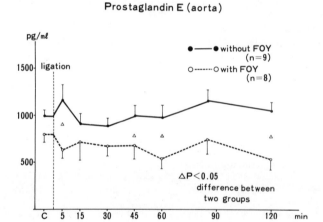

Fig. 4.   Changes in prostaglandin E levels in aorta after coronary
artery ligation in two groups with and without FOY treatment.

Changes in PGE in aorta are illustrated in figure 4. No significant change occurred after ligation in the group without FOY,
while it tended to decrease in FOY group and there were significant
differences between two groups at 5, 45, 60 and 120 minutes after
ligation.

Figure 5 indicates the changes in PGE in GCV after coronary
ligation. Marked increase in PGE was observed in the group without

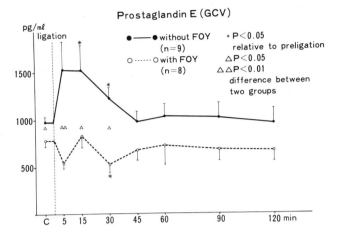

Fig. 5. Changes in prostaglandin E levels in great cardiac vein (GCV) after coronary artery ligation in two groups with and without FOY treatment.

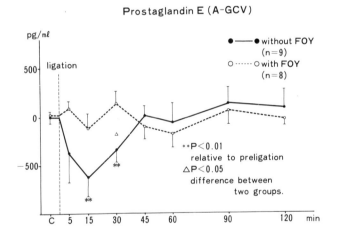

Fig. 6. Changes in A-GCV differences of prostaglandin E after coronary artery ligation in two groups with and without FOY treatment.

FOY until 30 minutes after ligation, while it tended to decrease in FOY group and there were statistically significant differences between two groups at 5, 15 and 30 minutes after ligation.

Transmyocardial PGE production calculated by PGE in aorta minus GCV was illustrated in figure 6. Marked decrease in A-GCV differences of PGE was observed in the group without FOY until 30 minutes after ligation, indicating that PGE was produced at myocardial is-

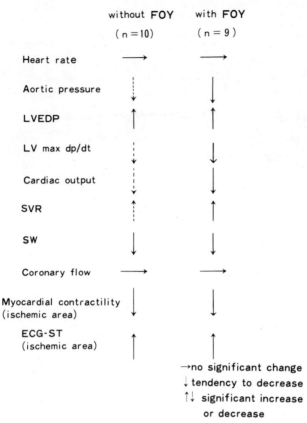

Fig. 7.   Summary of hemodynamic changes.

chemic area in the early phase of infarction. Contrarily, no significant change was observed in the group with FOY, which means that
FOY inhibited not only kinin formation but also PGE production during
myocardial ischemia.

Hemodynamic changes in both groups are summarized in figure 7.
Both groups showed similar changes. However, lowering of blood
pressure, LV max dp/dt and cardiac output and increase in systemic
vascular resistance were more prominent in the group with FOY than
without FOY, indicating that the inhibition of endogeneously released bradykinin and prostaglandin E during myocardial ischemia
has an effect to deteriorate cardiac function.

DISCUSSION

Release of bradykinin and prostaglandins during myocardial
ischemia have been reported by several investigators (1,2,3,5,6,7,

8,9,11,13,14), however, the role of and the interrelationships between bradykinin and prostaglandins in such pathological conditions have not yet been elucidated. As to the releasing mechanism, Needleman and coworkers (12) proposed the hypothesis that various stimuli such as myocardial infarction and angina pectoris cause an inappropriate cardiac oxygen balance that activates kinin synthesis, which in turn stimulates local prostaglandin production, and this, alone or in combination with kinins, causes pain and coronary vasodilation. In our present study, kinin and PGE were released from ischemic area soon after coronary artery ligation, and not only kinin but also PGE release were inhibited by a kinin forming enzyme inhibitor, FOY. This suggests that the activation of kinin is an initial event in acute myocardial ischemia, which is in accordance with the hypothesis of Needleman et al. However, our recent study (9) indicated that indomethacin, a prostaglandin synthetase inhibitor, also blocked not only PGE but also kinin release after coronary artery ligation in dogs. It may be speculated that myocardial ischemia induces both kinin and prostaglandin release, and either one can cause the release of the other.

As to the role of both substances during myocardial ischemia, Needleman and coworkers (12) stated that the induction of local kinin and prostaglandin synthesis would be expected to blunt part of the adverse effects of the myocardial ischemia, since the reflex bradycardia and hypotension would decrease cardiac oxygen demand, and coronary dilation would increase the oxygen supply. In our recent clinical study (8), we have observed the release of kinin from myocardial ischemic area concomitant with lowering of blood pressure and peripheral vascular resistance in patients with acute myocardial infarction who survived, while kinin was not detected in patients with acute myocardial infarction who died of cardiogenic shock or congestive heart failure. From these observations, we concluded that kinin might be of benefit for survivors by decreasing the afterload of the heart. In the present study, the inhibition of both kinin and prostaglandin release after coronary ligation induced the increase of afterload of the heart, which resulted in decrease in cardiac output and myocardial contractility.

The results suggest that kinin and prostaglandin release during myocaridal ischemia have an effect to protect the deterioration of the cardiac function.

ACKNOWLEDGEMENT

FOY-007 used in this study was kindly given by the Ono Pharmaceutical Company, Osaka, Japan.

REFERENCES

1. Attar, S.M.A., H.B. Tingey, J.S. McLaughlin and R.A. Cowley, 1967, Bradykinin in human shock, Surg. Forum 18, 46.

2. Berger, H.J., B.L. Zaret, L. Speroff, L.S. Cohen and S. Wolfson, 1976, Regional cardiac prostaglandin release during myocardial ischemia in anesthetized dogs, Circ. Res. 38, 566.

3. Berger, H.J., B.L. Zaret, L. Speroff, L.S. Cohen and S. Wolfson, 1977, Cardiac prostaglandin release during myocardial ischemia induced by atrial pacing in patients with coronary artery disease, Am. J. Cardiol. 39, 481.

4. Burch, G.E. and N.P. DePasquale, 1963, Bradykinin, Am. Heart J. 65, 116.

5. Dzizinskii, A.A. and A.D. Kuimov, 1972, Blood kinin system in pathogenesis and clinic of ischemic heart disease, Cor Vasa 14, 9.

6. Hashimoto, K., J. Wanka, R.N. Kohn, H.J. Wilkens, R. Steger and N. Back, The vasopeptide kinin system in acute clinical cardiac diseases, 1976, in:Advances in Experimental Medicine and Biology, Vol.70, eds. F. Sicuteri, N. Back and G.L. Haberland (Plenum Press, New York and London) p.245.

7. Hashimoto, K., M. Hirose, S. Furukawa, H. Hayakawa and E. Kimura, 1977, Changes in hemodynamics and bradykinin concentration in coronary sinus blood in experimental coronary artery occlusion, Jap. Heart J. 18, 679.

8. Hashimoto, K., H. Hamamoto, Y. Honda, M. Hirose, S. Furukawa and E. Kimura, 1978, Changes in components of kinin system and hemodynamics in acute myocardial infarction, Am. Heart J. 95,619.

9. Hashimoto, K., T. Takano, Y. Honda, H. Mitamura, S. Kawasumi, E. Kimura and M. Tsunoo, Changes in blood level of prostaglandin E and kininogen in acute experimental myocardial ischemia, and their relationships to the hemodynamics, 1978, in:Abstracts-I, VIIIth World Congress of Cardiology (Tokyo, Japan) p.133.

10. Jaffe, B.M., H.R. Behrman and C.W. Parker, 1973, Radioimmuno-assay measurement of prostaglandin E, A, and F in human plasma, J. Clin. Invest., 52, 398.

11. Kimura, E., K. Hashimoto, S. Furukawa and H. Hayakawa, 1973, Changes in bradykinin level in coronary sinus blood after the experimental occlusion of a coronary artery, Am. Heart J. 85, 635.

12. Needleman, P., S.L. Key, S.E. Denny, P.C. Isakson and G.R. Marshall, 1975, Mechanism and modification of bradykinin-induced coronary vasodilation, Proc. Nat. Acad. Sci. 72, 2060.

13. Sicuteri, F., G. Franchi, P.L. Del Bianco and E. Del Berne, 1967, A contribution to the interpretation of shock and pain in myocardial infarction, Malattie Cardiovasculari 8, 343.

14. Staszewska-Barczak, J., S.H. Ferreira and J.R. Vane, 1976, An excitatory nociceptive cardiac reflex elicited by bradykinin and potentiated by prostaglandins and myocardial ischemia. Cardiovascular Res. 10, 314.

15. Wilkens, H.J., and R. Steger, Agents with kinin-like activity, 1971, in:Screening Methods in Pharmacology, Vol.2, eds. R.A. Turner and P. Hebborn (Academic Press, New York) p.61.

Blood Pressure Regulation:
Kinin, Angiotensin, and Prostaglandin

PARTIAL PURIFICATION OF PRORENIN AND ACTIVATION BY KALLIKREINS:

A POSSIBLE NEW LINK BETWEEN RENIN AND KALLIKREIN SYSTEMS

T. Inagami, N. Yokosawa, N. Takahashi and Y. Takii

Department of Biochemistry, Vanderbilt University

Nashville, Tennessee 37232, U.S.A.

INTRODUCTION

Renin is a highly specific protease which serves for the single purpose of producing angiotensin I from the amino terminal portion of the α_2-globulin substrate angiotensinogen. Biochemical studies of pure renin by group specific reagents have revealed that renin belongs to the family of acid protease (1-3). However, structural basis has not been elucidated to explain its highly restricted substrate specificity limited solely to the cleavage of the single unique leucylleucine peptide bonds in the specific sequence Asp-Arg-Val-Tyr-Ile-His-Pro-Phe-His-Leu-Leu-Val-Tyr-Ser- which is located at the N-terminal region of the substrate molecule. Also, in contrast to other acid proteases renin is active in neutral pH ranges. Again we have no clear-cut explanation for this property deviant from those of general acid proteases.

Many of proteases are known to be formed from its zymogen. Although the presence of such a zymogen of renin has not been known, evidence for an activatable form of renin has been obtained with human amniotic fluid by Morris and Lumbers and Skinner et al (4,5). Renin activity in the amniotic fluid were shown to be markedly increased by dialysis against pH 3.3 or by proteases such as trypsin and pepsin.

Similar activation of renin by dialysis against acid and proteases was observed with human plasma both in hypertensive and normotensive subjects (6-10). Rat plasma shows similar activation though to a lesser extent than humans (11).

Not only proteases or acid treatment but mere storage of human plasma at a low temperature without freezing was found to cause activation (12, 13).

Renin activity in hog kidney were reported to undergo a similar activation upon acid treatment by Rubin (14). Leckie found that the activatable form of renin in rabbit kidney also has a higher molecular weight than the fully active enzyme (15). Boyd reported that the activatable form of renin in hog kidney has a molecular weight of 60,000 compared to the lower molecular weight (40,000) of the fully active renin (16). These investigators also reported that the activation can be realized in a reversible manner by the removal of a peptide by various treatments such as chromatography on DEAE cellulose (17) or exposure to high salt concentration (16). The discovery of the high molecular weight enzyme as the activatable form (designated variously as the inactive form, renin precursor or prorenin) was very important in identifying the prorenin as a distinct molecular species. Subsequently these high molecular weight forms of renin were partially purified by Levine et al (18) and completely purified by Inagami and Murakami (19). The high molecular weight form of human renal renin were also isolated by Slater and Haber (20). However, none of these investigators were able to demonstrate significant activation of the isolated high molecular weight form of renin (18, 20, 21).

Analogous to renin in crude extracts of animal kidney, the activatable form of renin (prorenin) in the human plasma was also identified with the high molecular weight form (60,000 vs. 40,000) by Day and Luetscher (22). Moreover, the high molecular weight forms were reported to be associated only with certain diseases such as Wilms' tumor, chronic renal failure or diabetes mellitis (6,23). Recently, however, Hsueh, Luetscher et al. have reported that plasma of normal humans also contain high molecular weight renin (24). Hollifield et al. claims that both low molecular weight form and the high molecular weight form are activatable (25). Thus, it looks as if the relationship of molecular weight and the activatability does not seem to be as clearcut as was initially thought. Furthermore, the terms such as prorenin, renin precursor, inactive renin, and activatable renin have always been applied to the renin with finite activity which also possesses a potential for further activation implying that the activation of prorenin is a mere quantitative augmentation of its activity presumably mediated by conformational changes. Such a partially active proenzyme clearly deviate from the classical concept of zymogen and seems to present a new form of enzyme regulation.

In order to investigate the unique property of prorenin Boyd attempted to partially purify it from human plasma by stepwise chromatography on a DEAE-cellulose column and obtained a partially active prorenin possessing potential for further activation by protease treatments (26). This prorenin was reported to have a molecular weight of 43,000 which is reduced by approximately 2,000 upon activation. Shulkes, Gibson and Skinner also made a similar attempt to partially purify prorenin from human amniotic fluid by a similar method and obtained a partially active prorenin whose molecular weight (46,000) was not much different from that of active renin (44,000) (27).

This brief review of prorenin shows the wide range of disagreement concerning the relationship of the molecular weight and the capacity for activation in the crude, partially purified and completely purified materials. The past studies have also failed to provide an unequivocal answer to the question as to whether prorenin is really a new type of enzyme precursor already possessing a considerable enzyme activity or a classical zymogen completely devoid of enzyme activity.

Our knowledge on the mechanism and factors involved in the activation of prorenin is even less clear. Obviously the extreme conditions used in laboratory studies on the activation of prorenin such as, acidic pH, cold temperature or treatments with digestive proteases, whose primary role is extensive digestion of proteins, will not be functional in the physiological activation mechanism. Since varying demands for renin seem to affect the ratio of active renin to prorenin secreted into plasma, the conversion of prorenin to active renin may be mediated by physiologically controlled mechanism presumably in the kidney. Although activation of prorenin in plasma under physiological conditions is not likely, evidence for the presence of enzymes or their precursors in the plasma capable of prorenin activation under some extreme conditions is accumulating. The activation of exposure to cold temperature or acid pH suggests the activation process by serine protease inhibitors (29,30) further supports the notion that serine proteases or possibly a kallikrein may be able to activate prorenin.

The whole plasma is a complex mixture of a large number of proteins, lipids and other substances. Particularly, the whole plasma contains various inhibitors of proteases and kallikreins. Use of such a complex system complicates the studies of molecular properties of prorenin and of the mechanism of its activation.

With a long range objective of studying the mechanism of renin formation we have initiated the isolation of human plasma prorenin and also preliminary studies on its activation. We wish to report our finding that prorenin in human plasma is a completely inactive zymogen of the classical type in contrast to the previous report that it is a partially active proenzyme.

METHODS AND MATERIALS

Chromatographic separation of inactive prorenin and active renin: Two steps of affinity chromatography were required for the complete separation of active renin and completely inactive prorenin. EDTA-plasma (2 ml) obtained from healthy, normotensive human subjects was fractionated by a column (2.5 x 4 cm) of Affigel-Blue (Bio-Rad, Los Angeles, California). The plasma sample, bufferized with 0.02 M phosphate buffer (pH 7.1) was applied to the column, washed exhaustively with 150 ml of the same buffer containing 0.2 M NaCl, then with the same buffer containing 1.4 M NaCl. Prorenin containing fractions were eluted by this last step.

This prorenin still exhibited a considerable amount of renin activity, suggesting the possibility of contamination with active renin. It was further fractionated by an affinity column consisting of pepstatin coupled to aminohexyl-Sepharose (31). The prorenin containing fractions from the Affigel-Blue column (Peak II) was equilibrated by dialyzing against 0.02 M acetate buffer (pH 6.0), applied to the pepstatin column (2.0 x 3.0 cm), washed in sequence with 40 ml of the same buffer, with 40 ml of the same buffer containing 1 M NaCl and with 0.5 M Tris buffer (pH 7.5). Fractions which did not adhere to the pepstatin column was designated Peak A, the peak eluted by 1 M NaCl Peak B and fractions eluted by the Tris buffer Peak C.

Renin activity assay: Renin activity was determined essentially by the method of Haber et al. (32) in which angiotensin I generated at pH 7.5 (0.2 M Tris buffer) and 37° for an appropriate period of time from partially purified renin-free hog substrate (Miles Laboratories, Elkhart, Indiana) was quantified by the radioimmuno-assay.

The renin activity of the prorenin containing fractions were determined before and after its activation. Trypsin (Worthington, TRL) was used as the standard catalyst for the activation. Fraction-ated plasma (0.1 ml) was treated for 30 min at 25°C with 5 μg of trypsin in the presence of 0.5 mg of bovine serum albumin (Sigma Chemical Co., 3 x crystallized) and 0.05 M Tris buffer (pH 7.5). The activation was terminated by the addition of 50 μg of limabean trypsin inhibitor (Sigma Chemical Co). Prorenin in the unfractionated plasma (0.1 ml) was activated with 100 μg of trypsin without additional bovine serum albumin. Acid activation was carried out by two successive dialysis of the plasma or fractionated plasma preparations first against 0.05 M glycine buffer (pH 3.2) containing 0.1 M NaCl for 20 hrs then against 0.1 M Tris buffer (pH 7.5) also containing 0.1 M NaCl for 20 hr. Cold activation was done by storing prorenin fractions at 0°C for 5 to 50 days.

Molecular weight: The molecular weight of renin and prorenin in plasma and fractionated preparations were estimated by gel filtration on a calibrated column (2.5 x 80 cm) of Sephadex G-100. In order to minimize run-to-run variations, radio-labeled internal standards were employed throughout this study. Bovine serum albumin labeled with [1-^{14}C]-iodoacetic acid was prepared by incubating 34 mg of bovine serum albumin, and 1.5 mg of [1-^{14}C]-iodioacetic acid (50 µCi) in 3.3 ml of 0.1 M Tris buffer (pH 7.5) containing 0.13 M KCl and 1.5 mM EDTA for 6 hr at room temperature followed by exhaustive dialysis. N-[^{14}C]-methylated ovoalbumin was prepared by treating 30 mg of crystalline ovoalbumin (Sigma Chemical Co) with 4 mM [^{14}C]-formaldehyde (100 µCi) in 30 ml of 0.2 M Na-borate buffer (pH 9.0) at 25° with 4 sequential additions of sodium borate every 30 sec to maintain pH 9.0 by the method of Rice and Means (33).

Hog pancreatic kallikreins purified to homogeneity were kind gifts of Dr. H. Fritz and Drs. E. Truscheit and G. Schmidt-Kastner of Baeyer AG. Pure human urinary kallikrein was kindly supplied by Dr. H. Fritz and Drs. J.J. Pisano. Pure human plasma kallikrein was supplied by Dr. J.J. Pisano, Drs. E. Shaw and G. Ketner. Pure bovine thrombin was supplied by Drs. M.R. Downing and K. Mann. Trasylol$^{(R)}$ was also supplied by Baeyer AG. ([R] Registered trade mark of Baeyer AG).

RESULTS

Isolation of prorenin from active renin: The Affigel-Blue column separated human plasma renin into 2 major fractions. As shown in Fig. 1, the breakthrough fractions (peak I) which exhibited little affinity to the affinity ligand Cibacron Blue F3GA was separated from another type of renin (peak II) with affinity to this dye. Peak II could be eluted only at a high salt concentration. Renin activity under peak I was greater than peak II (filled circles). Peak I renin could not be activated by the trypsin treatment or dialysis against acid pH as described in the method section. Rather, it was inactivated to a certain extent presumably due to general proteolytic action of trypsin (open circles).

Fractions under peak II (filled circles), on the other hand, could be activated by trypsin or dialysis at pH 3.3 as shown by open circles. The extent of the activation by these two different methods were comparable with 9 different plasma samples. Both peaks I and II contain a considerable amount of kallikrein inhibitory activity.

Plasma already activated by the trypsin treatment or dialysis against acid pH exhibited renin activity only in the peak I fractions. Little or no detectable renin activity was present in the peak II

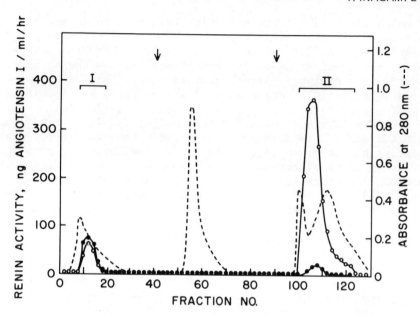

Figure 1.   Affinity chromatography of normal human plasma on Cibacron
            Blue F3GA-agarose column.   The column was eluted by step-
            wise increases of NaCl concentration to 0.6 M at the
            first arrow and to 1.4 M at the second arrow.   Closed
            circles indicate renin activity before trypsin activation,
            open circles represent renin activity after the activation.

fractions.   Further trypsin or acid activation of the peak I fractions
obtained from the trypsin treated plasma did not result in the
formation of additional renin activity.

    These obversations suggested that the peak II fractions
possessing the binding affinity to the Cibacron Blue dye represents
predominantly prorenin and peak I is active renin.   The proportion
of the renin activities under peak I and peak II (filled circles,
Fig. 1) were variable from individual to individual presumably
reflecting varying proportions of active renin and prorenin in
different individuals.

    These observations seemed to indicate that prorenin is a
partially active renin in agreement with previous observations made
by Boyd with human prorenin (26) and with recent reports of Shulkes
et al. on human amniotic fluid (27).   However, the extent of the
activation either by trypsin or acid dialysis was markedly variable.
This variability seemed to indicate that prorenin was not homogenous
suggesting that the separation of prorenin and active renin by the
single step of affinity chromatography by Affigel Blue was not

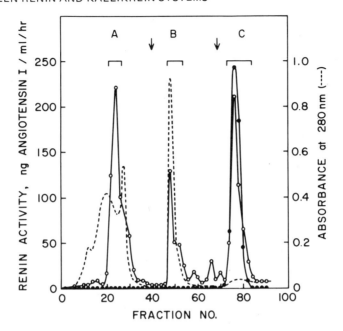

Figure 2. Affinity chromatography of peak II from the Cibacron Blue
column on a pepstatin-aminohexyl-agarose column. The
column was eluted by stepwise changes of the buffer to
0.02 M Na-acetate buffer, pH 6.0 (at the first arrow)
and to 0.5 M Tris-acetate buffer, pH 7.5 (at the second
arrow). Closed circles: renin activity before trypsin
activation, open circles: after the activation.

complete and that the peak II fractions contained both prorenin
and active renin to varying proportions.

    In order to separate these two components more completely the
peak II materials were subjected to an additional affinity chromatography on pepstatin-aminohexyl-agarose. Three major peaks A,B, and
C were separated (Fig. 2). Peak A which did not have affinity to
pepstatin contained most proteins but did not exhibit any measureable
renin activity before activation. Peak B eluted by a higher NaCl
concentration did not have renin activity either. However, these
two peaks contained prorenin which was transformed to active renin
upon the trypsin treatment or acid dialysis (open circles). A small
amount of additional proteins (peak C) was eluted out upon shifting
the buffer to a higher pH. This peak contained active renin (filled
circles) as expected from the affinity of renin to pepstatin. This
active form of renin did not increase its activity upon the usual
treatment known to increase renin activity. The result of the
trypsin treatment shown in open circles, indicated that even as small

an amount of trypsin as 1 µg destroyed active renin to a certain
extent.

Prorenins thus isolated (peaks A and B) are completely inactive.
This is in marked contrast to the numerous past reports (4-13, 26,
27) that prorenin is a partially active renin with a potential for
activation. Moreover, the prorenin isolated in the present studies
could not be activated by cold treatment at 0° for 5 to 15 days.
On the other hand, active renin isolated either by Affigel-Blue
(peak I) or peak C did not have potential for further activation.

Peak A fractions containing prorenin did not inhibit urinary
kallikrein activity to hydrolyze tosyl-L-arginine methyl ester as
tested with 0.42 m units (10 ng) of pure urinary kallikrein. On
the other hand, peak B fractions contained a large amount of
kallikrein inhibitors.

Activation of prorenin by kallikreins and other proteases: The
peak A substance without appreciable amount of the kallikrein inhibitors was used as the prorenin preparation to test the ability of
human urinary kallikrein to activate human plasma prorenin. As
summarized in Table I, the pure urinary kallikrein supplied by Dr.
J.J. Pisano and used at a concentration of 5 ~ 25 µg/100 µl did
not activate plasma prorenin unless prorenin has been previously
dialyzed against pH 3.3 Plasma prorenin pretreated by dialysis
at pH 3.3 already gained some activity due to this pretreatment.
However, it underwent a marked, additional activation by human
urinary kallikrein to the same level attainable by trypsin activation.
Trasylol added at 10-fold molar excess of the kallikrein inhibited
this activation completely. Pure hog pancreatic kallikrein were
also found to activate prorenin to the maximal level. Pure human
renin was also found to activate prorenin of peak II to a certain
extent. This activation was inhibited by Trasylol. Pure thrombine
used at 0.14 mg (84 units) ml did not show any activation.

Molecular weight: The apparent molecular weight of prorenin
determined on the calibrated Sephadex G-100 column using the radiolabeled bovine serum albumin and ovalbumin as internal standards
was found to be 57,000 ± 2,000.

                              DISCUSSION

Studies on prorenin in the past were conducted mostly with
unfractionated plasma or with partially fractionated samples in
which active renin, prorenin and kallikrein inhibitors were not
completely separated which caused uncertainty and confusion in
interpretation of experimental results. An attempt made by Boyd

TABLE I: ACTIVATION OF PARTIALLY PURIFIED
HUMAN PLASMA PRORENIN BY KALLIKREINS

Treatment	Renin Activity pg angiotensin I/100µl/2hr.	
	Before Dialysis	After Dialysis at pH 3.3
Control	22[a]	55
Trypsin Activation[b]	145	153
Kallikrein Activation[c]		
Human Urinary Kallikrein		
0.15 TAME unit	19	65
0.3	14	101
0.75	19	133
0.75 + Trasylol	–	33
Human Plasma Kallikrein		
0.02 TAME unit	39	68
0.02 + Trasylol	–	33
Hog Pancreatic Kallikrein		
0.22 TAME unit	31	104
1.08	35	167

[a] This base line activity is due to renin contaminating angio-tensinogen preparation.

[b] 1 µg in 2 min reaction at pH 7.5 and 22°C in 100 µl.

[c] 60 min reaction at pH 7.5 and 22°C in 100~125 µl.

to separate prorenin from human plasma by ion exchange chromato-graphy (26) and by Shulkes et al. (27) from human amniotic fluid produced prorenin fractions which had a considerable activity. These observations suggested that prorenin was a partially active and potentially activatable form of renin, a concept distinct from that of the classical inactive zymogen. This could have been due to incomplete separation and aroused continued question as to the validity of these separation methods.

The present results clearly indicate for the first time that human plasma prorenin is an inactive zymogen and that active renin has no potential for further activation, at least by currently available techniques. It was also shown that activatable renin with partial activity is a mixture of active renin and its zymogen. The widely variable extent of the activation of the Peak II sub-stance (Fig. 1) can be explained very well if it is a mixture of these two components in varying proportions. In light of these findings it is likely that the partially active prorenin isolated by Boyd (26) and Shulkes et al. (27) and the activatable prorenin reported by various investigators (4-13) are also similar mixtures. The fact that the renin zymogen (inactive prorenin) has a molecular weight close to 60,000 fits very well with the observation by Day and Leutscher (22) that it is "big renin" that can be activated. However, "big renin" may have been a mixture of zymogen and active renin with a similar molecular weight.

The molecular weight estimated as 57,000 is definitely higher than values assigned by previous reports (26,27). In order to ascertain the validity of our results the radio-labeled internal standard was used.

The diminished affinity of pepstatin to prorenin suggests that the active sites of these zymogens are of different forms from that of the active renin which has a much stronger affinity to pepstatin. The selective affinity of the Cibacron Blue F3GA dye to prorenin was discovered in our attempt to remove plasma albumin for which the dye has affinity (33). Although the molecular basis for such a selectivity is not clear, the affinity technique will be useful for the study of plasma prorenin.

Erdos and his collaborators have shown that the renin-angiotensin system and the kallikrein-kinin system are related through kininase II which also functions as angiotensin I converting enzyme (34,35). The present study suggests the strong possibility that the vasoconstricting system and the vasodilating system may be related by yet another link. The regulatory mechanism of prorenin activation must be closely linked to the regulation of renin activity and to the blood pressure regulation. Various relationships between urinary kallikrein levels and various conditions associated with blood pressure have been reported (36,37) although the intermediacy of prostaglandins in the action of kinin on renal blood flow (36) and renin release is another probable mechanism, the present study shows yet another, perhaps direct, action of kallikrein on the activation of prorenin to active renin as illustrated below.

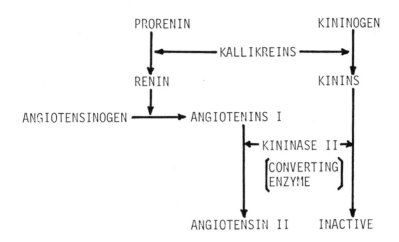

Prorenin in the plasma may not be activated to renin due to plasma inhibitors of kallikrein inhibitors. However, there exists ample evidence that prorenin-renin conversion takes place in the kidney in response to varying demands for renin. Urinary kallikrein is localized in epithelial cells lining distal tubules extending from juxtaglomerular apparatus (39,40). It is likely that this kallikrein interacts with prorenin in certain controlled manner in regulating the proportion of active renin to prorenin in the circulation. Since relatively large amounts of kallikrein are needed for the activation of prorenin, and since pretreatment at pH 3.3 is required, this leaves an element of doubt about the exact role of kallikrein in the activation of prorenin under physiological conditions. However, these can be explained by small amounts of kallikrein inhibitors remaining in peak A fractions. In fact, peak I fractions treated under similar conditions required much higher concentrations of kallikrein. Facilitation of activation by extensive removal of kallikrein inhibitor by an additional step of chromatography and acid treatment was observed. Furthermore, the activation was completely suppressed by Trasylol. These findings seem to lend further support to the possible involvement of kallikrein to the activation of prorenin. However, it is also possible that the acid treatment partially modifies prorenin to a form susceptible to kallikrein. Whichever the mechanism may be, it is extremely interesting that the highly specific kallikrein reacts with a molecule totally unrelated to kininogen.

SUMMARY

With the objective of identifying prorenin and its physiological activation mechanism, human plasma prorenin was completely separated from active renin for the first time. It was shown that prorenin has no activity whereas active renin has no potential for further activation. Urinary kallikreins were found to activate prorenin fractions freed from kallikrein inhibitors by affinity chromatography and treatment at pH 3.3. Human plasma kallikrein also exhibited weak activation.

ACKNOWLEDGMENT

The authors are greatly indebted to Drs. J.J. Pisano, H. Fritz, E. Truscheit, G. Schmidt-Kastner, E. Shaw and G. Ketner for their kind gifts of kallikreins, to Drs. M.R. Downing and K. Mann for thrombin, and to Dr. H. Umezawa and T. Aoyagi for their kind gift of pepstatin. The research was supported by U.S. Public Health Service research grants from N.I.H. HL-14192 and HL-22288.

REFERENCES

1. Inagami, T., K. Misono, and A.M. Michelakis, 1974. Definitive evidence for similarity in the active site of renin and acidic protease. Biochem. Biophys. Res. Communs. $\underline{56}$: 503.

2. McKown, M.M. and R.I. Greggerman, 1975. Human renin inhibition by diazoacyl reagent: relationship of the enzyme to other proteinases. Life Sci. $\underline{16}$: 77.

3. Workman, R.J. and T. Inagami, 1975. Characterization of a new class of renin inhibitors as potential affinity levels of the enzyme. Endocrinol. $\underline{95}$: Suppl. 138.

4. Morris, B.J. and E.R. Lumbers, 1972. The activation of renin in human amniotic fluid by proteolytic enzymes. Biochim. Biophys. Acta. $\underline{289}$: 385.

5. Skinner, S.L., E.J. Cran, R. Gibson, R. Taylor, W.A. Walters, K.J. Catt, 1975. Angiotensin I and II, active and inactive renin, renin substrate, renin activity and angiotensinase in human liquor amnii and plasma. Am. J. Obst. Gynecol. $\underline{121}$: 626.

6. Day, R.P. and J.A. Leutscher, 1974. Big renin: a possible prohormone in kidney and plasma of a patient with Wilms' tumor. J. Clin. Endocrinol. Metab., $\underline{38}$: 923.

7. Weinberger, M.H., W. Aoi and C. Grim, 1977. Dynamic responses of "big renin" in normal and hypertensive humans. Circulation Res., $\underline{41}$ (Suppl. II), 21.

8. Derkx, F.H.M., J.M.G.v. Gool, G.J. Wenting, R.P. Verhoeven, A.J. Manin't Veld and M.A.D.H. Schalenkamp, 1976. Inactive renin in human plasma. The Lancet I: 496.
9. Leckie, B.J., A. McConnell, J. Grant, J.J. Morton, M. Tree and J.J. Brown, 1977. An inactive renin in human plasma. Circ. Res. 40: (Suppl. I) 46.
10. Sealey, J.E. and J.H. Laragh, 1975. "Prorenin" in human plasma. Circ. Res. 36/37 (Suppl I), 10.
11. Oparil, S. and R. Lagocki, 1977. Acid activation of renin in the rat. Circulation 56: (Suppl. II), 832.
12. Osmond, D.H., L.J. Ross and K.D. Scaiff, 1973. Increased renin activity after cold storage of human plasma. Can. J. Physiol. Pharmacol. 51: 705.
13. Sealey, J.E., C. Moon, J.H. Laragh and M. Alderman, 1976. Plasma prorenin; cryoactivation and relationship to renin substrate in normal subjects. Am. J. Med. 61: 731.
14. Rubin, I., 1972. Purification of hog renin; properties of purified hog renin. Scand. J. Clin. Lab. Invest. 29: 51.
15. Leckie, B., 1973. Activation of a possible zymogen of renin in rabbit kidney. Clin. Sci. Mol. Med. 44: 310.
16. Boyd, G.W., 1974. Protein-bound form of porcine renal renin. Circ. Res. 35: 426.
17. Leckie, B. and A. McConnell, 1975. A renin inhibitor from rabbit kidney. Circ. Res. 36: 513.
18. Levine, M., K.E. Lentz, J.R. Kahn, F.E. Dorer and L.T. Skeggs, 1976. Partial purification of a high molecular weight renin from hog kidney. Circ. Res. 38 (Suppl. II) 90.
19. Inagami, T. and K. Murakami, 1977. Purification of high molecular weight forms of renin from hog kidney. Circ. Res. 41 (Suppl. II), 11.
20. Slater, E.E. and E. Haber, 1978. A large form of renin from normal human kidney. J. Clin. Endocrinol. Metab. 47: 105.
21. Inagami, T., S. Hirose, K. Murakami and T. Matoba, 1977. Native form of renin in the kidney. J. Biol. Chem. 252: 7733.
22. Day, R.P. and J.A. Leutscher, 1975. Biochemical properties of big renin extracted from human plasma. J. Clin. Endocrinol. Metab. 40: 1085.
23. Day, R.P., J.A. Leutscher and C.M. Gonzales, 1975. Occurence of big renin in human plasma, amniotic fluid and kidney extracts. J. Clin. Endocrinol. Metab. 40: 1078
24. Hsueh, W.A., J.A. Leutscher, E.J. Carlson and G. Grislis. Big renin in plasma of healthy subjects on high sodium intake. The Lancet, I: 1281.
25. Hollifield, J.W., D.L. Page, A.D. Glick, J.P. Wilson, R. K. Rhamy, V. Goncharenko and Clyde Smith, 1978. Acid activatable prorenin production by an angiolipoma. J. Clin. Endocrinol. Metab. in press.
26. Boyd, G.W., 1977. An inactive higher-molecular-weight renin in normal subjects and hypertensive patients. The Lancet, 1, 215.

27. Shulkes, A.A., R.R. Gibson and S.L. Skinner, 1978. The nature of inactive renin in human plasma and amniotic fluid. Clin. Sci. Mol. Med. 55: 41.

28. Laake, K., H. Gjønnaess, and M.K. Fagerhol, 1973. Components of the kallikrein-kinin system and the spontaneous cold activation of factor VII in human plasma. 33: 229.

29. Osmond, D.H., and A.Y. Loh, 1978. Protease as endogenous activator of inactive renin. The Lancet, 1, 102.

30. Atlas, S.A., J.E. Sealey, and J.H. Laragh, 1978. Protease as endogenous activator of inactive renin. The Lancet, 1, 555.

31. Murakami, K. and T. Inagami, 1975. Isolation of pure and stable renin from hog kidney. Biochem. Biophys. Res. Commun. 62: 757.

32. Haber, E., T. Koerner, L.B. Page, B. Kliman and A. Purnode, 1969. Application of a radioimmunoassay for angiotensin I to the physiologic measurements of plasma renin activity in normal human subjects. J. Clin. Endocrinol. Metab. 29: 1349.

33. Travis, J., J. Bowen, D. Tewksbury, D. Johnson and R. Pannel, 1976. Isolation of albumin from whole human plasma and fractionation of albumin-depleted plasma. Biochem. J. 157: 301.

34. Yang, H.Y.T., E.G. Erdös and Y. Levin, 1970. A dipeptidyl carboxypeptidase that converts angiotensin I and inactivates bradykinin. Biochim. Biophys. Acta. 214: 374.

35. Oshima, G., A. Gecse and E.G. Erdös, 1974. Angiotensin I converting enzyme of the kidney cortex. Biochim. Biophys. Acta. 350: 26.

36. Margolius, H.S., R. Geller, J.J. Pisano, A. Sjoerdsma, 1971. Altered urinary kallikrein excretion in human hypertension. Lancet 2: 1063.

37. Croxatto, H.R. and M. San Martin, 1970. Kallikrein-like activity in the urine of renal hypertensive rats. Experientia 26: 1216.

38. McGiff, J.C., N.A. Terragno, K.U. Malik and A.J. Lonigro, 1972. Release of a prostaglandin E-like substance from canine kidney by bradykinin. Circ. Res. 31: 36.

39. Ørstavik, T.B., K. Nustad, P. Brandtzaeg and J.V. Pierce, 1976. Cellular origin of urinary kallikreins, J. Histochem. Cytochem. 24: 1037.

40. Tyler, D.W., 1978. Localization of renal kallikrein in the dog. Experientia 34: 621.

Note added in proof: While this manuscript was in preparation, activation of human plasma by urinary kallikrein was reported by J.E. Sealey, S.A. Atlas, J.H. Laragh, N.B. Oza and J.W. Ryan, 1978. Nature 275: 144.

BLOOD PRESSURE REGULATION BY ANGIOTENSIN IN THE SPONTANEOUSLY

HYPERTENSIVE RATS

H. Sokabe, K. Kawashima and T.X. Watanabe

Department of Pharmacology, Jichi Medical School,

Minamikawachi, Tochigi-ken, 329-04 Japan

Plasma renin activity (PRA) was subnormal or normal in the main strain of spontaneously hypertensive rats (SHR). PRA increased greatly in the stroke-prone substrain of SHR (SHRSP) at 20-30 weeks of age. Captopril (SQ 14,225) is an orally active angiotensin-converting enzyme inhibitor. The drug acutely decreased blood pressure moderately in SHR, and markedly in SHRSP. Participation of the renin-angiotensin system in the pathogenesis of hypertension in SHR may be limited. Etiology of hypertension in connection with renal excretory function and the central and peripheral nervous system is discussed.

INTRODUCTION

The spontaneously hypertensive rats (SHR) which become hypertensive cardiovascular disease without manipulations or treatments, have been reported (Okamoto and Aoki, 1963). The stroke-prone SHR rats (SHRSP) are a substrain of SHR, which cause cerebral stroke in more than 80% of male individuals by 30 weeks of age (Okamoto et al., 1974).

The purpose of this article is to summarize the results from our laboratory on the renin-angiotensin system (RAS) in these hypertensive rats; to discuss the role of the system in blood pressure regulation; and to extend a speculation into the etiology of hypertension in SHR rats.

429

PLASMA RENIN ACTIVITY.   Sokabe (1965) found a decrease of renin
activity in the kidney of SHR at F8-9 generation, and suggested
that the decrease was a compensatory reaction to the blood pressure
elevation.   Plasma renin activity (PRA) may better reflect the
activity of the renin-angiotensin system.   However, difficulty
existed in obtaining the blood sample without inducing renin
release in the rat, and the results had been so unreliable.   A
method to obtain blood samples of 0.5 ml without anesthesia or
restraint through a cannula inserted into the abdominal aorta has
been devised (Shiono and Sokabe, 1976).   PRA was determined by a
modification of the method of Boucher et al.   SHR were the inbred
strain of F27-30 from the colony of the Department of Pharmacology,
Jichi Medical School.   PRA was lower in SHR than in normal rats of
Donryu strain at age of 5, 10, 20 and 30 weeks (fig. 1.)

We have extended the determinations into SHRSP and SHRSR (a stroke-
registrant substrain) rats (Kawashima et al., 1978.   Main strain
of SHR, F32, Wistar-Kyoto (WKY) from which SHR had been derived,
and normotensive Donryu strain rats (DON), were used as the controls.

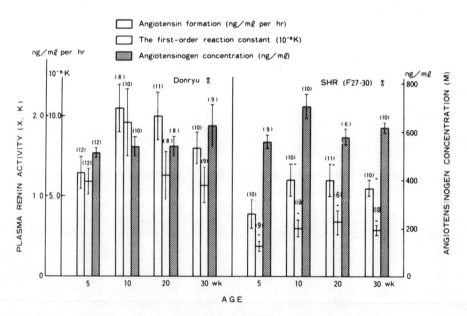

Figure 1.   Plasma renin activity in SHR.   Values are means ± S.E.,
             with number of rats in parentheses.   Asterisk indicates
             statistically significant difference (P < 0.05).
             (Shiono and Sokabe, 1976).

The rats were all male. Blood pressure (BP) in SHR, SHRSR, and SHRSP exceeded hypertensive levels of 150 mmHg by, at latest, 10 weeks of age. In SHR and SHRSR maximum BP levels were less than 200 mmHg. In SHRSP, BP reached to 250 mmHg by 28 weeks of age. BP in DON remained lower than 130 mmHg. BP in WKY showed a tendency to rise close to 150 mmHg by 30 weeks of age. PRA was determined by the method of Calvalho et al., (1975) in this series. No significant difference in PRA was observed among experimental groups at 5, 10, 20, and 30 weeks of age, except, in SHRSP in which PRA was markedly increased at 20 and 30 weeks of age. SHRSP at these ages are in a malignant phase, in which extremely high blood pressure, sodium and water loss, stroke etc. were seen.

In summary, PRA in SHR is basically unchanged or rather suppressed from those in normotensive control rats. No increase to explain the elevation of BP was seen except in SHRSP at a malignant phase.

EFFECT OF CAPTOPRIL. Captopril is a specific inhibitor of angiotensin-converting enzyme, developed by Ondetti et al., (1977) of the Squibb Institute for Medical Research. It has been called as SQ 14,225 by a code. Chemically, it is non-peptidic and orally active.

We determined the acute vasodepressor effect of captopril in DON, WKY, SHR and SHRSP rats (Watanabe et al., 1978). They were male, ca. 20 weeks of age. Aqueous solution of captopril was administered orally, 3 mg/kg, by gavage. Distilled water (5 ml/kg, p.o.) was given to the control group. BP was determined without anesthesia or restraint through a cannula inserted into the abdominal aorta via the femoral artery a day before. BP was recorded for each 15 min prior to and following 60 min. after the drug administration.

The results are shown in Table 1. Both net and % decrease are shown. We calculated % decrease, because the decrease was greater when BP levels was higher. Marked vasodepressor effect was observed in SHRSP. It was moderate in SHR. The effects of captopril were only slight in DON and WKY.

PRA in our colony of SHR rats was not high as shown above, when compared with WKY or DON rats. Therefore, the acute vasodepressor effect of captopril in the main strain of SHR can not be explained by inhibition of angiotensin converting enzyme. Some other mechanism, such as inhibition of kininase II, must be considered. The BP levels after captopril treatment were 165 ± 5 mmHg in SHRSP, which are about the same as those of 169 ± 3 mmHg in SHR. The results accord with the increased RAS in SHRSP at this age, which may partly participate in elevating BP. Bilateral nephrectomy 24 hr before attenuated the effect of captopril in SHRSP. BP decrease in SHRSP after the treatment became about the same as in SHR.

Table 1

Effect of captopril on mean blood pressure in SHR and SHRSP rats

Rat	Treatment	No. of rat	Blood pressure (mmHg)			Decrease (%)	P value*
			Control	1 hr after	Decrease		
DON	SOL	9	124 ± 2	122 ± 2	2 ± 1	1.3 ± 0.6	
	SQ	10	125 ± 3	120 ± 3	4 ± 1	3.4 ± 0.6	< 0.025
WKY	SOL	9	128 ± 2	126 ± 2	2 ± 1	1.7 ± 0.8	
	SQ	10	129 ± 2	121 ± 2	8 ± 1	5.9 ± 1.0	< 0.006
SHR	SOL	10	187 ± 6	182 ± 5	5 ± 1	2.5 ± 0.6	
	SQ	11	187 ± 4	169 ± 3	18 ± 3	9.5 ± 1.5	< 0.001
SHRSP	SOL	12	203 ± 6	200 ± 6	3 ± 2	1.4 ± 1.1	
	SQ	12	207 ± 3	162 ± 5	45 ± 6	21.6 ± 2.6	< 0.001

SOL: Distilled water 5 ml/kg, p.o. SQ: Captopril 3 mg/kg, p.o. Figures are means ± S.E. * Calculated from the decrease (%) in SQ against SOL by Student's t-test. (Watanabe and Sokabe, 1978)

These data shown above, and those from many other laboratories indicated that RAS in SHR rats is rather suppressed, and the system has only a limited role in BP regulation.

TABLE 2.

FUNCTIONAL CHANGES IN THE KIDNEY OF SHR RATS

1. Prohypertensive, when transplanted into the F1-hybrid between normotensive Wistar rats with lower BP.

2. Potentially impaired excretion of NaCl and water (renal function curve shifts to right).

3. Normal or suppressed renin-angiotensin system. Markedly elevated in SHRSP at a malignant phase.

4. Decreased excretion of urinary kallikrein.

5. Rather increased activity of prostaglandin system.

TABLE 3.

ETIOLOGY OF HYPERTENSION IN SHR RATS

1. Renal origin.

2. By the renal-body fluid mechanism.

3. Excretory disfunction of NaCl and water.

4. Possible intrarenal roles of the humoral factors.

5. Possible importance of central and peripheral system.

ETIOLOGY OF HYPERTENSION. According to Guyton et al., (1974), the blood pressure level is chronically determined by the renal-body fluid mechanism. The renin-angiotensin system are effective only with the short-term feedback gain and the limited operational range. If the renal-body fluid mechanism is important, we must look at the kidney in SHR. Table 2 summarizes the changes in the kidney

reported in SHR beside the morphological ones seen in the late
stage. The changes mean here the objective alterations seen in
SHR, without interpreting either as the cause or result. They are:
(1) BP regulating function, observed by the transplantation experiments. Kawabe et al., (1978) from our laboratory reported that the
kidney in SHR rat 10 or 20 weeks of age had a BP elevating action
when it was transplanted into the rats of lower BP:F1 hybrid between
SHR and normal Wistar rats; and (2) Renal excretory function of NaCl
and water was potentially impaired,as shown by Normal et al., (1978)
as the shifts to right of the renal function curve in SHR. Besides
the changes of RAS, it was reported that urinary excretion of kallikrein was decreased (Geller et al., 1975), while there were some
evidences for an increased activity of renal prostaglandins in SHR
rats (Dunn and Hood, 1977).

     Thus, the etiology of hypertension in SHR rats may be considered
as follows (Table 3): It is of renal origin. Hypertension caused
by the renal-body fluid mechanism, but not by the RAS except for an
additional rise at the malignant phase in SHRSP. The kidney of SHR
has an excretory disfunction of NaCl and water, which in turn raised
blood pressure to compensate for the fluid retention. Renal humoral
factors: angiotensins, kinins, or prostaglandins may possibly have
intrarenal action, regulating the excretory function. Thus these
factors possibly participate in the pathogenesis of hypertension
in SHR rats.

     Besides the causal role of the kidney, evidence suggests a
contribution of both central and peripheral nervous system in the
pathogenesis of SHR rats (Yamori, 1976). Although the afferent
paths from the kidney to the central nervous system (CNS) are not
known at present, it is possible that the kidney sends some signal
to the CNS, which elevates BP through activating the peripheral
sympathetic nervous system. (Fig. 2.).

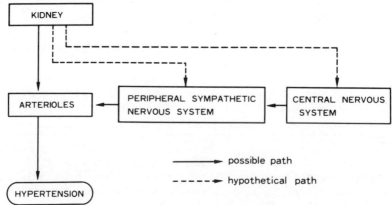

Figure 2. Possible participation of the peripheral and central
           nervous system in the etiology of hypertension in SHR rats.

REFERENCES

Carvalho, J.S., R. Shapiro, P. Hopper and L.B. Page, 1975. Methods for serial study of renin-angiotensin system in the unanesthetized rat. Amer. J. Physiol. 228: 369.

Dunn, M.J. and V.L. Hood, 1977. Prostaglandins and the kidney. Amer. J. Physiol. 233: F169.

Geller, R.G., H.S. Margolius, J.J. Pisano and H.R. Keiser, 1975. Urinary kallikrein excretion in spontaneously hypertensive rats. Circ. Res. 36-37: I 103.

Kawabe, K., T.X. Watanabe, K. Shiono and H. Sokabe, 1978. Influence on blood pressure by renal isografts between spontaneously hypertensive and normotensive rats, utilizing the Fl hybrids. Jap. Heart J. 19 (in press).

Kawashima, K., K. Shiono and H. Sokabe, 1978. Plasma renin activity and excretion of water and electrolytes in stroke-prone SHR rats. Jap. Heart J. 19: 657.

Norman, R.A., Jr., J.A. Enobakhare, J.W. DeClue, B.H. Douglas and A.C. Guyton, 1978. Arterial pressure-urinary output relationship in hypertensive rats. Amer. J. Physiol. 234: R98.

Okamoto, K. and K. Aoki, 1963. Development of a strain of spontaneously hypertensive rats. Jap. Circ. J. 27: 282.

Okamoto, K., Y. Yamori and A. Nagaoka, 1974. Establishment of the stroke-prone spontaneously hypertensive rats. Circ. Res. 34-35: I-143.

Ondetti, M.A., B. Rubin and D.W. Cushman, 1977. Design of specific inhibitors of angiotensin-converting enzyme: A new class of orally active antihypertensive agents. Science 196: 441.

Shiono, K. and H. Sokabe, 1976. Renin-angiotensin system in spontaneously hypertensive rats. Amer. J. Physiol. 231: 1295.

Sokabe, H., 1965. Renin-angiotensin system in the spontaneously hypertensive rat. Nature 205: 90.

Watanabe, T.X., and H. Sokabe, 1978. Acute vasodepressor effect of D-3-mercapto-2-methylpropanoyl-L-proline (SQ 14,225) in the stroke-prone substrain of spontaneously hypertensive rats. (SHRSP). Jap. J. Pharmacol. 28: (in press).

Yamori, Y., 1976. Interaction of neural and nonneural factors in the pathogenesis of spontaneous hypertension. In: The Nervous System in Arterial Hypertension. eds. S. Julius and M.D. Esler (C.C. Thomas, Springfield). p. 17.

EFFECT OF HYPOPHYSECTOMY UPON RENAL KALLIKREIN-KININ SYSTEM IN
RATS

H.R. Croxatto, B. Zamorano, M. Rojas and R. Arriagada

Laboratorio de Fisiologia, Instituto de Ciencias
Biologicas, Pontificia Universidad Catolica de Chile
Casilla 114-D, Santiago, Chile.

Preliminary data have shown that hypophysectomy in the rat,
is followed by a significant and persistent decrease in urinary
kallikrein activity (Croxatto, 1972). There is a growing evidence
implicating renal kallikrein in the development of different types
of hypertension (Croxatto et al., 1977) and according to Geller
et al. (1973) and Margolius et al. (1974), mineralocorticoid would
be the major factor regulating kallikrein excretory rate by the
kidney. In order to assess whether the fall in the kallikrein
level in the urine of hypophysectomized rats was secondary to
adrenal atrophy, urinary kallikrein was determined at regular
intervals before and after the daily administration of either ACTH,
corticosterone, aldosterone or pituitary anterior lobe extracts
in hypophysectomized rats. At the end of the experiment, kallikrein activity in the kidneys of the different groups of rats was
determined.

MATERIAL AND METHODS

Total hypophysectomy was carried out in two groups of female
Sprague-Dawley rats, weighing 170-180 and 145-155 g, respectively.
The operation was performed by para-pharyngeal route (Silva, H. et
al., 1950). In control groups (8 to 10 rats) similar surgical
procedure was performed including the drilling in the skull base,
but the pituitary was left untouched. Autopsy at the end of the
experiment allowed a careful inspection of the operated region;
kidneys and endocrine organs were weighed. Pituitary glands in
5 rats of the first series and in 3 rats of the second one, were
completely removed; in three of the first and in two of the second

series visible remnants of the anterior lobe were found, and these
animals were classified as partially hypophysectomized. In these
rats, endocrine organs exhibited normal or higher weight than in
control rats at the end of the experiment, excepting thyroid gland
which had significantly lower weight. Brometone 40 mg/kg was used
as anaesthetic before autopsy. For five days after the operation
all the animals received a daily dose of Cortisol (10 µg) and 10.000
units of Penicillin in 2 ml of .9% NaCl solution containing 9.4 mg
of glucose.

Kallikrein determinations in the urine were started seven days
after the operation. The animals were placed once or twice a week
in individual metabolic cages for eight hours without food and
with tap water "ad libitum". Urinary volume, Na and K were measured.
Urinary and renal kallikrein were determined by using two different
bioassays: a) direct oxytocic effect upon rats uterus (Croxatto and
Noe, 1972, Croxatto, et al., 1972), and b) indirect method, measuring
the kinin forming activity of the urine when acting upon low molecular weight kininogen obtained from the rat plasma (Jacobson and
Krisz, 1967). Formed kinins were measured using cat jejunum.
Because there was a good correlation between both methods, most of
the data given in the results were obtained by the direct method.
A freshly prepared bradykinin solution was used as standard and
kallikrein activity in the urine was expressed in ng of bradykinin
equivalent per hour and 100 g b.w.

Kallikrein activity in the kidneys was determined in the renal
extracts, prepared by the procedure described (Croxatto et al., 1974)
and tested by using the same bioassays employed for kallikrein
determinations in the urine. The activity was expressed in ng
or in µg of bradykinin equivalents per g and per total kidney mass.

ACTH. A commercial ACTH preparation (60 U/ml) was used: ACTH-
Zinc (Organon). Five hypophysectomized rats of the first series
were injected subcutaneously with 12.5 mU twice a day, for 8 weeks.
Injections were started 86 days after the operation and interrupted
10 days before an autopsy.

Corticosterone.   10 mg of Corticosterone (Sigma) dissolved in 1 ml
of pure ethanol, was diluted in .9% NaCl solution. 10µg in 0.1 ml
was injected twice a day for 9 days.

Aldosterone. d-Aldosterone (Sigma) was similarly dissolved as
Corticosterone. For 6 days, three hypophysectomized rats received,
twice a day 10µg of mineralocorticoid.

Anterior Pituitary Extracts. Anterior pituitary lobes extracts were
obtained from normal adult rats, and were homogenized in a little
mortar and suspended in a small volume of saline. The suspension
was given subcutaneously to the hypophysectomized rats, in such a

dose to provide an amount equivalent to one gland per rat/day. Injections were given for 19 days, interrupted for 8 days and re-assumed for 30 days.

RESULTS

Kallikrein excretion in the totally hypophysectomized rats was significantly lower than in partially and sham-operated controls (Table I and II). Kallikrein activity in the urine measured either by the direct or indirect methods, was 1/5 - 1/6 of the controls in both series, although the urine volume was constantly higher* in the hypophysectomized rats.

ACTH administration for a period of two months produced no significant changes in urinary kallikrein (Table 1). The mean values and s.e. in five hypophysectomized rats including the data of eight determinations during ACTH period, were 20.5 ± 4.3 ng Br per h/100 g b.w. During the pre-injection period lasting 25 days, the respective values for eleven determinations were 27.8 ± 3.7.

Neither corticosterone nor aldosterone injections were followed by significant changes in kallikrein excretion when compared to the respective values of the basal and post-injections period (Table II). Under corticosterone, kallikrein in the urine was 27 ± 4.8 ng Br (3 rats and 2 determinations), versus 23 ± 3.8 ng Br in the pre-injection period (11 determinations). The same animals during aldosterone injections excreted 23 ± 4.3 ng Br (2 determinations).

The administrations of fresh pituitary anterior lobe homogenates produced soon after the fourth day a significant increase in body weight and in urinary kallikrein excretion (Fig. 1). The mean value and s.e. of UK after 19 pituitary injections was 67 ± 10 ng b.w., significantly higher as compared to previous period when no injections were given; but still this value is only one half the amount of kallikrein excreted by controls. Treatment interruption was followed by a fall in body weight and kallikrein in the urine (39.4 ± 5.4 ng Br), but both parameters reached again higher values when injections were given (p <.05) (Fig. 1). During pituitary admini-stration, in four instances, the hypophysectomized rats showed vaginal smears characteristic of oestrus.

Renal kallikrein activity in hypophysectomized rats was con-siderably reduced as compared to either partially hypophysectomized or control rats. In the first series of hypophysectomized animals (5) renal kallikrein activity measured by their kininogenic effect was 2.24 ± 8 μg Br per g of renal tissue, and 1.6 ± 0.6 μg Br in total kidney mass (Fig. 2). In the sham-operated rats, renal kalli-krein activity per g of renal tissue was approximately 4 times higher

Table 1. Urinary Kallikrein in excretion in the three groups of rats expressed in ng of Bradikinin equivalent per hour and 100 g body weight. Mean rat body weight in each period is indicated in ( ). The 5 hypophysectomized rats, received every day 12.5 mU ACTH for 81 days.

Groups	n	Pre-Inject. Period (25 days)	ACTH Period (81 days)	Post-Inject. Period (20 days)
Total. Hypo- physect.	5	27.8±3.7	20.5±4.3	20±2.3
Body Weight g		(162)	(165)	(160)
Part. Hypo- physect.	3	119±11	137±14	125±7.1
Body Weight g		(262)	(281)	(274)
Sham- Operat.	8	115±7.2	119±9.4	112±9.7
Body Weight g		(252)	(290)	(278)

(8.6 ± 0.4 µg Br), and in partially hypophysectomized the respective value was even greater (14.5 ± 1.3 µb Br). In the three hypophysectomized rats of the second series, the kallikrein activity in the kidneys was significantly lower (3.4 ± 0.4 µg Br per g) than in the other groups (Fig. 3), but approximately 30% more than the mean value of the hypophysectomized rats of the first series.

Fig. 3 shows not only the striking difference in renal kallikrein between the hypophysectomized and the other two groups of rats, but also confirms the parallel results obtained with both methods of testing kallikrein.

Table II. Urinary kallikrein excretion in the three groups of rats, expressed in ng of Br equivalents per hours and 100 g body weight. Mean rat body weight is indicated in ( ). The upper part shows the effect of corticosterone, and the lower part the effect of aldosterone in the totally hypophysectomized rats.

Groups	n	Pre-Inject. Period (44 days)	Corticost. Period (9 days)	Post-Inject. Period (6 days)
Total. Hypo- physect.	3	23.4±3.8 (120)	27± 4.8 (120)	22±4.3 (118)
Part. Hypo- physect.	2	66±4.9 (260)	140±14 (265)	99±9 (275)
Sham- Operat.	8	106±8 (211)	138±12 (220)	108±7 (230)

Groups	n	Pre-Inject. Period	Aldosteron. Period (6 days)	Post-Inject. Period
Total. Hypo- physect.	3	22±6.3 (114)	23±4.3 (115)	22±2.9 (115)
Part. Hypo- physect.	2		91±9 (275)	101±8 (280)
Sham- Operat.	8		108±7 (230)	113±3 (230)

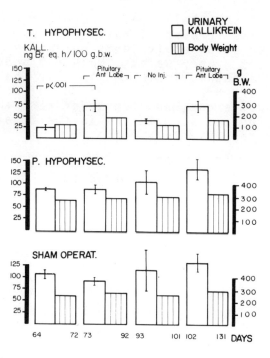

Figure 1.   Body weight and urinary kallikrein excretion (mean
            value and s.e.) in the three groups of rats: totally
            hypophysectomized (3 rats), partially hypophysecto-
            mized (2 rats) and sham-operated (10 rats). After
            a basal period, each totally hypophysectomized rat
            was given pituitary anterior lobe homogenate obtained
            from normal rats every day, during two separate
            periods.

DISCUSSION

      The results confirm that hypophysectomy produces a considerable
and persistent reduction in urinary kallikrein activity. In
addition, they demonstrate that kallikrein in the kidney of the
hypophysectomized rats is significantly lower than in the controls.
Although these data provide a further evidence that pituitary
hormones play a role on renal kallikrein system, they do not
clarify the mechanism involved in the pituitary hormone action.

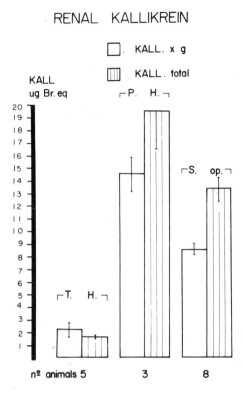

RENAL KALLIKREIN

☐. KALL. x g

▥ KALL. total

Figure 2. Body weight and kallikrein activity in the kidneys
of three groups of rats: totally hypophysectomized
(5 rats), partially hypophysectomized (3 rats) and
sham-operated (8 rats). Kallikrein activity was
measured by the indirect method. Mean values and
s.e. are expressed in μg of bradykinin per g and
per total kidney mass.

Apparently ACTH is unable to increase urinary kallikrein activity.
This negative result agrees with the lack of action of corticosterone and aldosterone, but contradicts Margolius et al (1974)
report about the important role of mineralocorticoids in urinary
kallikrein excretion in normal rats. It is possible that the
action of these steroids upon kallikrein in the hypophysectomized
rats is impaired by the complex endocrine and metabolic deficiencies
in these animals. The favorable effect of pituitary anterior lobe
homogenates increasing urinary kallikrein, suggests that hormones
other than ACTH are required for the synthesis of the enzyme.
Systemic studies by using purified pituitary hormones, single or
associated, could solve the pituitary involvement in kidney kalli-

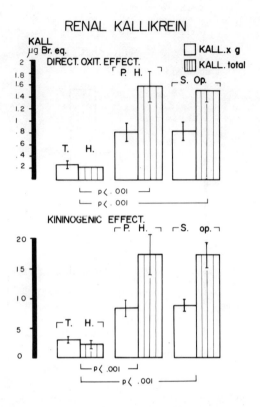

Figure 3. Kallikrein activity (k.a.) in the kidneys of three
           groups of rats: totally hypophysectomized (3 rats),
           partially hypophysectomized (2 rats) and sham-
           operated (10 rats). K.a. measured by the direct
           and indirect method (kininogenic effect) is expressed
           in µg of bradykinin per g and per total kidney mass.

krein. It is interesting to point out that small remnants of
anterior pituitary lobe are enough to keep the normal growth of
the body and endocrine glands (excluding thyroid) and also the
kallikrein levels in kidney and urine.

SUMMARY

     It is confirmed that urinary kallikrein is significantly
and persistently decreased in totally hypophysectomized rats.
In addition, kallikrein activity in the kidneys in these animals

is significantly reduced (p < .001) as compared to partially hypophysectomized and sham-operated rats.

The administration of 125 mU of ACTH twice a day for 2 months, did not modify urinary kallikrein excretion. Negative effects were also obtained in subsequent periods, by injection of 10 μg corticosterone and 10 μg aldosterone, twice a day for 9 and 6 days, respectively.

The administration of rat pituitary anterior lobe homogenates, freshly prepared, increased significantly urinary kallikrein level in hypophysectomized rats.

ACKNOWLEDGEMENTS

This work was supported by grants PNUD-UNESCO RLA 76-006 and 308-77 from the Catholic University Research Fund.

REFERENCES

Croxatto, H. 1972. Calicreina versus renina? Rev. Med. Chile, 100: 700.

Croxatto, H.R. and Noe, G., 1972. Kallikrein like enzyme in purified renal extracts containing renin. Commentarii Pontificia Academia Scientiarum, 40: 1.

Croxatto, H.R., San Martin, M. and Roblero, J., 1972. Kallikrein on arterial hypertension: kallikrein like activity in the urine of the figure-in-eight ligature in one kidney, in: "Vasoactive polypeptides". N. Back and F. Sicuteri, eds., Plenum Publishing Corp., New York, p. 457-475.

Croxatto, H.R., Albertini, R., Roblero, J. and Corthorn, J., 1974. Renal kallikrein (kininogenase activity) in hypertensive rats. Acta physiol. Lat. 24: 439-442.

Croxatto, H.R., Albertini, R., Corthorn, J. and Rosas, R., 1977. "Kallikrein and Kinins in Hypertension:, in: Genest, E. Koiw and O. Kuchel, eds., McGraw-Hill Book Co., New York. p. 364-373.

Geller, R.G., Margolius, H.S., Pisano, J.J. and Keiser, H.R., 1973. Effects of mineralocorticoids, altered sodium intake and adrenalectomy on urinary kallikrein in rats. Circul. Res., 31: 857-861.

Jacobson, S. and Krisz, M., 1967. Some data on two purified kininogens from human plasma. Brit. J. Pharmacol. Chemother. 29: 25.

Margolius, H.S., Horwitz, D., Geller, R.G., Alexander, R.W., Gill, J.R., Pisano, J.J. and Keiser, H.R., 1974. Urinary kallikrein excretion in normal man, Circul. Res. 35: 125.

Silva, M.W., Zamorano, B., Croxatto, H.R. and Becerra, M., 1956. Rate of displacement of oxytocic substances from the diencephalon to tuber cinereum in hypophysectomized rats. Proc. Soc. exp. Biol. Med. 92: 352-353.

RESPONSES OF THE RENIN-ANGIOTENSIN SYSTEM AND KALLIKREIN-KININ

SYSTEM TO SODIUM AND CONVERTING ENZYME INHIBITOR (SQ 14,225)

P. Geoffrey Matthews and Colin I. Johnston

Department of Medicine, Monash University

Prince Henry's Hospital, Melbourne 3004, Australia

INTRODUCTION

Several situations exist where the renin-angiotensin system and kallikrein-kinin system are concurrently influenced by endogenous or exogenous stimuli (Johnston et al., 1976; Wong et al., 1975; Mersey et al., 1977; Margolius et al., 1976). Both systems are known to be changed in the acute and chronic phases of altered sodium intake (Johnston et al., 1976). We have already shown that plasma renin levels are closely related to urinary kallikrein excretion. Little, however, is known of the circulating components of the kallikrein-kinin system and the relationship of these components to urinary kallikrein excretion or the activity of the renin-angiotensin system.

Angiotensin converting enzyme (kininase II) is a component common to both peptide hormonal systems. It converts angiotensin I to the active vasopressor hormone, angiotensin II and degrades the vasodepressor bradykinin to inactive fragments (Erdos, 1976, Figure 1). Specific blockade of converting enzyme activity can now be achieved with synthetic chemical inhibitors. The pharmacological effects of converting enzyme blockade may be a consequence of dual interference with the renin-angiotensin system and kallikrein-kinin system. Inhibition of converting enzyme prevents the vasopressor response of exogenously administered angiotensin I and potentiates the vaso-depressor response to exogenous bradykinin (Rubin et al., 1978).

To further elucidate the relationship of activity of the renin-angiotensin system to the kallikrein-kinin system, we have studied concurrent changes in endogenous hormone levels (plasma renin activity, blood angiotensin I, urinary kallikrein and blood bradykinin) in

447

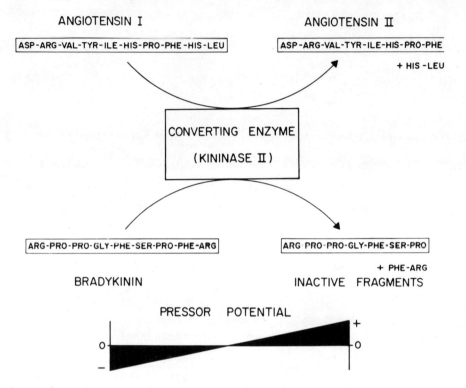

Figure 1.   Diagrammatic representation of the actions of converting
            enzyme (kininase II) on the peptide products of the renin-
            angiotensin system and the kallikrein-kinin system. Normal
            (uninhibited) action, associated with angiotensin II
            generation and bradykinin degradation, may lead to positive
            pressor response. Inhibition of activity may not only
            reduce this pressor potential but also induce a positive
            vasodepressor effect.

situations of varied sodium intake and after converting enzyme
inhibition with an orally active converting enzyme inhibitor,
SQ 14,225.

METHODS

     Three groups of normal male Sprague Dawley rats were placed
simultaneously in metabolic cages for a ten day period. During the
five day experimental period (days five to ten) groups were given
either a normal diet and tap water, a low-sodium diet and tap water
or a normal diet with 1% saline to drink. On day ten 24 h urine
collection was completed and rats were bled for plasma renin activity,
blood angiotensin I and blood bradykinin estimations.

Three paired groups of seven normal male Sprague Dawley rats were gavaged with converting enzyme inhibitor (SQ 14,225) at doses of 1 mg kg^{-1}, 3 mg kg^{-1} or 30 mg kg^{-1}, while the respective control groups were gavaged with vehicle alone. Thirty minutes after gavage, rats were bled for plasma renin activity, blood angiotensin I and blood bradykinin.

Plasma renin activity was measured by an enzyme kinetic technique using a radioimmunoassay for angiotensin I generated by the incubation of diluted rat plasma at 37°C and pH 6.2 (Johnston et al., 1975). Blood angiotensin I was measured by radioimmunoassay of an extract prepared from whole blood which had been added to 20 volumes of ethanol, washed with diethyl ether, evaporated to dryness and reconstituted in assay buffer. Plasma bradykinin was measured by radioimmunoassay after an extraction procedure similar to that of angiotensin I. The total amount of blood required for the assays for plasma renin activity, blood angiotensin I and blood bradykinin was 750 μl.

Urinary kallikrein in the rat was measured by an enzyme kinetic technique. Urine was incubated at 37°C and pH 8.5 with excess semipurified dog kallikrein substrate. The bradykinin generated was measured by radioimmunoassay (Johnston et al., 1976 and 1976a).

Angiotensin II crossreactivity in the angiotensin I radioimmunoassay was less than 0.01%. Lysyl-bradykinin displaced ^{125}I-labelled Tyr^{8}-bradykinin from 60-130% as effectively as the bradykinin standard in the bradykinin radioimmunoassay, depending on the antibody used. Methonyl-lysyl bradykinin showed 100% crossreactivity in this assay. The intra-assay coefficient of variation was 9% (n=10) and inter-assay coefficient of variation was also 9% (n=10).

RESULTS

The effects of 5 days of modification of dietary sodium intake on plasma renin activity, blood angiotensin I and blood bradykinin are depicted in Figure 2. Twenty-four hour urinary sodium excretion in the rats fed a normal diet was 0.74 mmole per day, whereas the high and low sodium regimens resulted in daily excretions of 5.25 ± 0.43 (mean ± s.e.m.) and 0.02 ± 0.01 mmoles of sodium, respectively. The low sodium diet resulted in a marked stimulation of plasma renin activity (15.81 ± 3.34 ng AI ml^{-1}h^{-1} compared to 3.80 ± 0.92 ng AI ml^{-1}h^{-1} in control animals, t=3.4629, p<0.0025, ν=12). A high sodium diet resulted in suppression of plasma renin levels compared to controls (3.06 ± 0.69 ng AI ml^{-1}h^{-1}) but this difference did not reach statistical significance. Blood angiotensin I levels followed the pattern of plasma renin activity (standard diet, 93 ± 8 pg ml^{-1}, low sodium diet 217 ± 12 pg ml^{-1}, t=8.3315, p<0.0005, ν=12 and high sodium diet 77 ± 10 pg ml^{-1}). There was a close linear correlation between plasma renin and blood angiotensin I in these rats (r=0.8215, p<0.001, ν=19).

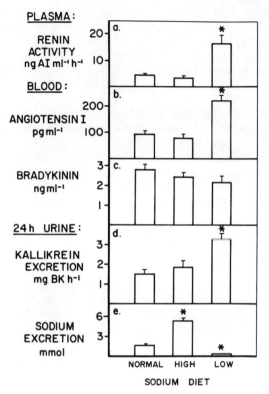

Figure 2.   The effect of normal, high and low sodium diets on plasma
             renin, blood angiotensin I, urinary kallikrein and blood
             bradykinin in simultaneously obtained samples, five days
             after commencing the experimental diet. The asterisk
             indicates values significantly different from the group
             on a normal diet (n=7, for each group).

        Blood bradykinin levels in rats fed the standard diet were
2.78 ± 0.28 ng ml^{-1}. Five days of dietary sodium variation did not
result in a significant change in bradykinin levels in the two
experimental groups (low sodium diet, 2.15 ± 0.29 ng ml^{-1}; high sodium
diet 2.45 ± 0.14 ng ml^{-1}). On the other hand, 24 h urinary kallikrein
excretion increased significantly after sodium depletion (3.28 ±
0.22 mg BK h^{-1} compared with 1.47 ± 0.22 mg BK h^{-1} in controls,
t=5.7907, p<0.0005, ν=12) although the high sodium regimen did not
change kallikrein excretion significantly from control animals.
Plasma renin levels were directly correlated with 24 h urinary
kallikrein excretion during dietary sodium manipulation (r=0.5850,
p<0.01, ν=20) and blood angiotensin I levels were similaraly related
(r=0.6432, p<0.01, ν=20).

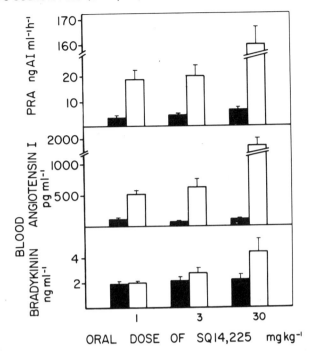

Figure 3.   The effect of inhibition of converting enzyme with
             SQ 14,225, at three dose levels, on plasma renin, blood
             angiotensin I and blood bradykinin, in rats, 30 minutes
             after gavage. The shaded bars represent values in
             control group. Responses, overall, were dose dependent.
             Significant differences were seen in the renin and
             angiotensin I levels at all doses. Blood bradykinin
             levels were significantly different from controls only
             at 30 mg kg^{-1}.

     The effect on plasma renin activity, blood angiotensin I and
blood bradykinin levels of 1, 3 and 30 mg kg^{-1} of the converting
enzyme inhibitor, SQ 14,225 given orally, is shown in Figure 3
together with the responses of control animals gavaged with vehicle
alone. The results are those observed 30 minutes after treatment.
Plasma renin activity was increased significantly above controls at
all dose levels of the inhibitor and showed a progressive rise with
increasing doses (1 mg kg^{-1}: $t=3.4952$, $p<0.0025$, $\nu=12$; 3 mg kg^{-1}:
$t=6.7257$, $p<0.0005$, $\nu=12$; 30 mg kg^{-1}: $t=28.4426$, $p<0.0005$, $\nu=11$).
The response of blood angiotensin I levels followed a similar pattern
to plasma renin, both rising at the highest dose to levels, an order
of magnitude greater than those seen in sodium depeletion. Blood
bradykinin levels, however, did not show the same responses. At
1 mg kg^{-1} of SQ 14,225, bradykinin values were not different to those
of the control group (1.91 ± 0.19 ng ml^{-1}). At 3 mg kg^{-1} bradykinin

levels were also not increased above their control groups. However, the levels in the 3 mg kg^{-1} group were significantly greater than in the 1 mg kg^{-1} group (t=2.1850, p<0.025, ν=12). Only with 30 mg kg^{-1} was a statistical difference from the control group demonstrated (t=2.0299, p<0.05, ν=12).

As was shown for the animals with varying sodium intake, plasma renin and blood angiotensin I were closely correlated in the animals given SQ 14,225 (r=0.9134, p<0.001, ν=12). However, this relationship is altered so that for any given level of plasma renin, there was a higher level of blood angiotensin I in the rats given the converting enzyme inhibitor. Table 1 shows the regression coefficients for the linear equation, $y = a_o + a_1x$, for angiotensin (y) on renin (x) in the two groups, where a_o = intercept on the y axis and a_1 = slope. Although the slopes were the same the intercepts for the untreated animals (75 pg ml^{-1}) was significantly different from the animals given converting enzyme inhibitor 411 pg ml^{-1}. This difference in angiotensin I may represent the contribution from converting enzyme inhibition independent of the concomitant rise in plasma renin.

Plasma renin activity and the blood levels of angiotensin I and bradykinin after the low sodium diet and during converting enzyme inhibition at 1 mg kg^{-1} are compared in Table 2. Similar values are seen in each group of animals.

DISCUSSION

A low sodium diet is well known to stimulate plasma renin levels (Gross et al., 1965). Circulating levels of the decapeptide, angiotensin I, have been measured less frequently, but have been correlated with the circulating renin levels (Waite, 1973). The observations in the present study emphasize this relationship over a wide range of varied sodium balance and extend it to the situation of inhibition of converting ensyme activity. We have previously found that plasma angiotensin II levels to be related to plasma renin in the rat during dietary sodium manipulation (Johnston et al., 1976, 1976a). It is of interest that the plasma angiotensin I levels are of a similar order to angiotensin II levels in the rat and both circulate at levels somewhat higher than in other species. Marieb and Mulrow (1965) reported corresponding changes in adrenal aldosterone secretion.

The studies of urinary kallikrein in altered sodium balance support our earlier finding of an inverse relationship between urinary kallikrein and sodium excretion (Johnston et al., 1976). In the present study, a diet of 5.25 mmoles of sodium per day was not sufficient, after five days, to cause any significant suppression of urinary kallikrein excretion. It has been suggested that aldosterone

Table 1. Relationship of Plasma Renin Activity
          To Blood Angiotensin I Levels.
          (Linear Regression Analysis).

	a_o	a_1	r	ν	p
Treated animals alone.	411	9.2	0.9134	12	<0.001
Animals on varied salt intake.	75	7.0	0.8215	19	<.001

(Equation to line of best fit: $y = a_o + a_1x$).

Table 2. Comparison of Low Salt Diet And
          Converting Enzyme Inhibition.

	Plasma renin activity* ($ng\ AI\ ml^{-1}h^{-1}$)	Blood angiotensin I* ($pg\ ml^{-1}$)	Blood bradykinin* ($ng\ ml^{-1}$)
5 Days of Low Salt Diet. (24 h sodium excretion = 0.02 mmole)	15.81 ±3.34 n=7	217 ±12 n=7	2.15 ±0.29 n=7
Converting Enzyme Inhibition. (30 min after SQ 14,225 at 1 mg kg^{-1})	18.30 ±4.18 n=7	517 ±56 n=7	1.98 ±0.18 n=7

* mean ± s.e.m.

may be responsible for the appearance of kallikrein in the kidney (and
by extrapolation in the urine), and the present study is consistent
with such a proposition (Margolius et al., 1976). However, alternative explanations also require evaluation.

This study has revealed a dissociation between the levels of
circulating bradykinin and urinary kallikrein. Although grouped data
suggested a possible inverse relationship between these two components
of the kallikrein-kinin system, statistical analysis did not support
this. The lack of relationship may indicate that renal kallikrein
may be compartmentalized and not have access to plasma substrate in
the circulation. Circulating bradykinin levels may therefore be

subject to different control mechanisms to renal components of the
kallikrein-kinin system.

SQ 14,225, given orally, in a range of doses has been shown to
be effective in modifying the circulating levels of angiotensin I
and bradykinin. Low dose converting enzyme inhibition resulted in
changes in renin and angiotensin that were of the same order as
those resulting from sodium depletion. Inhibition of converting
enzyme has been shown to lead to natriuresis (McCaa et al., 1978;
Bengis et al., 1978) however this was not measured in the present
experiments. It is possible that this phenomenon could contribute
to the rise in plasma renin.

Over the range of converting enzyme inhibition observed,
angiotensin I levels correlated closely with plasma renin activity,
confirming the association during sodium manipulation of the renin-
angiotensin system. It is of interest, that although the regression
lines of angiotensin I on plasma renin activity for treated and
untreated animals were similar in slope, the difference in y axis
intercepts represented a difference of some 350 pg of angiotensin I
per ml of blood. Since circulating blood levels of angiotensin I
are a function of both its generation and clearance, this difference
may represent that contribution to the circulating angiotensin I
levels made by the impaired clearance of angiotensin I due to
converting enzyme inhibition.

Blood bradykinin levels also showed a dose-related increase
after converting enzyme inhibition. The positive association
between high renin and angiotensin I levels and blood bradykinin is
consistent with inhibition of converting enzyme and implies a common
enzyme. On the other hand, it is clear that the responsiveness of
these two systems is different. At a dose of 1 mg kg^{-1} of SQ 14,225
there were clear rises in angiotensin I but no measureable effect
on blood bradykinin levels. Increased plasma renin levels which
would augment the generation rate of angiotensin I may be partly
contributed to by a decrease in angiotensin II negative feedback on
renal renin release (Blair-West et al., 1971). In addition, impaired
removal of angiotensin I from the circulation may further augment
the levels of this hormone, perhaps explaining why the angiotensin I
changes can occur at lower doses of the drug. Bradykinin levels, on
the other hand, were much less responsive, approximately two fold
less,than angiotensin I levels. These differences in responsiveness
of the two circulating peptide substrates, acted upon by presumably
the same enzyme, may relate to differing pool sizes for the
circulating component having access to the enzyme. This, in turn,
is a function of generation rates or, clearance rates which may also
differ. Different affinities of these two peptides for converting
enzyme may also explain the differential effect. It is also known
that converting enzyme is not the exclusive enzyme degrading
angiotensin I and bradykinin and that other specific and non-specifc

enzymes exist in vivo which may contribute to the process (Erdos and Yang, 1970; Page and Bumpus, 1974). Control of the functions of these other enzymes is poorly understood. In addition, high dose converting enzyme inhibition are known to be accompanied by haemo-dynamic alterations (Gavras et al., 1978) which may indirectly raise bradykinin.

For these reasons, neither circulating endogenous angiotensin I nor circulating bradykinin may accurately and directly reflect the inhibition of angiotensin converting enzyme. The rise in angiotensin I levels, however, seems to be a more sensitive index of converting enzyme inhibition.

SUMMARY

Plasma renin activity, blood angiotensin I, urinary kallikrein and blood bradykinin levels have been measured concurrently in rats over a range of daily sodium intake. Plasma renin activity, blood angiotensin I levels and urinary kallikrein were significantly increased by the low sodium diet (0.02 mmole per day). Bradykinin levels did not change. Plasma renin and blood angiotensin I were closely linearly related over the range of sodium intakes. Both were associated positively with urinary kallikrein excretion. Converting enzyme inhibition caused prompt, significant changes in plasma renin activity, endogenous circulating angiotensin I, and bradykinin. The changes in circulating hormone levels were dose dependent. Blood angiotensin I levels showed a greater responsiveness than blood bradykinin levels. Plasma renin activity and blood angiotensin I levels are closely related after converting enzyme inhibition. Both increased plasma renin, and impaired clearance of angiotensin I may contribute to blood angiotensin I levels. Difference in responsiveness of blood angiotensin I and blood bradykinin levels after inhibition suggests that other independent controls of the circulating levels of these hormones exist.

ACKNOWLEDGEMENTS

The excellent technical assistance of S.Lamont and B.Clappison is acknowledged. The project was supported by grants from the Life Insurance Medical Research Fund of Australia and New Zealand, and the National Heart Foundation. Dr. Matthews is a Fellow of the National Health and Medical Research Council of Australia. SQ 14,225 was donated by Dr.Z.P.Horowitz, Squibb Institute for Medical Research, Princeton, New Jersey.

REFERENCES

Bengis, R.G., Coleman, T.G., Young, D.B. and McCaa, R.E., 1978, Long-term blockade of angiotensin formation in various norm-otensive and hypertensive rat models using converting enzyme inhibitor (SQ 14,225), Circulation Res., Suppl.I, I:45.

Blair-West, J.R., Coghlan, J.P., Denton, D.A., Funder, J.W. Scoggins, B.A. and Wright, R.D., 1971, Inhibition of renin secretion by systematic and intrarenal angiotensin infusion, Amer. J. Physiol., 220:1309.

Erdos, E.G., 1976, Conversion of angiotensin I to angiotensin II, Amer. J. Med., 60:749.

Erdos, E.G. and Yand, H.Y.T., Kininases, in: "Handbook of Experimental Pharmacology, vol.XXV, Bradykinin, Kallidin and Kallikrein", Springer-Verlag, Berlin, 1970, p.289.

Gavras, H., Liang, C.-S. and Brunner, H.R., 1978, Redistribution of regional blood flow after inhibition of the angiotensin-converting enzyme, Circulation Res., Suppl.I, 43:1-59.

Gross, F., Brunner, H. and Ziegler, M., 1965, Renin-angiotensin system, aldosterone, and sodium balance, Recent Progr. Horm. Res., 21:119.

Johnston, C.I., Matthews, P.G., Davis, J.M., Morgan, T., 1975, Renin measurement in blood collected from the efferent arteriole of the kidney of the rat, Pflugers Arch., 356:277.

Johnston, C.I., Matthews, P.G. and Dax, E., Effects of dietary sodium, diuretics and hypertension on renin and kallikrein, in: "Systemic Effects of Antihypertensive Agents", ed. M.P. Sambhi, Symposia Specialists, Miami, 1976a, p.323.

Johnston, C.I., Matthews, P.G. and Dax, E., 1976a, Renin-angiotensin and kallikrein-kinin systems in sodium homeostasis and hyper-tension in rats, Clin. Sci. Mol. Med., 51:238s.

Margolius, H.S., Chao, J. and Kaizu, T., 1976, The effects of aldosterone and spirinolactone on renal kallikrein in the rat, Clin. Sci. Mol. Med., 51:279s.

Margolius, H.S., Horowitz, D., Pisano, J.J. and Keiser, H.R., 1976, Relationships among urinary kallikrein, mineralocorticoids and human hypertensive disease, Federation Proc., 35:203.

Marieb, N.J. and Mulrow, P.J., 1965, Role of the renin-angiotensin system in the regulation of aldosterone secretion in the rat, Endocrinology, 76:657.

Mersey, J.H., Williams, G.H., Hollenberg, N.H. and Dluhy, R.G., 1977, Relationships between aldosterone and bradykinin, Circulation Res., 40, Suppl.I, I-84.

Page, I.H. and Bumpus, F.M., eds., "Handbook of Experimental Pharmacology, Vol XXXVII, Angiotensin" Springer-Verlag, Berlin, 1974.

Rubin, B., Laffan, R.J., Kotler, D.G., O'Keefe, E.H., Demaid, D.A. and Goldberg, M.E., 1978, SQ 14,225 (D-3-Mercapto-2-methyl-propanoyl-L-proline), a novel orally active inhibitor of angiotensin I-converting enzyme, J.Pharmacol. Exptl. Ther., 204:271.

Waite, M.A., 1973, Measurement of concentrations of angiotensin I in human blood by radioimmunoassay, Clin. Sci. Mol. Med., 45:51.

Wong, P.Y., Talamo, R.C., Williams, G.H. and Coleman, R.W., 1975, Response of the kallikrein-kinin and renin-angiotensin systems to saline infusion and upright posture, J.Clin. Invest., 55:691.

RELATIONSHIP BETWEEN KININS AND PROSTAGLANDINS: CONTRIBUTION OF RENAL

PROSTAGLANDINS TO THE NATRIURETIC ACTION OF BRADYKININ IN THE DOG

M. Cynthia Blasingham and Alberto Nasjletti

Department of Pharmacology
University of Tennessee Center for the Health Sciences
Memphis, Tennessee 38163

Intrarenal infusion of bradykinin stimulates production of a prostaglandin E-like substance by the canine kidney (Terragno et al, 1972; McGiff et al, 1972) through liberation of non-esterified arachidonic acid, the precursor of the endoperoxide intermediate. The effects of intrarenal bradykinin, PGE_2, and arachidonic acid are similar- augmentation of renal blood flow and water and electrolyte excretion. The effects of arachidonic acid infusion are thought to be a consequence of enhanced renal prostaglandin production since they can be blocked by inhibition of cyclo-oxygenase which converts arachidonic acid to the endoperoxide intermediate (Tannenbaum et al, 1975).

To study the effects of stimulation of renal prostaglandin biosynthesis by bradykinin in vivo, we assessed the changes in canine renal hemodynamics and excretory functions induced by intrarenal infusion of bradykinin before and during inhibition of cyclo-oxygenase, and hence prostaglandin synthesis, by sodium meclofenamate. A modification in the renal actions of bradykinin during prostaglandin biosynthesis inhibition would suggest withdrawal of a prostaglandin-mediated component.

METHODS

Experiments were performed on male mongrel dogs, mean weight 21.6 ± 2.6 kg (S.D.), anesthetized with 30 mg/kg sodium pentobarbital i.v. Arterial blood pressure was monitored continuously. Following a priming dose, a solution of inulin in 2.5% dextrose and 0.45% saline was infused i.v. at 5 ml/min throughout the experiment. A volume load of 10 ml/kg 5% dextrose was administered i.v.

459

The ureter was cannulated through a left flank incision and a needle placed in the renal artery for infusions at 0.2 ml/min. A flow transducer was placed on the renal artery, and renal blood flow was monitored on a square wave electromagnetic flowmeter (Carolina Medical Electronics). Arterial blood was sampled through a femoral arterial catheter.

Blood samples containing 0.1 ml 15% ammonium EDTA were centrifuged at 4°C. The sodium concentrations in plasma and one aliquot of collected urine were determined by flame photometry (Instrumentation Laboratory, Inc.) Glomerular filtration was estimated by the clearance of inulin (Davidson and Sackner, 1963).

One aliquot of collected urine from six dogs in Series 1 was frozen for later determination of the content of PGE-like material by bioassay after extraction and separation by thin-layer chromatography (TLC). Ten ml of urine were acidified to pH 3.0 and the lipids extracted first with ethyl acetate and subsequently with 0.1 M potassium phosphate buffer, pH 8.0. Following acidification of the aqueous layer to pH 3.0, the lipids were extracted with chloroform, concentrated in a vacuum at 35°C, dissolved in chloroform:methanol (4:1 by volume), and applied to TLC plates which were developed with chloroform:methanol:acetic acid (18:2:1 by volume). Following elution of the PGE_2 zone by chloroform:methanol (4:1 by volume), eluates were dried under nitrogen and reconstituted in 0.15 M NaCl (Nasjletti et al, 1978).

With PGE_2 as a reference standard, the concentration of PGE-like material in the reconstitued eluate was determined by bioassay on rat stomach strips superfused with Krebs solution.

The excretion of sodium (μEq/min) was calculated by urinary concentration of sodium (mEq/L) x urine flow (ml/min). The excretion of PGE-like material (ng/min) was calculated by (ng "PGE"/ml urine) x urine flow (ml/min). The clearance of inulin was calculated by urinary mg % x urine flow (ml/min)/plasma mg %.

Three protocols were used. In Series 1, the effects of blockade of prostaglandin synthesis on the renal effects of bradykinin infusion were determined in 8 dogs. Following a control period of intrarenal saline infusion, bradykinin triacetate (Sigma) was infused at 10 ng/min/kg. Saline was reinfused during a recovery period. The cyclo-oxygenase inhibitor sodium meclofenamate (Parke-Davis) was then administered i.v. at 5 mg/kg and allowed 20-30 minutes to effect blockade of prostaglandin synthesis. The saline control, bradykinin, and saline recovery periods were then repeated. Periods of infusion and simultaneous urine collection lasted from 15 to 60 minutes depending on urine flow. Arterial blood was drawn at the midpoint of each period.

In Series 2, any effects of prostaglandin synthesis inhibition on the renal actions of PGE_2, the major renal prostaglandin, were noted. The protocol was identical to that of Series 1 except that PGE_2 was infused intrarenally at 5 ng/min/kg instead of bradykinin.

Control Series 3, was identical to that of Series 1 except that the saline vehicle for meclofenamate was administered i.v.

Results are expressed as mean $\pm$ S.E.M. Data within a group were compared by either the Student t-test for paired observations or the Signed Rank Test. Data between groups were compared by the Student t-test for unpaired comparisons.

RESULTS

In Figure 1, bradykinin infusion (10 ng/min/kg) increased urinary "PGE" excretion from 1.00 $\pm$ 0.25 to 3.88 $\pm$ 1.09 ng/min (p<.05). After meclofenamate however, urinary "PGE" excretion decreased to 0.11 $\pm$ 0.06 ng/min (p<.05) and remained depressed, indicating prostaglandin synthesis inhibition.

Before meclofenamate, bradykinin increased sodium excretion (p<.01), urine flow (p<.05), and renal blood flow (p<.001). However, it had no effect on mean arterial pressure or glomerular filtration rate.

After inhibition of prostaglandin synthesis by meclofenamate, bradykinin again increased urine flow (p<.02) and renal blood flow (p<.01). However, the natriuretic effect of the kinin was markedly reduced (p<.05). Before meclofenamate, sodium excretion increased by 64.8 $\pm$ 18.0 µEq/min with bradykinin; after meclofenamate it was not significantly increased. Thus, inhibition of prostaglandin synthesis by meclofenamate reduced the natriuretic effect of intrarenal bradykinin without reducing the vasodilatory and diuretic effects. On the other hand, in Series 3, neither the natriuretic nor the renal vasodilatory and diuretic actions of bradykinin were affected by administration of the meclofenamate vehicle.

Figure 2 illustrates the effects of intrarenal PGE_2 infusion (5 ng/min/kg) before and during prostaglandin synthesis inhibition by meclofenamate. Before meclofenamate, PGE_2 increased sodium excretion, (p<.01), urine flow (p<.05), and renal blood flow (p<.01) as did bradykinin in Series 1. Again, there was no change in arterial blood pressure or glomerular filtration rate. These effects of intrarenal PGE_2 infusion were unaltered by prostaglandin synthesis inhibition by meclofenamate, in contrast to the results of Series 1 in which the natriuretic effect of the kinin was blocked by prostaglandin synthesis inhibition.

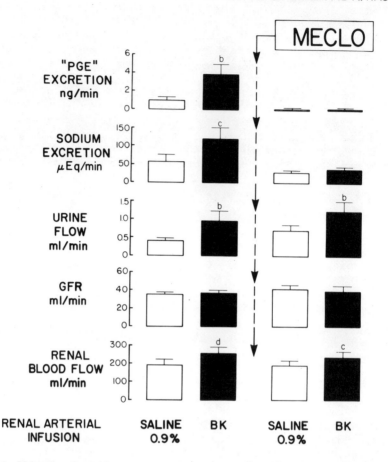

Figure 1 illustrates the changes in renal "PGE" excretion (ng/min), sodium excretion (µEq/min), urine flow (ml/min), glomerular filtration rate (GFR, ml/min), and renal blood flow (ml/min) induced by intrarenal infusion of bradykinin (BK, 10 ng/min/kg) before and after i.v. administration of sodium meclofenamate (MECLO, 5 mg/kg), a cyclo-oxygenase inhibitor, n = 8. (a = $p<0.1$, b = $p<0.05$, c = $p<0.01$, d = $p<0.001$).

DISCUSSION

Intrarenal infusion of bradykinin concurrently increased renal production of a PGE-like material and augmented sodium excretion, both of which effects were blocked during inhibition of prostaglandin cyclo-oxygenase activity by meclofenamate. In contrast, the ability of bradykinin to increase renal blood flow and urine flow was not affected by prostaglandin synthesis inhibition. From this evidence, we conclude first that intrarenal arterial infusion of bradykinin stimulates synthesis of a product of prostaglandin cyclo-

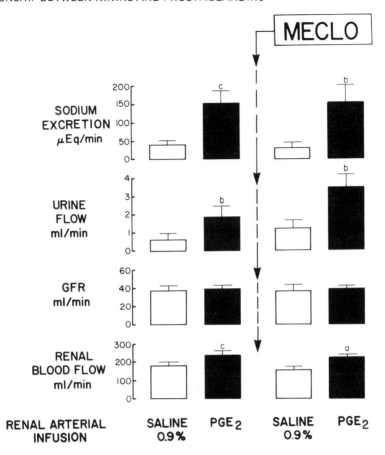

Figure 2 illustrates the changes in sodium excretion (µEq/min), urine flow (ml/min), glomerular filtration rate (GFR, ml/min), and renal blood flow (ml/min) elicited by intrarenal infusion of PGE_2 (5 ng/min/kg) before and after i.v. administration of sodium meclofenamate (MECLO, 5 mg/kg), n = 5. (a = p<0.1, b = p<0.05, c = p< 0.01, d = p<0.001).

oxygenase activity, probably PGE_2, which augments urinary sodium excretion and mediates the natriuretic action of the kinin. Second, prostaglandins produced by the kidney during bradykinin infusion do not appear, under these experimental conditions, to contribute to either the vasodilatory or the diuretic actions of the kinin. Furthermore, the possibility of a nonspecific inhibition of sodium excretion by meclofenamate is minimized since the natriuretic action of PGE_2, was not impaired by the cyclo-oxygenase inhibitor.

Since intrarenally infused arachidonic acid is converted to

products which cause renal vasodilation, diuresis, and natriuresis
(Tannenbaum et al, 1975), it appears inconsistent that the arachidonic acid liberated by bradykinin infusion is converted to products which contribute to the natriuresis of bradykinin, but not
the vasodilation or diuresis. The explanation may be that infused
arachidonic acid is converted to both PGE_2 and PGI_2, whereas endogenous arachidonic acid released from tissue phospholipids by
bradykinin is converted to PGE_2 only (Needleman et al, 1978).
Since PGI_2 is produced primarily in the renal cortex (Whorton et
al, 1978), it is feasible that it produces renal vasodilation during
arachidonic acid infusion. In contrast, PGE_2, which is produced
primarily in the medulla (Larsson and Anggard, 1973) and is elevated
during bradykinin infusion, may not augment renal blood flow because
the amount reaching the blood vessels of the cortex, via the tubular
route (Williams et al, 1977), may be insufficient.

Renal arterial infusion of either bradykinin (Stein et al,
1972; Strandhoy et al, 1974) or PGE_2 (Strandhoy et al, 1974) into
the canine kidney has been reported to augment sodium excretion by
interfering with sodium reabsorption in distal nephron segments.
Further, PGE_2 effects inhibition of sodium transport in the distal
nephron of the rat (Kauker, 1977) and in the cortical and outer
medullary collecting tubules of the rabbit (Stokes and Kokko, 1977).
Thus, PGE_2 produced by cellular elements of the renal medulla during
bradykinin administration may mediate the kinin-induced natriuresis
by reducing sodium reabsorption in the distal nephron.

Kinins are generated continuously within the kidney and may
influence renal hemodynamic and excretory functions (Nasjletti and
Colina-Chourio, 1976). Recent studies showed interrelations between
the renal kallikrein-kinin and prostaglandin systems which suggest
that a product of renal kallikrein activity is instrumental in
regulating renal prostaglandin production (Nasjletti and Colina-
Chourio, 1976; Nasjletti et al, 1978). Assuming that kinins formed
intrarenally stimulate production of a natriuretic prostaglandin,
these studies and our observations suggest that the renal kallikrein-
kinin and prostaglandin systems may be integral parts of a mechanism
that promotes excretion of sodium.

Davidson, W.D., and M.A. Sackner, 1963, Simplification of the
    anthrone method for the determination of inulin in clearance
    studies, J. Lab. Clin. Med. 62:351-356.
Kauker, M., 1977, Prostaglandin E_2 effect from the luminal side on
    renal tubular ^{22}Na efflux: tracer microinjection studies, Proc.
    Soc. Exptl. Biol. Med. 154:274-277.
Larsson, C. and E. Anggard, 1973, Regional differences in the
    formation and metabolism of prostaglandins in the rabbit kidney,
    Eur. J. Pharmac. 21:30-36.

McGiff, J.C., N.A. Terragno, K.U. Malik, and A.J. Lonigro, 1972,
  Release of a prostaglandin E-like substance from canine kidney
  by bradykinin, Circulation Res. 31:36-43.
Nasjletti, A., and J. Colina-Chourio, 1976, Interaction of mineralocorticoids, renal prostaglandins and the renal kallikrein-kinin
  system, Federation Proc. 35:189-193.
Nasjletti, A., J.C. McGiff, and J. Colina-Chourio, 1978, Interrelations of the renal kallikrein-kinin system and renal prostaglandins in the conscious rat, Circulation Res. in press.
Needleman, P., S.D. Bronson, A. Wyche, and M. Sivokoff, 1978,
  Cardiac and renal prostaglandin I_2. Biosynthesis and biological
  effects in isolated perfused rabbit tissues, J. Clin. Invest.
  61: 839-849.
Stein, J.H., R.C. Congbalay, D.L. Karsh, R.W. Osgood, and T.F.
  Ferris, 1972, The effect of bradykinin on proximal tubular
  sodium reabsorption in the dog: evidence for functional nephron
  heterogeneity, J. Clin. Invest. 51:1709-1721.
Stokes, J.B. and J.P. Kokko, 1977, Inhibition of sodium transport
  by prostaglandin E_2 across the isolated, perfused rabbit collect-
  ing tubule, J. Clin. Invest. 59:1099-1104.
Strandhoy, J.W., C.E. Ott, E.G. Schneider, L.R. Willis, N.P. Beck,
  B.B. Davis, and F.G. Knox, 1974, Effects of prostaglandins E_1
  and E_2 on renal sodium reabsorption and Starling forces, Am. J.
  Physiol. 226:1015-1021.
Tannenbaum, J., J.A. Splawinski, J.A. Oates, and A.S. Nies, 1975,
  Enhanced renal prostaglandin production in the dog: effects on
  renal function, Circulation Res. 36:197-203.
Terragno, N.A., A.J. Lonigro, K.U. Malik, and J.C. McGiff, 1972,
  The relationships of the renal vasodilator action of bradykinin
  to the release of a prostaglandin E-like substance, Experientia
  28:437-439.
Whorton, A.R., M. Smigel, J.A. Oates, and J.C. Frolich, 1978,
  Regional differences in prostacyclin formation by the kidney.
  Prostacyclin is a major prostaglandin of renal cortex, Biochim.
  Biophys. Acta 529:176-180.
Williams, W.M., J. Frolich, A.S. Nies, and J.A. Oates, 1977,
  Urinary prostaglandins: site of entry into renal tubular fluid,
  Kidney Intern. 11:256-260.

Supported by USPHS Grant HL-18579 and AHA Grant 76 781. M.C.B.
is the recipient of a Research Fellowship from the Kidney Foundation
of West Tennessee. A.N. is the recipient of National Heart and Lung
Institute Career Research Development Award 1 K04 HL 00163.

PURIFICATION AND PROPERTIES OF ANGIOTENSIN I-CONVERTING ENZYME IN HUMAN LUNG AND ITS ROLE ON THE METABOLISM OF VASOACTIVE PEPTIDES IN PULMONARY CIRCULATION

Tatsuo Kokubu, Einosuke Ueda, Tadafumi Joh and
Kazutaka Nishimura

The 2nd Department of Internal Medicine
Ehime University School of Medicine
Shigenobu, Onsen-gun, Ehime 791-02, Japan

Purification of angiotensin I-converting enzyme from human
lung and characteristics of the enzyme was studied. Experimental
pneumonitis was produced in rabbits and the change of the activity
of angiotensin I-converting enzyme was studied in purpose to
clarify the role of this enzyme in the metabolism of vasoactive
peptides in the lung. Purification was performed using trypsin
treatment, acid treatment, DE52-cellulose column chromatography,
hydroxyapatite chromatography and Sephadex G-200 gel filtration.
The enzyme after final step showed a single band on disc gel
electrophoresis. Experimental pneumonitis was produced by injection of Complete Freund's adjuvant(acute pneumonitis) and of N-
nitroso-N-methylurethane(chronic pneumonitis). In acute experiment, angiotensin I-converting enzyme activity in pulmonary tissue
and in plasma was significantly decreased. In perfusion experiment, conversion of angiotensin I to angiotensin II and inactivation of bradykinin were also significantly decreased. In case
of decreased activity of angiotensin I-converting enzyme in the
lung, less angiotensin II will be released into systemic circulation and bradykinin will pass through the pulmonary circulation
into systemic circulation, thus this may result in the decrease
of systemic blood pressure.

INTRODUCTION

The metabolism of vasoactive substances in the lung has been
interested in recent years. Especially we interested in the
metabolism of vasoactive peptides related to renin-angiotensin and
kallikrein-kinin system. Angiotensin I-converting enzyme(ACE),
dipeptidyl carboxypeptidase(EC 3.4.15.1) converts inactive angiotensin I(AI) to angiotensis II(AII), a potent vasopressor peptide,

by releasing the C-terminal dipeptide, and also inactivate bradykinin, a potent depressor peptide(Yang and Erdős, 1967; Yang et
al., 1971; Ueda et al., 1972; Nishimura et al., 1976; Nishimura et
al., 1977). This enzyme is thought to work mainly in the lung in
physiological conditions(Ng and Vane, 1968, 1976; Bakhle et al.,
1969; Oparil et al., 1971; Ryan et al., 1971). To elucidate the
physiological role of ACE in the lung, (1) the purification of
this enzyme from human lung was done to make clear the characteristics of the enzyme, (2) the change of the activity of this
enzyme in the lung and in plasma of the rabbits with experimental
pneumonitis was examined.

MATERIALS AND METHODS

Hippuryl-His-Leu-OH, angiotensin I, angiotensin II, bradykinin
were purchased from the Institute for Peptide Research, Suita,
Osaka, Japan. Trypsin and Complete Freund's Adjuvant were from
Difco Lab., Detroit, U.S.A. The molecular weight marker kit was
obtained from Boehringer Mannheim, West Germany and Sephadex G-
200, Hydroxyapatite and Dextran Blue 2000 from Pharmacia, Uppsala,
Sweden. DE-52 cellulose was from Whatman, Kent, England. Chemicals used for acrylamide gel electrophoresis were from Wako Pure
Chemicals, Osaka, Japan.

Human cadaveric lung were obtained from a patient who died
from a traffic accident.

Measurement of AI, AII and BK:
Radioimmunological assay, which had been proven that the cross
reaction between AI and AII with antibodies was less than 10 %,
was employed for perfusion experiment. Biological assay using
isolated rat uterus was employed for ACE assay when AI, AII or BK
was used as the substrate.

Measurement of ACE activity in purification step:
ACE activity was measured by the spectrophotometric method of
Cushman and Cheung, 1971. One unit of the enzyme activity was
defined as that amount of the enzyme which hydrolyzed 1 μmol of
Hippuryl-His-Leu-OH per min at 37 C under the conditions described
by them.

Measurement of ACE activity in rabbit lung tissue:
Whole lung was chopped and homogenized with 25 mM borate buffer,
pH 8.3 using Potter homogenizer, then an aliquot of the homogenate
was homogenized again with Polytron(Kinematica, Luzern, Switzerland) for 1 min. The homogenate was centrifuged at 700 x g for
10 min and the supernatant was used as the material. Activity of
the enzyme was expressed as nmol/wet weight g/min or nmol/mg prot/
min.

Angiotensinase activity: Angiotensinase activity was determined by using AII as substrate, and remained AII was assayed in
the isolated rat uterus.

Purification of ACE from human lung: The lung(36 g) was
chopped into small pieces and suspended in 20 mM of potassium

phosphate buffer, pH 7.8, containing 0.25 M sucrose. The suspension was homogenized in a Waring blender and centrifuged for 20
min at 700 x g. The supernatant was adjusted to pH 5.2 with
acetic acid and centrifuged at 15000 x g for 30 min. The pellet
was suspended in 10 mM potassium phosphate buffer, pH 7.8 and
adjusted to pH 7.8 with 1 M NaOH. This acid precipitated fraction
was incubated with trypsin(1 mg/500 mg protein) for 120 min at 37
C at the presence of 0.1 mM of $CaCl_2$. The solution was readjusted
to pH 5.2 with acetic acid and centrifuged at 15000 x g for 30 min.
The supernatant was used for next step. DE-52 cellulose column
(2.6 x 30 cm) was equilibrated with 10 mM potassium phosphate
buffer, pH 7.8, the linear gradient elution of NaCl(0-0.5 M) was
used for enzyme elution. Hydroxyapatite column(2.6 x 8.5 cm) was
equilibrated with 1 mM potassium phosphate buffer, pH 6.8. A
linear gradient of phosphate buffer increasing in molarity from 1
to 30 mM elution was employed for enzyme elution. Sephadex G-200
column(2.6 x 89 cm) was equilibrated with 10 mM potassium phosphate buffer, pH 7.8, and the gel filtration was performed as the
last step of the purification.

Disc gel electrophoresis: Analytical disc gel electrophoresis
was performed on 7.5 % acrylamide gel at pH 8.6 with current of
2.5 mA per tube for 4 h. For determination of the molecular weight
of the enzyme which was incubated with 1 % sodium dodecyl sulfate
and 1 % 2-mercaptoethanol for 2 h at 50 C, disc gel electrophoresis on 7.5 % acrylamide gel was performed with 0.1 M sodium phosphate buffer, pH 7.2, containing 0.1 % sodium dodecyl sulfate.
A current of 8 mM per tube was used for 5 h. Gels were stained
0.05 % Coomasie Blue in 12.5 % trichloroacetic acid.

Production of acute experimental pneumonitis: 0.5 ml of
Complete Freund's Adjuvant was injected intravenously two times
with one week interval, and the rabbits were used as acute pneumonitis on 3rd, 7th, and 14th day.

Production of chronic experimental pneumonitis: 0.5 ml of N-
nitroso-N-methylurethane(NMU)(100 x dilution) was injected intravenously four times with one week intervals, and the rabbits were
used as chronic pneumonitis on 30th day after fourth injection.

Perfusion experiment: Rabbits were anesthetized with pento-
barbital-Na and were breathed with Harvard Respirator. Then the
lungs were perfused with Tyrode's solution at a constant rate of
5.6 ml/min from pulmonary artery without taking out the lung from
thorax, then after ligation of the aorta, perfusate were collected
from left ventricle. 5 µg of AI(1 ml of 5 µg/ml), 5 µg of AII(1
ml of 5 µg/ml), or 5 µg of BK(1 ml of 5 µg/ml in saline) were
perfused and a total of 20 ml of perfusate was collected for each
experiment. AI and AII in the perfusate were measured radioimmunologically and BK in the perfusate was measured by biologically in a isolated rat uterus.

Table 1.   Purification step of angiotensin I converting enzyme
from human lung

Purification step	Volume (ml)	Total protein (mg)	Total activity (units)	Specific activity	
				Hip-His-Leu (U/mg)	Angiotensin I (nmol/min/mg)
A The homogenate, supernatant centrifuged at $700 \times g$	81.4	2296.4	3.215	0.0014	
B Sediment from the pH 5.2 precipitation, resuspended in 10mM phosphate buffer, pH 7.8	40.4	1066.5	1.813	0.0017	
C After trypsin treatment and acidification to pH 5.2, the supernatant centrifuged at $15000 \times g$	149.0	448.3	4.93	0.011	
D DE 52 eluate	48.0	15.4	10.50	0.684	47.9
E Hydroxylapatite eluate (conc.)	3.0	1.0	8.13	8.13	568.6
F Sephadex G-200 filtrate (conc.)	5.0	0.7	6.75	9.50	665.0

RESULTS

Purification of ACE from human lung: Purification steps of
ACE from human lung using trypsin were summarized in Table 1.   ACE
which is considered to be a membrane-bound enzyme was sedimented
in the acidification step of pH 5.2 with acetic acid.   After
trypsin treatment of the sediment, most of ACE activity was found
in the supernatant.   After the acidification step, specific
activity increased about 10 folds of the initial step(from 0.0014
to 0.011 u/mg).

In DE 52-cellulose column chromatography, ACE activity was
eluted at the concentration of 0.09 M of NaCl.   The enzyme was
purified about 60 folds by this step(from 0.011 to 0.684 u/mg).
After the Hydroxyapatite column, the specific activity increased
13 folds, from 0.684 u/mg to 8.13 u/mg.   After final step of
Sephadex G-200 gel filtration, the specific activity was 9.50 u/mg
, means about 700 folds increase from initial material(Fig. 1).
The specific activity for AI was increased parallely with the
increase for Hippuryl-His-Leu-OH.

Disc gel electrophoresis: The sample after final step showed
a single protein band after disc gel electrophoresis(Fig. 2).

Characteristics of the enzyme after final step: The enzyme
inactivated bradykinin as well as conversion of AI.   The specific
activity of the enzyme was 9.5 u/mg prot. for H-H-L, 0.665 μmol/min
for AI, and 9.5 μmol/min for BK.   The molecular weight of the
enzyme by gel filtration of Sephadex G-200 was calculated for
290000, and more than 200000 by disc gel electrophoresis in the
presence of sodium dodecyl sulfate.   The optimal pH was 8.3, Km
for Hippuryl-His-Leu-OH was 1.1 mM.   The enzyme was inactive in
the Cl^- free medium, inhibited by EDTA($I_{50}=5 \times 10^{-5}$ M), Arg-Pro-
Pro($I_{50}=1.2 \times 10^{-8}$ M), Bradykinin potentiating peptide C($I_{50}=5 \times$

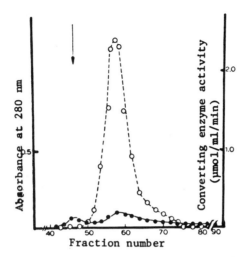

Fig. 1. Sephadex G-200 column chromatography. The arrow indicates the void volume of the column as determined with Blue Dextran 2000. Applied sample: Hydroxylapatite eluate. ●——● : absorbance at 280 nm   o——o : enzymic activity

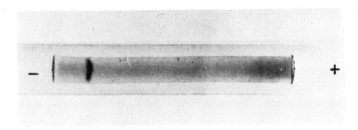

Fig. 2. 7.5 % polyacrylamide disc gel electrophoresis. Applied sample: 10 ug of the purified enzyme. The line on the lower portion of the gel indicates migration of the marker dye.

10^{-6} M), SQ 14225(I_{50}=2.7 x 10^{-8} M) and SQ 20881(I_{50}=7.5 x 10^{-8} M). Inactivated 90 % at 50 C for 10 min. No angiotensinase activity was found in this enzyme after 12 h incubation with AII.

Production of acute experimental pneumonitis: A massive cell infiltration including polymorphnuclear cells, monocytes, lymphocyte, eosinocytes and histiocyte was observed in alveolar space and interstitial tissue. Desquamation of endothelium of small artery was observed.

Production of chronic experimental pneumonitis: The thickening of alveolar septa with lymphocyte infiltration was prominent. Desquamation of endothelial cell was not observed.

ACE activity in lung tissue and in plasma in rabbits with experimental pneumonitis: Results were shown in Table 2. Plasma ACE and lung ACE were significantly decreased in acute pneumonitis , namely, from 57.23 ± 3.21 to 42.41 ± 4.20 nmol/ml/min in plasma, and from 54.46 ± 46 to 5.55 ± 0.79 nmol/mg prot/min in lung tissue, respectively.

On the other hand, there was no significant change in chronic pneumonitis.

Conversion of AI and inactivation of BK in perfusion experiment: Conversion rate of AI to AII in perfusion experiment of the isolated lung with acute pneumonitis was significantly decreased, from 81.65 ± 2.84 to 70.76 ± 2.88 %. Rate of inactivation of BK also significantly decreased in acute pneumonitis, from 92.2 ± 2.46 to 85.92 ± 1.12 %. On the other hand, there was no significant deviation of conversion activity and inactivation activity in

Table 2. Angiotensin I-converting enzyme activity in plasma and lung homogenate of rabbits with experimental pneumonitis.

		Days or months after treatment						
		Before	1 – 2 D	4 D	7 D	10 D	14 D	1 M
FA Group[1] (Acute)	Plasma ATCE[3]	57.23[7] ±3.21	42.41[4]* ±4.20	47.30[4] ±4.21	58.20[4] ±2.43	58.95[4] ±4.45	71.40[4]** ±7.79	
	Lung ATCE[4]	54.46[5] ±4.02	5.55*** ±0.79		21.62[5]*** ±2.55		24.74[5]*** ±3.46	
	Lung ATCE[4]	6940[5] ±323.4	2997[4]*** ±311.4		4930[5]* ±728.6		4630[5]* ±867.7	
NMU Group[2] (Chronic)	Plasma ATCE[3]	57.23[7] ±3.21						59.98[4] ±3.90
	Lung ATCE[4]	54.46[5] ±4.02						49.70[5] ±4.69

1) Treated with Complete Freund's Adjuvant
2) Treated with N-Nitroso-N-methylurethan
3) n mole/ml/min
4) n mole/mg protein/min
5) n mole/wet weight g/min
    * $P < 0.05$ ( )=n
   ** $P < 0.01$
  *** $P < 0.001$

Table 3. Perfusion experiment in isolated normal and pathological lung of rabbits.
(Conversion of AT I to AT II and inactivation of BK)

	Rate of conversion (%) of AT I to AT II	Inactivation rate (%) of BK	Perfusion pressure (cmH$_2$O)
Control Group	81.65±2.84 (n=4)	92.2 ±2.46 (n=5)	10.66±0.36 (n=24)
FA group[1] (Acute)	70.76±2.88* (n=6)	85.92±1.12* (n=5)	13.45±1.09** (n=18)
NMU Group[2] (Chronic)	83.4 ±3.52 (n=5)	94 ±2.02 (n=6)	5.92±0.58** (n=15)

(1) Treated with Complete Freund's Adjuvant
(2) Treated with N-Nitroso-N-methylurethan
  * $P < 0.05$
 ** $P < 0.001$

chronic pneumonitis. The results obtained in perfusion experiment were compatible to the results obtained in in vitro experiment using lung homogenate(Table 3).

DISCUSSION

ACE has been considered to have a dual action, namely conversion of AI to AII and inactivation of BK since Yang et al., 1971, suspected this character. We showed clearly this fact in this experiment directly using purified ACE from human lung. Highly purified enzyme which was single band in disc gel electrophoresis converted AI to AII and inactivated BK. The specific activity for BK was 15 folds higher than that for AI. The molecular weight of 290000 was consistent to the result of Lieberman, 1975, Silverstein et al., 1965 from human plasma, but not to the result of Nakajima et al., 1973 from human lung. This difference might be resulted from the difference of the purification method.

In experimental pneumonitis, the conditions were non-physiologic because we tried to produce the condition that the ACE activity was decreased in plasma and in the lung. In rabbit with acute pneumonitis, the activity of ACE was significantly decreased in lung homogenate and the result was compatible to the perfusion experiment in which the conversion of AI to AII and inactivation of BK was significantly decreased in the lung with acute pneumonitis. Several factors affecting the level of serum ACE were reported in experimental conditions, such as chronic hypoxia(Molteni et al., 1974) and serum Na level(Allen and Gilmore, 1975; Molteni et al., 1976). In addition to these factors, it appeared that the direct injury of pulmonary tissue caused a decrease of serum ACE level. In this condition of acute pneumonitis, the conversion of AI to AII would be reduced and less AII would be flooded out into systemic circulation than in normal condition,

and much BK might passed through the pulmonary circulation into
systemic circulation. It will be supposed that in patients with
some pulmonary disease, vasoactive peptides and their metabolites
might pass through the pulmonary circulation into systemic circulation, resulting by induction or modification of some pathological conditions.

REFERENCES

Allen, F.B. and J.P. Gilmore, 1975, Influence of altering total
    body sodium on angiotensin I systemic converting activity,
    Proc. Soc. Exp. Biol. Med. 148, 511.
Bakhle, Y.S., A.M. Reynard and J.R. Vane, 1969, Metabolism of the
    angiotensins in isolated perfused tissue, Nature 222, 956.
Cushman, D.W. and H.S. Cheung, 1971, Spectrophotometric assay and
    properties of the angiotensin-converting enzyme of rabbit
    lung, Biochem. Pharmacol. 20, 1637.
Lieberman, J., 1975, Elevation of serum angiotensin-converting
    enzyme(ACE) level in sarcoidosis, Am. J. Med. 59, 365.
Molteni, A., K.B. Mullis, R.M. Zakheim and L. Mottioli, 1976, The
    effect of change in dietary sodium on lung and serum angio-
    tensin converting enzyme in the rat, Lab. Invest. 35, 569.
Molteni, A., R.M. Zakheim, K.B. Mullis and L. Mottioli, 1974, The
    effect of chronic alveolar hypoxia on lung and serum angio-
    tensin converting enzyme activity, Proc. Soc. Exp. Biol. Med.
    147, 263.
Nakajima, T., G. Oshima, H.S.J. Yeh, R. Igic and E.G. Erdös, 1973,
    Purification of the angiotensin I-converting enzyme of the
    lung, Biochim. Biophys. Acta 315, 430.
Ng, K.K.F. and J.R. Vane, 1976, Conversion of angiotensin I to
    angiotensin II, Nature 216, 762.
Ng, K.K.F. and J.R. Vane, 1968, Fate of angiotensin I in the
    circulation, Nature 218, 144.
Nishimura, K., K. Hiwada, E. Ueda and T. Kokubu, 1976, Solubili-
    zation of angiotensin I converting enzyme from rabbit lung
    using trypsin treatment, Biochim. Biophys. Acta 452, 144.
Nishimura, K., N. Yoshida, K. Hiwada, E. Ueda and T. Kokubu, 1977,
    Purification of angiotensin I-converting enzyme from human
    lung, Biochim. Biophys. Acta 522, 229.
Oparil, S., G.W. Tregear, T. Koerner, B.A. Barnes and E. Haber,
    1971, Mechanism of pulmonary conversion of angiotensin I to
    angiotensin II in the dog, Circul. Res. 29, 682.
Ryan, J.W., J. Robles, J.M. Stewart and W.P. Leary, 1971, Metabo-
    lism of vasoactive polypeptides in the pulmonary circulation,
    Chest 59(suppl.), 8s.
Silverstein, E., J. Friedland, H.A. Lyons and M. Kitt, 1965, Serum
    angiotensin converting enzyme in sarcoidosis, Clin. Res. 23,
    352 A.
Ueda, E. T. Kokubu, H. Akutsu and T. Ito, 1972, Angiotensin I
    converting enzyme and kininase, Jap. Circul. J. 36, 583.

Yang, H.Y.T. and E.G. Erdӧs, 1967, Second kininase in human blood
    plasma, Nature 215, 1402.
Yang, H.Y.T., E.G. Erdӧs and Y. Levine, 1971, Characterization of
    dipeptidyl hydroxylase(Kininase II; angiotensin I converting
    enzyme), J. Pharmacol. Exp. Therap. 177, 292.

INHIBITION OF KININASE II (ANGIOTENSIN I CONVERTING ENZYME) BY HUMAN SERUM ALBUMIN AND ITS FRAGMENTS

Rainer J. Klauser, Carol J.G. Robinson and Ervin G. Erdös

Departments of Pharmacology and Internal Medicine

University of Texas Health Science Center @ Dallas, Texas

Commercial 5% plasma protein preparations, and human serum albumin and its fragments inhibit in vitro purified peptidyl dipeptidase of human lung or hog kidney. Fragment C of albumin (sequence 124-298) is a more potent inhibitor (K_i = 1.7 x 10^{-5}M) than albumin itself. Reduction and carboxymethylation of five of the six S-S bridges in fragment C increase the inhibitory potency (K_i = 3 x 10^{-6} M) but reduction of the sixth bridge raises the K_i. This suggests the importance of the secondary structure in fragment C for inhibition of the enzyme. Albumin and fragment C are not substrates of the enzyme. Fragment C and its derivative also inhibit the inactivation of bradykinin in vitro by the human enzyme as shown by bio-assay. Inhibition of peptidyl dipeptidase may contribute to the hypotension caused by infusion of plasma protein preparation, by potentiating the effects of bradykinin and blocking the release of angiotensin II.

Peptidyl dipeptidase (angiotensin I converting enzyme or kininase II, E.C. 3.4.15.1; CE) cleaves dipeptides from the C-terminal end of peptides such as angiotensin I, bradykinin (Yang et al., 1970, 1971) or enkephalins (Erdös et al., 1978). The enzyme is present in blood of man and animals (Skeggs et al., 1956; Yang and Erdös, 1967) probably only in partially active form because plasma contains one or more inhibitors of CE (Yang et al., 1971; Oshima et al., 1974).

Because of the obvious biological importance of CE we have studied its inhibition by plasma proteins. Here we report on the inhibition of human CE by human albumin and its fragments.

MATERIALS AND METHODS

Human serum albumin essentially fatty acid free was obtained
from Sigma Chemicals (St. Louis, Mo.). Five % plasma protein
preparations (Plasmatein, Protenate and Plasmanate) were obtained
from Abbott Laboratories, Hyland Laboratories and Cutter Laboratories
respectively. CE was prepared from swine kidney by the method of
Oshima et al. (1974). Human lung CE was prepared by gel filtration
on a Sephadex G-200 column followed by chromatography on DEAE-
Sephadex A-50 and hydroxyapatite columns (Klauser and Erdös, to
be published). Human endothelial cells were cultured according
to Johnson and Erdös (1977). Antibody to human lung CE and to
human albumin was elicited in the goat.

CE was assayed using tert-butyloxycarbonyl-Phe(NO_2)-Phe-Gly
(BPPG) or hippuryl-glycyl glycine (Hip-Gly-Gly) as substrate (Yang
et al., 1971). One unit of enzyme (U) cleaved 1 µmole of substrate
per min. When inhibitors were used they were preincubated for
10-15 min with the enzyme. The best lung CE preparation contained
8 U per mg and showed a single protein band in polyacrylamide gel
electrophoresis.

The inactivation of bradykinin by CE was followed by measuring
the decrease in activity on the isolated rat uterus (Yant et al.,
1971; Oshima et al., 1974).

Amino acid analysis was performed in a Durrum Amino Acid Analyzer after hydrolyzing the peptides at 110°C for 16 hr with
6 N HCl in sealed evacuated tubes. Values for residues of amino
acids per mol fragment were calculated by using amino acid determinations of McMenamy et al (1971) and amino acid sequence data
of Meloun et al. (1975) for comparison.

The concentration of protein in the solutions was determined
either by the method of Lowry et al. (1951) or by measuring the
absorption at 280 nm using fragment C as a standard.

Human serum albumin was cleaved to fragments A, B and C with
CNBr and the fragments were separated and purified by the sequential
use of gel filtration and column chromatography according to McMenamy
et al. (1971).

The reduction (and carboxymethylation) of the disulfide bridges
of the fragment was performed according to Crestfield et al. (1963)
with slight modifications. Mercaptoethanol was added to fragment
C under nitrogen 25-fold excess over the 12 possible SH-residues
of fragment C. Iodoacetic acid was then added dropwise at pH 8.7
(Method 1).

Alternatively the reduction was carried out in 8 M urea (Method 2) or with only a 4-fold excess of mercaptoethanol over the possible SH-groups (Method 3).

Immunodiffusion was carried out on Ouchterlony plates using antiserum to human albumin and to purified human lung CE.

RESULTS

Inhibition by Albumin

First we tested commercially prepared plasma protein preparations which contained over 83% albumin. Different preparations of three manufacturers inhibited purified CE of hog kidney. Thirty-five ul of the 5% protein solution inhibited the hydrolysis of BPPG by 50%.

Because commercial plasma protein preparations contain 4×10^{-3} M acetyltryptophan added as stabilizer, we tested this compound for inhibition of CE. The I_{50} with Hip-Gly-Gly substrate and with either human or hog CE was 5×10^{-4} M.

Since, during purification of human CE (Oshima et al., 1974; Nishimura et al., 1977), crude preparations exhibit low enzymic activity, we examined human lung CE preparations during the various stages of purification for the presence of albumin. CE of homogenized human lung extracted with detergent and purified with gel filtration on Sephadex G-200 column still contained albumin as shown by immunodiffusion. On immunodiffusion plates the preparation of CE formed a precipitin band with antibody to human lung CE but also with antibody to human serum albumin. Albumin, which has a molecular weight of 66,500 eluted in gel filtration on a Sephadex G-200 column with CE which has a much higher molecular weight; thus CE probably forms a complex with albumin.

After additional steps of purification on ion exchange columns CE did not react with antibody to human albumin indicating that albumin was removed from the preparation during purification (Stewart, to be published). CE, in the preparation, however, still formed a precipitin band with antibody to the human lung enzyme.

Commercially prepared plasma protein preparations contain over 83% albumin (FDA, 1977) thus we studied the inhibition of CE by purified, fat free albumin. We found that purified CE of human lung and hog kidney are equally inhibited by albumin. The I_{50} values with Hip-Gly-Gly substrate were 2×10^{-4} M and 1.9×10^{-4} M. The inhibition of human lung enzyme was non-competitive. The K_i determined in the Dixon plot was 3×10^{-4} M.

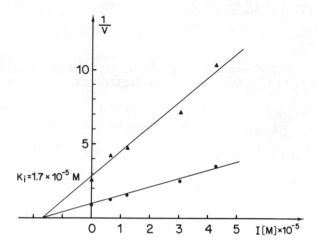

Fig. 1. Dixon plot of inhibition of human lung CE by fragment C.
▲————▲ 2 x 10^{-4} M Hip-Gly-Gly, ●————● 10^{-3} M Hip-Gly-Gly.
K_i = 1.7 x 10^{-5} M.

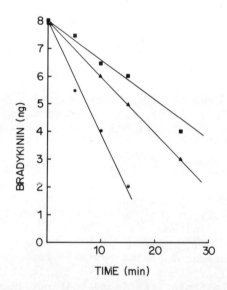

Fig. 2. Inhibition of the inactivation of bradykinin of human
lung CE by fragment C and by its reduced and carboxymethylated derivative (CMFC 3). Bio-assay on the isolated rat uterus, ●————●
inactivation of bradykinin, ▲————▲ inhibition by 7.5 x 10^{-5} M
fragment C, ■————■ inhibition by 4.5 x 10^{-5} M CMFC 3.

Inhibition by Fragments

Since the commercial plasma protein solutions inhibited CE relatively more than accounted for by albumin content, we investigated whether fragments of human albumin may be more potent inhibitors than the native protein. Human albumin was cleaved to three fragments at the methionine residues with CNBr and the fragments were separated by column chromatography (McMenamy et al., 1971; Meloun et al., 1975). Following their nomenclature we called fragment B the residues 1-123 of albumin, fragment C residues 124-298 and fragment A residues 299-585. All three fragments inhibited CE. The I_{50} values were 2.2×10^{-5}M, 7.4×10^{-5}M, 2.5×10^{-5}M for fragments A, B and C respectively.

The inhibition of CE by homogeneous fragment C and its derivatives was studied further. In order to establish the structural features of fragment C important for inhibition of CE, we reduced and carboxymethylated the disulfide bridges in fragment C formed by 12 cysteine residues (CM-cysteine) and denatured the peptide. Three different conditions were used for reduction. Method 1: mercaptoethanol was used in 25-fold excess over the theoretically available SH groups to obtain fragment CMFC 1. Method 2: mercaptoethanol was used in 25-fold excess with the addition of 8 M urea (CMFC 2). Method 3: mercaptoethanol was used in 4-fold excess (CMFC 3). Thus, with each method the conditions of denaturing fragment C differed. With methods 1 and 2 all disulfide bridges of fragment C were derivatized in CMFC 1 and CMFC 2. In addition, method 2 disrupted the secondary structure of the peptide. Method 3 left one of the 6 bridges intact in CMFC 3. Accordingly amino acid analysis of fragment C indicated 12.1 and 12.8 CM-cysteine residues obtained with methods 1 or 2 but only 9.6 with method 3, since 2 CM-cysteines are formed after reduction of each bridge. All three reduced fragments inhibited purified human CE non-competitively, but to a different degree. The calculated K_i values for non-competitive inhibition of CE by fragment C and CMFC 1, CMFC 2 and CMFC 3 are shown in Table I. Mild reduction which leaves one disulfide bridge intact (method 3) lowered the K_i of fragment C from 1.7×10^{-5}M to 3×10^{-6}M (Fig. 1). Carboxymethylation of all cysteine residues (method 1) decreased the inhibition, $K_i = 7.5 \times 10^{-6}$M. When fragment C was completely denatured by urea and by reducing all the disulfide bridges (method 2) the resulting fragment inhibited less than fragment C, $K_i = 8 \times 10^{-5}$M.

In separate experiments it was established that the inhibition by fragment C and CMFC 3 was not due to binding a metal cofactor and that neither albumin nor fragment C were substrates of the enzyme. Fragment C and CMFC 3 inhibited the inactivation of bradykinin by human lung CE as assayed on the isolated rat uterus (Fig. 2).

Fragment C also inhibited the inactivation of bradykinin by the enzyme on the surface of intact suspended cultured human endothelial cells. CMFC 3 was a better inhibitor of CE on the endothelial cells than fragment C was, because CMFC 3 inhibited 58% at 10^{-5}M concentration while fragment C (10^{-4}M) inhibited 49%.

Table I

Inhibition of Human Lung CE by Fragment C and its Derivatives

Inhibitor	CM-Cysteine (mol/mol)	K_i (M)
Fragment C	---	1.7×10^{-5}
CM Fragment C (Method 1; CMFC 1)	12.1	7.5×10^{-6}
CM Fragment C (Method 2; CMFC 2)	12.8	8×10^{-5}
CM Fragment C (Method 3; CMFC 3)	9.6	3×10^{-6}

DISCUSSION

Commercial plasma proteins are prepared by harsh methods which include alcohol precipitation and heating over ten hr at 60°C (Mulford et al., 1955; Hink et al., 1957). They contain over 83% albumin, plus acetyltryptophan and other additives. These protein preparations may have bradykinin (Izaka et al., 1974) and a pre-kallikrein activator, Hageman factor fragment, as contamination (Alving et al., 1978). Infusion of such proteins may cause severe hypotensive reactions in patients (Harrison et al., 1971; Bland et al., 1973; FDA, 1977; Alving et al., 1978). The reactions are particularly severe in patients with cardiopulmonary bypass.

In plasma, bradykinin is inactivated mainly by kininase I or carboxypeptidase N Kininase II, CE, which is identical with the angiotensin I converting enzyme (Yang et al., 1970; 1971; Igic et al., 1972) has low activity in plasma; it is a more active kininase on the surface of endothelial (Bakhle and Vane, 1974) and epithelial cells (Erdös, 1977).

Inhibition of CE prolongs the hypotensive effects of kinins and abolishes the vasoconstrictor effect of renin by blocking the release of angiotensin II (Erdös, 1977).

The low activity of CE in plasma may be due in part to its inhibition by albumin. Because the concentration of albumin is 5 to 8 x 10^{-4}M in plasma hypothetically it is sufficiently high enough to inhibit much of the activity of CE. Albumin may interfere with assaying of CE activity in plasma of in crude extracts. Although in gel filtration CE exhibits a molecular weight about three times as high as albumin, albumin was eluted in the peak containing CE, indicating binding. Albumin present in partially purified human CE preparations may account for the low CE activity of these preparations.

Our experiments have shown that albumin and its fragments inhibit CE noncompetitively, without being substrates of the enzyme. This inhibition may be enhanced by the presence of acetyltryptophan, an additive in commercial preparations. In general, fragments of albumin were more potent inhibitors than albumin itself. All three fragments obtained by cleaving human serum albumin with CNBr have lower K_i values than albumin. Fragment C which contains residues 124-298 of albumin is of particular interest because it has most of the ligand binding potency of albumin (Gambhir and McMenamy 1973).

Changes in the secondary and tertiary structure of fragment C can change its inhibitory action as shown by carboxymethylation and denaturation of this fragment. The K_i of CMFC 3, which has only 5 reduced and carboxymethylated bridges, is much lower than that of fragment C. In fragment CMFC 1 all the cysteine residues were derivatized (Method 1). Its K_i is half of that of fragment C. These experiments suggest that introduction of carboxyl groups increases the inhibition of CE by fragment C, especially when one intact disulfide bridge preserves the original conformation. When derivatization is carried out under denaturing conditions in urea, the fragments (CMFC 2) inhibits less than fragment C itself. Because the CM-cysteine content of fragments CMFC 1 and CMFC 2 is identical but CMFC 2 has a K_i ten times as high as CMFC 1, preservation of the secondary structure appears to affect the inhibition constant more than the incorporation of carboxyl groups.

In conclusion, inhibition of CE on vascular endothelial cells and in plasma by albumin and its fragments may enhance the hypotensive effects of kinins if they are present in, or liberated by, infused plasma protein preparations. Hypotension may be most marked when the lung is excluded from the circulation since the pulmonary vascular bed is very rich in CE (Bakhle and Vane, 1974). In addition the inhibition of CE can also block the release of angiotensin II from angiotensin I by the same enzyme.

ACKNOWLEDGEMENTS

We are grateful for the collaboration of Dr. C.M. Herman of the University of Washington, Seattle, Wash., and for the assistance of Katy Hammon and Tess Stewart of U.T.H.S.C.D. Endothelial cells were supplied by Dr. A.R. Johnson and fragment C by Drs. D.V. Marinkovic and J. Kato. Amino acid analysis was done by Dr. J. Capra and Miss P. Frank.

These studies were supported in part by the Department of the Navy N00014-75-C-0807 and by NIH USPHS HL 16320 and HL 14187. Dr. Rainer J. Klauser received a travel grant from Deutsche Forschungsgemeinschaft.

REFERENCES

Alving, B.M., Hojima, Y., Pisano, J.J., Mason, B.L., Buckingham, Jr., R.E.,Mozen, M.M., Finlayson, J.S.: Hypotension associated with prekallikrein activator (Hageman-factor fragments) in plasma protein fraction. New Eng. J. Med. 299: 66-70, 1978.

Bakhle, Y.S., Vane, J.R.: Pharmacokinetic function of the pulmonary circulation. Physiol. Rev. 54: 1007-1045, 1974.

Bland, J.H.L., Laver, M.B., Lowenstein, E.: Vasodilator effect of commercial 5% plasma protein fraction solutions. J. Amer. Med. Assoc. 224: 1721-1724, 1973.

Crestfield, A.M., Moore, S., Stein, W.H.: The preparation and enzymatic hydrolysis of reduced and S-carboxymethylated proteins. J. Biol. Chem. 238: 622-627, 1963.

Erdös, E.G., Johnson, A.R., Boyden, N.T.: Hydrolysis of enkephalin by cultured human endothelial cells and by purified peptidyl dipeptidase. Biochem. Pharm. 27: 843-848, 1978.

Erdös, E.G.: The angiotensin I converting enzyme. Fed. Proc. 36: 1760-1765, 1977.

F.D.A. Bulletin: Adverse reactions to plasma protein fraction. 7: 20-21, 1977.

Gambhir, K.K., McMenamy, R.H.: Location of the indole binding site in human serum albumin. Characterization of major cyanogen bromide fragments with respect to affinity labeling positions. J. Biol. Chem. 248: 1956-1960, 1973.

Harrison, G.A., Robinson, M., Stacey, R.V., McCulloch, C.H., Torda, T.A., Wright, J.S.: Hypotensive effects of stable plasma protein solution (SPPS): a preliminary communication. Med. J. Australia 2: 1040-1041, 1971.

Hink, Jr., J.H., Hidalgo, J., Seeberg, V.P., Johnson, F.F.: Preparation and properties of a heat-treated human plasma protein fraction. Vox Sanguinis 2: 174-186, 1957.

Igic, R., Erdös, E.G., Yeh, H.S.J., Sorrells, K., Nakajima, T.:
    Angiotensin I converting enzyme of the lung. Circul. Res. 31:
    II-51-II-61, 1972.

Izaka, K., Tsutsui, E., Mima, Y., Hasegawa, E.: A bradykinin-like
    substance in heat-treated human plasma protein solution.
    Transfusion 14: 242-248, 1974.

Johnson, A.R., Erdös, E.G.: Metabolism of vasoactive peptides by
    human endothelial cells in culture: angiotensin I converting
    enzyme (kininase II) and angiotensinase. J. Clin. Invest. 59:
    684-695, 1977.

Lowry, O.H., Rosenbrough, N.J., Farr, A.L., Randall, R.J.: Protein
    measurement with the Folin phenol reagent. J. Biol. Chem. 193:
    265-275, 1951.

McMenamy, R.H., Dintzis, H.M., Watson, F.: Cyanogen bromide fragments
    of human serum albumin. J. Clin. Invest. 246: 4744-4750, 1971.

Meloun, B., Moravek, L., Kostka, V.: Complete amino acid sequence
    of human serum albumin. FEBS 58: 134-137, 1975.

Mulford, D.J., Mealey, E.H., Welton, L.D.: Preparation of a stable
    human plasma protein solution. J. Clin. Invest. 34: 983-986,
    1955.

Nishimura, K., Yoshida, N., Hiwada, K., Ueda, E., Kokubu, T.:
    Purification of angiotensin I-converting enzyme from human lung.
    Biochim. Biophys. Acta. 483: 398-408, 1977.

Oshima, G., Gecse, A., Erdös, E.G.: Angiotensin I converting enzyme
    of the kidney cortex. Biochim. Biophys. Acta 350: 26-37, 1974.

Skeggs, L.T., Kahn, J.R., Shumway, N.P.: Preparation and function
    of the hypertensin-converting enzyme. J. Exp. Med. 103: 295-
    299, 1956.

Yang, H.Y.T., Erdös, E.G., Levin, Y.: A dipeptidyl carboxypeptidase
    that converts angiotensin I and inactivates bradykinin.
    Biochim. Biophys. Acta 214: 374, 1970.

Yang, H.Y.T., Erdös, E.G., Levin, Y.: Characterization of a dipeptide
    hydrolase (kininase II; angiotensin I converting enzyme). J.
    Pharmacol. Exper. Therap. 177: 291-300, 1971.

Yang, H.Y.T., Erdös, E.G.: Second kininase in human blood plasma.
    Nature 215: 1402-1403, 1967.

RENAL KALLIKREIN-KININ SYSTEM AND PROSTAGLANDIN IN HYPERTENSION:

THEIR RELATION TO RENIN-ANGIOTENSIN-ALDOSTERONE SYSTEM

Keishi Abe, Minoru Yasujima, Satoru Chiba, Makito Sato, Nobuo Irokawa, Yutaka Imai and Kaoru Yoshinaga

Department of Internal Medicine, Tohoku University School of Medicine, 1-1, Seiryocho, Sendai 980, Japan

ABSTRACT

The present study was done to investigate the interrelationships between renal kallikrein-kinin, renal prostaglandin E and renin-angiotensin-aldosterone systems in normal subjects and in essential hypertension by means of measuring urinary excretion of kallikrein and prostaglandin E, plasma renin activity and plasma aldosterone concentration before and after stimulation or inhibition of the renin-angiotensin-aldosterone system and inhibition of renal prostaglandin E generation. Urinary kallikrein excretion was increased after the stimulation of the renin-angiotensin-aldosterone system by low Na diet or the administration of furosemide and upright posture, while it decreased after the inhibition of the action of aldosterone by spironolactone. These data show that the change in urinary kallikrein excretion was related to that in the renin-angiotensin-aldosterone system following various stimuli, suggesting that renal kallikrein-kinin system may regulate blood pressure by opposing the action of the renin-angiotensin-aldosterone system. Urinary PGE excretion was decreased after sodium depletion and increased after the administration of furosemide in spite of the augmentation of the renin-angiotensin-aldosterone system. The change in urinary PGE excretion was closely related to that in urinary Na output after various stimuli, and a significant positive correlation was found between basal levels of urinary PGE and those of urinary Na, suggesting that renal prostaglandin E may be involved in the regulation of blood pressure by affecting renal sodium handling. The present data show that basal level of urinary excretion of PGE and kallikrein was lower in essential hypertension than in normal subjects and that the release of renal kallikrein and PGE after the furosemide administration was also suppressed in patients with essential hypertension compared with that in normal subjects, suggesting that there exists, in this disease, an impaired defense mechanism against the renin-angiotensin-aldosterone system resulting in sodium retention.

INTRODUCTION

It is now generally accepted that kidney has both pressor and depressor mechanisms and that hypertension occurs when the former is stimulated or the latter is suppressed. Kallikrein and prostaglandin (PG) E are vasodilating substances naturally generated in the kidney. Recently, Margolius and his coworkers (1974, 1975) have reported that renal generation of kallikrein is regulated by aldosterone or other sodium-retaining steroid hormones. Johnston and his coworkers (1976) also reported that there was a close relationship between plasma renin activity (PRA) and urinary kallikrein excretion in rats after the sodium loading or depletion. On the other hand, recent reports by McGiff and his coworkers (1970, 1975) have shown that there are close interrelationships between renal PGE and renin-angiotensin system or between renal PGE and renal kallikrein-kinin system in animal experiments. Thus, the possibility exists that renal PGE and kallikrein-kinin system may regulate blood pressure by opposing the action of renin-angiotensin-aldosterone system in human subjects.

To investigate this possibility, we examined interrelationships among renal kallikrein-kinin, renal PGE and the renin-angiotensin-aldosterone systems in normal volunteers and in patients with essential hypertension by means of measuring urinary excretion of kallikrein and PGE, PRA and plasma aldosterone concentration (PAC) before and after stimulation or inhibition of the renin-angiotensin-aldosterone system and inhibition of renal PGE generation.

MATERIALS AND METHODS

Subjects.

Eighty-four healthy subjects, 55 patients with essential hypertension and 10 patients with primary aldosteronism were included in this study. Normal subjects were 61 men and 23 women ranging in age from 18 to 66 years with an average of 40.0 ± 1.6 (SE). Essential hypertensives were 35 men and 20 women ranging in age from 15 to 63 years with an average of 37.1 ± 1.8. The diagnosis of essential hypertension had been made by history, physical examination, radioisotope renography, renoscintigraphy, angiography and determinations of 11-OHCS, aldosterone and urinary catecholamines or vanillyl mandelic acid. Patients with primary aldosteronism were 3 men and 7 women ranging in age from 30 to 47 years with an average of 35.0 ± 3.0. They had persistent hypokalemia, suppressed plasma renin activity and increased plasma aldosterone level, and 8 patients out of them were cured later by removal of adrenal adenoma. Hypertensive patients had blood pressures of 150 mmHg in systolic and 90 mmHg in diastolic or higher on repeated measurements. They were allowed to take unrestricted ad libitum Na diet, and antihypertensive medications had been discontinued at least for 2 weeks before the study. Sampling of blood was done in the patients, after overnight fasting, kept in recumbent position for 1 hr in the morning, and urine was collected for 24 hrs in a bottle kept in a refrigerator. Basal levels of PRA, PAC and urinary excretion of PGE and kallikrein were measured.

Method.

Measurement of urinary kallikrein. Urinary kallikrein activity was measured as kininogenase activity using radioimmunoassay of kinin, bioassay and TAME esterolytic activity. After urine was dialysed against tap-water, it was concentrated and measured by the esterolytic assay using TAME as a substrate or bioassay measuring the autoperfused dog femoral arterial blood flow. A significant correlation between urinary kallikrein determined by TAME esterolytic activity and bioassay in 24 subjects ($r = 0.91$, $p < 0.001$) was obtained. Kininogenase activity was measured as follows: an aliquot of urine (0.05~0.1 ml) was incubated with 4 µg of low molecular weight kininogen (supplied by Dr. Kato, Protein Research Institute, Osaka) dissolved in 0.4 ml of 0.1 M phosphate buffer pH 8.4 containing 0.1% neomycin, 3 mM 8-hydroxy-quinoline and 30 mM disodium ethylene diamine tetraacetic acid (EDTA) at 37°C for 20 min. After the incubation, the mixture was diluted with distilled water and heated at 80°C for 15 min to stop the enzymatic reaction and stored at -20°C until the measurement. The generated kinin during the incubation was determined radioimmunologically. In the present method, the extraction procedure was not necessary, because low molecular weight kininogen had no cross-reaction to the antiserum. The values of urinary kallikrein determined by the radioimmunoassay in 31 subjects showed a highly significant correlation with the values determined by the TAME esterolytic activity ($r = 0.78$, $p < 0.001$).

Measurement of prostaglandin. Urinary PGE was measured radioimmunologically by the method already described (Abe et al., 1977). A urine sample (5~10 ml) was lyophilized. After the residue had been dissolved in 1 ml of 0.05 M phosphate buffer, pH 7.4, urinary PGE was converted to PGB by alkaline treatment according to Zusman's method (Zusman, 1972). Then, the sample was acidified to pH 3 to 4 with hydrochloric acid and extracted with ethyl acetate. The organic phase was dried, and the residue was applied to a silicic acid column; PGB was eluted by a mixture of benzene-ethyl acetate (60:40) according to the method of Jaffe (Jaffe et al., 1973).

The PGB fraction was dried and measured radioimmunologically using PGB antiserum (CA501, Clinical Assay) which does not distinguish PGB_1 from PGB_2. The endogeneous PGB was also measured by the same procedure without alkaline treatment. The urinary PGE value was calculated by subtracting the PGB value before alkaline treatment from that after alkaline treatment. The ratio of the endogenous PGB to PGE was 8~25%. Prior conversion of PGE to PGB precluded dehydration of PGE to PGA during the extraction procedure. The overall recovery rate of added PGE (1 to 3 ng) was 54.8 ± 0.7% (mean ± SE, n=15). The estimated value was corrected for this loss.

Urinary $PGF_2\alpha$ was measured radioimmunologically. Urine, 3~5 ml, was acidified to pH 3 to 4 with hydrochloric acid and extracted with ethyl acetate. The organic phase was dried, and the residue was applied to a silicic acid column, and $PGF_2\alpha$ was eluted by a mixture of benzene-ethyl acetate methanol (60:40:20). The $PGF_2\alpha$ fraction was dried and measured radioimmunologically using $PGF_2\alpha$ antiserum.

Main urinary metabolite of prostaglandin $F_2\alpha$, $F\alpha$, 7α-dihydroxy-11-keto tetranor prostan-1, 16-dioic acid was measured by Ohki's method (Ohki et al., 1974). Diluted urine was directly measured radioimmunologically using $PGF_2\alpha$-MUM antiserum.

Measurement of plasma renin activity and aldosterone concentration. PRA was determined by means of radioimmunoassay of angiotensin I. Plasma, 1.0 ml was adjusted to pH 5.5 and incubated at 37°C for 6 hours with EDTA and diisopropyl fluorophosphate. After the incubation, the sample was diluted 10-fold with physiological saline and heated in a boiling water bath for 5 minutes. After centrifugation, angiotensin I in the supernatant extract was assayed radioimmunologically. PRA was expressed in terms of nanograms of generated angiotensin I per milliliter of plasma per hour of incubation. This method was approximately 4 times more sensitive than Haber's method (Haber et al., 1969).

Aldosterone concentration in plasma and urine was measured with a commercial radioimmunoassay kit (Cer Ire Sorin). This method was sensitive to 10 pg of aldosterone.

Urinary Na and K were measured using an autoanalyzer. All results were expressed as mean ± SEM. The significance of differences between mean values were evaluated by student's t-test. The level of significance was taken as 0.05.

RESULTS

Urinary excretion of kallikrein and prostaglandin E. Basal levels of urinary excretion of kallikrein and PGE in 84 normal

subjects, in 55 patients with essential hypertension and in 10
patients with primary aldosteronism were shown in Figure 1 and 2.
The estimated values of urinary kallikrein output were 34.5 ± 4.0
μg/day in normal subjects, 18.3 ± 2.8 μg/day in essential hypertension and 80.8 ± 10.0 in primary aldosteronism. The excretion
rate was significantly lower in essential hypertension (p < 0.05)
than in control subjects, whereas it was higher in primary aldosteronism (p < 0.05). Urinary PGE excretion was 737 ± 32 ng/day
in normal subjects, 394 ± 29 ng/day in essential hypertension and
369 ± 44 ng/day in primary aldosteronism. A significant decrease
in urinary PGE output was found in essential hypertension (p <
0.001) and in primary aldosteronism (p < 0.001) compared with that
in control subjects.

Interrelationships between urinary kallikrein, urinary PGE
and renin-angiotensin-aldosterone system.
Ad libitum diet. Among basal levels of PRA, PAC, urinary
kallikrein and urinary PGE, there was a significant correlation
between PAC and urinary kallikrein in essential hypertension.
However, there were no significant correlations between urinary
excretion of PGE and PRA or PAC, and between urinary excretion of
kallikrein and that of PGE or PRA in normal subjects and in patients
with essential hypertension. There were significant correlations
between urinary excretion of PGE and that of Na (normal r=0.39,
hypertension r = 0.62) or urine flow (normal r = 0.30, hypertension
r = 0.38) in normal subjects and in patients with essential hypertension.

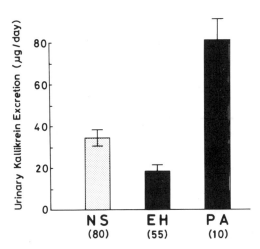

Figure 1. Urinary kallikrein excretion in normal subjects (NS),
           patients with essential hypertension (EH) and patients
           with primary aldosteronism (PA).

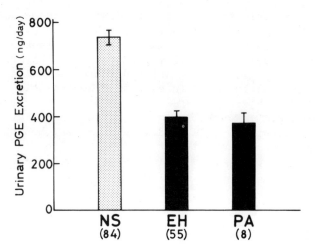

Figure 2.   Urinary prostaglandin E excretion in normal subjects
            (NS), patients with essential hypertension (EH) and
            patients with primary aldosteronism (PA).

Influence of low Na diet. Ten patients received first a diet
containing 200 mEq of Na daily for a week and then 100 mEq of Na
and finally 30 mEq of Na each for 3 days, and the 24 hours' urine
was collected in the last day of each period, and the blood sampling was done in the next morning. As shown in Table 1, PRA, PAC
and urinary kallikrein excretion increased after dietary sodium
depletion. On the contrary, urinary Na and PGE excretion decreased. The changes in urinary kallikrein excretion were closely
related to those of renin-angiotensin-aldosterone system after
sodium depletion, whereas a dissociation   occured between
urinary PGE excretion and renin-angiotensin-aldosterone system
or urinary kallikrein excretion.

Effect of furosemide. Sixteen normal subjects were allowed
to take unrestricted ad libitum Na diet. After they, fasted overnight, were kept supine position for 1 hour, sampling of blood and
urine during control period was done. Then, furosemide (1 mg/kg)
was injected intravenously, and the subjects were asked to assume
an upright posture for 120 minutes. At 30 (F30) and 120 (F120)
minutes after furosemide administration, blood and urine samples
were taken. As shown in Figure 3, PRA and PAC were continuously
increased up to 120 minutes after the administration of furosemide,
and maximum values were found at F120. On the other hand, urinary
excretion of kallikrein, PGE and $PGF_2\alpha$ rapidly increased during
the first 30 minutes after the furosemide injection. Subsequently
it decreased and returned to the control level at 120 minutes.

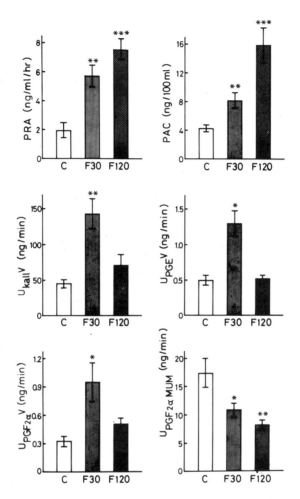

Figure 3. Mean changes in plasma renin activity (PRA), plasma
aldosterone concentration (PAC), and urinary excretion
of kallikrein ($U_{Kall}V$), prostaglandin E ($U_{PGE}V$), prostaglandin $F_2\alpha$ ($U_{PGF_2\alpha}$) and prostaglandin $F_2\alpha$ main
urinary metabolite ($U_{PGF_2\alpha}$ MUM) in 19 normal subjects
(mean ± SEM). c=control period, F30=30 minutes after
the furosemide injection, and F120=120 minutes after
the furosemide injection. *Values significantly different from control values ($p < 0.05$), ** $P < 0.01$,
*** $p < 0.005$.

Table 1.
Changes in plasma renin activity, urinary excretion of
aldosterone ($U_{Ald}V$), prostaglandin E ($U_{PGE}V$) and kallikrein ($U_{Kall}V$) after the sodium depletion in 10 patients
with essential hypertension. (mean ± SEM).

	200 mEq/day	100 mEq/day	30 mEq/day
PRA (ng/ml/hr)	4.0 ± 0.9	--	9.4 ± 1.4**
$U_{Ald}V$ (μg/day)	2.1 ± 0.4	3.4 ± 0.6	5.8 ± 1.2*
$U_{PGE}V$ (ng/day)	529 ± 26	451 ± 40	305 ± 33***
$U_{Kall}V$ (EU/day)	3.1 ± 0.4	3.2 ± 0.4	4.8 ± 0.6*

* p <0.05, ** p <0.01, *** p <0.001; Values significantly different
from the values on 200 mEq/day Na intake.

On the contrary, urinary excretion of $PGE_2\alpha$-metabolite decreased
continuously after the furosemide administration. There were
significant correlations between urinary excretion of PGE and that
of kallikrein (r=0.65) or $PGF_2\alpha$ (r=0.56). However, no significant
correlation was found between urinary excretion of PGE and PRA or
PAC, between urinary excretion of kallikrein and PRA or PAC, and
between urinary excretion of $PGF_2\alpha$ and PRA or PAC after the admi-

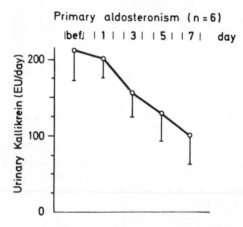

Figure 4.   Effect of spironolactone on urinary excretion of kallikrein in 6 patients with primary aldosteronism. bef. =
before spironolactone administration.

nistration of furosemide. There were significant correlations
between urinary excretion of Na and that of PGE (r=0.71) or kallikrein (r=0.61), and urine flow and urinary excretion of PGE (r=0.72)
or kallikrein (r=0.62).

    Effect of spironolactone.   Six patients with primary aldo-
steronism and 3 patients with essential hypertension were given
spironolactone (100 mg/day) for a week, and the sampling of urine
was done before and during the spironolactone administration. In
patients with primary aldosteronism, urinary kallikrein excretion
continuously decreased (Figure 4). The changes in urinary excretion of PGE and kallikrein was studied after the spironolactone
administration in 3 patients with essential hypertension. Urinary
excretion of kallikrein gradually decreased while urinary excretion
of PGE and Na increased on the first day of the spironolactone
administration and then, decreased gradually to control level.

    Effect of indomethacin. Two patients with renovascular
hypertension and 11 patients with essential hypertension receiving
unrestricted ad libitum Na diet were given a diet 90 mEq/day of
Na with the oral administration of furosemide (80 mg/day) for 3
days, and then, the oral administration of indomethacin (150 mg/day)
was added for additional 3 days. Sampling of blood and urine was

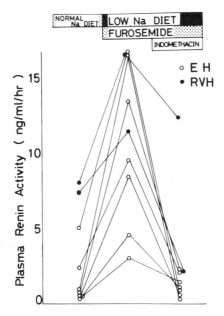

Figure 5.   Effect of indomethacin on plasma renin activity (PRA)
            in 11 patients with essential hypertension and 2
            patients with renovascular hypertension.

done before and during the indomethacin administration. As shown
in Figure 5, PRA was markedly increased after the administration
of furosemide with low Na diet in all subjects.

However, PRA was completely decreased after the addition of indomethacin in all subjects except one with renovascular hypertension.
The changes of PAC were similar to those of PRA (Figure 6).
Urinary excretion of PGE was also significantly decreased, and
that of kallikrein and Na tended to decrease, respectively,
following the indomethacin administration, while blood pressure
tended to elevate.

Release of renal kallikrein and PGE in essential hypertension.

An intravenous administration of furosemide (1 mg/kg) following
2 hours upright posture was loaded in 19 normal subjects and in 16
patients with essential hypertension, and then the release of renal
kallikrein and PGE in essential hypertension was compared with that
in normal subjects. The increments of PRA and PAC were similar
in normal subjects and in patients with essential hypertension.
However, the increments of urinary kallikrein and PGE excretions
after furosemide administration were greater in normal subjects
than in patients with essential hypertension (Figure 7).

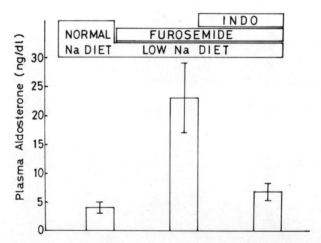

Figure 6.   Effect of indomethacin on plasma aldosterone concen-
            tration (PAC) in 11 patients with essential hypertension
            and 2 patients with renovascular hypertension.
            INDO=Indomethacin.

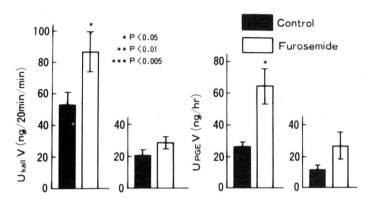

Figure 7.   Effect of furosemide and upright posture on urinary
            excretion of kallikrein ($U_{Kall}V$) and prostaglandin E
            ($U_{PGE}V$) in 19 normal subjects (left panel) and 16
            patients with essential hypertension (right panel).

DISCUSSION

     In 1975, Margolius and his coworker have reported that the
release of kallikrein in the rat renal cortical cell suspension
is increased by aldosterone and reduced by spironolactone and
proposed a hypothesis that the biosynthesis of renal kallikrein
is regulated by aldosterone or other sodium retaining steroid
hormones. In the present experiment, urinary kallikrein excretion
increased after the stimulation of the renin-angiotensin-aldosterone system by low Na diet or the administration of furosemide
and upright posture and decreased after the administration of
spironolactone in primary aldosteronism and in essential hypertension. These results support their hypothesis.

     In 1970, McGiff and coworkers reported that intrarenal arterial
infusion of angiotensin II induces a marked release of PGE in
renal venous effluent in the dog. Frolich (1975) also reported
that urinary PGE_2 excretion was increased in the urine obtained
from an ipsilateral ureter after the intrarenal arterial infusion
of angiotensin II in the dog. In our experiment, however, urinary
PGE excretion was decreased after sodium depletion in spite of an
augmentation of the renin-angiotensin system. There was no correlation between urinary PGE excretion and PRA or PAC under normal
sodium intake. The urinary excretion of PGE was closely related
to urinary Na output after low Na diet and after the administration

of furosemide or spironolactone. A significant positive correlation was also found between basal levels of urinary PGE and
those of urinary Na in normal volunteers and in patients with
essential hypertension. On the other hand, urinary PGE excretion
was concimitantly increased with PRA after the administration of
furosemide and upright posture. However, the time course of PRA
alteration following furosemide administration and upright posture
was different from that of urinary PGE excretion. In addition,
urinary excretion of $PGF_2\alpha$-metabolite was decreased after the
furosemide administration in spite of an increase in urinary PGE
and $PGF_2\alpha$ excretion. The augmentation of urinary PGE excretion
following furosemide administration was independent of the
enhanced renin-angiotensin system, but might be due to the inhibition of 15-hydroxy-PG dehydrogenase induced by furosemide itself.
Thus, the present data that urinary excretion of PGE was decreased
after dietary Na depletion whereas PRA increased indicate that
urinary PGE excretion may not be regulated by renin-angiotensin
system but may depend on urinary Na excretion in human subjects.

A number of recent papers (Zusman and Keiser, 1977; Berl et
al., 1977) have described that antidiuretic hormone stimulates
renal PGE release whereas there may exist a feedback mechanism
between PGE in the renal tubular compartment and antidiuretic
hormone and that renal PGE may also participate in the renal water
regulation. Indeed, a significant correlation was also found between urinary PGE excretion and urine flow in our data. Our
results concerning relationships between urinary excretion of PGE
and sodium or water suggest that renal PGE may be involved in the
regulation of blood pressure by the mechanism of renal sodium and
water handling.

There are several studies showing that renal prostaglandin
system participates in the release of renin. Weber and coworkers
(Larsson et al., 1974; Weber et al., 1976) have reported that renin
release can be stimulated by the PG precursor, arachidonic acid,
or PG endoperoxides in rabbits and rats. Recently, Gerber and
coworkers (1978) have reported that PGI_2 and PGE_2 can also stimulate
the renin release in dog kidney and that the former is more potent
than the latter. On the other hand, a number of observations
indicate that PG synthetase inhibitor, indomethacin, inhibits the
increase of renin secretion following furosemide injection or
other simuli (Patak et al., 1975; Romero et al., 1976; Frolich et
al., 1976). In the present experiment, an augmented PRA induced
by the furosemide administration with low Na diet was suppressed
by the addition of indomethacin and this result supports the intrarenal mechanism of PG besides PGE_2, possibly PGI_2, mediated renin
release, since urinary excretion of PGE was decreased after
dietary Na depletion whereas PRA increased.

McGiff and coworkers (1975) have reported that there is coupling between the kallikrein-kinin system and PGE within the kidney. In the present experiment, urinary excretion of PGE and kallikrein was increased after the administration of furosemide, and decreased after the administration of indomethacin. However a dissociation between urinary kallikrein and PGE was found after dietary Na depletion. A reversed alteration   also occured after this stimulus between urinary Na excretion and the renin-angiotensin-aldosterone system. There was positive correlation between urinary PGE excretion and urinary Na excretion or between urinary kallikrein excretion and PRA or PAC. Thus, it is possible that urinary PGE excretion depends on urinary Na excretion rather than kallikrein and that urinary kallikrein excretion depends on the renin-angiotensin-aldosterone system rather than PGE. This could be the explanation for the dissociation between urinary excretion of kallikrein and PGE in our experiment.

In 1934, Elliot and Nuzum found that the excretion of urinary kallikrein was decreased in patients with essential hypertension. In 1971 a similar result was reported by Margolius and coworkers. The present data that the decreased urinary output of kallikrein and PGE was found in essential hypertension indicate that the biosynthesis of the release of these vasodilator substances in the kidney is impaired in this disease. In addition, the data that the increase in urinary excretion of kallikrein and PGE after the furosemide administration and upright posture was less in essential hypertension than in normal volunteers in spite of the similar degree of augmentation in the renin-angiotensin-aldosterone system in both groups, support that the responses of renal kallikrein and PGE to any stimuli are also suppressed in essential hypertension when compared with that in normal volunteers.

The recent paper regarding oral active angiotensin I converting enzyme inhibitor, SQ 14225 indicate that the major antihypertensive effect of this drug is dependent on the inhibition of renin-angiotensin-aldosterone system (Laffan et al., 1978). However, a previous paper by Romero and Strong (1977) was revealed that renin-angiotensin-aldosterone system   also inhibited by the administration of indomethacin in experimental hypertensive rabbits, whereas hypertension advanced progressively in the animal with the impaired renal function. In the present experiment, blood pressure elevated slightly after the administration of indomethacin whereas the renin-angiotensin-aldosterone system was inhibited. Why does not the blood pressure reduce in spite of the suppression of renin-angiotensin-aldosterone system after the administration of indomethacin? This is a big puzzle in which a key may be held by the depressor system. Thus, our data indicate that the suppression of renal PGE and renal kallikrein-kinin system in essential hypertension may be the impairment of defense mechanism against the renin-angiotensin-aldosterone system and sodium retention and may participate in the pathogenesis of the hypertension in this disease.

ACKNOWLEDGMENTS

We thank Dr. O.A. Carretero of Henry Ford Hospital, Detroit for the supply of kallidin antiserum and Dr. C.I.Johnston of Manash University, Melbourne for the supply of bradykinin antiserum.

REFERENCES

Abe, K., M. Yasujima, S. Chiba, N. Irokawa, T. Itoh, K. Yoshinaga and T. Saito, 1977. Effects of furosemide on urinary excretion of prostaglandin E in normal volunteers and patients with essential hypertension, Prostaglandins 14, 513.

Berl, T., A. Raz, H. Wald, J. Horowitz and W. Czaczkes, 1977. Prostaglandin synthesis inhibition and the action of vasopressin: Studies in man and rat. Am. J. Physiol. 232, F529.

Elliot, A.H. and F.R. Nuzum, 1934. Urinary excretion of a depressor substance (kallikrein of Frey and Kraut) in arterial hypertension. Endocrinology 18, 462.

Frolich, J.C., T.W. Wilson and B.J. Sweetman, 1975. Urinary prostaglandin: Identification and origin. J. Clin. Invest. 55, 763.

Frolich, J.C., J.W. Hollifield, J.C. Dormois, B.L. Frolich, H. Seyberth, A.M. Michelakis and J.A. Oates, 1976. Suppression of plasma renin activity by indomethacin in man. Circ. Res. 39, 447.

Gerber, J.G., R.A. Branch, A.S. Nies, J.F. Gerkens, D.G. Shand, J. Hollifield and J.A. Oates, 1978. Prostaglandins and renin release: II. Assessment of renin secretion following infusion of PGI_2, E_2 and D_2 into the renal artery of anesthetized dogs. Prostaglandin. 51, 81.

Haber, E., T. Koerner, L.B. Page and A. Purnode, 1969. Application of a radioimmunoassay for angiotensin I to the physiologic measurement of plasma renin activity in normal human subjects. J. Clin. Endocrinol. Metab. 29, 1349.

Jaffe, B.M., H.R. Behman and L.W. Parker, 1973. Radioimmunoassay measurement of prostaglandin E, A and F in human plasma. J. Clin. Invest. 52, 398.

Johnston, C.I., P.G. Matthews and E. Dax, 1976. Renin-angiotensin and kallikrein-kinin system in sodium homeostasis and hypertension in rats. Clin. Sci. Mol. Med. 51, 283s.

Kaizu, T. and H.S. Margolius, 1975. Studies on rat renal cortical cell kallikrein I. Separation and measurement. Biochim. Biophys. Acta. 411, 305.

Laffan, R.J., M.E. Goldberg, J.P. High, T.R. Schaeffer, M.H. Waugh and B. Rubin, 1978. Antihypertensive activity in rats of SQ 14,225, and orally active inhibitor of angiotensin I -

converting enzyme. J. Pharmacol. Exp. Ther. 204, 281.

Larsson, C., P.C. Weber and E. Anggard, 1974. Arachidonic acid increases and indomethacin decreases plasma renin activity in the rabbit. Eur. J. Pharmacol. 28, 291.

Margolius, H.S., R.G. Geller, J.J. Pisano and A. Sjoerdsma, 1971. Altered urinary kallikrein excretion in human hypertension. Lancet II, 1063.

Margolius, H.S., D. Horwitz, R.G. Geller, R.W. Alexander, J.R. Gill Jr., J.J. Pisano and H.R. Keiser, 1974. Urinary kallikrein excretion in normal man: Relationships to sodium intake and sodium-retaining steroids. Circ. Res. 35, 812.

McGiff, J.C., K. Crowshaw, N.A. Terragno and A.J. Lonigro, 1970. Release of a prostaglandin-like substance into renal venous blood in response to angiotensin II. Circ. Res. 26(suppl I), I-121.

McGiff, J.C., H.D. Itskovitz and N.A. Terragno, 1975. The actions of bradykinin and eledoisin in the canine isolated kidney: relationship to prostaglandin. Clin. Sci. Mol. Med. 49, 125.

Ohki, S., T. Hanyu and K. Imaki 1974. Radioimmunoassays of prostaglandin $F_2\alpha$-main urinary metabolite with prostaglandin ^{125}I-tyrosine methyl ester amide. Prostaglandins. 6, 137.

Patak, R.V., B.K. Mookerjee, C.J. Bentzel, P.E. Hysert, M. Baber and J.B. Lee, 1975. Antagonism of the effects of furosemide by indomethacin in normal and hypertensive man. Prostaglandins 10, 649.

Romero, J.C., C.L. Dunlap and C.G. Strong, 1976. The effect of indomethacin and other anti-inflammatory drugs on the renin-angiotensin system. J. Clin. Invest. 58, 282.

Romero, J.C. and C.G. Strong, 1977. The effect of indomethacin blockade of prostaglandin synthesis on blood pressure of normal rabbits with renovascular hypertension. Cir. Res. 40, 35.

Weber, P.C., C. Larsson, M. Hamberg, E. Anggard, E.J. Corey and B. Samuelsson, 1976. Effects of stimulation and inhibition of the renal prostaglandin synthetase system on renin release in vivo and in vitro. Clin. Sci. Mol. Med. 51, 271s.

Zusman, R.M., 1972. Quantitative conversion of PGA or PGE to PGB. Prostaglandins. 1, 167.

Zusman, R.M. and H.R. Keiser, 1977. Prostaglandin biosynthesis by rabbit renomedullary interstitial cells in tissue culture: Stimulation by angiotensin II, bradykinin, and arginine vasopressin. J. Clin. Invest. 60, 215.

RELATIONSHIP OF HUMAN URINARY AND PLASMA KININS TO SODIUM-RETAINING STEROIDS AND PLASMA RENIN ACTIVITY

J.M. Vinci, R.M. Zusman, J.L. Izzo, Jr., R.E. Bowden,
D. Horwitz, J.J. Pisano, and H.R. Keiser

Hypertension-Endocrine Branch, Section on Experimental
Therapeutics, National Heart, Lung, and Blood Institute,
National Institutes of Health, Bethesda, Maryland 20014

INTRODUCTION

We have shown previously that urinary kallikrein excretion is regulated by the level of sodium-retaining steroid (Margolius, H.S., et. al., 1974a and Margolius, H.S., et. al. 1974b) and by the level of renal blood flow ((Keiser, H.R., et. al., 1976). Recently in our laboratory we have developed a radio-immunoassay for the kinin peptides, bradykinin, and lysyl-bradykinin in both blood and urine. We therefore studied normal volunteers and patients with Bartter's Syndrome to determine what physiologic factors would affect blood and urinary kinin levels.

METHODS

Thirty-six normal Caucasian women, aged 19 to 59 years and 7 women with Bartter's Syndrome aged 9 to 46 years were studied while hospitalized at the Clinical Center, NIH. The normal subjects were studied according to one or more of 4 protocols: a) diets with variable sodium and constant potassium (100 mEq/day), b) diets with variable potassium and constant sodium (109 mEq/day), c) administration of fludrocortisone, and d) administration of ACTH (corticotropin). The patients with Bartter's syndrome were studied before, during, and after administration of either indomethacin or ibuprofen. These patients were reported previously in greater detail (Vinci, et. al., 1978).

Venous blood was obtained for the determination of plasma renin activity, aldosterone concentration, bradykinin, and prekallikrein when the patient had been recumbent overnight and again when the patient had been upright for 3 hours. Urine was collected daily in 24-hour periods with each voiding split by a funnel equally into 2 containers (one with 20 ml. 6N HCl and 200 µg pepstatin and the other without preservative) (Vinci, J.M., et. al. 1978). Aliquots were taken for measurement of $[Na^+]$, $[K^+]$, aldosterone, kallikrein, and kinins. Plasma renin activity and aldosterone in plasma and urine were radioimmunoassayed by Hazelton Laboratories, Inc., Vienna, Va., under a special contract. Urinary kallikrein was determined by the radiochemical esterolytic method with TAMe (N^α-tosyl-L-arginine-^{3}H-methyl ester) as substrate (Vinci, J.M., et. al., 1978). Values are expressed in TAMe esterase units (TU) excreted per 24 hours. Whole blood and urine were collected and processed as previously reported (Vinci, J.M., et. al., 1978). Both urinary kinin (bradykinin and lysyl-bradykinin) and plasma bradykinin were determined by the same radioimmunoassay recently reported (Vinci, J.M., et. al., 1978). Values for urinary kinins are expressed as ng/24 hr. and those for plasma bradykinin (corrected for recovery of 45 nCi bradykinin triacetate [2-prolyl-3,4-^{3}H(N)], specific activity, 50 Ci/mmole) as ng/ml.

Values are reported as mean ± SEM unless stated otherwise. The student's t-test was used to determine statistical significance and p = 0.05 was considered the upper level of significance. Regression lines, which are depicted graphically, and correlation coefficients that relate any two variables under more than one condition are derived from the regression line and correlation coefficients between these two variables for each patient. The mean slope, intercept and correlation coefficient, where N is the number of patients, is then computed (Rao, C.R., 1965).

TABLE I

Dietary Na K mEq/d		N	UNaV mEq/d	UKV mEq/d	AER µg/d	UKaV TU/d	UKiV µg/d
9	100	17	1±0.5**	93±4	56.3±5.5**	18.4±1.4**	12.5±1.3
109	100	29	94±3	98±3	12.4±1.1	8.7±0.7	13.4±0.9
259	100	8	241±7**	101±6	4.8±1.1**	7.4±1.0	14.7±2.1

**Differs from 109 mEq/d Na with p<.005. N is number of subjects. Urinary sodium (UNaV), potassium (UKV), kallikrein (UKaV), kinin (UKiV) excretion and aldosterone excretion rate (AER) were measured when subjects consumed 9, 109, and 259 mEq/d sodium and 100 mEq/d potassium. Excretion values are means ± SEM of the average value for each subject on the last 2 or 3 days of each diet.

TABLE II

Dietary Na K mEq/d	PRAR ng/ml/hr	PRAU ng/ml/hr	PACR ng/100ml	PACU ng/100ml	PBKR ng/ml	PBKU ng/ml
9 100	3.8±0.5*	8.8±1.0**	39.9±6.0**	165±14.3**	5.4±0.7**	8.3±0.7**
109 100	2.1±0.4	5.2±0.5	5.5±0.5	44.4±3.1	3.3±0.3	4.5±0.5
259 100	0.6±0.1*	2.9±0.4*	4.0±0.5	13.3±3.8**	2.9±0.3	4.0±0.6

Differs from 109 mEq/d Na with $p < .05$*, .005**. See legend Table I. Plasma renin activity (PRA), plasma aldosterone concentration (PAC) and plasma bradykinin (PBK) were measured on the last day of each diet when subjects were recumbent (R) and in the upright position (U).

RESULTS

Effects of Sodium Intake

When normal subjects were fed diets with 9, 109 or 259 mEq/d sodium and constant potassium (100 mEq/d) excretion of sodium and aldosterone changed as expected and urinary kallikrein was significantly higher in subjects fed 9 mEq/d sodium (Table I). However, regardless of the level of excretion of sodium, aldosterone, or kallikrein the excretion of kinins was unchanged. Mean plasma bradykinin (subjects recumbent) of subjects fed 9 mEq/d sodium was significantly higher than that of subjects fed either 109 or 259 mEq/d sodium (Table II). Mean plasma bradykinin was increased after the subjects had been upright for 3 hours. Intersubject correlations between basal levels of plasma renin activity and bradykinin were significant in the 17 sodium-deplete recumbent subjects as well as in the 29 sodium-replete recumbent and upright subjects. There was poor correlation between levels of plasma aldosterone and plasma bradykinin. Intrasubject correlations between plasma bradykinin and plasma renin activity were also significant [mean correlation coefficient $(\bar{r}) \pm$ SEM was $0.88 \pm .07$, $p < 0.001$] in each of eleven subjects who were fed both diets with 109 and 9 mEq/d sodium (Fig. 1).

Effects of Potassium Intake

Five subjects were fed 185 mEq/d and then 25 mEq/d potassium for 7 days respectively (Fig. 2). Sodium was constant at 109 mEq/d. By the third day of low potassium diet urinary potassium equalled

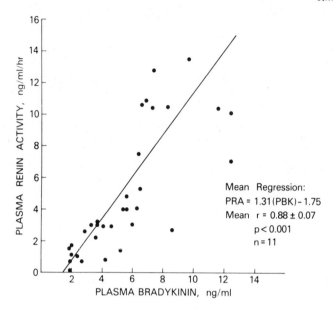

Figure 1. Highly significant correlation between plasma renin
activity and plasma bradykinin concentration for eleven
subjects fed diets containing either 9 (recumbent and
upright) or 109 mEq/d (recumbent) sodium and 100 mEq/d
potassium. These are the only subjects who received
both diets.

dietary intake and aldosterone excretion had decreased by 78%.
Both values remained unchanged for the rest of the study. Urinary
kallikrein excretion decreased in a stepwise fashion during low
potassium intake but kinin excretion was unchanged. Urinary kallikrein was highly correlated with aldosterone excretion ($\bar{r}$ = 0.57 ±
.11, p <.01) and plasma renin activity in recumbent ($\bar{r}$ = .85 ± .06,
p <.001) and upright subjects ($\bar{R}$ = .80 ± .08, p <.001). There were
no significant correlations between urinary kallikrein and kinin
excretion, or between urinary kinin and aldosterone excretion.

Effects of Fludrocortisone

During fludrocortisone administration (0.5 mg/d x 6 days, diet
109 mEq/d sodium, 100 mEq/d potassium) kallikrein excretion increased
in a stepwise fashion yet kinin excretion was unchanged (Fig. 3).
Plasma renin activity (subjects recumbent or upright) decreased
significantly and progressively and plasma bradykinin also decreased
20% (N.S.) when subjects were recumbent and 38% (p<0.02) when subjects were upright. When fludrocortisone administration ceased
urinary kallikrein decreased but urinary kinin excretion, remained
unchanged.

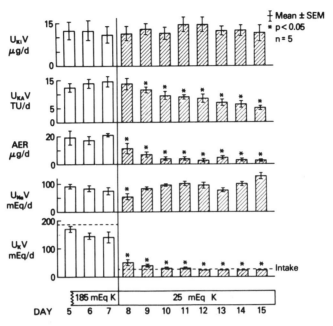

Figure 2.   Effect of dietary potassium intake on (mean ± SEM)
            urinary potassium (UKV), sodium (UNaV), kallikrein (UKaV),
            and kinin (UKiV) excretion and aldosterone excretion rate
            (AER) in five subjects who were fed diets with 185 mEq/d
            potassium and 109 mEq/d sodium for 7 days and 25 mEq/d
            potassium and 109 mEq/d sodium for the next 8 days.
            * is p<0.05.

Effects of ACTH

Eleven subjects were given ACTH (Corticotropin 80 units/d
intravenous infusion) for 48 hours (9 mEq/d sodium and 100 mEq/d
potassium diet (Fig. 4). Excretion of sodium decreased while
excretion of aldosterone and kallikrein increased but kinin
excretion was unchanged. On the second day of ACTH, plasma renin
activity increased significantly (subject recumbent or upright)
but plasma bradykinin was not changed.

There was a highly significant correlation between urinary
kallikrein and aldosterone excretion for the eleven subjects who
participated in at least 3 studies (Fig. 5). There were no correlations between kinin excretion and urinary kallikrein or aldosterone
excretion in these same subjects and studies.

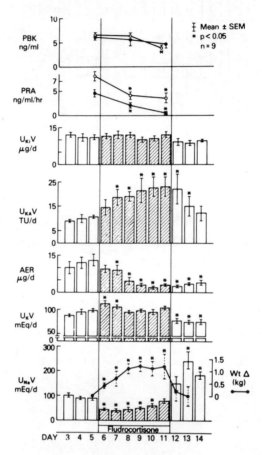

Figure 3.   Effect of 0.5 mg/day fludrocortisone on (mean ± SEM)
            urinary sodium (UNaV), potassium (UKV), kallikrein (UKaV),
            and kinin (UKiV) excretion, aldosterone excretion rate
            (AER), plasma renin activity (PRA) (subjects recumbent
            (0) and upright (0)), and weight change (WT Δ) in nine
            subjects fed 109 mEq/d sodium and 100 mEq/d potassium.
            * is p<0.05.

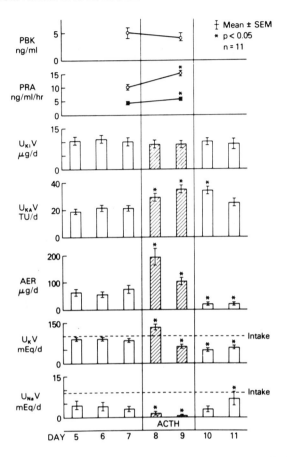

Figure 4. The effects of an intravenous infusion of ACTH
(Corticotropin, 80 units/d for 2 days) in 11 subjects
fed diets with 9 mEq/d sodium and 100 mEq/d potassium.
See legend Fig. 3. * is p <0.05.

Patients with Bartter's Syndrome

Under basal conditions the seven patients with Bartter's
Syndrome had the expected marked increases in plasma renin activity
and aldosterone excretion and the expected decrease in serum
potassium. In addition their urinary kallikrein excretion and plasma
bradykinin were much greater than normal while their urinary kinin
excretion was much less than normal (Table III). When either indomethacin or ibuprofen was administered orally for 7 to 9 days
urinary prostaglandin E excretion decreased (48%) as did urinary
aldosterone and sodium excretion and plasma renin activity (Fig. 6).
At the same time the abnormalities in the kallikrein-kinin system

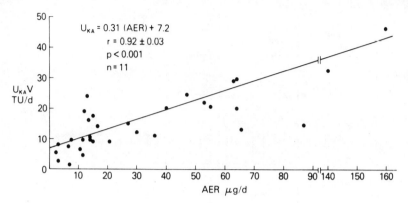

Figure 5.   Highly significant correlation between urinary
            kallikrein excretion (UKaV) and aldosterone excretion
            rate (AER) for 11 subjects during any 3 of the following
            dietary intakes or studies: when subjects were fed diets
            with 9 or 109 mEq/d sodium and 100 mEq/d potassium;
            25 or 195 mEq/d potassium and 109 mEq/d sodium; when
            given ACTH while being fed a diet with 9 mEq/d sodium
            and 100 mEq/d potassium.   Each point represents the
            mean of at least 2 days in a study when a subject had
            reached hormonal equilibrium.

returned to or toward normal; i.e., urinary kallikrein excretion and
plasma kinin decreased while urinary kinin excretion increased
(Fig. 7).

DISCUSSION

In this series of studies urinary kallikrein was positively
correlated with the level of sodium-retaining steroid but plasma
and urinary kinins were not. Levels of plasma bradykinin increased
in response to sodium-depletion and upright posture and were positively correlated with the level of plasma renin activity. Urinary
kinin excretion was unresponsive to changes in the level of sodium-
retaining steroid or plasma renin activity. In patients with
Bartter's Syndrome plasma renin activity and bradykinin were elevated
in the basal state and were decreased by prostaglandin synthetase
inhibitors. In these same patients urinary aldosterone and kallikrein excretion were elevated while urinary kinin excretion was
decreased in the basal state. Prostaglandin synthetase inhibitors
decreased both urinary aldosterone and kallikrein excretion while
urinary kinin excretion increased. Those patients who excreted the
least kinins had the greater basal hormonal derangements and they
showed the greater response to prostaglandin synthetase inhibitors.
Thus in patients with Bartter's Syndrome the low kinin excretion

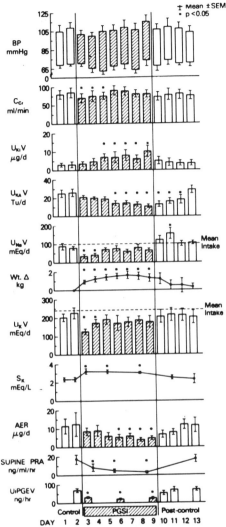

Figure 6. Effects of prostaglandin synthetase inhibition (PGSI)
in seven patients with Bartter's Syndrome on blood
pressure (BP), creatinine clearance (Ccr), kinin excretion (UKiV), kallikrein excretion (UKaV), urinary
sodium excretion (UNaV), weight change (WT. Δ), urinary
potassium excretion (UKV), serum potassium (SK), aldosterone excretion rate (AER), plasma renin activity (PRA),
and urinary immunoreactive prostaglandin E excretion
(UiPGEV). * is p<0.05.

TABLE III

	NORMALS (N)	B.SYNDROME(7)	P
SK (mEq/L)	3.9 ± 0.1 (16)	2.4 ± 0.2	0.001
PRAR (ng/ml/hr)	1.4 ± 0.2 (16)	17.3 ± 5.3	0.005
AER (μg/d)	4.5 ± 0.5 (19)	12.0 ± 5.1	N.S.
UiPGEV (ng/hr)	29 ± 5 (25)	70 ± 11	0.005
UKaV (TU/d)	8.2 ± 0.7 (25)	24.8 ± 0.6	0.001
UKiV (μg/d)	13.3 ± 0.9 (25)	4.3 ± 0.2	0.001
PBKR (ng/ml)	2.95 ± 0.2 (19)	13.2 ± 0.8	0.001

Mean ± SEM basal values for serum potassium (SK), plasma renin activity subject recumbent (PRAR), urinary aldosterone excretion rate (AER), urinary excretion of immunoreactive prostaglandin E (UiPGEV), kallikrein (UKaV) and kinin (UKiV) and plasma bradykinin, subject recumbent (PBKR) in normal subjects and 7 patients with Bartter's Syndrome fed 109 mEq/d sodium.

appears to be mediated by the level of renal prostaglandin E and not by the level of urinary kallikrein.

These studies confirm the observation that urinary kallikrein is dependent on aldosterone and extend the observation to encompass an eighty-fold range in aldosterone excretion and a thirty-fold range in kallikrein excretion (Fig. 5). It is clear that urinary kinin excretion is independent of kallikrein excretion since the former remained unchanged while the latter changed thirty-fold. In the patients with Bartter's Syndrome prostaglandin synthetase inhibitors produced a decrease in urinary kallikrein while urinary kinins increased. It is well established that our radioimmunoassay for kinins measures accurately bradykinin and lysyl-bradykinin present in urine samples collected into acid and pepstatin.

However, we now question the physiologic significance of measurements of kinins in 24-hour collections of urine for several reasons. First, the substrate kininogen, has been found in urine. Second, there is also kininase activity in urine. The factors which control the release of kininogen into the urine and the activity of the kininases in urine are unknown. Preliminary data from our laboratory indicate that kininase activity varies considerably from subject to

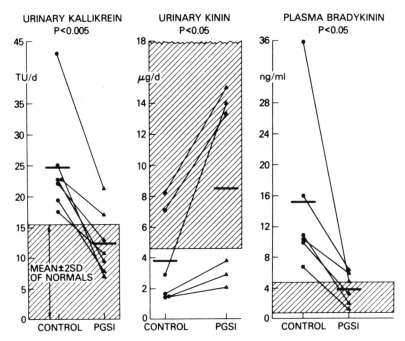

Figure 7.   Effect of prostaglandin synthetase inhibition (PGSI)
             on urinary kallikrein excretion (UKaV) on the 7th day
             of treatment in seven patients, on urinary kinin
             excretion (UKiV) on the 7th day of treatment in six
             patients, and on mean plasma bradykinin (PBK) on the
             4th and 7th days of treatment in six patients. The
             shaded area is the mean ± SD for normal subjects fed
             109 mEq/d sodium. Horizontal bars represent the mean
             for each group.

subject and that levels of urinary kinins are higher in urines
voided frequently.

    Plasma bradykinin is highly correlated with plasma renin
activity in all situations studied except for administration of
ACTH. This discrepancey was most likely due to the effect of ACTH-
stimulated cortisol which increased renin substrate concentration
and thus plasma renin activity while plasma bradykinin was unchanged.
In all of the other situations studied.the changes in both plasma
bradykinin and plasma renin activity appear related to changes in
extracellular fluid volume.

In these studies we have shown that: 1. urinary kallikrein is an index of sodium-retaining steroid activity and may participate in the anti-natriuretic and kaliuretic effects of these hormones; 2. urinary kinin excretion is independent of changes in urinary kallikrein excretion; 3. levels of plasma bradykinin are highly correlated with levels of plasma renin activity probably because both respond to changes in extracellular fluid volume; and, 4. plasma bradykinin may act to antagonize angiotensin II to maintain normal blood pressure in hyper-reninemic states.

REFERENCES

Margolius, H.S., D. Horwitz, J.J. Pisano, and H.R. Keiser, 1974a. Urinary kallikrein in normal man: Relationships to sodium intake and sodium retaining steroids. Circ. Res. 35: 812-819.

Margolius, H.S., D. Horwitz, J.J. Pisano, and H.R. Keiser, 1974b. Urinary kallikrein excretion in hypertensive man: Relationships to sodium intake and sodium-retaining steroids. Circ. Res. 35: 820-825.

Keiser, H.R., M.J. Andrews, Jr., R.A. Guyton, H.S. Margolius, and J.J. Pisano, 1976. Urinary kallikrein in dogs with constriction of one renal artery. Proc. of the Exper. Biol. and Med. 151: 53-56.

Vinci, J.M., J.R. Gill, Jr., R.E. Bowden, J.J. Pisano, J.L. Izzo, Jr., N. Radfar, A.A. Taylor, R.M. Zusman, F.C. Bartter, and H.R. Keiser, 1978. The kallikrein kinin system and its response to prostaglandin synthetase inhibition. J. Clin. Invest. 61: 1671-1682.

Rao, C.R., 1965. The theory of least squares when parameters are stochastic and its application to the analysis of grown curves. Biometrika 52: 447-458.

SOME ASPECTS OF URINARY KALLIKREIN IN A PATIENT WITH BARTTER'S

SYNDROME

Y. Tamura, Y. Matsuda*, K. Yamada, T. Takagi, T. Nishikawa,
M. Watanabe, K. Mikami, H. Moriya* and A. Kumagai

The 2nd Dept. of Medicine, Chiba Univ. Hosp., Chiba,
Japan. *Faculty of Pharmaceutical Sciences, Science
Univ. of Tokyo, Japan

INTRODUCTION

Bartter's syndrome is a disorder characterized by enhancement
of renin-angiotensin-aldosterone system with normal blood pressure,
hypokalemia, metabolic alkalosis, J.G. cell hyperplasia and vascular-
insensitivity to angiotensin II and an abnormality in the renal
handling of electrolytes (Solomon and Brown, 1975; Tomko et al.,
1976).

Recently it was reported that the overproduction of two vasoactive substances, e.g., prostaglandin and kallikrein in Bartter's
syndrome, both of which are vasodepressive and natriuretic, could
be intimately related to the pathogenesis of Bartter's syndrome
(Gill et al., 1976; McGiff, 1977).

Here we have investigated the character of urinary kallikrein
in one patient with Bartter's syndrome and found its properties
were somewhat different from those of normal subjects.

Case Report

A 48-year-old woman was admitted with a history of progressive
muscular weakness, polydypsia and polyuria. A few months before
admission, she noticed progressive fatigability, muscular weakness
and occasional attacks of nausea and vomiting. Hypokalemia was
found and the patient was referred to our hospital for the evaluation of hypokalemia. Ten years ago, hypokalemia was noted and she
received potassium supplements for a short period. Since then

polydypsia and polyuria has been noted. She did not have any
medication inducing hypokalemia. Her past and family history were
otherwise non-contributory. On admission, she appeared to be
emaciated, slightly dehydrated and could not walk without assistance.
She had a height of 155 cm and a weight of 30 kg. The blood pressure
was 98/58 mmHg and the pulse rate 86/min and regular. The examination
of chest, heart and abdomen were normal. Neurological examination
showed generalized muscular weakness. On the first hospital day,
plasma sodium was 131 mEq/l and plasma potassium was 1.9 mEq/l.
Creatinine clearance was 50-58 ml/min. Plasma calcium and phosphorus
concentrations were normal. Liver, pancreatic functions and glucose
tolerance test were normal. On a regular hospital diet (sodium
200-250 mEq/day) with potassium supplement (potassium 180 mEq),
the patient excreted 3-6 liters urine containing about 320-410 mEq
sodium and 175-260 mEq potassium. The urine specific gravity was
1.006-1.008.

Urinalysis were negative for protein or sugar and urine pH
ranged from 6.0 to 9.0. Urine culture was negative. Ammonium
chloride acidification test showed a decrease in urine below pH
6.0. Thyroid function, 17OHCS and 17 KS were normal. Intravenous
pyelogram demonstrated somewhat delayed appearance of dye in both
kidneys and slight bilateral dilation of the collecting system.
Renal biopsy showed a marked hyperplasia of the juxtaglomerular
apparatus.

MATERIALS AND METHODS

Sephadex G-75, G-100 and QAE-Sephadex A-50 (3.0104 mEq/g)
were obtained from Pharmacia Fine Chemicals, Uppsala, Sweden.
DEAE-cellulose (0.92 mEq/g) were purchased from Brown Chemicals,
U.S.A. Carrier Amphorite (pH range 3.5 to 5.0) was purchased from
LKB Produkter AB, Sweden. BAME (N-α-benzoyl-L arginine methyl
ester) and TAME (N-α-tosyl-L-arginine methyl ester) were supplied
from Peptide Institute Co., Ltd., Osaka, Japan. Angiotensin II
(Hypertensin Ciba) was a gift from Chiba Geigy Co., Ltd., Tokyo.

Plasma renin activity and plasma aldosterone concentration
was measured by radioimmunoassay (CEA-IRE-SORIN, France).

Esterolytic Activity

Esterolytic activities of HUK were measured by the three
methods, e.g., fluorometry (Matsuda, et al., 1976a), colorimetry
(Moriwaki et al., 1971) and spectrophotometry (Schwert and Takenaka,
1955; Hummel, 1959), using BAME and TAME as substrate. All of the
esterolytic activities were expressed in terms of esterase unit
(E.U.) which is identical in terms of μ moles substrate hydrolyzed
per min.

Vasodilator Activity

This was assayed by the method reported previously (Moriya et al., 1965), by measuring the increase in arterial blood flow in dogs. This activity was expressed in terms of kallikrein units (K.U.).

Purification of Urinary Kallikrein

Purification was carried out under the methods and experimental conditions as previously reported (Matsuda et al., 1976b) with slight modification. Briefly the extraction and purification were performed by the following procedures, e.g., DEAE-cellulose adsorption, DEAE-cellulose chromatography, Sephadex G-100 gel filtration, QAE-sephadex A-50 chromatography and Sephadex G-75 gel filtration in this order. Final preparation of urinary kallikrein was used for the investigations.

Isoelectric Focusing Fractionation

Isoelectric focusing fractionation was performed as reported previously (Matsuda et al., 1976b). Briefly isoelectric focusing was performed with carrier ampholyte (pH 3-5) on LKB8100 equipment. Electrophoresis was carried out at 500 volts and 6-8° for 40 hr.

Determination of Protein Concentration

Protein concentration was determined spectrophotometrically by measuring the absorbance at 280 nm, using a Hitachi spectrophotometer, model 124 with a cell of 1 cm light path, and the amount of protein was calculated taking a value for the extinction coefficient of HUK, $E_{280}^{1\%}$ of 14.1.

RESULTS

Hospital Course

When the patient was put on regular hospital diet (sodium 200-250 mEq/day) with potassium gluconate (180 mEq potassium), there was noted a gradual return of serum potassium up to 2.8 - 3.2 mEq/l from 1.9 mEq/l. Then her muscle strength returned and she was able to be up and about. Subsequently potassium supplements were discontinued. Serum potassium again fell to 1.6 mEq/l. At this time urinary kallikrein ranged from 27.3 to 50.1 E.U./day (normal range 8.60 ± 3.8 E.U./day) and plasma renin activity 26.04-45.47 ng/ml/hr (normal range 1.68 ± 1.18) and plasma aldosterone 2282.5-2839.7 pg/ml (normal range 147.1 ± 81.6 pg/ml). Then 75 mg of indomethacin was

administered. There was noted an increase in serum potassium to
2.8 - 3.2 mEq/1, which was accompanied by a decrease in plasma
renin activity to 4.6 - 8.2 ng/ml/hr, plasma aldosterone to 380.5 -
420.7 pg/ml and urinary kallikrein to 12.6-14.5 E.U./day. Since
then she has been treated with 75 mg of indomethacin and 180 mEq of
potassium gluconate. Serum potassium has ranged between 3.2-3.8 mEq/1
and the patient gained weight about 11 kg during her hospitalization.

Angiotension II Infusion Test

The pressor response to angiotensin II was measured at a rate
of infusion of 10 ng/kg/min of angiotensin II for 60 min, when the
patient was receiving potassium supplements alone and also indomethacin together with potassium supplements. Without indomethacin,
there was virtually no response to angiotensin II. However.when
indomethacin was given, a marked improvement of the blood pressure
response to angiotensin II (50 mmHg rise in systolic pressure and
30 mmHg in diastolic pressure) was demonstrated.

Purification of Urinary Kallikrein in the
Patient with Bartter's Syndrome

A summary of the purification procedures and the esterolytic
activity of the purified kallikrein are shown in Table 1. From the
starting materials, 8090 fold purification was achieved with 16%
activity recovery. The specific activity of the final preparation

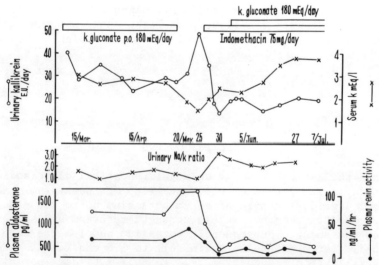

Figure 1.   Effect of 75 mg/kay of indomethacin administration on
urinary kallikrein, urinary Na/K ratio, serum K,
plasma renin activity and plasma aldosterone.

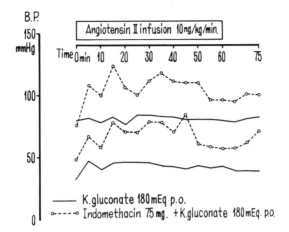

Figure 2.   Effect of indomethacin administration on pressor
             response to angiotensin II.

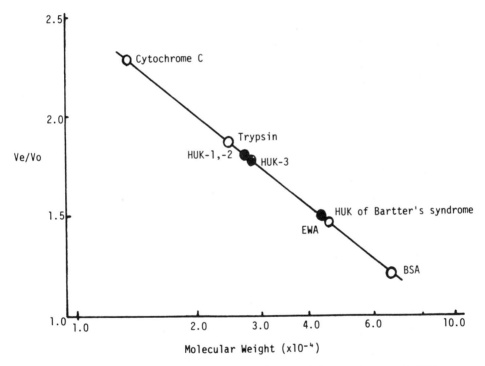

Figure 3.   Estimation of the molecular weights of normal HUK
             and urinary kallikrein in the patient with Bartter's
             syndrome.

Table 1. Summary of purification of urinary kallikrein in the
          patient with Bartter's syndrome

	Protein		Esterolytic activity (EU*)		
	Total A280	Total EU	EU/A280	Recovery	P.F.
Original urine (12.7 1)	235,000	614	0.0026	100	1
DEAE-cellulose absorption	900	230	0.26	38	99
DEAE-cellulose chromatography	88	207	2.4	34	905
Sephadex G-100 gel filtration	58	188	3.2	31	1230
QAE-Sephadex A-50 chromatography	16	139	8.8	23	3350
Sephadex G-75 gel filtration	4.7	100	21.1	16	8090

* EU: 1 μmole TAME hydrolyzed per min at pH 8.0, at 30°

P.F.: Purification factor

was 20.1 E.U. per A 280 (esterolytic assay) and 550 KU per A 280
(vasodilator assay).

Estimation of the Molecular Weight

The molecular weight of the components of normal HUK and urinary
kallikrein in the patient with Bartter's syndrome was estimated by
gel filtration on a Sephadex G-100 column. The approximate molecular
weight of urinary kallikrein in the patient with Bartter's syndrome
was 4.2×10^4, which was greater than those of normal HUK (HUK-1
and HUK-2 2.7×10^4, and HUK-3 2.9×10^4) as previously reported
by Matsuda et al. (1976b). The molecular weights of the three
components of normal HUK and urinary kallikrein from the patient
with Bartter's syndrome were estimated by gel filtration on a
Sephadex G-100 column, as previously reported by Matsuda et al.,
(1976). Cytochrome C (M.W. 1.3×10^4), trypsin (M.W. 2.37×10^4), egg
white albumin EWA (M.W. 4.45×10^4) and bovine serum albumin BSA,
(M.W. 6.7×10^4) were used as marker protein.

Estimation of Km Values

Km values towards synthetic N-substituted arginine esters (TAME and BAME) were determined. As demonstrated in Table 2, Km values of the purified urinary kallikrein in our patient with Bartter's syndrome was not correspondent with any of those three components of normal HUK.

Table 2. Km values of urinary kallikreins in normal subjects and patient with Bartter's syndrome

Urinary kallikrein	Substrate	
	TAME	BAME
HUK-1	750	330
HUK-2	490	190
HUK-3	330	230
Bartter's syndrome	410	710

Km: μM at pH 8.0
Km values of urinary kallikreins from normal subjects (Matsuda et al, 1976) and the patient with Bartter's syndrome towards TAME and BAME were determined by Lineweaver-Burk plots. Esterolytic activities were assayed spectrophotometrically, measuring the increase in absorbancy at 247 nm (TAME) and 254 nm (BAME).

Isoelectric Focusing Fractionation

The purified urinary kallikrein in our patient with Bartter's syndrome was applied to an Ampholine column. As shown on the left side, one component of urinary kallikrein was obtained in our patient, of which the isoelectric point was pI 4.3. On the contrary, as shown on the right side, three components of urinary kallikrein purified from the urine collected on a large scale from normal male persons were separated by isoelectric focusing and were named HUK-1 (Human Urinary Kallikrein I, pI 3.9), HUK-2 (pI 4.0) and HUK-3 (pI 4.2), respectively.

DISCUSSION

Excessive urinary kallikrein excretion and the restoration of pressor response to angiotensin II infusion after the administration of indomethacin in our patient with Bartter's syndrome were consistent

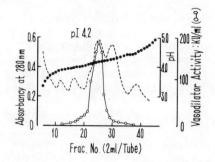 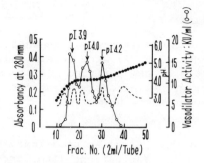

Figure 4.   Isoelectric focusing fractionation of urinary
     kallikrein in normal subjects and the patient with
     Bartter's syndrome using an Ampholine system.

     As shown on the right side, three components of normal
     HUK were separated by this process and named as HUK-1
     (pI 3.9), HUK-2 (pI 4.0) and HUK-3 (pI 4.2).

     As shown on the left side, urinary kallikrein in the
     patient with Bartter's syndrome had one component (pI
     4.3).

     ● ● ● ●   pH value, o——o vasodilator activity using
     dogs, -------   concentration of protein.

with the reports of Lechi et al. (1976) and Halushka et al. (1977).
Though indomethacin, an inhibitor of prostaglandin synthesis,
suppressed the renin-angiotensin-aldosterone system, decreased
urinary kallikrein excretion and increased serum potassium concentration, they were not reversed to normal range, which were similar
with the report of Gill et al. (1976a).

    As excessive urinary kallikrein excretion reported not only in
Bartter's syndrome, but also in primary aldosteronism, so the
stimulation and the suppression of the renin-angiotensin-aldosterone
system, though opposite in direction, are associated with an increase
in aldosterone production and urinary kallikrein excretion. In
addition, spironolactone, aldosterone antagonist is reported to
decrease kallikrein excretion (Lechi et al. 1976; Margolius et al.
1974).

    From these evidences described above, it can be thought that
urinary kallikrein excretion is primarily controlled by mineralocorticoids such as deoxycorticosterine or aldosterone. Then one
of the most likely explanations for a decrease in urinary kallikrein excretion by indomethacin in our patient with Bartter's
syndrome is that indomethacin inhibited a prostaglandin mechanism
which participated in the regulation of renin-angiotensin system,
leading to a decrease in aldosterone production followed by a

decline of urinary kallikrein excretion, though there remains mechanisms which are different from those mentioned above.

From the present data, it can be said that isoelectric point, molecular weight and Km value in this patient did not correspond to those in any of the three types of urinary kallikrein, indicating that the character of urinary kallikrein of our patient with Bartter's syndrome was qualitatively different from normals.

Moriya and co-workers demonstrated that the molecular weight of dog renal kallikrein was larger than that of dog urinary kallikrein (Moriwaki et al., 1976). Porcelli et al. (1975) showed also a similar finding in the rat. They suggested that the urinary kallikrein might be a partial degradation of renal kallikrein. Then it may be speculated that the urinary kallikrein in our patient with Bartter's syndrome was renal kallikrein which was not degraded.

A renal tubular dysfunction has been thought to be at least in part responsible for the pathophysiology of Bartter's syndrome (Tomko et al., 1976; Gill et al., 1977b). Nustad et al.(1975) indicated that urinary kallikrein is of renal origin, so our present finding might reflect a renal tubular dysfunction in this patient with Bartter's syndrome. Nevertheless. finding that the urinary kallikrein in our patient was still under the influence of renin-angiotensin-aldosterone system or renal prostaglandins system was interesting. Whether this derangement is a primary or secondary phenomenon in Bartter's syndrome is still undetermined.

This work was supported by grants from Ministry of Education (248187 and 257542), Japan.

REFERENCES

Gill, J.R., et al. 1976a. Bartter's syndrome: A disorder characterized by high urinary prostaglandins and a dependence of hyperreninemia or prostaglandin synthesis. Amer. J. Med. 61: 43.

Gill, J.R., et al., 1977b. Impaired tubular chloride reabsorption as a proximal cause of Bartter's syndrome. Clin. Res. 25: 526A.

Halushka, P.V., et al., 1977. Bartter's syndrome: Urinary prostaglandin E-like materials and kallikrein: indomethacin effects. Ann. Int. Med. 87: 281.

Hummel, B.C.W., 1959. A modified spectrophotometric determination of chymotrypsin, trypsin and thrombin. Can. J. Biochem. Physiol. 37: 1393.

Lechi, A., et al., 1977. Urinary kallikrein excretion in Bartter's syndrome. J. Clin. Endo. & Metab. 43: 1175.

Margolius, H.S., et al., 1974. Urinary kallikrein in normal man:
    relationship to sodium intake and sodium retaining steroids.
    Cir. Res. 35: 820.

Matsuda, Y., et al., 1976a. Fluorometric methods for assay of kalli-
    krein-like arginine esterases. J. Biochem. 79: 1197.

Matsuda, Y., et al., 1976b. Studies on urinary kallikreins I:
    purification and characterization of human urinary kallikreins.
    J. Biochem. 80: 671.

McGiff, J.C., 1977. Bartter's syndrome results from an imbalance
    of vasoactive hormones. Ann. Int. Med. 87: 369.

Moriwaki, C., et al., 1971. A new assay method for esterolytic
    activity of kallikreins with chromotropic acid. Yakugaku-
    Zashi (in Japanese) 91: 413.

Moriwaki, C., et al., 1976. Dog renal kallikrein: Purification and
    some properties. J. Biochem. 80: 1277.

Moriya, H., et al., 1965. Biochemical studies on kallikreins and
    their related substances. J. Biochem. 58: 208.

Nustad, K., et al., 1975. Synthesis of kallikreins by rat kidney
    slices. Brit. J. Pharmacol. 53: 229.

Procelli, G., et al., 1975. Preliminary data on purified kallikrein
    from rat kidney. Life Science 16: 788.

Schwert, G.W. and Y. Takenaka, 1955. A spectrophotometric deter-
    mination of trypsin and chymotrypsin. Biochem. Biophys. Acta.
    16 570.

Solomon, R.J. and R.S. Brown, 1975. Bartter's syndrome: New insight
    into pathogenesis and treatment. Amer. J. Med. 59: 575.

Tomko, D.J., et al., 1976. Bartter's syndrome. Amer. J. Med. 61: 111.

Yamada, K., et al., 1979. Quantitative and qualitative estimation
    of urinary kallikrein in a patient with Bartter's syndrome.
    Endocrinol. Japa. (in press).

Kinins, Renal Function and
Blood Pressure Regulation

DEPENDENCE OF UROKALLIKREIN EXCRETION ON THE PERFUSION PRESSURE

IN EXPLANTED PERFUSED KIDNEYS

M. Maier and B.R. Binder

Department of Physiology, School of Medicine, Univ.

Vienna, Austria, A 1090, SchwarzspanierstraBe 17

All animals investigated so far excrete urokallikrein into the urine (Frey et al., 1968). An interrelationship between urokalli- krein excretion and blood pressure was first shown in 1934 by Elliot (Elliot and Nuzum 1934) who demonstrated that urokallikrein excretion is significantly reduced in patients with essential hypertension. In contrast, in most other forms of hypertension, the level of urokallikrein is normal or raised (Adetuyibi and Mills 1972). Urokallikrein excretion is also influenced by sodium- and potassium-load, by water-load, and by infusion of some prostaglan- dins and of vasoactive drugs. Such findings as well as those from studies with specific inhibitors suggest connections between uro- kallikrein, the renal prostaglandin system (Abe et al., 1978) and the renin-angiotensin system (Sealey et al., 1978). Up to now only one investigation has dealt with the relationship of perfusion pressure to excretion of urokallikrein. By means of in situ perfusion of dog kidneys and with variation of the perfusion pres- sure through clamping of the renal artery, this study demonstrated that urokallikrein excretion into the urine is dependent on the kidney perfusion pressure (Bevan et al., 1974).

In order to avoid uncontrolled systemic effects on urokalli-

ABBREVIATION

KGA - kinin generating activity; PAA- plasminogen activating activity; BK - bradykinin; BAEE - N-α-benzoyl-L-arginin ethyl ester hydro- chloride; MW - molecular weight; CTA - comity on thrombolytic agents; GOT - glutamic oxaloacetic transaminase; GPT - glutamic pyruvic transaminase; LDH - lactic dehydrogenase.

krein excretion, we used explanted hog kidneys perfused at 4-6°C
with an albumin-containing balanced salt solution to study the
urokallikrein excretion. We found that the urokallikrein excreted
by these kidneys is identical with normal pig urokallikrein and that
its excretion at any given time is dependent on the perfusion
pressure employed.

MATERIALS AND METHODS

Kidneys of normal pigs were removed and immediately rinsed
with icecold physiological saline containing heparin and xylocain
until the effluent from the renal vein was visually bloodfree.
Within 100-120 minutes kidney perfusion with an electrolyte
solution containing 2.5% albumin was started (Fig. 1).
A pulsatile perfusion pressure from the renal artery to the renal
vein was employed. In 15 experiments the mean pressure was kept
constant at 80 mm Hg (10.7 kPa) and in the remaining 4 experiments
the mean pressure was stepwise varied between 50 and 130 mm Hg (6.7
and 17.3 kPa) by altering perfusion volume per minute. In all
experiments the urine was collected in 3 ml portions. In experiments
with constant pressure perfusate samples were taken at one hour
intervals. In the experiments with altered pressure the perfusate

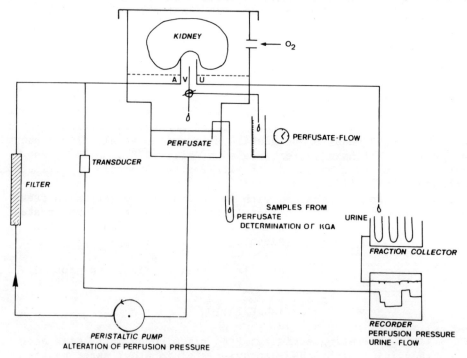

Figure 1.   Kidney Perfusion System (4°C). Diagram of perfusion
system and experimental procedure.

samples were taken 30 minutes after and immediately before the pressure changes.

In the course of 5 of the experiments the functioning of the perfused kidneys was determined. In urine and perfusate samples obtained during the first hour of perfusion, and between the 20th and the 30th hour, the following evaluations were done: Na^+, K^+, pH, GOT, LDH, GPT, lactate, pyruvate, and glucose (Table 1). Only the concentrations in both urines and perfusates of GOT and LDH increased significantly with a high degree of variation during the time of perfusion. The micromorphology of the perfused kidneys determined at the end of the perfusion experiments, did not differ significantly from that of control kidneys. The control kidneys were taken from the same animal at the same time as the perfused kidneys, rinsed in icecold saline and stored at 4°C without perfusion. In the perfused kidneys and in the non-perfused controls, deterioration of the brush border membranes was seen – a finding which is consistent with the high amount of GOT and LDH in the urine and perfusate samples. The changes observed in the integrity of the kidneys in our experiments were considered to be of minimal consequence for the in vitro evaluation of definitive kidney functions.

TABLE 1.   ASSESSMENT OF KIDNEY FUNCTION.

	URINE		PERFUSATE	
	after 1 hour	after 20-30 hours	after 1 hour	after 20-30 hours
NA^+ mval/l	168.7 ± 7.3	172.0 ± 8.1	176.2 ± 8.2	176.2 ± 3.7
K^+ mval/l	11.3 ± 1.2	12.5 ± 0.8	11.3 ± 0.9	13.1 ± 0.7
pH	7.16 ± 0.04	7.0 ± 0.1	7.25 ± 0.09	7.19 ± 0.1
GOT mU/ml	56.2 ± 53.0	275 ± 25	15.2 ± 10.8	240 ± 60
GPT mU/ml	8.6 ± 4.1	7.0 ± 3.3	7.0 ± 4.9	8.3 ± 1.6
LDH mU/ml	272 ± 251	503.3 ± 111.4	134 ± 111	351.6 ± 211
LACTATE mg %	24.2 ± 3.6	22.05 ± 0.8	15.7 ± 14.4	9.3 ± 8.6
PYRUVATE mg %	0.32 ± 0.16	0.38 ± 0.02	0.31 ± 0.06	0.26 ± 0.04
GLUCOSE mg %	54.0 ± 10.9	49 ± 14.8	48.5 ± 1.5	54.0 ± 13.3

Values represent means and standard deviations for 5 kidneys.

In the urine and perfusate samples, kinin generating activities (KGA) were determined by bioassay on the guinea pig ileum using heat inactivated plasma as a cource of kininogen (Webster and Prado, 1970), and expressed as ng's bradykinin equivalent per ml. Esterolytic activities were determined through use of the BAEE-ADH method of Trautschold (Trautschold et al., 1977). The results of these kallikrein determinative methods correlated with an r = 0.87 (p < 0.001). Fibrinolytic activities were measured as diameters of lytic zones on plasminogen-containing fibrin-agarose plates and expressed in CTA units per ml. Proteolytic activities were estimated on plasminogen-free fibrin-agarose plates.

Proteins with kinin generating activities from pooled urines and pooled perfusates were isolated by means of aprotinin-affinity chromatography according to the method of Ole-Moi Yoi (Ole-Moi Yoi 1978). This method was modified by omission of the step involving ion-exchange chromatography on DE-52 cellulose and induction of the use of Blue Sepharose CL-6B (Pharmacia, Sweden) as follows: after gel filtration on Sephadex G-100 the eluates containing KGA's were concentrated 10-fold and equilibrated with an equal amount of Blue Sepharose CL-6B for 30 minutes at room temperature. After removal of the gel material by centrifugation for 10 minutes at 2500 x g, the supernatants were concentrated 10-fold and subjected to alkaline disk electrophoresis on 7.5% acrylamid gels at pH = 9.3 in replica gels (Maurer, 1971). One gel was stained with Coomassie blue, the other gel was cut into 2 mm slices. Each slice was eluted with 0.1 ml of buffer and aliquotes of the eluates were used to determine KGA. Molecular weight determinations of the purified materials with and without reduction (Maurer, 1971) performed with SDS gel electrophoresis in 10% acrylamid gels and 0.1% SDS. Normal pig urine was treated in the same way in order to isolate control pig urokallikrein. Transferin, human serum albumin, ovalbumin and chymotrypsinogen were used as molecular weight marker proteins for the Sephadex G-100 gel filtration and for the SDS gel electrophoresis.

RESULTS

UROKALLIKREIN EXCRETION AT CONSTANT PERFUSION PRESSURE

Fifteen kidneys were perfused at constant perfusion pressure with a mean of 80 mm Hg (10.7 kPa). The perfusion volume was 140± 15 ml/minute and the resulting urine flow was between 60-90 ml/hour. KGA values of all urine and perfusate samples obtained during the first hour of perfusion were calculated for their means and standard deviations. The same was done with the values from samples obtained during each subsequent five-hour perfusion period (Fig. 2).

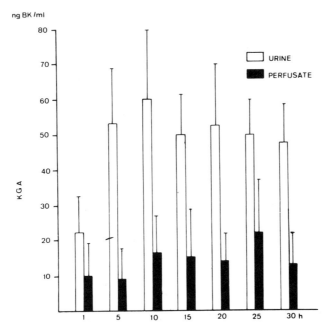

Figure 2. Kidney Perfusion with Constant perfusion pressure of
           80 mm Hg. Concentration of kinin generating activity
           in urines and perfusates of kidneys perfused with
           constant perfusion pressure. Mean and SD of 15
           experiments, 5 hour intervals.

The mean urine KGA was initially 22± 11 ng BK equivalent/ml and
increased to 53± 15 ng BK equivalent/ml between the second and the
fifth hour. Thereafter, the KGA remained at 48–60 ng BK equivalent/
ml. Total excretion of KGA in this period was 4350± 1950 ng BK
equivalent per hour. The mean urine esterolytic activity on BAEE
was 0.125 U per ml during the first hour, and increased to a level
of 0.15 U/ml resulting in an excretion of 11.83± 3.45 U per hour.
The mean KGA in the perfusate samples was 10± 9 ng BK equivalent/ml
after one hour of perfusion and remained at a mean level of 16± 10
ng BK equivalent/ml during the subsequent perfusion period.

ISOLATION OF KGA

     60–80% of KGA originally present in the concentrates of normal
pig urine, pooled test urines and pooled test perfusates were eluted
from an aprotinin-sepharose affinity resin by 0.1 molar acetate
buffer pH = 3.5 containing 1 molar NaCl. Gel filtration on Sephadex
G-100 of concentrated, active material eluted from the affinity
resin effected separation of the contained proteins in two OD peaks

at 280 nm (Fig. 3), one free of KGA in the exclusion volume, and
the other corresponding to the one activity peak of KGA, in the
included eluates. The KGA containing eluate, following concentration,
was incubated with Blue Sepharose CL-6B to yield 100% recovery of
KGA in the unbound supernatant. The latter product was subjected
to alkaline polyacrylamide gel electrophoresis. The only one
Comassie blue stainable band corresponding to the one KGA band
given by replicate gels was observed immediately behind the buffer
front when the material was derived from normal pig urine (Fig. 4).

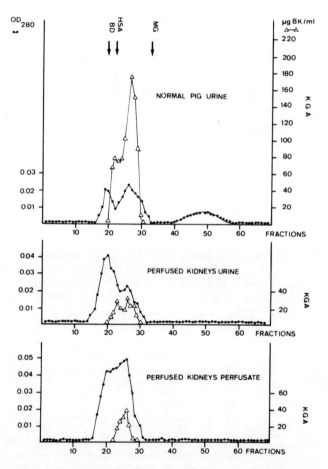

Figure 3.   Gel filtration (Sephadex G-100) of aprotinin-Sepharose
            purified proteins. Vv = 72 ml, bed volume 200 ml,
            flow rate 10 ml/h, 3 ml fractions collected.

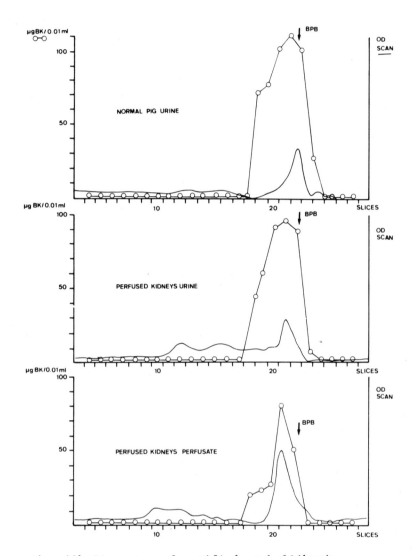

Figure 4. Alkaline page of purified urokallikrein.
Alkaline polyacrylamide gel electrophoresis of concentrated purified urokallikreins. Anode to the right, 7.5% gels. KGA's of eluates from replicate gels in ng BK/0.01 ml.

Similarly, the material from test urines gave an identical protein
and KGA band, plus 2 faintly stained bands in the middle of the gel.
KGA isolated from test perfusates showed a slightly lower mobility
in the gel corresponding to the predominant stainable band. The
same two minor contaminating bands were again observed. The alkylated unreduced urokallikrein purified from normal pig urine presented as a single stained band with a molecular weight of 43.000
on SDS gel electrophoresis. After reduction and alkylation the
protein was again present as a single stainable band with the same
molecular weight. Similar results were obtained when material
derived from test urines was subjected to SDS gel electrophoresis.
The one predominant stainable band in the alkylated unreduced sample
showed a molecular weight of 43.000 which remained unchanged after
reduction followed by alkylation. In unreduced as well as in
reduced samples faintly stainable bands with higher molecular weights
were observed. SDS-polyacrylamide gel electrophoresis from materials
derived from test perfusates was not performed, because of the
minimal amount of purified material available.

EXCRETION OF UROKALLIKREIN AT ALTERED PERFUSION PRESSURES

     Perfusion of kidneys with varied perfusion pressure resulted
in a change of the KGA-excretion pattern. The results of a typical
experiment are given in Fig. 5. Starting with a mean perfusion
pressure of 50 mm Hg (6.7 kPa), excretion of KGA into the urine
increased within 40 minutes from zero to a level of 70 ng BK
equivalent/ml (0.17 U/ml esterolytic activity on BAEE). When the
perfusion pressure was maintained at this level, the KGA slowly
reached a plateau level of 73 ng BK equivalent/ml within two hours.
Later stepwise in simultaneous increases of KGA. Thirty minutes
after the perfusion pressure reached 130 mm Hg (17.3 kPa), KGA
excretion was 141 ng BK equivalent/ml (0.24 U/ml). Each step
increase of the perfusion pressure effected a sharp alteration of
KGA excretion reaching a constant value 2-3 hours after the pressure
change. The initial change in KGA excretion was $71\pm 15\%$ of the
total change achieved by the pressure alteration. Lowering the
perfusion pressure led to a decreased excretion of KGA, following
a time lag of 30-90 minutes. Plasminogen-activating-activity (PAA)
in urines showed an initial decrease from 2.0 CTA units/ml at the
beginning of perfusion to 0.4 CTA units/ml after 2-3 hours. Thereafter, PAA excretion remained at this lower level during the whole
experiment.

     KGA in the samples from the perfusates was detectable only
after one hour of perfusion at a mean pressure of 60-70 mm Hg (8-
9.3 kPa) and was altered thereafter only to a minor extent to give
a mean activity of 22 ± 12 ng BK equivalent/ml (0.12 U/ml). PAA in
the perfusion fluids increased from an initial level of 0.2 CTA units/
ml after one hour of perfusion to a value of 0.38 CTA units/ml after
3 hours of perfusion and remained constant thereafter. No proteo-

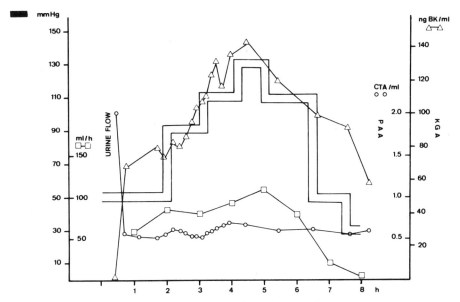

Figure 5. Kidney perfusion with altered perfusion pressure.
Urinary excretion pattern of kinin generating activity
(KGA) and plasminogen activating activity (PAA) in a
kidney perfused with altered pressure. Every 5th urine
sample is shown.

lytic activity could be detected either in the urines or in the
perfusates. Urine flow was affected by the perfusion pressure but
was not linearly dependent.

In all experiments with altered perfusion pressure, the KGA
excretion into the urines showed a significant dependence on the
pressure employed (Fig. 6). From the 4 experiments the KGA's
correlated with the perfusion pressure with an r-value of 0.80
(p << 0.001). There was no significant correlation observed between
the perfusion pressure and the KGA's in the perfusates (r = 0.19,
p > 0.1). PAA in the urines and in the perfusates showed no
significant correlation with the perfusion pressures.

DISCUSSION

Urokallikrein isolated from normal pig urine by aprotinin
affinity chromatography followed by gel filtration on Sephadex G-100
revealed a preparation contaminated with hog albumin. Removal of

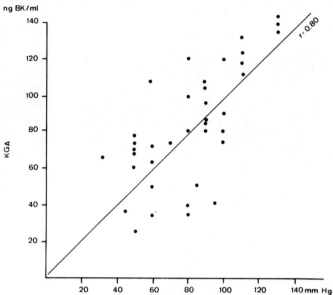

Figure 6.   Correlation of KGA to perfusion pressure in urines.
Correlation between kinin generating activity (KGA) in
urines and perfusion pressure. The correlation is
highly significant (p << 0.001).

the albumin by batch affinity chromatography using Blue Sepharose[R]
CL-6B resulted in a urokallikrein preparation showing a single band
on alkaline disc electrophoresis corresponding to KGA eluted from
replicate gels. The MW on the preparation assessed on polyacrylamide
gel electrophoresis was 43.000, a value which was only slightly
higher than that obtained by gel filtration on Sephadex G-100.
Since reduction of the purified protein did not alter the molecular
weight assessed by SDS polyacrylamide gel electrophoresis, hog urinary
kallikrein is a single polypeptide chain. These data are consistent
with the molecular weight of hog urokallikrein reported in the
literature and also with the single polypeptide chain structure of
all other urokallikreins investigated (Fritz et al., 1977).

Isolation of urokallikrein from pooled urines of kidneys
perfused at 4-6°C revealed a protein with the same characteristics
on alkaline disc electrophoresis as pig urokallikrein. The two minor
contaminating protein bands on alkaline gels as well as the faint
high molecular weight bands on SDS polyacrylamide gel electrophoresis
are most likely due to the way the fractions had been pooled after
gel filtration. Reduction and alcylation followed by SDS gel

electrophoresis and did not effect the molecular weight of the protein which was 43.000 and the same for the unreduced sample. Therefore the KGA excreted into the urine of perfused hog kidneys is also a single polypeptide chain with a molecular weight of 39.000-43.000.

Isolated urokallikrein from pooled perfusates of perfused kidneys revealed also one major protein band corresponding to KGA eluted from replicate gels on alkaline disc gels. Its mobility was slightly lower than that of KGA's isolated from both urinary sources. In all cases the amount of purified material obtained was not large enough to determine specific activities on a protein basis. From the intensity of the stain of the protein band and from the amount of KGA eluted from that region of the acrylamide gels it is suggested that the specific activity of the KGA from the perfusate is lower than that of KGA's isolated from urines. Therefore, KGA excreted into the urine of explanted and perfused hog kidneys at 4-6°C is most likely identical to urokallikrein isolated from normal pig urine whereas KGA isolated from perfusates might be slightly different from that excreted into the urine.

At constant perfusion pressure urokallikrein excretion into the urine plateaued after 2-3 hours and remained constant thereafter over a period of up to 30 hours. Stepwise increase of the perfusion pressure resulted in a concomitant increase of urokallikrein excretion within a pressure range of 50-130 mm Hg (6.7-17.3 kPa). Decreasing the perfusion pressure led to a decreased excretion of urokallikrein whereby the time lag was slightly greater than in the case of pressure increase. To determine whether the pattern of KGA excretion under conditions of varied perfusion pressure is peculiar to it or shared by PAA, the excretion of the latter was simultaneously investigated. PAA excretion at altered perfusion pressure was not different from that at constant perfusion pressure. In experiments with constant perfusion pressure of 80 mm Hg (10.7 kPa) a constant urine flow of 60-90 ml per hour was observed. In experiments with altered perfusion pressure changes in urine flow followed pressure changes. Within a range of 70-130 mm Hg (9.3-17.3 kPa) the resulting changes in urine flow were only minimal and the same perfusion pressure did not cause a comparable urine flow in the same kidney. At perfusion pressure of 50 mm Hg (6.7 kPa) or less, the urine flow was significantly altered. Calculation of the dependence of urokallikrein excretion into the urine, into the perfusate and of PAA excretion into the urine and into the perfusate on the perfusion pressure and on the urine flow resulted in only one highly significant correlation between urokallikrein excretion into the urine and perfusion pressure (Fig. 6) Alteration of the perfusion pressure in the kidney perfusion system is effected by changing the perfusion volume per time. Therefore urokallikrein excretion might be dependent not only on the perfusion pressure but also on the perfusion volume per time. From our experiments we conclude that perfusion pressure and/or perfusion flo influence urokallikrein excretion.

REFERENCES

Abe, K., N. Irokawa, M. Yasujima, M. Seino, S. Chiba, Y. Sakurai,
    K. Yoshinaga, T. Saito, 1978. The The Kallikrein-Kinin System
    and Prostaglandins in the Kidney. Circulation Res. 43: 254-260.

Adetuyibi, A., I.H. Mills, 1972. Relation Between Urinary Kallikrein
    and Renal Function, Hypertension and Excretion of Sodium and
    Water in Man. The Lancet II, p. 203-207.

Bevan, D.R., N.A.A. MacFarlane, I.H. Mills, 1974. The Dependence of
    Urinary Kallikrein Excretion on Renal Artery Pressure. J.
    Physiol. 241: 34P-35P.

Elliot, A.H., F.R. Nuzum, 1934. The Urinary Excretion of a Depressor
    Substance (Kallikrein of Frey and Kraut) in Arterial Hyper-
    tension. Endocrinology, 18: 462-474.

Frey, E.K., H. Kraut, E. Werle, 1968. Das Kallikrein-Kinin-System
    und seine Inhibitoren. p. 18-28, Ferdinand Enke Verlag, Stutt-
    gart.

Fritz, H., F. Fiedler, T. Dietl, M. Warwas, E. Truscheit, H.J.
    Kolb, G. Mair, H. Tschesche, 1977. On the Relationships
    between Porcine Pancreatic, Submandibular, and Urinary Kalli-
    kreins. Ed. G.L. Haberland, J.W. Rohen, T. Suzuki. Kinino-
    genases 4, Kallikrein. Physiological Properties and Pharmaco-
    logical Rationale. F.K. Schattauer Verlag Stuttgart - New York.

Maurer, H.R., 1971. Disc Electrophoresis and Related Techniques of
    Polyacrylamide Gel Electrophoresis. Walter de Gruyter Verlag.

Ole Moiyoi, O., J. Spragg, K.F. Austen, 1978. Inhibition of Human
    Urinary Kallikrein (Urokallikrein) by Anti-enzyme Fab. J.
    Immunol. 121:No. 1., 66.

Sealey, J.E., S.A. Atlas, J.L. Laragh, N.B. Oza, J.W. Ryan, 1978.
    Human Urinary Kallikrein Converts Inactive to Active Renin
    and is a Possible Physiological Activator of Renin. Nature,
    275: 144-145.

Webster, M.E., E.S. Prado, 1970. Glandular Kallikreins from Horse
    and Human Urine and from Hog Pancreas. Meth. Enz. 19: 681-706.

DEFECT IN KALLIKREIN-KININ-SYSTEM IN ESSENTIAL HYPERTENSION AND REDUCTION OF BLOOD PRESSURE BY ORALLY GIVEN KALLIKREIN

A. Overlack, K.O. Stumpe, W. Zywzock, C. Ressel and F. Drück

Medizinische Universitäts-Poliklinik, Bonn Wilhelmstr. 35, 5300 Bonn, Fed. Rep. of Germany

INTRODUCTION

Kallikrein is a proteolytic enzyme which catalyses the formation of the vasodilatory and natriuretic kinins, kallidin and bradykinin, from an alpha-2-globulin substrate, kininogen.

Urinary kallikrein appears to be derived from the kidney (9). It has been proposed that kallikrein exists in the renal cortex and may occupy a location that is juxtaposed to the enzyme renin (4). Systemic or intrarenal infusion studies indicate that the kinins, the enzymatic products of kallikrein, have both natriuretic and vasodilatory properties and increase renal blood flow (3, 10).

It has been suggested that increased renal vascular resistance as well as diminished sodium excretion play an important role in the pathogenesis of essential hypertension (6). Therefore, intrarenal kallikrein activity could not only be of physiological but also of pathophysiological importance in blood pressure regulation. This concept is supported by studies demonstrating decreased urinary kallikrein excretion in patients with essential hypertension (1, 7, 8).

In the present study, urinary kallikrein excretion was measured in normotensive persons and in patients with borderline or established essential hypertension on different sodium intake. Also, the relationship between the kallikrein-kinin-system, the renin-angiotensin-aldosterone-system, and renal blood flow was investigated.

MATERIALS AND METHODS

The patients and the normotensive persons ranged in age from
23 to 35 years. There was no significant difference between the
three groups in age, body weight and sex. Arterial blood pressure
in patients with borderline hypertension ranged from 140/90 to
160/95 mm Hg, although occasional values were sometimes greater
than 160/100 mm Hg and sometimes less than 140/90 mm Hg. In all
patients with established hypertension average blood pressure
was greater than 160 mm Hg systolic or 95 mm Hg diastolic or both.
Kallikrein was measured by a modification of the assay procedure
described by Amundsen et al. (2). In this assay a chromogenic
substrate (H-D-Val-Leu-Arg-pNA) is used. It is split by glandular
kallikrein. The rate of p-nitroaniline (pNA) formation, the absorbance of which is read in a photometer at 405 nm, increases
linearly with an increasing concentration of kallikrein. We used
highly purified porcine pancreatic kallikrein as standard. To
validate this enzymatic method, a bioassay on an anesthetized dog
was performed, as described by Frey et al. (5). Correlation
between the two methods was highly significant. Data were analysed
by Student's t-test.

RESULTS

Urinary kallikrein excretion was related to 24-hour sodium
excretion in normotensive persons and in patients with borderline
or established hypertension (fig. 1). The normotensive subjects
had significantly higher urinary kallikrein excretion than the
hypertensive patients. In the normotensives there was an inverse
correlation between urinary kallikrein and sodium excretion. No
such correlation could be demonstrated in the hypertensive
patients who, on a low salt diet, showed only a slight or no increase in kallikrein excretion. In the borderline hypertensives,
on an unrestricted and high salt diet, urinary kallikrein was
within the normal range. However, only a small increase in kallikrein excretion was observed on a low sodium diet.

Endogenous creatinine-clearance was similar in the three
groups. Thus, the decrease in urinary kallikrein excretion observed in the hypertensive patients cannot be explained by a diminished glomerular filtration rate. No significant day night
variation in kallikrein excretion was observed in the normotensive
and hypertensive groups.

Mean values of kallikrein excretion obtained on different
sodium intake are summarized in figure 2. On an unrestricted
sodium diet, urinary kallikrein in patients with established hypertension was significantly lower as compared to normotensive controls.
This defect in kallikrein excretion became still more pronounced

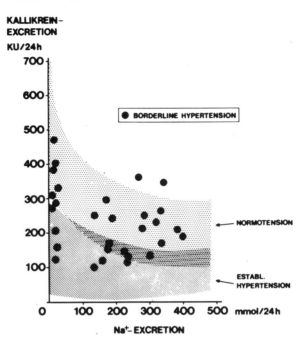

Fig. 1. Relationship between 24-hour urinary kallikrein and
sodium excretion in patients with borderline or
established essential hypertension and in normotensive
controls on different sodium intake.

after six days of a low salt diet containing 10 mmoles sodium per
day. Under these conditions urinary kallikrein rose markedly in
the normotensive group. In contrast, no or only a slight increase
in enzyme excretion occurred in the hypertensive patients.
Similarly, following six days of a high salt diet containing 350
mmols sodium per day, the hypertensives exhibited a relatively
fixed rate of renal kallikrein excretion, whereas a pronounced
decrease in enzyme excretion was observed in the normotensives.
Although the patients with borderline hypertension had almost
normal kallikrein excretion on an unrestricted salt diet, sti-
mulatory or suppressing effect of low or high sodium intake,
respectively, was blunted. These data point to an already present
but latent defect in renal kallikrein excretion in the borderline
hypertensive patients.

Because kallikrein appears to originate in the renal cortex
near the distal tubule at a site close to the site of renin
formation, an interrelated antagonism between the two enzyme-
systems has been discussed (11).

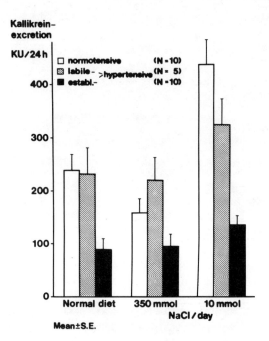

Fig. 2. Effect of different sodium intake on urinary excretion
of kallikrein in patients with borderline and established
hypertension and normotensive controls.

In figure 3, kallikrein excretion is related to plasma renin
activity and plasma aldosterone concentration in normotensives and
established hypertensives. In the normotensives, there was a positive correlation between urinary kallikrein and plasma renin
activity and plasma aldosterone concentration, respectively. Such
a correlation could not be demonstrated in patients with essential
hypertension. These findings suggest that the proposed antagonism
between the renin-angiotensin-aldosterone system and the kallikrein-
kinin system is not present in essential hypertensive patients.
It may therefore be assumed that the absence of the interrelated
modulation between the two enzyme systems in the hypertensive
patients may influence renal hemodynamics.

On a high salt intake PAH-clearance was comparable in the
hypertensive patients and the normotensive controls. However, when
the high salt diet was replaced by a low salt intake, a significantly greater fall in PAH-clearance occurred in the hypertensive
patients than in the normotensive controls, as it is shown in
figure 4.

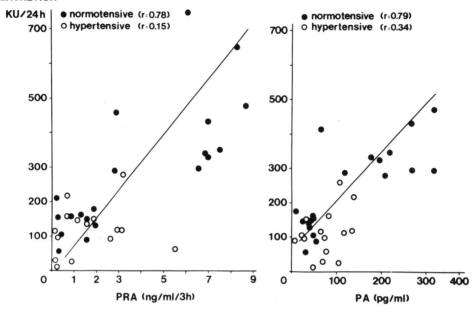

Fig. 3. Relationship between urinary kallikrein excretion and
plasma renin activity (PRA) as well as plasma aldosterone
concentration (PA) in normotensives and patients with
established hypertension.

In the second part of our study the influence of an orally
given dose of kallikrein on blood pressure and urinary kallikrein
excretion was investigated. Following a placebo period of two
weeks, 19 patients with mild to moderate essential hypertension
were treated with 200 kallikrein units (Padutin 100[R]) three times
daily. At the end of the second week, blood pressure had significantly decreased from 160/106 mm Hg to 146/95 mm Hg in the supine
and from 154/107 mm Hg to 142/97 mm Hg in the upright position.
After 8 weeks of therapy there was a further fall in supine and
standing pressure levels to 142/86 mm Hg and 138/94 mm Hg, respectively. Continuation of therapy up to a period of 15 weeks
did not produce any further change in blood pressure. When the
patients, who had responded to therapy, were given placebo again,
blood pressure increased only slowly and reached its pretreatment
level after 2 months (fig. 5).

In 17 patients the relation of the antihypertensive effect
of oral kallikrein to pretreatment levels of urinary kallikrein
excretion was evaluated (fig. 6). It became evident that patients
with markedly reduced urinary kallikrein exhibited after treatment

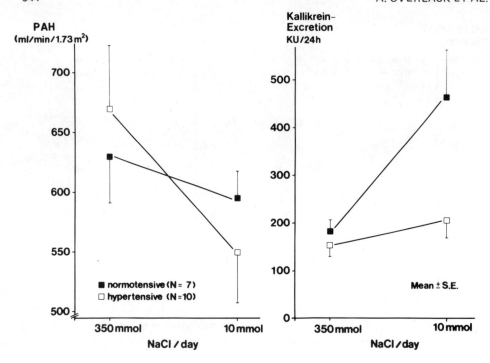

Fig. 4. Relationship between PAH-clearance and urinary kallikrein
excretion in normotensives and patients with established
hypertension on high and low sodium intake.

a more pronounced decrease in arterial pressure than patients
with normal or only slightly reduced kallikrein excretion. Also,
enzyme excretion rate appeared to increase only in the low group,
but not in the normal kallikrein group after 6 weeks of therapy.

There were almost no side-effects, although in one patient
therapy had to be interrupted after 5 days because of diarrhea.
Two patients complained of transitory epigastric pain and two
others of temporary headache.

DISCUSSION

Patients with established essential hypertension excrete
significantly less kallikrein in urine than normotensive persons.
The decrease in urinary kallikrein activity may indicate a defect
in the formation of intrarenally active kinins. If one assumes
that the kallikrein-kinin system functions as a regulator of
renal blood flow, the detection of impaired renal kallikrein
activity in the hypertensive patients would suggest that deficiency
of enzyme activity may be involved in increased vascular resistance,

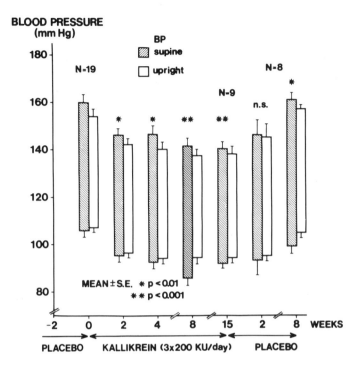

Fig. 5. Blood pressure response to orally given
         kallikrein in 19 patients with established
         essential hypertension.

an alteration that has been proposed to be an important factor
in the genesis of hypertension (6).

The observation that borderline hypertensives exhibited only a
blunted rise in urinary kallikrein excretion after sodium restric-
tion does suggest that deficient enzyme activity may already be
present in the early stage of blood pressure elevation and may
contribute to the development of essential hypertension.

    The mechanisms underlying the blood pressure lowering effect
of orally given kallikrein remain to be elucidated. The drug
appeared to exert its antihypertensive effect only in those
patients who showed a markedly reduced renal kallikrein excretion
and who exhibited a rise in enzyme excretion following treatment.
From these results it is tempting to speculate that the blood
pressure lowering effect was due to a normalization of reduced
renal kallikrein-kinin activity. Interpretation of these
results, however, is tempered by the fact that the number of
patients so far studied is still relatively small.

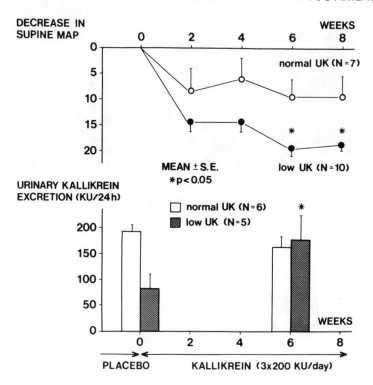

Fig. 6.   Effect of orally administered kallikrein on mean arterial
          blood pressure (MAP) and on urinary kallikrein excretion
          in hypertensive patients with low or normal kallikrein
          excretion.

ACKNOWLEDGEMENTS

     We are indebted to Prof. Haberland and Prof. Pütter for many
helpful suggestions, and to Prof. Fritz for carrying out the bioassay.

     We are grateful for the supply of the purified enzyme and
Padutin 100[R] by Bayer A.G., Fed. Rep. of Germany, and for the
chromogenic substrate supplied by Kabi Ltd. Sweden.

REFERENCES

1.   Abe, K., Seino, M., Sakurai, Y., Irokawa, N., Miyazaki, S.,
     Yasujima, M., Chiba, S., Saito, K., Otsuka, Y., Yoshinaga,
     K.: Studies on urinary kallikrein and kinin in essential
     hypertension. In: Kininogenases 4, Haberland, G.L., Rohen,
     J.W., Suzuki, T. (ed.), Stuttgart-New York: Schattauer
     1977, p. 351 ff.

2. Amundsen, E., Pütter, J., Friberger, P., Claeson, G.: Methods for the determination of glandulary kallikrein by means of a chromogenic tripeptide substrate, in press.

3. Barraclough, M.A., Mills, I.H.: Effect of bradykinin on renal function. Clin. Sci. 28: 69, (1965).

4. Carretero, O.A., Scicli, A.G.: Renal kallikrein: its localization and possible role in renal function. Fed. Proc. 35: 194 (1976).

5. Frey, E.K., Draut, K., Werle, E., Vogel, R., Zickgraf-Rüdel, G., Trautschold, I.: Das Kallikrein-Kinin-System und seine Inhibitoren. Stuttgart, Ferdinand Enke Verlag, 1968.

6. Guyton, A.C., Coleman, T.G., Cowley, A.W., Scheel, K.W., Manning, R.D., Norman, R.A.: Arterial pressure regulation. Overriding dominance of the kidneys in long-term regulation and in hypertension. Amer. J. Med. 52: 584, (1972).

7. Levy, S.B., Lilley, J.J., Frigon, R.P., Stone, R.A.: Urinary kallikrein and plasma renin activity as determinants of renal blood flow. The influence of race and dietary sodium intake. J. Clin. Invest. 60: 129, (1977).

8. Margolius, H.S., Horwitz, D., Pisano, J.J., Keiser, H.R.: Urinary kallikrein excretion in hypertensive man. Relationship to sodium intake and sodium-retaining steroids. Circ. Res. 35: 820, (1974).

9. Nustad, K., Vaaje, K., Pierce, J.V.: Synthesis of kallikreins by rat kidney slices. Brit. J. Pharmacol. 53: 229, (1975).

10. Willis, L.R., Ludens, J.H., Hook, J.B., Williamson, H.E.: Mechanism of natriuretic action of bradykinin. Amer. J. Physiol. 217: 1, (1969).

11. Wong, P.Y., Talamo, R.C., Williams, G.H., Colman, R.W.: Response of the kallikrein-kinin and renin-angiotensin systems to saline infusion and upright posture. J. Clin. Invest. 55: 691, (1975).

A CLINICAL STUDY ON URINARY KALLIKREIN IN PATIENTS WITH RENAL
DISEASES

Kaname Kimura, Kogo Onodera* Yasuburo Oike, Hideaki
Yamabe, Hiroo Numahata, Kinihiko Kikuchi and Shigeko
Hanada
The 2nd Dept. of Internal Medicine*, Hirosaki Univ.
School of Medicine, Hirosaki, Japan. 5 Zaifucho,
Hirosaki, Aomori Prefecture, Japan

ABSTRACT

The urinary kallikrein activity (KA) was measured to investigate
its significance in the renal diseases by using tosyl-arginine
methyl ester (TAME) as a substrate.

The examinees were 94 patients with renal diseases and 25
normal persons.

The daily urinary kallikrein excretion (KE, KE=KAxdaily urinary
volume) is less in chronic glomerulonephritis and outstandingly
less in chronic renal failure than in the normal controls. The KE
also shows a positive correlation moderately to 15-min PSP excretion
and relatively to creatinine clearance. KE is closely related to
renal function and decreases with the degree of renal damage.

KA has no relation to the concentration of urine protein, but
it was parallel, in general, to the urokinase activity.

In nephrotic syndrome, KA tends to show a negative correlation
to the urinary α_1-antitrypsin.

α_1-antitrypsin may have a function as an inhibitor to the
urinary kallikrein.

INTRODUCTION

Kallikrein-kinin system is considered as one of the regulatory factors in an organism, and is researched physiologically and pathophysiologically for its function. Urinary kallikrein is proved to be different from plasma kallikrein, and has similarities to the renal kallikrein in its properties.

From these studies, the origin of urinary kallikrein is considered to be the kidney.

Studies on the urinary kallikrein in patients with renal diseases are few. We measured the urinary kallikrein in patients with renal diseases, and investigated the significance in renal diseases.

MATERIALS AND METHODS

Ninety-four patients with renal diseases were studied (55 males and 39 females: mean age 31.8, range 16 -56 years). There were 56 patients with nephrotic syndrome (19 with acute stage, 37 with non-acute stage), 17 with chronic glomerulonephritis, 21 with renal failure (9 with dialysis, 12 without dialysis). In these patients, blood pressure was controlled within normal range, but in renal failure blood pressure was not stable. The patients with heavy heamaturia, urinary tract infection and diabetes mellitus, were omitted.

The controls were 25 healthy persons (19 males and 6 females; mean age 28.6, range 18-40 years). As test material, dialysed urine collected for 24 hours with toluene was used. Before measurement, the test material was dialysed against running water for 6 hours and then against distilled water for 2 hours.

Urinary kallikrein activity was measured by the fluorometric method of Matsuda (1) using tosyl-arginine methyl ester (TAME as a substrate.

As shown in Fig. 1, we added a little modification. Fluorometric density was measured as calculation of free methanol (n mole/min/ml). Urokinase activity was measured by fibrin plate method. α_1-antitrypsin and α_2-macroglobulin were measured by immunodiffusion method (M-Partigen, Gehringwerke). As a renal function, 15-min PSP excretion and creatinine clearance were used, and serum urea nitrogen and creatine were measured as parallel.

```
              0.1 M Phosphate Buffer (pH 8.0)        0.1 ml
                │  5 mM TAME                          0.1 ml
                │  "Dialysed Urine"                   0.2 ml
              30°C, 90 min, Incubation
                │  10% (v/v) HClO₄                    0.2 ml
                │  0.2%(v/v) KMnO₄                     0.2 ml
                │  0.2%(v/v) NH₂OH HCl                 0.2 ml
                │  0.2%(v/v) Acetylacetone
                │     in 0.5 M Ammonium Malate
                │              (pH 6.0)  3.0 ml
              56°C, 10 min, Incubation
              Fluorometry
                  Wave Length at Extinction: 410 nm
                  Wave Length at Emission:   510 nm
```

Figure 1. Fluorometric Method for Kallikrein Activity.

RESULTS

Influence of urokinase activity to this method: In human urine, urokinase which has esterase activity is excreted, so, we must consider the influence of urokinase to this method. As shown in Table 1, urokinase activity which is generally excreted in urine of healthy persons, had no influence on the kallikrein activity in this method. The data measured by this method might show almost all urinary kallikrein activity.

Urinary kallikrein in patients with renal diseases: Daily urinary kallikrein excretion (KE) in renal diseases is shown in Table 2. Average value of daily urinary excretion is 98.7 ± 68.6 KU/day in healthy persons, 86.0 ± 90.7 KU/day in nephrotic syndrome (acute stage), 68.0 ± 74.0 KU/day in nephrotic syndrome (non-acute stage), 42.7 ± 34.5 KU/day in chronic glomerulonephritis, 8.0 ± 13.3 KU/day in renal failure without dialysis and 1.3 ± 2.6 KU/day in renal failure with dialysis. Kallikrein excretion was significantly decreased in patients with chronic glomerulonephritis and renal failure compared with that in normal subjects.

Relation between KE and renal function: As shown in Figures 2 and 3, the exretion of KE in renal diseases positively correlated to the values of 15-min PSP test ($r = 0.48$, $P < 0.01$), and relatively correlated to the values of creatinine clearance ($r = 0.32$, $0.02 <$

TABLE 1.   FIBRINOLYTIC ACTIVITY (LYSIS AREA)
                  AND ESTEROLYTIC ACTIVITY OF UROKINASE

Ploug Unit/ml	5	10	20	30	40
Fibrinolytic Activity (mm^2/18 hr)	126	210	320	372	510
Esterolytic Activity (nmole/min/ml)	N.D.	N.D.	N.D.	N.D.	N.D.

N.D. = Not Detectable

TABLE 2.   DAILY URINARY KALLIKREIN IN PATIENTS
                  WITH RENAL DISEASES

		Case	Kallikrein (KU/day)
Control		25	98.7 ± 68.6
Nephrotic Syndrome	Acute Stage	19	86.0 ± 90.7
	Latent Stage	37	68.0 ± 74.0
	Total	56	74.0 ± 79.4
Chronic Glomerulonephritis		17	42.7 ± 34.5
Chronic Renal Failure	Hemodialy (−)	12	8.0 ± 13.3
	Hemodialy (+)	9	1.3 ± 2.6
	Total	21	5.3 ± 10.7

P<0.05). This result suggested the interrelationship between KE
and renal function. Then we observed the relationship between KA
and urinary protein, in each group of the same degree of 15-min
PSP test. As shown in Fig. 4, there was no significant difference
of KA by concentration of urinary protein in the same degree of
15-min PSP.

Correlation between kallikrein activity (KA) and urokinase activity:
It is generally said that the origin of urokinase is the kidney
and urokinase activity decreases with the decrease of renal function,
so the correlation of KU and KA was examined. As shown in Fig. 5,
positive correlation was generally obtained in renal diseases
except in nephrotic syndrome with acute stage and in renal failure.
In renal failure, both urokinase and KA are very low, thus, the
correlation might not be obtained. In nephrotic syndrome with
acute stage, no correlation was obtained. This might suggest the
influence of the urinary kallikrein inhibitor excreted with the
urinary protein.

The inhibitor of urinary kallikrein: There are many studies on plasma
kallikrein inhibitor, and α_1-antitrypsin as well as α_2-macroglobulin
are known as inhibitory factors of plasma kallikrein. But the
studies on urinary kallikrein inhibitor are few. As shown in Fig.
6, negative correlation was obtained in nephrotic syndrome between
KA and α_1-antitrypsin (r = -0.45, 0.05>P>0.10). But no correlation
was obtained between KA and α_2-macroglobulin as shown in Fig. 7.

Excretory pattern of KE in patients with renal diseases: Excretory
pattern of KE in 15 renal diseases, whose clinical feature changed
rapidly, were illustrated. As shown in Figures 8 and 9, excretory
pattern changed every moment in those patients whose clinical feature changed rapidly, but in patients with relatively fixed state,
KU was relatively constant.

                              DISCUSSION

     Urinary kallikrein was first reported by Frey in 1926 as a
hypotensive substance in urine. (2). Recently, the origin of
urinary kallikrein is considered to be the kidney from many experiments. (3,4,5,6). For studying the significance of urinary
kallikrein in patients with renal diseases, we measured urinary
kallikrein using tosyl-arginine methyl ester as a substrate.
According to the report of Seino, (7) this method is in good
correlation to bioassay test and the kininogenase activity estimated
by the radioimmunoassay of kinin. In this method, we must consider
the influence of other esterolytic enzymes in urine such as urokinase, but there was no significant influence of urokinase activity
contained in normal human urine. So this method is suitable for
measuring the human urinary kallikrein.

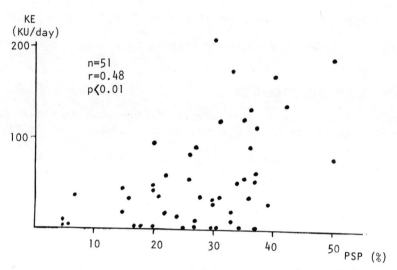

Figure 2.   Correlation between kallikrein excretion (KE) and 15-
            minute PSP excretion in patients with renal diseases.

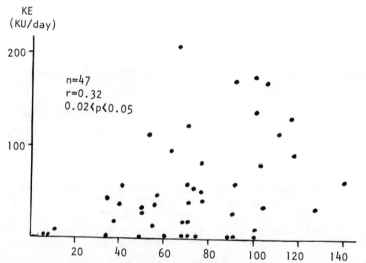

Figure 3.   Correlation between kallikrein excretion (KE) and Ccr
            in patients with renal diseases.

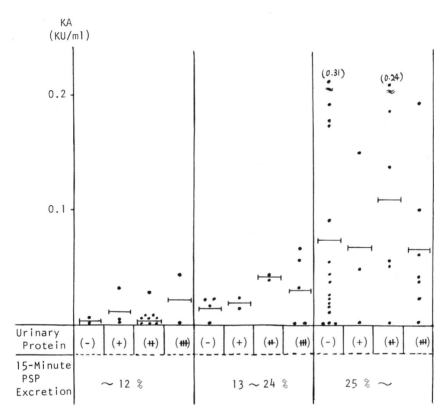

Figure 4.　Kallikrein activity and urinary protein by PSP groups.

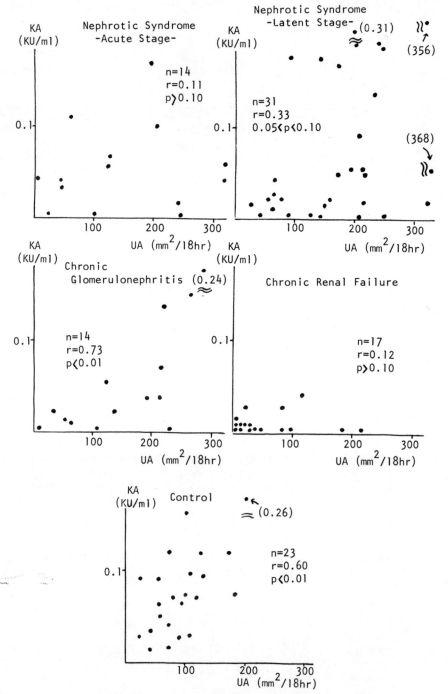

Figure 5.   Correlation between kallikrein activity (KA) and
Urokinase activity (UA) in patients with renal diseases.

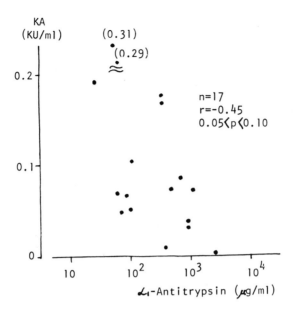

Figure 6.   Correlation between kallikrein activity and α_1-anti-
trypsin in nephrotic syndrome urine in logarithmic
expression

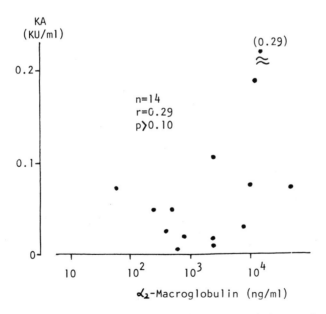

Figure 7.   Correlation between kallikrein activity and α_2-macro-
globulin in nephrotic syndrome urine in logarithmic
expression.

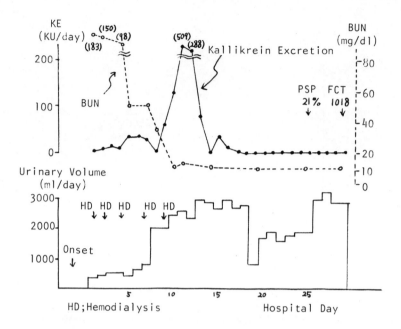

Figure 8.   CASE 1: 45 year old male.   Acute renal failure due to
DIC in a case with acute cholecystitis

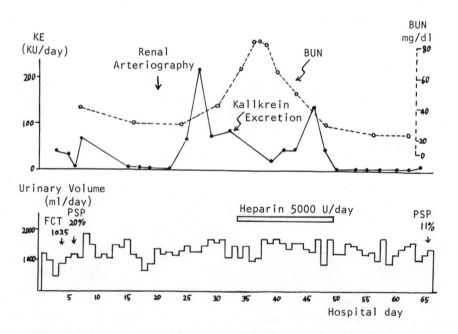

Figure 9.   CASE 2: 46 year old male. Chronic glomerulonephritis.

In patients with renal diseases, the kallikrein excretion was significantly decreased in chronic glomerulonephritis and renal failure compared with that in normal subjects. These data might indicate that KE depends upon the renal function. The KE in renal diseases correlated moderately to 15-min PSP excretion and relatively to creatinine clearance. Recently, the existance of urinary kallikrein was reported to be from the distal portion of renal tubules. KE may decrease with the damage of kidney and is not influenced by the concentration of urinary protein. The origin of urokinase is said to be renal tubulus, and is excreted in urine. The correlation between urokinase and KA was generally observed in patients with renal diseases, but not in nephrotic syndrome with acute stage and renal failure. Inhibitor of plasma kallikrein is studied, but the reports of urinary kallikrein inhibitor are few. In our report, Ka tended to show a negative correlation to urinary α_1-antitrypsin (8), and this might suggest that α_1-antitrypsin has a function as an inhibitor to the urinary kallikrein.

KE excretion of six cases with various renal diseases were continuously observed from the acute stage to the recovery stage. No definite tendency was found in the excretory pattern of KE, but in the fixed stage KE was excreted constantly in the same degree.

REFERENCES

1. Matsuda, Y. et al, 1976. Fluometric method for kallikrein-like arginine esterases. J. Biochem., 79: 1197-1200.
2. Frey, E.K., 1926. Zusammenhänge zwischen Herzarbeit und Nierentätigkeit, 50 Tagung der Deut. Ges. Chir. Arch. Klin. Chir. 142: 663-669.
3. Nustard, K., 1976. The relationship between kidney and urinary kininogenase. Br. J. Pharma. 39: 73-86.
4. Nustard, K. and Vaaje, K., 1976. Synthesis of kallikreins by rat kidney slices. Br. J. Pharmac., 53: 229-234.
5. Carretero, O.A. and Scicli A.G., 1976. Renal kallikrein; its localization and possible role in renal function. Fed. Proc., 35: 194-198.
6. Orstabik, T.A., Nustard, K., Brandtzaeg, P. and Pierce, J.V. 1976. Cellular origin of urinary kallikreins. J. Histochem. Cytochem., 24: 1037-1039.
7. Masahide, Seino et al., 1978. Studies of Urinary Kallikrein in Patients with VariousTypes of Hypertension (Relationship to Renin-Angiotensin-Aldosterone System). Japanese J. Nephrology. 20: 877.
8. Fritz, H. et al., 1969. Zur Identität des Progressiv-Antikallikre kreins mit α_1-Antitrypsin aus Humanserum. Hoppe-Seylers Z. Physiol. Chem., 350: 1551-1555.

INTERACTION BETWEEN ARTERIAL PRESSURE AND VASOACTIVE HORMONES IN THE RELEASE OF RENAL KALLIKREIN

Ivor H. Mills, Pamela A. Newport and Leonard F.O. Obika

Department of Medicine, University of Cambridge

Addenbrooke's Hospital, Cambridge CB2 2QQ, England

INTRODUCTION

Urinary kallikrein closely resembles renal kallikrein (Nustad, 1970). Labelled glandular kallikrein is largely destroyed before being excreted in the urine (Mills et al, 1975). The excretion of kallikrein in the urine, therefore, reflects the release of renal kallikrein from its inactive precursor.

The physiological control of renal kallikrein release has been studied in a series of experiments on dogs.

MATERIALS AND METHODS

The studies were all carried out on dogs anaesthetized with sodium pentobarbitone. Both ureters were catheterised and the left renal artery was cleared without denervation for injection of drugs, measurement of renal artery pressure or application of a constriction to the artery.

Infusions of inulin and para-aminohippurate (PAH) were given for clearance determination and measurements were made by an auto-analyser technique. Sodium and potassium were determined by Eppendorf flame photometer, chloride by a chloride titrator (Radiometer Copenhagen) and osmolality by freezing point depression.

Kallikrein was measured by its esterase activity as described by Mills and Obika (1977a). It depends upon the release of (^{3}H) methanol from the synthetic substrate p-tosyl-L-arginine-(^{3}H) methyl ester ((^{3})TAMe). One esterase unit is equivalent to the hydrolysis of 4.8 μmole (^{3}H)TAMe per hour at pH 8.5 and 37°C.

The results are given as the mean ± its standard error.

RESULTS

The Effect of Changes in Renal Artery Pressure

This was studied by Bevan et al (1974). Decrease in renal artery pressure lowered the excretion of kallikrein and release of renal artery constriction raised the kallikrein excretion. There was a very high correlation between the renal artery pressure measured beyond the point of constriction and the rate of kallikrein excretion per minute: r was between 0.685 and 0.824 in a series of experiments and p < 0.001 in each case. The changes in kallikrein excretion and in sodium excretion were significantly correlated, p < 0.01. The changes in urinary osmolality were negatively correlated with kallikrein excretion, p < 0.001.

The Effect of Vasodilators

The infusion of a variety of vasodilators directly into the renal artery is associated with an increase in kallikrein excretion and sodium excretion: in many cases there is also a decrease in urinary osmolality.

Substance P is natriuretic when infused into the renal artery, down to a dose of 1 ng per min (Mills et al, 1974; Macfarlane et al, 1974b). At this dose the increase in kallikrein excretion was not statistically significant but it was highly significant when 10 ng per min was infused. The increase in PAH and inulin clearances and fall in urinary osmolality were highly significant (Table 1).

Larger doses of substance P lose their natriuretic effect. At 1 μg per min there was consistently a fall in blood pressure (-16.6 ± 1.5 mmHg, p < 0.001), a rise in packed cell volume (3.3 ± 0.38, p < 0.001) and no significant change in sodium or water excretion. However, the changes in the latter two were always highly correlated with the excretion of kallikrein (Macfarlane et al, 1974c).

Prostaglandin E$_1$ is also natriuretic at very low doses when given into the renal artery in the dog (Mills and Obika, 1977a); 1 ng per min increased the excretion of kallikrein and sodium but was insufficient to lower the urinary osmolality.

TABLE 1. Changes (±S.E.) produced by substance P infusions

	1 ng.min^{-1} (N = 12)	10 ng.min^{-1} (N = 13)	100 ng.min^{-1} (N = 12)
C_{PAH} (ml..min^{-1})	2.0 ± 2.6	5.2 ± 1.7	17.1 ± 5.9
p	N.S.	< 0.01	< 0.02
C_{in} (ml..min^{-1})	2.0 ± 2.0	5.1 ± 1.6	6.7 ± 4.0
p	N.S.	< 0.01	N.S.
Urine flow (ml..min^{-1})	0.06 ± 0.08	0.70 ± 0.13	1.69 ± 0.28
p	N.S.	< 0.001	< 0.001
Osmolality (m-osmole.kg^{-1})	-355 ± 78	-266 ± 4	-120 ± 56
p	< 0.001	< 0.001	N.S.
Sodium excretion (μ-equiv.min^{-1})	8.3 ± 2.9	80.4 ± 16.0	129.2 ± 19.2
p	< 0.02	< 0.001	< 0.001
Kallikrein (m-E.U..min^{-1})	29 ± 31	127 ± 33	218 ± 55
p	N.S.	< 0.005	< 0.005

N = number of collection periods

After Macfarlane et al, 1974b

At 10 ng per min the effect was greater (see Table 2), the urinary osmolality fell, the renal plasma flow rose and the inulin clearance increased.

Bradykinin increases the excretion of both kallikrein and sodium and these are highly correlated (Mills et al, 1976). A dose of 100 ng per min into the renal artery increased sodium and kallikrein excretion and lowered urinary osmolality (Table 2) (Mills and Obika, 1977b).

Eledoisin is a vasodilator which is not associated with release of renal prostaglandin (Dressler et al, 1975). However, it has a similar effect to the other vasodilators in increasing sodium and kallikrein excretion in a dosage of 20 ng per min (Table 2). It does not lower urinary osmolality (Mills and Obika, 1977b).

Isoprenaline produces sodium retention when given intravenously but when given into the renal artery at a dose of 100 ng per min it caused natriuresis and increased kallikrein excretion (Table 2)

TABLE 2. The effect of vasodilators intra-arterially
on sodium and kallikrein excretion in the dog[a]

Drug and dose		Control	Experimental
Prostaglandin E_1	Sodium	63.9 ± 1.9	122.5 ± 1.9**
10 ng/min	Kallikrein	137 ± 2.4	196 ± 11.6****
	Osmolality	1280 ± 21	970 ± 50*
Bradykinin	Sodium	8.8 ± 0.35	18.5 ± 0.94**
100 ng/min	Kallikrein	120 ± 1.0	151 ± 4.6*
	Osmolality	1132 ± 10	901 ± 66*
Eledoisin	Sodium	82.1 ± 1.6	98.8 ± 4.7***
20 ng/min	Kallikrein	182 ± 6.9	210 ± 1.5****
	Osmolality	1222 ± 19	1128 ± 28*****
Isoprenaline	Sodium	86.9 ± 2.9	129.7 ± 2.1**
100 ng/min	Kallikrein	212 ± 7.3	268 ± 11.3**
	Osmolality	875 ± 15	698 ± 8**
Dopamine	Sodium	67.7 ± 3.5	111.6 ± 6.4*
5 µg/min	Kallikrein	183 ± 11.3	245 ± 3.0*
	Osmolality	1366 ± 73	1389 ± 33*****
After α and β	Sodium	96.9 ± 1.6	125.7 ± 49*
blockade	Kallikrein	172 ± 1	193 ± 3.1*
	Osmolality	773 ± 13	676 ± 15*
Acetylcholine	Sodium	67.6 ± 15.6	309.3 ± 19.5*
10 µg/min	Kallikrein	168 ± 45	407 ± 67**
	Osmolality	1724 ± 17	787 ± 58**

[a] The values represent mean ± S.E. values for sodium
as µ.equiv./min and kallikrein as milliesterase units/min

* $p < 0.01$;   ** $p < 0.001$;   *** $p < 0.05$;
**** $p < 0.005$;   ***** N.S.

(Mills et al, 1978b). A significant fall in urinary osmolality also
occurred.

Acetyl choline in highly unphysiological doses intra-arterially
also caused natriuresis, increased kallikrein excretion (Table 2) and
lowering of urinary osmolality (Mills et al, 1978b).

Dopamine differs from other vasodilators in two respects.   In

large enough doses the α-adrenergic action overcomes the renal
vasodilating effect of the dopaminergic receptor stimulation
(Mills and Obika, 1976). Secondly, although at 1 and 5 µg per min
intra-arterially it increases sodium and kallikrein excretion, it
does not lower urinary osmolality until its α-adrenergic action is
antagonised with phentolamine (Table 2).

The Effect of Vasoconstrictors

Angiotensin when infused into the renal artery at 0.1 or
1.0 µg per min caused decreased sodium excretion (Klein et al,
1971). At doses of 5 or 10 µg per min it is natriuretic after the
first 10 min (Klein et al, 1971; Macfarlane et al, 1974a; Mills
et al, 1978a). When sodium retention occurred in the first ten
minutes of infusion a fall in kallikrein excretion was seen: when
natriuresis occurred there was a correlated rise in kallikrein
excretion (Macfarlane et al, 1974a; Mills and Newport, 1978)
(Table 3).

Noradrenaline when given intra-arterially at 10 ng per min
produces a small natriuresis and increased kallikrein excretion.
However, on stopping the infusion the responses both became
greater (Mills and Obika, 1977c). When prostaglandin synthesis was
inhibited no significant response to noradrenaline occurred either
during the infusion or after stopping it. However, the urinary
osmolality fell before prostaglandin synthesis was inhibited with
indomethcain whereas after inhibition the noradrenaline caused a
highly significant rise in urinary osmolality (Table 4).

TABLE 3. The effect of angiotensin intra-arterially on
sodium and kallikrein excretion and urinary osmolality
and with renal artery pressure lowered 5-10 mmHg
(Units as in Table 1)

Drug and dose		Control	Experimental
Angiotensin	Sodium	43.2 ± 7.5	192.2 ± 19.1
5 µg/min	Kallikrein	171 ± 19	306 ± 19
	Osmolality	1055 ± 208	455 ± 29
With renal	Sodium	15.2 ± 1.5	7.0 ± 1.3
artery pressure	Kallikrein	52.6 ± 5.0	26.5 ± 5.5
85-90 mmHg	Osmolality	963 ± 74	1093 ± 103

* p < 0.001;   ** p < 0.005;   *** N.S.

After Mills and Newport, 1978

TABLE 4. Effects of infusion of 10 ng min^{-1} noradrenaline intra-arterially (mean ± S.E.) left kidney only (Units as in Table 1)

Urinary excretion	Without PGE inhibition			After PGE synthesis inhibition		
	C	E	R	C	E	R
Kallikrein (m-esterase u.min^{-1})	199 ± 6	207 ± 7	243*** ± 9	151 ± 3	150 ± 6	150 ± 4
Sodium (μequiv min^{-1})	108 ± 3	126* ± 6	148*** ± 3	121 ± 2	119 ± 3	115 ± 8
Urinary osmolality (m-osmole kg^{-1})	643 ± 5	592* ± 22	495*** ± 31	1138 ± 41	1357*** ± 33	1363*** ± 4

C = control, E = experimental, R = recovery
* $p < 0.05$; *** $p < 0.001$

Noradrenaline superimposed upon angiotensin reverses the natriuretic effect of 5 µg per min of the latter drug. It does so in doses of 1 µg per min (Mills et al, 1978a; Mills et al, 1978b) and in 2 µg per min. In the latter studies, not only was the natriuresis reversed but the elevated kallikrein excretion was also decreased (Mills and Newport, 1979) (Table 5).

The Effect of Reduced Renal Artery Pressure

When bradykinin was infused at 100 ng per min and the renal artery pressure was lowered to 85-90 mmHg, there was no natriuresis and no increase in kallikrein excretion (Mills and Obika, 1977b).

The renal artery pressure was lowered by 5-10 mmHg while angiotensin was infused at 5 µg per min intra-arterially. There was decreased sodium and kallikrein excretion and no significant change in urinary osmolality (Mills and Newport, 1978) (Table 3).

DISCUSSION

Although all the vasodilators tested have produced a natriuresis and an increased excretion of kallikrein, they probably do not all operate in the same way. In the rat intra-aortic infusion of substance P at 50 pg per min above the renal arteries produced a natriuresis, increased urine flow and decreased reabsorption in the proximal tubule, as assessed by micropuncture. There was no increase in renal plasma flow, inulin clearance or the pressures in the various vascular and tubular lumina. It seems possible, therefore, that substance P might release kallikrein

TABLE 5. The effect of 5 µg per min angiotensin alone
and angiotensin plus 2 µg per min noradrenaline i.a.
(Units as in Table 1)

Drug and dose		Control		Experimental	
Angiotensin	Sodium	44.4 ±	9.3	189 ±	47.6***
5 µg/min i.a.	Kallikrein	45 ±	3.6	96 ±	20.3*
	Osmolality	1410 ±	143	415 ±	117**
Angiotensin 5 µg/min	Sodium			† 44.4 ±	15.5***
plus noradrenaline	Kallikrein			† 43 ±	8.7*
2 µg/min i.a.	Osmolality			†496 ±	119****

† p values for comparison with angiotensin 5 µg/min
alone in the same dog

* p < 0.01; ** p < 0.001; *** p < 0.005; **** N.S.

directly.   Since the peptide also stimulates salivary secretion
which is associated with a fall in glandular kallikrein (Gautvick
et al, 1972) and caused nasal secretion, which is a kallikrein
related process (Eccles and Wilson, 1973), the effect of high doses
of substance P may be due to generalised stimulation of kallikrein
release.   The effects on blood pressure and vascular permeability
closely resemble the effects seen with kallikrein infusions
(Macfarlane et al, 1973).

The effect of prostaglandin E_1 in releasing kallikrein into
the urine is of particular interest.   The natriuretic action of
prostaglandin may be due to kallikrein release.   The lowering of
urinary osmolality may not be a direct effect of the infused
prostaglandin E_1 but may be due to prostaglandin E_2 released in
the medulla in response to the (lysyl-) bradykinin (McGiff et al,
1972) released by the kallikrein.

The effect of dopamine is blocked by haloperidol (Mills and
Obika, 1976) which blocks the specific dopamine receptors in the
renal vessels.   This is known to involve the activation of
adenylate cyclase which must is some way lead to the release of
kallikrein.   In the case of bradykinin it seems clear that lowering
renal arterial pressure abolishes the release of kallikrein.   It
does so also in the case of natriuretic doses of angiotensin (Mills
and Newport, 1978).   In both situations the pressure change
per se is of importance in the release of kallikrein.   The
natriuretic dose of angiotensin must normally cause some kallikrein
to be released into the interstitial fluid (de Bono and Mills, 1974).
The kinin released would then make the renal vessels resistant to
angiotensin and as the blood pressure rises, the direct pressure
stimulation of further kallikrein release (Bevan et al, 1974) would
produce the rise in urinary kallikrein and the related natriuresis.

Precisely how eledoisin, isoprenaline and acetyl choline cause
release of kallikrein is not clear but they could all do so in
response to the pressure change in the renal vessels as a result of
vasodilatation.

The inhibiting effect of noradrenaline on the natriuretic
action of angiotensin might be a direct pressure effect as a result
of afferent arteriolar constriction but it is perhaps more likely
that it acts to inhibit the release of kallikrein by the PGE
released by angiotensin, as suggested by Mills et al (1978a).   The
natriuretic action of very low doses of noradrenaline is clearly
due to the prostaglandin it releases since it is blocked by
indomethacin.   The greater kallikrein release after stopping
noradrenaline, as well as from the right kidney during the infusion
(Mills and Obika, 1977c) (the concentration of noradrenaline
reaching the right kidney must be lower than that reaching the left),
is in support of the view that noradrenaline has two actions, one

to release prostaglandin (in very low doses) at a site where it can stimulate kallikrein release and, secondly, in larger doses, to inhibit the release of kallikrein by prostaglandin.

The mechanisms by which the kallikrein/kinin system facilitates natriuresis are not clearly known but may involve release of natriuretic substances from the kidney itself (for discussion of this see Mills et al, 1978a).

This work was supported by the National Kidney Research Fund and the Medical Research Council. L.F.O.O. was a Junior Research Fellow of the University of Nigeria.

REFERENCES

Bevan, D.R., N.A.A. Macfarlane and I.H. Mills, 1974, The dependence of urinary kallikrein excretion on renal artery pressure, J.Physiol. 241, 34P.

de Bono, E. and I.H. Mills, 1974, Simultaneous increases in kallikrein in renal lymph and urine during saline infusion,J.Physiol.241,127P.

Dressler, W.E., G.V. Rossi and R.F. Orzechowski, 1975, Evidence that renal vasodilation by dopamine in dogs does not involve release of prostaglandin,J.Pharm.Pharmac.27,203.

Eccles,R. and H. Wilson, 1973, A kallikrein-like substance in cat nasal secretion,Brit.J.Pharmacol.49,712.

Gautvik, K.M., K. Nustad and J. Vystyd, 1972, Kininogenase activity in the stimulated submandibular salivary gland in cats, Acta physiol.scand.85,438.

Klein,G.L., I.H. Mills and R.J. Wilson, 1971, Changes in renal function associated with the development of resistance of the renal vasculature to the arterial infusion of angiotensin, J.Physiol.215,43P.

McGiff, J.C., N.A. Terragno, K.U. Malik and A.J. Lonigro, 1972, Release of a prostaglandin E-like substance from canine kidney by bradykinin, Circulation Res.31,36.

Macfarlane, N.A.A., A. Adetuyibi and I.H. Mills, 1974a, Changes in kallikrein excretion during arterial infusion of angiotensin, J.Endocr.61,lxxii.

Macfarlane, N.A.A., I.H. Mills and P.E. Ward, 1974b, The diuretic and natriuretic effects of arterial infusions of substance P and their relationship to kallikrein excretion,J.Physiol.239,28P.

Macfarlane, N.A.A., P.E. Ward and I.H. Mills, 1974c, Kallikrein-like actions of arterial infusion of microgram doses of substance P, J.Endocr.63,40P.

Macfarlane, N.A.A., I.H. Mills and E.P. Wraight, 1973, Increased vascular permeability produced by kallikrein infusions and its enhancement by nephrectomy,J.Physiol.231,45P.

Mills, I.H., N.A.A. Macfarlane and P.E. Ward, 1974, Increase in kallikrein excretion during the natriuresis produced by arterial infusion of substance P,Nature,Lond.247,108.

Mills, I.H., N.A.A. Macfarlane, P.E. Ward and L.F.O. Obika, 1976,
The renal kallikrein-kinin system and the regulation of salt and
water excretion,Fed.Proc.35,181.

Mills, I.H. and P.A. Newport, 1978, The dependence of the natriuretic
and kallikrein responses to intra-arterial angiotensin on renal
artery pressure,J.Physiol.in press.

Mills, I.H. and P.A. Newport, 1979, Inhibition of the natriuretic
and kallikrein response to angiotensin by simultaneous intra-
arterial infusion of noradrenaline,J.Physiol.,in press.

Mills, I.H. and L.F.O. Obika, 1976, The effect of adrenergic and
dopamine-receptor blockade on the kallikrein and renal response
to intra-arterial infusion of dopamine in dogs,J.Physiol.263,150P.

Mills, I.H. and L.F.O. Obika, 1977a, Increased urinary kallikrein
excretion during prostaglandin E_1 infusion in anaesthetized dogs
and its relation to natriuresis and diuresis,J.Physiol.273,459.

Mills, I.H. and L.F.O. Obika, 1977b, Urinary kallikrein excretion
during bradykinin and eledoisin infusions and its relationship
to urinary osmolality,J.Physiol.269,72P.

Mills, I.H. and L.F.O. Obika, 1977c, A novel effect of intrarenal
infusion of a non-vasoconstrictor dose of noradrenaline on renal
function: relationship to renal kallikrein and prostaglandin,
J.Physiol.267,21P.

Mills, I.H., L.F.O. Obika and P.A. Newport, Stimulation of the
renal kallikrein-kinin system by vasoactive substances and its
relationship to the excretion of salt and water, 1978a, in:
Contributions to Nephrology,Vol.12,eds. G.M. Eisenbach and
J. Brod (S. Karger,Basel) p.132.

Mills, I.H., P.E. Ward, N.A.A. Macfarlane and L.F.O. Obika, The role
of renal kallikrein in diuresis and natriuresis, 1978b, in:
Natriuretic Hormone,eds. H.J. Kramer and F. Krück (Springer-Verlag,
Berlin) p.77.

Mills, I.H., C.L. Paterson and P.E. Ward, 1975, The role of the kidney
in the inactivation of injected ^{125}I-kallikrein,J.Physiol.251,281.

Nustad, K., 1970, Relationship between kidney and urinary kininogenase,Br.J.Pharmac.39,73.

BLOOD KININ SYSTEM IN RENAL HYPERTENSIVE PATIENTS

ADMINISTERED WITH SQ 20881

Habib Edery[1], Talma Rosenthal[2], Giora Amitzur[1] and
Naftali Stern[2]

[1]Israel Institute for Biological Research, Ness Ziona
[2]Chaim Sheba Medical Center, Tel Hashomer, Sackler
School of Medicine, Tel Aviv University, Tel Aviv,
Israel

ABSTRACT

The i.v. administration of 0.25 mg/kg SQ 20881 to eight renal
hypertensive patients caused blood pressure fall and in five of
them also reduced heart rate. The latter was attributed to increase in vagal tone. Peripheral and renal blood samples taken at
the nadir of the hypotensive response showed considerable inhibition of plasma kininase activity, rise in free kinin level and reduced kininogen content. This reduction was not due to increased
consumption as shown by in vitro experiments. PGE_2 and PGF_2alpha
levels in kidney blood of three patients remained practically unchanged. Plasma renin activity was augmented to a larger extent
in blood of kidney with stenotic artery than in the one with patent
vessel. It is concluded that the action of SQ 20881 on human blood
kinin system, besides inhibition of kininase, involves also reduction of kininogen, the mechanism of which remains to be clarified.

INTRODUCTION

SQ 20881 (BPP_{9a}) a synthetic nonapeptide drug has been extensively administered for diagnostic purposes including renal artery
stenosis in hypertensive patients (Drayer et al.,1977; Re et al.,
1978; Rosenthal et al., 1978). In the present work the influence
of the drug on the blood kinin system of a number of such patients
has been studied.

SUBJECTS AND METHODS

Eight hypertensive patients (six males and two females) were
included in this study. Renal artery stenosis, either of the left,
right or intrarenal branches was diagnosed in seven subjects and in
one unilateral parenchymal disease. A probing dose of 0.25 mg/kg
SQ 20881 was administered i.v. as a bolus. Blood pressure was
monitored (Arteriosond 1011, Roche, U.S.A.) every 2 min and pulse
rate obtained manually. On the next day both renal arteries of six
patients were catheterized separately for blood sampling and the
injection of SQ 20881 was repeated. In two patients the drug was
administered only once. In all cases peripheral blood samples were
taken from the antecubital vein and in some also from the inferior
vena cava. Sampling was performed before injection of the drug and
at the nadir of the hypotensive response elicited. To prevent arti-
facts, syringes (fitted to siliconized needles), pipettes and tubes
of plastic material were used.

The following determinations were performed: total plasma
kininase activity (Edery and Lewis, 1962) expressed as T_{50} i.e.
time required for disappearance of half the amount of synthetic
bradykinin incubated with 0.2 ml plasma; plasma kininogen (Uchida
and Katori, 1978); blood free kinin (after ethanol extraction and
subsequent evaporation under reduced pressure); kinin activity was
evaluated on isolated rat uterus or sensitized guinea pig ileum
using synthetic bradykinin as standard   (Edery and Grunfeld, 1969).
Plasma renin activity was determined by radioimmunoassay using New
England Nuclear kit and aldosterone as described by Buhler et al.,
1974. In three patients, PGE_2 and PGF_2alpha levels of renal blood
were determined by radioimmunoassay. Results of all these determinations were expressed as mean$\pm$ S.E. and refer to the combined
values obtained for peripheral and renal blood samples, if not
otherwise stated.

SQ 20881 was kindly provided by E. R. Squibb & Sons, Inc.,
Princeton, U.S.A.

RESULTS AND DISCUSSION

In all cases, after administration of SQ 20881 blood pressure
began to fall, nadir occurring within 35 min of injection. Blood
pressure recovered 3-5 h post injection. In five patients the
hypotensive response was accompanied by reduced heart rate. Bradycardia was particularly notable in two patients. One of these also
showed flushing and moderate sweating and the other complained of
nausea and weakness. Heart rate returned to baseline values either
at about the same time as blood pressure recovery or 15-40 min afterwards.

The three parameters of the kinin system examined were greatly affected by the administration of the drug. Plasma kininase activity before and after injection was 10'±42" and 14'54"±1'24" respectively (difference 4'54"±1'12" $p < 0.01$). In addition kininase activity was more inhibited in blood of affected kidneys than in peripheral one. Pre-drug kininogen value (µg BK/ml) was 2.65±0.75 being reduced to 1.34±0.4 after injection (difference 1.31±0.7 $p < 0.05$). In a series of in vitro experiments an attempt was made to see whether or not the kininogen diminution could be due to its increased transformation by SQ 20881. Under the conditions studied the results showed that kininogen underwent partial spontaneous activation but the process was not increased in the presence of the drug. Concomitant to kininase inhibition and kininogen reduction, the free kinin levels were augmented. Pre-and post injection values (ng/ml) were 2.99±0.51 and 9.22±1.74 respectively (difference 6.23±1.65 $p < 0.005$).

Plasma renin activity (ng Ang.I/ml/h) before injection was 8.37±1.89 as compared with 22.94±5.34 post drug (difference 14.57 ±4.31 $p < 0.005$). Furthermore it was noted that plasma renin activity increased more markedly in the kidney with stenotic artery than in the one with patent circulation. Practically no changes in peripheral and renal blood levels of PGE_2 and PGF_2alpha occurred after drug administration. This contrasted with the releasing effect of SQ 20881 in isolated muscle preparations (Edery and Shemesh, 1978a,b).

Aldosterone secretion (ng/dl) before and after drug administration was 44.87±17.8 and 18.6±6.0 respectively, thus showing a considerable reduction.

The present study showed that SQ 20881 elicited the expected blood pressure fall in all cases and in most of them concomitant bradycardia. The mechanism of this latter is difficult to explain. It could be speculated that it originated from increased vagal tone brought about by either (a) direct drug action on neurons regulating vagal activity or (b) reflexly, after stimulation of aortic sensory receptors by accumulated angiotensin. In this regard it has been reported (Ueda et al., 1969) that intra-aortic injection of angiotensin into human subjects caused bradycardia, whereas increase in heart rate occurred when injected into a vertebral artery.

Two factors could be held responsible for the increase in blood free kinin occurring after SQ 20881 administration namely (a) inhibition of kininase and (b) reduction of kininogen. The former effect is readily understood as it has been repeatedly shown that the drug inhibited the angiotensin converting enzyme identified as kininase II (Erdos, 1977), which in the present case must have contributed to the total kininase activity. The kininogen decrease was unexpected. Most likely this reduction stems from its increased conversion to kinin thus raising the latter's blood level. The reduction cannot be attributed to activation of plasma kallikrein and consequent consumption because <u>in vitro</u> experiments were negative in this respect. Neither could it have been the result of hemodilution (Uchida and Katori, 1978) because it was noted that hematocrit values remained virtually unchanged after drug administration. Thence, the mechanism whereby SQ 20881 reduces kininogen remains to be elucidated.

REFERENCES

Buhler, R.F., J.E. Sealey and J.H. Laragh, Radioimmunoassay of plasma aldosterone, 1974, in: Hypertension Manual, ed. J.H. Laragh (Yorke Medical Books, New York) p.655.

Drayer, J.I.M., M.A. Weber, S.A. Atlas and J.H. Laragh, 1977, Phentolamine testing for alpha adrenergic participation in hypertensive patients: independence from renin profiles, Clin. Pharmac. Ther. 22,287.

Edery, H. and Y. Grunfeld, 1969, Sensitization of smooth muscle to plasma kinins: effects of enzymes and peptides on various preparations, Br. J. Pharmac. 35,51.

Edery, H. and G.P. Lewis, 1962, Inhibition of plasma kininase activity at slightly acid pH, Br. J. Pharmac. 19,299.

Edery, H. and M. Shemesh, 1978a, Release of prostaglandins mediating the potentiation of bradykinin by BPF and chymotrypsin in rat isolated ileum, Agents and Actions 8,159.

Edery, H. and M. Shemesh, Interaction of smooth muscle endogenous prostaglandins with kinins-potentiators, 1978b, in: Current concepts in kinin research, eds. G.L. Haberland and U. Hamberg (Pergamon Press, Oxford) in press.

Erdos, E.G., 1977, The angiotensin I converting enzyme, Fed.Proc. 36,1760.

Re, R., R. Novelline, M.T. Escourrou, C. Athanasoulis, J. Burton and E. Haber, 1978, Inhibition of angiotensin-converting enzyme for diagnosis of renal-artery stenosis, N. Eng. J. Med. 298,582.

Rosenthal, T., R. Adar, N. Stern, E. Kissin, E.T. Jacob and Z. Rubinstein, 1978, Use of converting enzyme inhibitor, SQ 20881 for lateralizing renal venous renin activity, Isr. J. Med. Sci. 14,388.

Uchida, Y. and M. Katori, 1978, An improved method for determination of the total kininogen in rabbit and human plasma, Biochem. Pharmac. 27,1463.

Ueda, H., Y. Uchida, K. Ueda, T. Gondaira and S. Katayama, 1969, Centrally mediated vasopressor effect of angiotensin II in man, Jap. Heart J. 10,243.

ISOLATION OF PROKALLIKREIN FROM HUMAN URINE

J. Corthorn, T. Imanari, H. Yoshida, T. Kaizu,
J. V. Pierce, and J. J. Pisano

Section on Physiological Chemistry, Laboratory of
Chemistry, National Heart, Lung, and Blood Institute,
National Institutes of Health, Bethesda, Maryland 20014

INTRODUCTION

During the course of reinvestigating the conditions of the
radiochemical assay for human urinary kallikrein, Dr. Imanari in
our laboratory noted that incubation of urine with trypsin increased
the total kallikrein activity (Corthorn et al., 1977; Pisano et al.,
1978). By means of DEAE-cellulose chromatography he found two nearly
separated peaks of TAME esterase activity: the first was trypsin-
activatable kallikrein and the second was already active kallikrein.
Although our earlier experiments indicated that inactive (or bound)
kallikrein was a proenzyme and not an enzyme-inhibitor complex, our
purest fraction at that time required at least stoichiometric amounts
of trypsin for complete activation. This led us to consider that the
prokallikrein activation peptide was a trypsin inhibitor. Recently,
however, we have succeeded in obtaining more highly purified prokallikrein fractions which require only catalytic amounts of trypsin
for activation. Trypsin activation of prokallikrein purified by
immunoaffinity chromatography yields an enzyme with the same ratio
of biological activity to TAME esterase activity as that found for
the naturally occurring active kallikrein.

METHODS

Assay

Kallikrein was assayed by the radiochemical esterolytic method
described previously by Imanari et al. (1976) which employs [3H]-TAME.
The same method was used to measure prokallikrein after trypsin activation (Table I).

Table I.   ASSAY OF TOTAL KALLIKREIN IN HUMAN URINE

Gel-filtered Urine	10 μl
Tris.HCl Buffer, 0.2 M pH 8.0	30 μl
Trypsin, 1 μg	10 μl

Let stand at R.T. for 20 min

Lima Bean Trypsin Inhibitor, 20 μg	10 μl
[^3H] TAME	10 μl

Incubate 30 min at R.T.

Active kallikrein was determined in the absence
of trypsin and prokallikrein was obtained by
difference.

Purification

Normal male urine was collected over an 8-hr period at room
temperature. Sufficient 25 percent NaN_3 was added periodically to
yield a final concentration of ca 0.025 percent. All subsequent
steps were performed at 4°. Urine was concentrated 100-fold in a
DC-2 Amicon hollow fiber apparatus containing an HIP8 cartridge.
The Tamm-Horsfall glycoprotein was precipitated with sodium chloride
and the supernatant solution was concentrated and desalted in the
DC-2 apparatus. Subsequent steps in the purification included DEAE-
cellulose chromatography, Sephadex G-100 gel filtration, Bio-Gel
A-15m gel filtration in 6M guanidine HCl, hydroxyapatite chromatography, and immunoaffinity chromatography employing urinary kallikrein antibody immobilized on agarose and Ultrogel AcA-44 gel filtration.

RESULTS

Analysis of twenty freshly voided urine samples showed that
prokallikrein constituted 64 ± 3 percent (mean ± SEM) of the total
kallikrein excreted. No sex difference was observed. When normal
male urine previously dialyzed, concentrated, and freed of the Tamm-
Horsfall glycoprotein was chromatographed on a column of DEAE-
cellulose, one peak of prokallikrein, one peak of active kallikrein,
and no other free esterase were observed (Fig. 1). Greater than catalytic amounts of trypsin were required for prokallikrein activation.
When fraction 3a in Figure 1 was fractionated on a hydroxyapatite
column, two trypsin inhibitors were separated from prokallikrein which

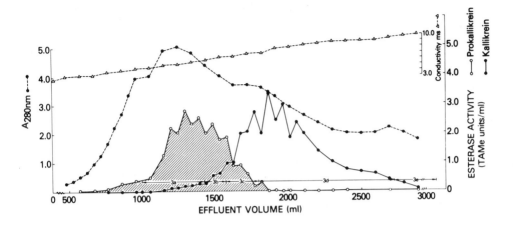

Fig. 1.   DEAE-cellulose chromatography (4°). Column: 5.6 x 26 cm.
Sample: 35,100 A_{280} units; 2,400 ml. Eluents: 3.4 liters
of 0.08 M NaP_i, pH 6.0; 3.0 liters of linear gradient of
0.08 M to 0.35 M NaP_i, pH 6.0. Fraction volume: 9.6 ml.
Flow rate: 60 ml/h.

could now be activated with catalytic amounts of trypsin. Another
aliquot of fraction 3a was used for estimating the molecular weight
on a column of Ultrogel AcA-44. The molecular weight determined for
prokallikrein in fraction 3a was 50,000, and that of kallikrein in
fraction 3d was 37,500. It is interesting to note that in a preliminary observation, kallikrein spontaneously generated from prokallikrein and kallikrein generated by trypsin had molecular weights
very similar to that of the proenzyme.

Although hydroxyapaptite chromatography removed trypsin inhibitors and along with the 6M guanidine HCl column step provided strong
evidence that inactive urinary kallikrein was a proenzyme, the yield
of enzyme from the hydroxyapatite column was only about 30 percent
and the purification only 2-fold. Another aliquot from the DEAE-
cellulose step, fraction 3b, was applied to an experimental column
of monospecific urinary kallikrein antibody immobilized on agarose
(Bio-Gel A-50m). Two prokallikrein fractions, 4b(1) and 4b(2), were
obtained which accounted for 60 percent of the applied proenzyme.
Fraction 4b(1) contained 21 percent of the applied activity, 96
percent of which was prokallikrein, and was 15-fold purified over
fraction 3b. It was further fractionated on a column of Ultrogel
AcA-44. Prokallikrein was purified 1.4-fold (specific activity =
14 TU/A_{280}) in 80 percent yield. Prokallikrein from a peak tube of
the Ultrogel gel filtration could be activated with a catalytic
amount of trypsin (Table II).

Table II. TIME COURSE OF TRYPSIN ACTIVATION[1] OF PROKALLIKREIN:

GENERATION OF TAME ESTERASE AND KININOGENASE ACTIVITIES

Time	Activation[2]	Bioassay[3] TAME Assay
Min	Percent	
15	53	135
30	64	157
60	75	206
120	95	183

[1] 0.025 mol trypsin/mol prokallikrein (M_r=50,000) at pH 8.0 and 25°.

[2] Measured by TAME hydrolysis.

[3] μg Lys-bradykin per min/nmol TAME/min. Purified kallikrein
assayed at 4 levels gave a mean value of 222 (range 187-275).

                              DISCUSSION

     It has been assumed that kallikrein in urine occurs entirely
as the free active enzyme and that the proenzyme is found only in
pancreatic juice (Webster, 1970). Little has been reported on porcine pancreatic prokallikrein (see the review by Nustad et al., 1978)
since it was first announced (Fiedler et al., 1970). Using fluorescent antibodies to rat submandibular kallikrein, Proud et al. (1978)
located prokallikrein in the acini of the rat pancreas.

     Human urinary prokallikrein has been purified by the following
steps: ultrafiltration, salt precipitation of the Tamm-Horsfall
glycoprotein, DEAE-cellulose chromatography hydroxyapatite chromatography, Sephadex G-100 gel filtration and Bio-Gel A-15m gel filtration in 6M guanidine HCl. In view of the very encouraging results
obtained by immunoaffinity chromatography, it appears that in the
future it will be possible to obtain highly purified prokallikrein
in three steps: ultrafiltration, removal of the Tamm-Horsfall glycoprotein and immunoaffinity chromatography. The third step separates
the active enzyme from the proenzyme in high yield. An additional
step(s) will be necessary to obtain a homogeneous preparation.

     All prokallikrein preparations have had detectable free TAME
esterase activity which can be reduced but not totally eliminated
by DFP treatment. Although it is possible that this activity is
inherent in the proenzyme, contamination with an activating enzyme

is likely, since esterase activity always increases as the prokallikrein samples age. Reactivation after DFP treatment could occur
during the assay which is very sensitive and able to detect traces
of activity. The proenzyme is not activated by urinary kallikrein,
plasmin, urokinase, acid treatment or 6M guanidine HC1. Trypsin
is very effective; thus, it seems likely that a trypsin-like enzyme
is the physiological activator.

The trypsin-activated proenzyme was indistinguishable from the
active enzyme isolated from urine in its ability to hydrolyze TAME
and release kinin from human kininogen. Studies are in progress to
further purify and characterize the proenzyme. Knowledge of factors
controlling its synthesis, excretion and activation are especially
relevant to understanding the pathophysiological significance of
renal kallikrein.

We gratefully acknowledge the expert technical assistance of
Kerin N. Yates and Patricia F. Highet.

REFERENCES

Corthorn, J, Imanari, T., Yoshida, H., Kaizu, T., Pierce, J., and
    Pisano, J., 1977, Inactive kallikrein in human urine, Fed. Proc.
    (Abs.), 36:893.
Fiedler, F., Hirschauer, C., and Werle, E., 1970, Enrichment of Pre-
    kallikrein B from Swine Pancreas and Properties of Different
    Forms of Pancreatic Kallikrein, Hoppe-Seyler's Physiol. Chem.,
    351:225.
Imanari, T., Kaizu, T., Yoshida, H., Yates, K., Pierce, J. V., and
    Pisano, J. J., 1976, Radiochemical Assays for Human Urinary,
    Salivary, and Plasma Kallikreins, in: "Chemistry and Biology
    of the Kallikrein-Kinin System in Health and Disease,"
    J. J. Pisano and K. F. Austen, eds., U. S. Government Printing
    Office, Washington, D. C.
Nustad, K., Orstavik, T. B., Gautvik, K. M., and Pierce, J. V., 1978,
    Glandular Kallikreins, Gen. Pharmac., 9:1.
Pisano, J. J., Corthorn, J., Yates, K., and Pierce, J. V., 1978,
    The Kallikrein-Kinin System in the Kidney, Contr. Nephrol.,
    12:116.
Proud, D., Bailey, G. S., Orstavik, T. B., and Nustad, K., 1977,
    The Location of Prekallikrein in the Rat Pancreas, Biochem.
    Soc. Trans. 5:1402.
Webster, M. E., 1970, Kallikreins in Glandular Tissues, in "Handbook
    of Experimental Pharmacology XXV," E. G. Erdos and A. F. Wilde,
    eds., Springer-Verlag, New York.

POTENTIATION OF BRADYKININ BY A FACTOR PRESENT IN THE SALIVARY

GLAND OF THE RAT

R.A.S. Santos, J.R. Cunha Melo, I.F. Heneine, Namir S. Lauar and W.T. Beraldo

Department of Physiology and Biophysics, Institute of Biological Sciences, UFMG, Brazil
Av. Alfredo Balena, 190

In the course of experiments on the effect of scorpion toxin on the secretion of kallikrein by parotid and submandibular gland of rats, it was observed that saliva of these glands, besides the ability to cause contraction of the isolated rat uterus had a strong potentiating effect upon the contractions elicited by bradykinin. A similar potentiation was observed when the saliva was collected by stimulation with pilocarpine and isoproterenol or when submandibular and parotid glands extract of non-treated rats were tested.

This paper is an attempt to isolate this factor and study its chemical and pharmacological properties.

MATERIAL AND METHODS

As submandibular gland presented a potentiating activity about 1000 times greater than that found in the parotid it was decided to use submandibular gland extract for isolation of the bradykinin potentiating factor.

Male Wistar rats (180 to 200 g) were used. The glands were homogenized in 0.15 M NaCl and centrifuged; the supernatant was precipitated with 70% ethanol and centrifuged at 6.000 rpm, for 15 min. The alcoholic supernatant was dried under reduced pressure. The dried residue was washed with anhydrous ether and kept in a desiccator. This powder will be referred to as salivary gland bradykinin potentiating factor (SBPF) for analogy with the bradykinin-potentiating factor (BPF) isolated from the venom of Bothrops jararaca (Ferreira and Rocha e Silva, 1963; Ferreira, 1965).

Biological assay. The activity of SBPF was assayed on the
isolated guinea-pig ileum, rat uterus, ileum and duodenum. It was
used as one arbitrary potentiating unit the amount of SBPF which
increases the effect of one single dose of bradykinin to that of a
double dose, a similar evaulation as used for BPF described by
Ferreira (1965).

For the biological assay on the blood pressure, rats were
anesthetized with sodium pentobarbital (30 mg/kg, i.p.). Arterial
blood pressure was measured through a cannula inserted into the
carotid artery, using a pressure transducer and recorded on an
E&M Physiograph. One of the femural veins was cannulated for
injections.

Kininase activity. Inhibition of kininase activity by SBPF
was tested incubating bradykinin with homogenates of guinea-pig
ileum or heparinized rat plasma.

Perfusion of isolated rat lungs. Under sodium pentobarbital
anesthesia (30 mg/kg, i.p.) the trachea and lungs were exposed, a
cannula tied into the trachea and the pericardium opened. The
lungs were insuflated through the tracheal cannula and the abdominal
aorta was cut. The lungs were perfused from the pulmonary artery
with Tyrode solution and collecting the venous outflow for assay
from a cannula into the left auricle.

                                 RESULTS

When 200 to 400 ug SBPF were added to the organ bath containing
rat uterus or guinea-pig ileum the preparation elicited no contraction at all. However, when bradykinin was added to the bath,
after previous addition of SBPF, the contractions evoked by bradykinin were enhanced. On the repetition of the same dose of SBPF
a similar potentiation was observed.

To ascertain whether SBPF sensitized the rat uterus or guinea-
pig ileum to other agonists besides bradykinin, acetylcholine,
histamine, oxytoxin, angiotensin and KCl were tested. Figure 1
shows the results of experiments in which some of these agonists
were used.

SBPF also sensitized the uterus to oxytoxin and in minor extended to acetylcholine and angiotensin; notwithstanding bradykinin
appeared to be more susceptible to the SBPF effect than the others.
The spasmogenic action of KC 1 was not affected.

Guinea-pig ileum is more specific for bradykinin-potentiating
factor than rat uterus; acetylcholine and histamine were not potentiated; however angiotensin was potentiated in some experiments.

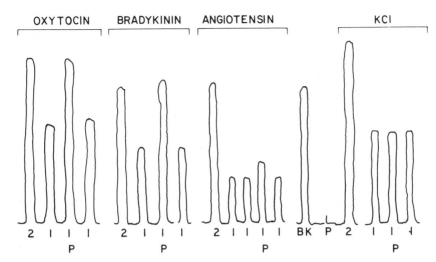

Figure 1. Contraction of rat uterus suspended in 10 ml Jalon
solution. 1 and 2, a single and a double dose of
agonists. BK, 1 ng bradykinin; P, 200 ug SBPF;
the single doses were 5 ng (oxytoxin); 0.5 ng (Bradykinin); 5 ng (angiotensin) and 2 mg (KCl). The
agonist was added to the bath 30 to 45 sec after
the addition of SBPF.

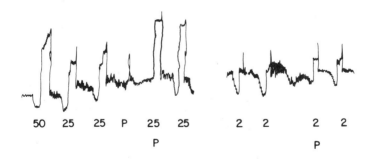

SBPF = 500 μg

Figure 2. Rat terminal ileum suspended in 10 ml Tyrode
solution. The numbers represent ng bradykinin.
P, 500 ug potentiating factor (SBPF). The
agonist was added to the bath 30 to 45 sec
after the addition of SBPF.

On the rat terminal ileum, the SBPF potentiated the contraction of bradykinin (25 to 100 ng); if a small dose of bradykinin (2 to 5 ng) were added to the bath, the relaxation was the predominant effect and the bradykinin potentiating factor in this condition, induced the appearance of contractions (Figure 2).

Potentiation of the hypotensive effect of bradykinin. When 5 to 15 mg/kg SBPF are injected into the veins of rats no alteration in the arterial blood pressure was observed. However, if brady-kinin is injected 10 to 30 sec following previous injection of SBPF a potentiation of the hypotensive effect of bradykinin was observed, as shown in Figure 3.

Inhibition of kininase activity. Used were homogenates of ileum of guinea-pig or plasma of the rat incubated with bradykinin with or without SBPF. The factor inhibited the destruction of bradykinin.

The salivary gland bradykinin-potentiating factor inhibits the inactivation of bradykinin when perfused through rat lungs. However, it has no effect on the angiotensin-converting process.

Kato and Suzuki (1974) showed that potentiator B and C isolated from the venom of Agkistrodon Halys Blomhoffii inhibited the conver-sion of angiotensin I to angiotensin II and degradation of brady-kinin. In addition, these peptides inhibited the contraction of angiotensin I on the isolated rat uterus; this activity was parallel to the ability to inhibit the angiotensin I converting enzyme.

In view of these data we decided to verify if SBPF presented such a parallelism. Our results showed that the salivary gland potentiator had no effect on either the angiotensin I conversion or the contraction evoked by angiotensin I on the rat uterus.

Some physical and chemical properties. Salivary gland brady-kinin potentiating factor is soluble in water and absolute ethanol and insoluble in ethyl ether and acetone. It is thermostable and dialysable. Boiling with 0.1 N NaOH, for 60 min destroys its activity; it resists a similar treatment with 0.1 N HCl. It is resistent to the action of chymotrypsin, but papain destroys its activity. So, it is probable that we are dealing with a peptide.

As far as the action of trypsin is concerned, the potentiating effect of this enzyme (Edery, 1964) could not be abolished by heat or by Trasylol, so we used a Biogel P-6 column to separate trypsin from SBPF after 1 hour incubation. Even after this treat-ment both the trypsin and SBPF showed potentiating activity.

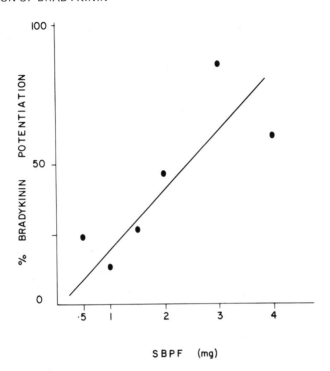

Figure 3.   Dose-response curve of the action of bradykinin-
            potentiating factor (SBPF) on the blood pressure
            of the rat. The animals were anesthetized with
            sodium pentobarbital (30 mg/kg, i.p.). Each
            point represents the mean of three experiments.

   Species differences. Bradykinin-potentiating activity was
found in the rabbit and guinea-pig, but not in the dog. However,
the salivary glands of the rat showed to be the most active.

DISCUSSION

   It is not a surprise that a bradykinin-potentiating factor
was found in the salivary gland of the rat and other animals,
for it was first described in the saliva of a snake, that is, in
the snake venom.

   We found a positive correlation between the amount of kallikrein and bradykinin-potentiating effect in the salivary glands
of the rat. The submandibular gland which presents higher concentration of kallikrein also shows a greater potentiating activity

when compared with the parotid gland.

The possibility of the SBPF being a kallikrein can be ruled out since its activity is not influenced by TRASYLOL; SBPF is dialysable and thermostable. However, we cannot exclude the possibility that more than one bradykinin-potentiating peptide is present in the SBPF preparation.

As far as the bradykinin-potentiating mechanism is concerned, it is suggested that the inhibition of kininases plays an important part. Another possible mechanism would be allosteric transition of the pharmacological receptor, as suggested by Camargo and Ferreira (1971).

The fact that the SBPF inhibits the inactivation of bradykinin when perfused through rat lungs, and has no effect on the angiotensin I conversion, is according to Ferreir (1974) and Stewart (1974) suggesting the existence of two enzymes or only one presenting two active centers.

ACKNOWLEDGEMENTS

Aided by CNPq, CAPES and CPq (UFMG). We are indebted to Sandoz Pharmaceuticals for bradykinin and to Dr. Mina Fichman, Butantan Institute, Sao Paulo, Brazil for the angiotensin.

REFERENCES

Camargo, A. and Ferreira, S.H., 1971. Action of bradykinin potentiating factor (BPF) and dimercaprol (BAL) on the responses to bradykinin of isolated preparations of rat intestines. Brit. J. Pharmacol. 42: 305-307.

Edery, H., 1964. Potentiation of the action of bradykinin on smooth muscle by chymotrypsin, chymotrypsinogen and trypsin. Brit. J. Pharmacol. 22: 371-379.

Ferreira, S.H., 1965. A bradykinin-potentiation factor (PBF) present in the venom of Bothrops Jararaca. Brit. J. Pharmacol. 24: 163-169.

Ferreira, S.H. The relative role of peptidase in the metabolism of peptides. 1974. In: Chemistry and Biology of the Kallikrein-Kinin system in Health and Disease. Eds. Pisano, J.J. and Austen, K.F., DHEW, p. 295-297.

Ferreira, S.H. and Rocha e Silva, M., 1963. Potenciacao de polipeptideos por um fator presente no veneno de B. Jararaca. Cienc. e Cult. 15: 276.

Kato, H. and Suzuki, T., Bradykinin-potentiating peptides from the venom of <u>Agkistrodon halys blomhoffii</u>: their amino-acid sequence and inhibitory activity on angiotensin I converting enzyme from rabbit lung. 1974. <u>In</u>: Chemistry and Biology of the Kallikrein-Kinin system in Health and Disease. Ed. Pisano, J.J. and Austen, K.F., DHEW, p. 299-303.

Stewart, J.M., Modifiers of the response to kinins and their interactions with other systems, 1974. <u>In</u>: Chemistry and Biology of the Kallikrein-Kinin system in Health and Disease. Ed. Pisano, J.J. and Austen, K.F., DHEW, p. 287-294.

PURIFICATION AND CHARACTERIZATION OF A KININASE FROM HUMAN URINE

Amintas F.S. Figueiredo and A.J. Marquezini

Depto. De Bioquimica, Inst. Cien. Biol. Universidade

Federal De Minas Gerais, CP 2486 30.000 Belo Horizonte

Brazil

ABSTRACT

A kininase has been purified from male human urine which splits the C-terminal arginyl residue from bradykinin, but does not split hippuryl-L-arginine or converts Angiotensin I into Angiotensin II. It contains cadmium ion in its active center, and has a molecular weight of 210,000 by ultracentrifugation.

INTRODUCTION

A highly active kininase was purified from human urine by a procedure that involves desalting by gel filtration, adsorption onto anion-exchange bed, elution and a chromatography on Sephadex G-150. The highly active fraction was obtained by the fixed partition technique, in the ultracentrifuge. Efforts are now under way to prepare the same activity by ammonium sulfate fractionation.

METHODS

Enzymatic activities were determined as described under Table 1. Acrylamide electrophoresis was carried out at pH 8.3, using 7.5% acrylamide and applying 200 µg protein to each tube. Coomassie-blue was used for dyeing, according to Laemmli (1970).

Electrofocussing on acrylamide gels was based on a modification by Barroso (1975) of the procedure of Colin (1968).

Cadmium characterization as the metallic ion that participates in catalysis was based on inhibition by EDTA and reactivation by Cd^{2+} in concentration equivalent to the inhibition.

Arginine liberation from the C-terminal sequence in bradykinin, as well as the lack of action on hippuryl-L-arginine were based on dansylation of the reaction mixtures followed by chromatography on silica gel plates, according to Seiler and Wiechman (1964). Rat uterus preparation was used for assays involving the action of purified kininase on angiotensin I.

RESULTS

Six hundred and thirty liters of male human urine, collected under toluene and stored at 4°C, were filtered and passed through 3 columns, 16 liter each, packed with Sephadex G-25. Each 16 liter eluate was applied to a 16 liter column packed with DEAE-Sephadex A-50, equilibrated with 0.10 M ammonium acetate, pH 7.0. After adsorbing all the material contained in the original 650 liters of urine, the ion-exchange column was washed with 12 liters of equilibration buffer, followed by the same containing 0.20 M NaCl, whereby inactive components were eluted. When the ionic strength was raised to that of 0.35 M NaCl in the same buffer, a protein fraction was eluted that contained both kinin-releasing and kininasic activities (Fig. 1). The fractions (500 ml each) were pooled, dialyzed, and freeze-dried. This material was then subjected to gel filtration on Sephadex G-150, on a 5 x 100 cm column equilibrated and eluted with 0.010 M ammonium acetate, 0.20 M NaCl, at pH 7.0. Three peaks were observed, the first one containing kininasic activity, the second rich in kallikrein activity, and the third peak inactive (Fig. 2).

The active fractions were pooled, dialyzed and freeze-dried. When submitted to analytical ultracentrifugation, this material displayed two peaks with s = 3.50 and s = 9.32, corresponding to molecular weights of approximately 60,000 and 210,000 daltons. When submitted to the technique of fixed partition at the ultracentrifuge the two components could be separated. The high molecular weight fraction, corresponding to 16.4% of the area in the photographs contained all the kininasic activity (Fig. 3). The purified kininase hardly penetrates acrylamide gels, even at 5% (w/v); the small amount that does penetrate the gel migrates very slowly. A pI - 4.45 could be measured using electrofocussing on acrylamide gels (Fig. 4).

TABLE I - PURIFICATION OF HUMAN URINARY KININASE

STEP	PROTEIN[a] TOTAL (mg)	REC	SPECIFIC ACTIVITY[b] g INACT. Bk/(min.mg)	TOTAL ACTIVITIES KININ INACTIVATING	REC	KININASE UNITIES U/mg[c]	PURIFICATION FACTOR
SEPHADEX G-25(630L)	64575	100	0.033	2131	100	0.98	1.0
DEAE SEPHADEX A-50	9945	15.4	0.176	1750	82.7	5.16	5.3
SEPHADEX G-150	211.7	0.34	2.136	452.2	21	62.60	64.1
FIXED PARTITION	34.7	0.05	12.985	452.2	31	381.60	389.9

a - protein was determined according to Lowry et al. (1951)

b - at pH 7.4, 37°C, according to Trautschold (1970). Bk = bradykinin

c - determined according to Trautschold (1970).

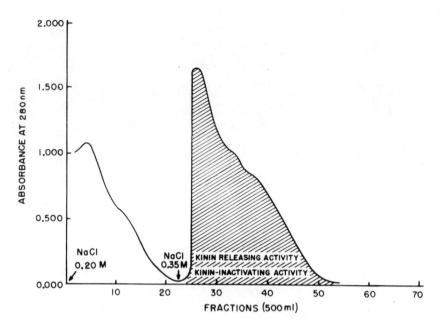

Figure 1. DEAE Sephadex A-50 chromatography: 630 L of male human
urine was applied to a 16 L column. Elution: ammonium
acetate 0.10 M (pH 7.0), 0.35 M in NaCl. Each fraction
contained 500 ml. Temperature, 4°C.

The kininasic activity is inhibited by 3 mM EDTA (Fig. 5A).
Cadmium ion gives the best recovery, as shown in Fig. 5B. The
purified kininase releases the C-terminal arginine of bradykinin.
It does not liberate arginine from hippuryl-L-arginine neither
does the enzyme convert Angiotensin I into Angiotensin II (Fig. 6).

DISCUSSION

Erdös et al. (1974) described a partial purification of human
urinary kininase together with experiments that pointed to a similarity with carboxypeptidase-N, a plasma kininase. The present
work was undertaken with the purpose of obtaining purified enzyme
in quantity sufficient to carry out experiments that extended to
evaluation of physiological activities of the enzyme.

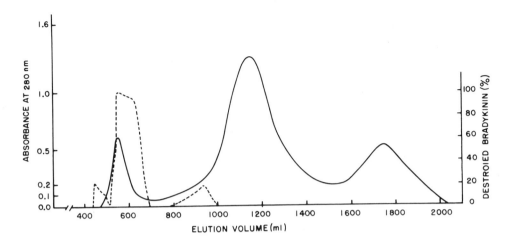

Figure 2. Sephadex G-150 chromatography: 500 mg of protein was
applied to a 5.0 x 100 cm column. Elution: ammonium
acetate 0.01 M (pH 7.0), 0.05 M in NaCl. Flow rate was
20.0 mL/hr, and each fraction contained 10 mL, temp.:4°C.

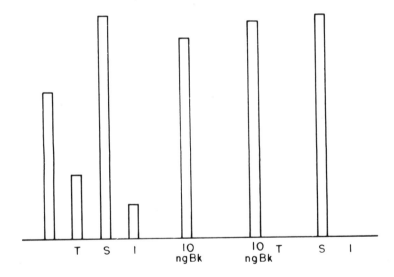

Figure 3. Kininase activity of the peaks obtained from the fixed
partition by ultracentrifugation in NaCl 0.16 M. Each
peak was incubated with bradykinin in Tris 0.20 M pH 7.4,
for 11 min, at 37°C. The activity was determined by biological assay using ileum of guinea pig according to
Trautschold (1970). T= solution of kininase before ultracentrifugation; I = fraction of higher P.M.; S=fraction
of smaller P.M.

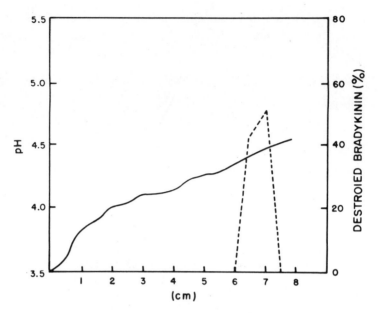

Figure 4. Electrofocussing of kininase in 7.5% acrylamide and
1.0% ampholine; pH range 3-6; 3 hr at 400 v and 3°C.
One gel was cut on fractions of 0.5 cm that were
macerated with 0.5 mL of distilled water and filtered.
The other gel was dyed by Coomassie-blue. The filtrates
were incubated with bradykinin in Tris 0.20 M (pH 7.4),
for 11 min, at 37°C. The activity was determined by
biological assay according to Trautschold (1970).

        The objective was partially attained, for a pure fraction was
isolated, its metallic ion was identified, and its molecular weight
and amino acid analysis could be determined. Although a single
band has been consistently observed on acrylamide gels, a considerable
amount of inactive material could be eliminated by fixed partition
ultracentrifugation. The activities on bradykinin, hippuryl-L-
arginine and angiotensin I demonstrate that this kininase is a
carboxypeptidase different from carboxypeptidase B from pancreas or
from carboxypeptidase N from plasma, given its lack of reaction
upon hippuryl-L-arginine. It is similar however, to the enzyme
described by Rugstad (1967) purified from Pseudomonas aeruginosa,
given similar behavior of the latter toward bradykinin and hippurly-
L-arginine.

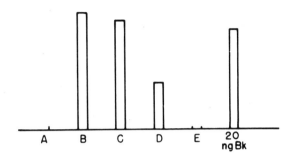

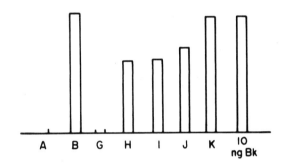

Figure 5A. Inhibition of kininase by EDTA. The enzyme was incubated with EDTA 2 hr at 37°C. A = enzyme; B = enzyme + 3 x 10^{-3} M of EDTA; C = enzyme + 3 x 10^{-4} M of EDTA; D = enzyme + 3 x 10^{-5} M of EDTA; E = enzyme + 3 x 10^{-6} M of EDTA; F = 10 ng of bradykinin.

Figure 5B. Restoration of the kininase activity. The enzyme was inhibited by 3 x 10^{-3} M of EDTA and 3 x 10^{-3} M of several ions were added. A = enzyme; B = enzyme + 3 x 10^{-3} M of EDTA; G = B + 3 x 10^{-3} M of Cd^{2+}; H = 3 x 10^{-3} M of Co^{2+}; I = B + 3 x 10^{-3} M of Mg^{2+}; J = B + 3 x 10^{-3} M of Mn^{2+}; K = B + 3 x 10^{-3} M of Ni^{2+}; L = 10 ng of bradykinin.

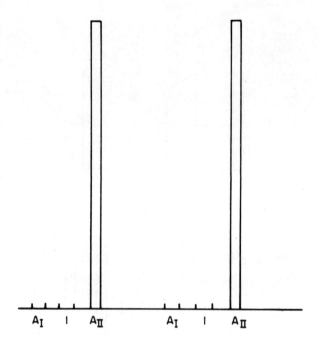

Figure 6.   Action of kininase on angiotensin I.   Incubation
             mixture: 1,5 µg of angiotensin I + 40 µg kininase in
             Tris-maleate 0.05 M pH 7.4 at 37°C.   Biological assay
             on rat uterus.   AI = angiotensin I; AII = angiotensin II;
             I = reaction mixture.

ACKNOWLEDGEMENTS

     The authors acknowledge the help of Drs. Armando Neves and
Marcelo Santoro in the experiments with the ultracentrifuge.

REFERENCES

Barroso, J. (1975).   Purification of dog kininogen. M. Sci. Thesis.
     Fed. University of Minas Gerais.
Colin, W. (1968).   Electrofocussing on acrylamide Gels.   Sci.
     Tools, 15: 21, 17-22.

Erdös, E.G., E.M. Sloane, and I.M. Wohler (1964). Carboxypeptidase
    in blood and other fluids. I. Properties, distribution and
    partial purification of the enzyme. Biochem. Pharmacol. 13:
    893.

Laemmli, U.K. (1970). Cleavage of structural proteins during the
    assembly of the head of bacteriophage T₄. Nature. 227: 680.

Lowry, O.H., J. Rosenbrough, A.F. Lewis and R.J. Randall (1951).
    Protein measurement with the folin phenol reagent. J. Biol.
    Chem. 193: 265-275.

Rugstad, H.E. (1967). Degradation of plasma kinins by an enzyme
    from Pseudomonas aeruginosa. B. J. Pharmacol. Chemother. 31:
    401-406.

Seiler, N. and J. Wiechman (1964). Zum Nachweis von Aminosäuren
    in 10^{-10} Molmabstad. Trennung von 1-dimethylamino-naphtalin-
    5-sulfonyl-Aminosäuren auf Dünnschicht-Chromatogrammen.
    Experientia 20: 559

Trautschold, I. (1970). Assay methods in the kinin system. In:
    Handbook of Experimental Pharmacology. 25: 67-69.

MAMMALIAN INHIBITORS OF ANGIOTENSIN CONVERTING ENZYME (KININASE II)

James W. Ryan, Larry C. Martin, Alfred Chung and
Guillermo A. Pena

Department of Medicine, University of Miami School
of Medicine, Miami, Florida 33101, USA

ABSTRACT

Urines and sera (human, guinea pig and rat) contain low molecular weight inhibitors of angiotensin converting enzyme (ACE).
The urines contain ACE, but the enzyme is scarcely measurable without prior ultrafiltration or dialysis. The activity increases
strikingly through three ultrafiltration steps using a membrane
with a 10,000 MW retention limit. As implied, the ultrafiltrates
contain inhibitory activity and can prevent the hydrolysis of
[^{3}H]benzoyl-Gly-His-Leu by ACE from any source, including lung and
serum. Human urinary ultrafiltrate contains at least three inhibitors separable on Bio-Gel P-2. The inhibitors are acidic and can
be partially purified on Bio-Rex 70 developed with an acetic acid
gradient. The smallest of the inhibitors can be purified to apparent homogeneity by partition chromatography (sephadex G-25;
butanol, acetic acid, H_2O; 4:1:5). The excretion of inhibitory
activity varies in response to dietary salt: Activity is low when
rats are maintained on a high NaCl diet and is high (3 x's control)
on a low NaCl diet. Thus, the activity of ACE may be modulated in
vivo by naturally-occurring enzyme inhibitors. Whether some hypertensive patients are deficient in ACE inhibitory activity remains to be determined.

INTRODUCTION

In October, 1974, Lieberman presented data which showed that
some patients with active sarcoidosis have unusually high levels of
serum angiotensin converting enzyme. Further, he showed that among
those patients treated beneficially with glucocorticoids or those who

underwent spontaneous remission, serum angiotensin converting enzyme
levels returned to within the normal range (presentation at Proceedings of the 5th International Symposium at Davos, Switzerland, 1974;
Lieberman, 1975, 1976). These findings have been confirmed by several different laboratories (e.g., Silverstein et al., 1976; Zorn
et al., 1977; and Rohatgi et al., 1978)

All of Lieberman's work was accomplished with a relatively
cumbersome assay; namely, that in which hippuryl-His-Leu is used
as substrate and enzyme is measured in terms of the rate of formation of hippuric acid (Cushman and Cheung, 1969; 1971). Hippuric
acid, after solvent extraction, is measured spectrophotometrically
(at 228 nm).

Because of the potential importance of the findings of Lieberman,
we set out to develop a simpler, more accurate and sensitive assay for
angiotensin converting enzyme; an assay that would facilitate clinical and epidemiologic studies. In addition, we were interested in
finding means of measuring angiotensin converting enzyme as it occurs
in urine; a measurement that we had been unable to make using the
Hip-His-Leu assay as originally described. Finally, we wanted a
simple, highly sensitive assay for measuring the enzyme as it occurs
in association with endothelial cells in culture (cf. Chiu et al.,
1975; Ryan et al., 1976a & b, 1978a & b).

Our experience with the assays developed in this laboratory led
to the finding that both blood and urine contain large amounts of
small molecular weight inhibitors of angiotensin converting enzyme.
These inhibitors appear to solve a puzzle: Plasma and urine contain
abundant angiotensin converting enzyme, but there is little or no conversion of angiotensin I into angiotensin II in blood (cf. Ng and
Vane, 1967; Boucher et al., 1970) and essentially no degradation of
bradykinin in voided urine (J. Pisano, personal communication).

MATERIALS AND METHODS

Preparation of Urine

Bio-Gel P-2 and Bio-Rex 70 were from Bio-Rad Laboratories, Inc.
Sephadex G-25 was from Pharmacia Fine Chemicals, Inc. Kinins and
angiotensins were synthesized in this laboratory. Low Na^+-rat chow
was from ICN.

Urine was collected and ultrafiltered as described in an accompanying paper (Ryan et al., this volume). The ultrafiltrand was used
to study protein components of the kallikrein-kinin system, and the ultrafiltrate was used to prepare inhibitors of angiotensin converting
enzyme and urinary kallikrein.

Assays

Except where noted, angiotensin converting enzyme was measured using [^{3}H]Hip-His-Leu as substrate (Ryan et al., 1978b). Early studies used [^{3}H]Hip-Gly-Gly (Ryan et al., 1977). Kallikrein was assayed using Pro-Phe-Arg-[^{3}H]anilide or the -[^{3}H]benzylamide as described by Chung et al. (this volume).

RESULTS AND DISCUSSION

Non-linearity of Angiotensin Converting Enzyme Assays

Our first radioassay for angiotensin converting enzyme (ACE) used [^{3}H]benzoyl-Gly-Gly-Gly ([^{3}H]hippuryl-Gly-Gly) as substrate (Ryan et al., 1977). As we began to develop a protocol for the use of the substrate to measure human serum enzyme, it became clear that the assay was linear over a rather limited range. There were two problems. The first was demonstrable using highly purified angiotensin converting enzyme, and was found to be caused by product inhibition. The dipeptide Gly-Gly inhibits the enzyme, and the inhibition is severe when Gly-Gly achieves concentrations much above 1 mM.

The second problem arose from the occurrence of small molecular weight inhibitors in plasma and serum. We found that human sera could be used in dilutions of 1/7 to 1/25 in the final reaction mixture to yield linear reactions, so long as less than 15% of substrate was used. However, at lower dilutions (e.g., 1/5 to 1/3, the reaction rates were markedly reduced. This observation is not unlike that of Yang et al., (1971), who found that guinea pig plasma assayed at high dilution appears to have much more kininase II activity in comparison with plasma assayed at low dilution; a phenomenon thought to be owing to a dissociable enzyme-inhibitor complex.

We found that dialysis of sera against H_2O or 0.9% NaCl suffices to eliminate the discrepancy: Dialyzed serum at a 1/4 dilution hydrolyzes [^{3}H]Hip-Gly-Gly at a rate five times faster than that of the same serum at a 1/20 dilution. Further, the supernatant prepared by centrifugation of plasma (or serum) heated at 100°C for 5 min contains inhibitory activity against ACE.

Bradykinin, angiotensin I, angiotensin II and angiotensin III can, as alternative substrates, inhibit ACE (cf. Chiu et al., 1976). However, these polypeptides do not occur in blood (or urine) in concentrations adequate to effect such inhibition.

Efforts to Assay ACE in Urine

As one of our first efforts to assess the components of the Kallikrein-kinin system in urine (Ryan, J.W. et al., this volume), we examined for kininase II. Erdos and Yang, (1970) had stated that

a kininase II-like enzyme may occur in urine, but no data were presented.

In prolonged incubations (3-6 h) of rat urine with [^{3}H]Hip-
Gly-Gly, we found evidence of weak hydrolytic activity. Dialysis
of urine increased the activity 3- to 6-fold. Further, we found
that the activity increases among rats on a high salt diet (normal
rat chow plus 1 or 2% NaCl in drinking H_2O, ad lib), and decreased
to vanishingly low levels on low salt diet (H_2O plus ICN low Na$^+$
pellets, ad lib).

Even in 16-24 h incubations, human urine showed little reactivity with [^{3}H]Hip-Gly-Gly. However, if urinary proteins were
concentrated with $(NH_4)_2SO_4$ (at 90% of saturation) or by ultrafiltration (see Ryan, J.W. et al., this volume; Ryan et al., 1978b),
vigorous ACE activity could be found. If the human urinary proteins were concentrated and then washed with H_2O by ultrafiltration,
the net activity increased even more (up to 30fold greater activity
after 4 washes than in the first ultrafiltrand).

When, however, samples of the first or second ultrafiltrate
were added back to the washed urinary proteins, the activity of ACE
disappeared. Like the plasma inhibitor(s), the urinary ACE inhibitory activity was found to be stable to heating at 100°C for 5 min.

One can find concentrations of urea that inhibit and inactivate ACE (e.g., Das et al., 1977), but the concentrations required
for inhibition are not obtained in urine. Urea would be required at
>16M in urine ultrafiltrate to achieve readily detectable inhibition
in our assay.

Characterization

The experiments that follow used concentrated urine ultrafiltrate. Typically, 500 to 1,000 ml of ultrafiltrate was reduced in
volume on a rotary evaporator and maintained at >45°C. As salts began to precipitate, they were removed by vacuum filtration, and the
resulting filtrate was returned to the rotary evaporator. No inhibitory activity was lost by co-precipitation.

The concentrated inhibitor was then extracted with butan-2-ol
(see below), or applied to a Bio Gel P-2 column (5 x 50 cm) developed
with H_2O. In the latter case, inhibitory activity was eluted in two,
and sometimes three, fractions (apparent molecular sizes: 1200, 800,
500). None of the inhibitory activity was excluded from Bio-Gel P-2,
and none co-chromatographed with urinary salts.

Purification of the Inhibitor, MW-500

Concentrated ultrafiltrate was acidified with 4% trifluoro-acetic acid, saturated with butan-2-ol and then extracted twice with two volumes of butan-2-ol saturated with 4%-trifluroroacetic acid. The butanol extract was evaporated to a small volume and urea was precipitated with acetone and H_2O. The precipitate was removed by filtration, and then the filtrate was evaporated to dryness.

The residue was dissolved in 1% acetic acid and was applied to a column (2.5 x 45 cm) of Bio Rex 70 equilibrated with 1% acetic acid. The column was washed with 5 column volumes of 1% acetic acid. The inhibitory activity was eluted shortly after the break-through fraction.

The active fraction from Bio Rex 70 was evaporated to dryness, dissolved in H_2O, and then applied to the Bio-Gel P-2 column. Three fractions contained inhibitory activity; the major fraction behaving like a substance having a MW of 500.

The major fraction was evaporated to dryness and then dissolved in butan-1-ol previously equilibrated in the system: butanol, acetic acid, H_2O (4:1:5). The solution was applied to a column (1 x 100 cm) of Sephadex G-25 prepared for partition chromatography in the same system. The fraction containing inhibitory activity was eluted with lower phase.

The active fraction behaved as a single substance on high performance liquid chromatography (reversed-phase ODS column developed with methanol-H_2O, 20-80%).

Properties of the Inhibitor

Activity of the inhibitor was lost on reaction with 6N HCl at 110°C for 20 h. The products formed by acid hydrolysis reacted strongly with ninhydrin, whereas the intact inhibitor did not appear to be reactive with ninhydrin. One ug of hydrolysate yielded ninhydrin color equivalent to 7 nmoles of leucine. The inhibitor was reactive with o-tolidine/Cl_2. If it is assumed that the molecule has a MW of 500, that no salts were formed during purification, and that the final compound was not hydrated, the I_{50} of the inhibitor was 10^{-6} M ([^{3}H]Hip-His-Leu assay using guinea pig urinary angiotensin converting enzyme; Ryan et al., 1978b). The inhibitor does not affect the activity of urinary kallikrein. The urinary kallikrein inhibitor is eluted from Bio-Gel P-2 just after the smallest ACE inhibitor.

The inhibitor behaved as an acidic substance on electrophoresis at pH 5.0, and as a neutral substance at pH 2.0. Its uv spectrum showed maximum absorbance at 295 nm.

Biological Implications

Although angiotensin converting enzyme is not generally regarded as a rate-limiting enzyme, there are circumstances in which
the enzyme is likely to be rate-limiting. Ng and Vane (1967) have
reported that angiotensin I is not converted into angiotensin II by
blood circulated, at 37°C, through silastic tubing. In contrast,
Boucher et al., (1970), have shown that ACE occurs abundantly in
dialyzed plasma. Similarly, it has been reported by workers using
a functional assay, that rabbit plasma may not contain kininase II
(Erdos and Yang, 1970), yet Soffer and colleagues have purified to
homogeneity the ACE of rabbit serum. Further, our computations of
their data indicate that ACE occurs in rabbit serum at the surprisingly high concentration of 1.23 mg/ml (~9.5 nM). Perhaps the rate-
limiting nature of ACE is more readily appreciated by the fact that
concentrations of angiotensin I in blood generally exceed those of
angiotensin II. If the enzyme were not rate-limiting (in a functional sense), angiotensin I should not be measurable.

Major questions arising from our studies bear on the variability
of ACE inhibition in blood and urine. Does the inhibitory activity
vary in normal function? In response to dietary factors? We have
found that rats on high NaCl diets have very little inhibitory
activity in their urines, whereas their litter mates on low salt
diets have increased concentrations (>2.5 of controls). Do patients
with some forms of hypertensive cardiovascular disease or secondary
hyperaldosteronism have unusually low levels of the ACE inhibitory
activity? Our ability to answer these questions will require
further characterization of the inhibitors and further development
of relevant assays.

ACKNOWLEDGEMENTS

This work was supported in part by grants from the U.S. Public
Health Service (HL22896 and HL22087), and the John A. Hartford
Foundation, Inc. The radioassays for angiotensin converting enzyme
were developed through support by the Council of Tobacco Research--
U.S.A., Inc.

REFERENCES

Boucher, R., H. Kurihara, C. Grise and J. Genest, 1970. Measurement
    of plasma angiotensin I converting enzyme activity, Section II,
    Conversion of Angiotensin I. Circ. Res. Suppl. 1, XXVI and
    XXVII: I-83--I-91.

Chui, A.T., J.W. Ryan, U.S. Ryan and F.E. Dorer, 1975. A sensitive radiochemical assay for angiotensin-converting enzyme (Kininase II). Biochem. J., 149: 297.

Chiu, A.T., J.W. Ryan, J.M. Stewart and F.E. Dorer, 1976. Formation of angiotensin III by angiotensin-converting enzyme. Biochem. J. 155: 189.

Cushman, D.W. and H.S. Cheung, 1969. A simple substrate for assay of dog lung angiotensin converting enzyme. Fed. Proc. 28: 799. Abstract.

Cushman, D.W. and H.S. Cheung, 1971. Spectrophotometric assay and properties of the angiotensin-converting enzyme of rabbit lung, Biochem. Pharmac., 20: 1637.

Das, M., J.L. Hartley and R.L. Soffer, 1977. Serum angiotensin-converting enzyme; isolation and relationship to the pulmonary enzyme. J. Biol. Chem., 252(4): 1316.

Erdos, E.G. and H.Y.T. Yang, 1970. Kininases, Vol. XXV, Handbuch der exp. Pharmak. Title: Bradykinin, Kallidin and Kallikrein. Ed. E.G. Erdos, Springer-Verlag, N.Y., p. 289.

Lieberman, J., 1975. Elevation of serum angiotensin-converting enzyme (ACE) level in sarcoidosis. Amer. J. Med., 59: 365.

Lieberman, J., 1976. The specificity and nature of serum-angiotensin-converting enzyme (serum ACE) elevations in sarcoidosis. Ann. N.Y. Acad. Sci., 278: 488.

Ng, K.K.F. and J.R. Vane, 1967. Conversion of angiotensin I to angiotensin II. Nature, 216: 762.

Rohatgi, P.K., T.H. Massey and J.W. Ryan, 1978 (Abstract). Serum angiotensin converting enzyme and sarcoidosis. Clin. Res., 26: 453A.

Ryan, J.W., A. Chung, C. Ammons and M.L. Carlton, 1977. A simple radioassay for angiotensin converting enzyme. Biochem. J., 167: 501.

Ryan, J.W., A. Chung, L.C. Martin and U.S. Ryan, 1978. New substrates for the radioassay of angiotensin converting enzyme of endothelial cells in culture. Tissue & Cell. 10: 555.

Ryan, J.W., A.R. Day, U.S. Ryan and A. Chung, 1976. Localization of angiotensin converting enzyme (kininase II). I. Preparation of antibody-heme-octapeptide conjugates. Tissue & Cell. 8: 111.

Ryan, J.W., N.B. Oza, L. C. Martin and G.A. Pena. (this volume). Components of the kallikrein-kinin system in urine.

Ryan, U.S., E. Clements, D. Habliston and J.W. Ryan, 1978. Isolation and culture of pulmonary artery endothelial cells. Tissue & Cell. 10: 535.

Ryan, Una S., J.W. Ryan, C. Whitaker and A. Chiu, 1976. Localization of angiotensin converting enzyme (kininase II). II. Immunocytochemistry and immunofluorescence. Tissue & Cell, 8: 125.

Silverstein, E.J. Friedland, H.A. Lyons and A. Gourin, 1976. Elevation of angiotensin-converting enzyme in granulomatous lymph nodes and serum in sarcoidosis: clinical and possible pathogenic significance. Ann. N.Y. Acad. Sci., 278: 498.

Yang, H.Y.T., E.G. Erdos and Y. Levin, 1971. Characterization of a
    dipeptide hydrolase (kininase II: angiotensin I converting
    enzyme), J. Pharmac. Exp. Therapeutics. 177(1): 291.
Zorn, S.K., M.R. Littner, C.E. Putman and J.B. Gee, 1977.
    Comparison of serum lysozyme and angiotensin convertase in
    the diagnosis and therapy of sarcoid. Clin. Res., XXIV:552A.

THE VASOTOXICITY OF THE LYSOSOMAL CONTENTS FROM THE RENAL CORTEX

Mieko Kai, Motoomi Nakamura, Hideo Kanaide,
Takeshi Kurozumi* and Kenzo Tanaka*

Research Institute of Angiocardiology and Department of
Pathology*, Kyushu University, Fukuoka, Japan

The retained proteins (fraction B: rich in renin) and the
not retained proteins (fraction A: no renin activity) were
obtained from the concanavalin A affinity column chromatography
of the lysosomal contents from the hog renal cortex. Intraperitoneal injection of fraction A, B and highly purified renin produced
angionecrosis of fibrinoid type of the small arteries and arterioles
in the bilaterally nephrectomized rats. The angionecrosis producing
activity (vasotoxicity) as well as vasopressor activity of fraction
B were prevented completely by the oral administration of SQ14225.
Although fraction A demonstrated no renin activity, intraperitoneal
injection of fraction A produced gradual and transient elevation
of blood pressure and fibrinoid necrosis which was milder and less
consistent as compared with fraction B. The vasotoxicity as well
as the transient vasopressor activity of fraction A were completely
abolished also by the previous administration of oral SQ14225.

INTRODUCTION

It is well known that malignant hypertension produces fibrinoid necrosis in the small arteries and arterioles as well as a
marked elevation of plasma renin activity. It was repeatedly
confirmed that an injection of renal extracts produced fibrinoid
necrosis in the arterioles and small arteries in the bilaterally
nephrectomized rats (Winternitz et al., 1940; Nairn et al., 1956;
Giese, 1963; Onoyama et al., 1971; Nakamura et al., 1975). However
whether fibrinoid necrosis brought about by renal extracts is
produced by elevation of blood pressure per se, or by any other

biochemical changes without hemodynamic effects remains unknown.

Previously we demonstrated that the lysosomal contents (Ly-C) from the hog renal cortex produced fibrinoid necrosis of the small arteries and arterioles in the bilaterally nephrectomized rats (Nakamura et al., 1975). Substances responsible for this vasotoxic activity in the Ly-C were partially purified by use of concanavalin A affinity column chromatography (Nakamura et al., 1975; Nakamura et al., 1978). Both the retained proteins (fraction B, rich in renin) and the not retained proteins (fraction A: no renin) for concanavalin A affinity column possessed the vasotoxic activity (Nakamura et al., 1978). Fraction B, like renin, produced a rapid, marked and sustained elevation of blood pressure but fraction A did not (Nakamura et al., 1978). In order to elucidate the role of renin in the production of fibrinoid necrosis, effects of oral ad- ministration of SQ14225, an inhibitor for the converting enzyme, were studied.

MATERIAL AND METHODS

Preparation of Ly-C

The Ly-C was prepared freshly from the hog renal cortex by use of differential centrifugation and osmotic shock treatment as reported previously (Nakamura et al., 1978). A degree of contami- nation of Ly-C with the other subcellular fractions was determined by measurement of enzyme profiles as reported previously (Nakamura et al., 1975). The Ly-C was further purified with the concanavalin A-Sepharose 4B affinity column chromatography. The column was equilibrated and eluted with phosphate buffer (0.02M)-NaCl(1M) at pH7.0 to obtain fraction A and then followed by the elution with methyl-α-D-glucoside (0.2M)-NaCl (1M) at pH7.0 to obtain fraction B as reported previously (Nakamura et al., 1975).

Measurement of blood pressure and vascular lesions

Three ml of the fraction A or B dissolved in physiological saline containing 5 to 15 mg of protein were injected intraperitone- ally into the conscious rats 6 hours after bilateral nephrectomy. Mean blood pressure of the conscious rats was continuously recorded for 18 hours in polygraphic recorder with a pressure transducer through the polyvinyl tube inserted into the carotid artery. Twenty four hours after nephrectomy, the rats were sacrificed and various organs such as the brain, lungs, heart, pancreas and mesenterium were removed, fixed in 10% formalin and stained with HE and PAS. The vasotoxic activity of substances producing fibrinoid necrosis was expressed arbitrarily as (-) to (+++) according to the severity and the frequency of vascular lesions as seen under microscopy.

SQ14225 (100 mg/kg/BW) was administered orally through stomach tube, in case when necessary, 60 min before the intraperitoneal injection of fraction A or B.

Purification of hog renin

Renin was purified from 20 kg wet weight of hog kidneys by the modification of the method described by Inagami and Murakami (1977). Briefly, the freshly obtained and frozen hog kidneys were partially thawed at room temperature, freed from fat and medulla by excision, minced in a meat grinder, freeze-dried, pulverized, defatted in ethyl ether and air-dried at room temperature. The dried powder weighing 2380g was then extracted with ethylene glycol monomethyl-ether-water mixture containing the protease inhibitors. Renin in the extract was absorbed to DEAE-Cellulose and eluted with acetate buffer (0.1M)-NaCl (0.2M) at pH4.8. The eluate was dialyzed against acetate buffer (0.01M) at pH5.5 for overnight at 4°C and applied to the pepstatin agarose column. The column was eluted by stepwise changes in pH and ionic concentration. The fractions containing renin were then subjected to gel filtration with Sephadex G-150. Fractions with the renin peak were purified on a DEAE-Cellulose column at pH6.2 with a concentration gradient of KCl. The active fractions were further purified on isoelectrofocusing between pH of 4 and 6.

Renin activity was determined by the method of Conradi and Jelinek (1969).

Sodium dodecyl sulfate (SDS) polyacrylamide gel electro-phoresis

SDS-10% polyacrymide gel electrophoresis was performed according to the method of Fairbanks et al (1971).

RESULTS

Preparation and partial purification of Ly-C

A contamination of Ly-C by the microsomal and mitochondrial fractions was about 1% in terms of specific activities of marker enzymes as reported previously (Nakamura et al., 1975; Nakamura et al., 1978). The renin activity was detected mainly in Ly-C. When Ly-C was applied to concanavalin A affinity column, glycoprotein fractions containing renin were retained completely by the column and eluted with methy-α-D-glucoside as fraction B.

Renin purification

Renin was purified about 11,000 fold over the kidney powder in terms of the specific activity. The purified renin showed a single band on SDS-polyacrylamide gel electrophoresis. A molecular weight of 37,500 was obtained for renin by the calculation using

the relative mobility of the standard proteins (Boehringer Mannheim)
in the SDS-polyacrylamide gel.

(a)

(b)

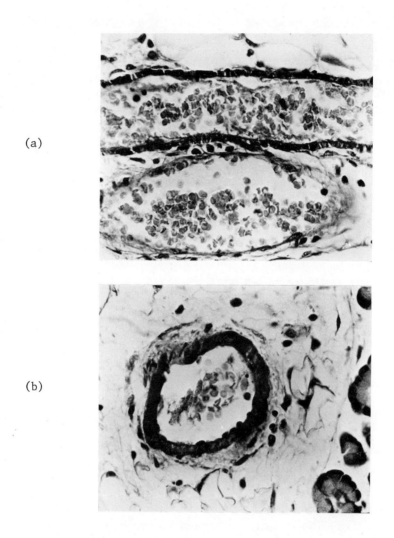

Fig. 1.
(a) Photomicrograph of pancreatic artery from a nephrectomized
rat fixed 18h after intraperitoneal injection of 14 mg of fraction A.
PAS stain, x440
(b) Photomicrograph of pancreatic artery from a nephrectomized
rat fixed 18h after intraperitoneal injection of 5 mg of fraction B.
PAS stain, x470

Effects of fraction A, B and the highly purified renin on blood pressure and production of vascular lesions

Both fraction B, rich in renin, and fraction A having no renin activity produced similar fibrinoid necrosis of the small arteries and arterioles in the pancreas, mesenterium and heart, but not in the brain (Fig 1). Much greater severity and frequency of fibrinoid necrosis on the basis of per mg of injected proteins were observed in the rats treated with fraction B than those with fraction A. When fraction B was injected intraperitoneally into three conscious bilaterally nephrectomized rats, mean blood pressure immediately elevated from 117+4 mmHg to 184+8 mmHg (mean+SD), which was maintained for several hours and decreased gradually thereafter, but was maintained more than 150 mmHg for 18 hours (Fig 2).

The elevation of blood pressure as well as fibrinoid necrosis of the pancreas, mesenterium and heart produced by fraction B was prevented almost completely when SQ14225 was administrated one hour prior to the intraperitoneal injection of fraction B (Table 1).

On the other hand, when fraction A having no renin activity was injected intraperitoneally, the mean blood pressure gradually elevated from 99+7 mmHg to 151+9 mmHg during the course of one hour after the injection, and then decreased gradually and returned to the control level within 18 hours after the injection as shown in Fig 3. The histological examinations of these rats revealed fibrinoid necrosis as in the cases of fraction B, but slightly milder and less consistent as compared with fraction B. The gradual elevation of blood pressure and fibrinoid necrosis of the arteries by fraction A were also abolished completely by the oral administration of SQ14225 one hour prior to the injection of fraction A.

When 200 µg of the highly purified renin (specific activity of 11,000 fold over the kidney powder) were injected intraperitoneally into the bilaterally nephrectomized rats (n=4), mean blood pressure elevated from 96+15 mmHg to 167+10 mmHg with a time course similar to fraction B, and fibrinoid necrosis was produced in all rats.

Effects of SQ14225 on the vasotoxic activity of fraction A and B were summarized in Table 1.

DISCUSSION

Although it was repeatedly confirmed by various investigators that an injection of extracts of the rat renal cortex produced fibrinoid necrosis in the small arteries and arterioles, the isolation and the characterization of the active substances which produce fibrinoid necrosis have not yet been accomplished. We have reported that the characteristic vascular lesions produced by intraperitoneal injection of Ly-C of the renal cortex into the bilaterally nephrectomized rats were fibrinoid necrosis and were similar to the one in malignant hypertension (Nakamura et al., 1975; Nakamura et al., 1978). The Ly-C contained a large amount of renin,

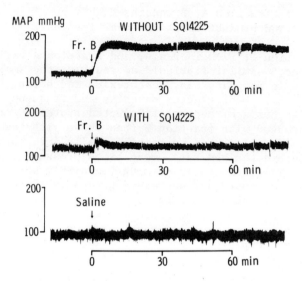

Fig. 2.   The effect of fraction B on the arterial pressure
MAP: mean arterial pressure

which was supposed to have the property of elevating blood pressure,
increasing vascular permeability and producing fibrinoid type lesions in the studies using crude preparations (Giese, 1963; Masson et
al., 1966).   However, vasotoxicity of the isolated renin has not
been examined yet.   In the present study, fraction B rich in renin

TABLE 1.   Angionecrosis produced by fraction A, B and renin, and
its inhibition by SQ14225

| Sample | Angionecrosis/(case) | |
	Without SQ14225	With SQ14225
Fraction A	5 / (9)	0 / (11)
Fraction B	3 / (3)	0 / (6)
Renin*	4 / (4)	----
Saline	0 / (2)	0 / (4)

* highly purified renin (specific activity of 11,000 fold over
the kidney powder   --- not performed

as well as the highly purified renin produced fibrinoid necrosis
consistently in the bilaterally nephrectomized rats. The development of fibrinoid necrosis as well as rapid and persistent elevation
of blood pressure after intraperitoneal injection of fraction B was
completely abolished by the previous oral administration of SQ14225,
inhibitor for converting enzyme. These results may strongly suggest
that renin produces fibrinoid necrosis through an elevation of blood
pressure. Since kininase II is known to be inhibited after SQ14225,
we must take account for the participation of kinin in the prevention of elevating blood pressure and fibrinoid necrosis (Erdos, 1975).

In the present study, as in the previous reports (Nakamura et
al., 1978), fraction A demonstrated no renin activity and yet produced fibrinoid necrosis as in the fraction B.

Fraction A demonstrated a slow, transient and mild pressor
activity which was completely different from the one of fraction B
and the purified renin in the intensity and the time course. An
increment of circulating volume, possibly produced by the intraperitoneal injection of 3 ml of saline containing vasotoxic substances, might not be responsible for the elevation of blood pressure by fraction A because the injection of 3 ml of saline as a
control did not change blood pressure and did not produce any vascular changes. Although fraction A did show no renin activity,

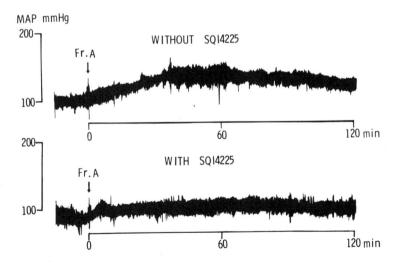

Fig. 3. The effect of fraction A on the arterial pressure
MAP: mean arterial pressure

the administration of SQ14225 prior to the injection of fraction A also prevented the elevation of blood pressure and fibrinoid necrosis. The exact mechanisms for SQ14225 to prevent elevation of blood pressure and fibrinoid necrosis produced by fraction A remains unknown although a potentiation of kinins must be taken into account.

The present study suggested that the Ly-C of the hog renal cortex contained at least more than two substances to produce fibrinoid necrosis. One is renin in fraction B and the others are in fraction A.

Nakao et al. (1966) demonstrated nonpressor substances capable of producing vascular injury independent of renin in ischemic kidney cortex. Shimomura (1971) demonstrated that fibrinoid necrosis was produced by the fraction of the kidney having very weak pressor activity. The identity of the substances of those investigators and the substances in fraction A remained to be studied more precisely.

ACKNOWLEDGEMENTS

This investigation was supported by grants from the Ministry of Education, Japan (No. 187072) for 1977 and 1978. SQ14225 was kindly donated from the Squibb Institute of Medical Research, Princeton, New Jersey.

REFERENCES

Conradi, K. and J. Jelinek, 1969, Strain and sex differences in renin content of rat kidneys, Proc. Soc. exp., Biol. Med. 132, 984.

Erdos, E.G., 1975, Brief review: angiotensin I converting enzyme, Circulation Res. 36, 247.

Fairbanks, G., T.L. Steck and D.F.H. Wallach, 1971, Electrophoretic analysis of the major polypeptides of the human erythrocyte membrane, Biochemistry 10, 2606.

Giese, J., 1963, Pathogenesis of vascular disease caused by acute renal ischemia, Acta path. microbiol. scand. 59, 417.

Inagami, T. and K. Murakami, 1977, Pure renin (Isolation from hog kidney and characterization), J. Biol. Chem. 252, 2978.

Masson, G.M.C., C. Kashii, M. Matsunaga and I.H. Page, 1966, Hypertensive vascular disease induced by heterologous renin, Circulation Res. 18, 219.

Nairn, R.C., G.M.C. Masson and A.C. Corcoran, 1956, The production of serous effusions in nephrectomized animals by the administration of renal extracts and renin, J. Path. Bact. 71, 155.

Nakao, K., M. Ikeda, J. Fujii, F. Terasawa, H. Kurihara, S. Kimata, S. Matsushita and H. Yamaguchi, 1966, Acute vascular lesions produced by selected nonpressor renal cortical extracts, Jap. Circul. J. 30, 539.

Nakamura, M., I Ezaki, A. Sumiyoshi, M. Kai, H. Kanaide, S. Naito
    and K. Kato, 1975, Renal subcellular fractions producing angio-
    necrosis and increased vascular permeability, Brit. J. exp. Path.
    56, 62.

Nakamura M., M. Kai, H. Kanaide, T. Kurozumi, Y. Yamamoto, H.
    Yamamoto and K. Kato, 1978, Partial purification of renal
    lysosomal substances producing angionecrosis and increased
    vascular permeability, Blood Vessels 15, 119.

Onoyama, K., N. Hattori, T. Omae and S. Katsuki, 1971, Vascular
    lesions produced in bilaterally nephrectomized rats by injection
    of fractionated renal cortical extracts, J. Jap. Coll. Angiol.
    11, 163 (in Japanese)

Shimomura, A., 1971, Experimental studies on pathogenesis of angio
    necrosis produced by administration of renal extracts, Acta med
    Nagasaki, 15, 58.

Winternitz, M.C., E. Mylon, L.L. Waters and R. Katzenstein, 1940,
    Studies on the relation of the kidney to cardiovascular disease,
    Yale J. Biol. Med. 12, 623.

ISOLATION AND CHARACTERIZATION OF RENIN AND HIGH MOLECULAR WEIGHT

FORMS OF RENIN FROM VARIOUS SPECIES

Kazuo Murakami and Tadashi Inagami*

Institute of Applied Biochemistry, University of Tsukuba
Ibaraki-ken, 300-31, JAPAN
* Department of Biochemistry, Vanderbilt University
School of Medicine, Nashville, TN 37232, U. S. A.

Research on the kinin-kallikrein system has been greatly
benefited by highly dependable results contributed from superb
biochemical studies which have been developed vigorously in the
last generation. Development of these rigorous enzymological
studies is now beginning to make us to realize the physiological
significance of this system which seems to be far more extensive
than we have thought earlier. In contrast, the major effort on
the study of the renin-angiotensin system has been concentrated in
the physiological and pharmacological areas. This was partly due
to several serious barriers which defied repeated attempts by
biochemists to approach this problem. As the results of these
difficulties, this field has long been deprived of access to pure
preparation of renin (EC 3.4.99.19) and to informations concerning
its molecular and enzymological properties, which are requisite
for rational approach to research of any system.

PURIFICATION OF RENAL RENIN

In the last decade some of the most serious technical difficulties have been gradually eliminated. In 1969, Haber and his
associates developed radioimmunoassay method of angiotensin I, and
Reinharz and Roth developed fluorometric assay for the determination of renin activity. These methods have provided biochemists
ready access to renin assay which is needed for the purification
and characterization of renin. Secondly, the concept of affinity
chromatography developed by Cuatrecasas, Wiltcheck and Anfinsen
has revolutionized our approach to renin purification. Thirdly,
discovery of pepstatin and its inhibitory action against renin
(Umezawa et al., 1972 and Aoyagi et al., 1972) have provided an

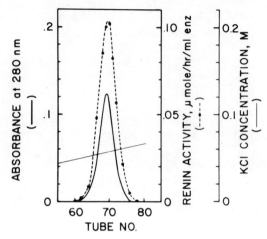

Fig. 1. Final purification of hog renal renin on a CM-
          cellulose column.
          (Inagami and Murakami, 1977[a])

TABLE I : Purification of renin from the hog kidney
          (Inagami & Murakami, 1977(a))

Purification Step	Total Protein mg	Specific* Activity	Purification	Yield %
Hog Kidney	18 kg**			
Kidney Powder	1,417,000***	0.002	1.0	100
Crude Extract	300,000	0.009	4.3	92
DEAE-batch	83,300	0.025	13	74
Affinity Column	167	9.3	4,700	55
Sephadex G-75	16.7	85	42,000	50
DEAE-Cellulose	2.9	260	130,000	31
CM-Cellulose	2.0	267	133,000	19

*   µg angiotensin I formed/µg protein/hr at pH 6.0
**   Total wet weight
*** Total weight 3,200 g

important handle to the initial attempts for the purification of
renin. Fourthly, examination of difficulties encountered in
numerous attempts to purify renin has led us to realize that co-
purification of proteases with renin destroys partially purified
renin and inclusion of protease inactivators can improve the
situation.

These technological developments set the stage for the completion
of the purification of renin almost 80 years after the initial
discovery of renin in the kidney (Tigerstedt and Bergman, 1898).
An affinity gel for renin, pepstatin-aminohexyl-Sepharose, was
prepared by coupling the N-acylated pentapeptide pepstatin to
aminohexyl-Sepharose (Murakami and Inagami, 1975) via N-hydroxy-
succinimide ester of pepstatin. Combination of affinity chromatography using this gel with 3 more steps of conventional chromatography has produced a pure and stable renin from the kidney for
the first time. As summarized in Table I, greater than 100,000-
fold purification has been achieved at an overall yield of 20 %.
The purified renin was shown to be homogeneous as judged by a
number of criteria such as the symmetrical peak of the chromatographic elution pattern of the last step of chromatography (Fig I),
single bands obtained by polyacrylamide gel electrophoresis, SDS-
polyacrylamide gel electrophoresis, isoelectric focusing, and by
sedimentation equilibrium ultracentrifugation. The specific
activity of 2,000 units/mg was obtained and the broad plateau of
its pH-activity profile covered the neutral physiological region.

    A similar method was applied to the purification of rat renal
renin (Matoba et al., 1978). Rat renin was far more difficult
than hog renin by some unknown reasons. The final products eluted
from a CM cellulose column by a NaCl gradient emerged in 4 peaks,
each one of which was homogeneous as judged by the similar
criteria of purity as those applied to the hog renin (Fig. 2, 3
and 4).

    Analogous to hog renin activity, the pH-activity profiles of
the rat renins I, II and III covered neutral pH region (Fig. 5) in
contrast to numerous previous observations in which pH optimum of
crude renin was in the vicinity of pH 5.5. Amino acid compositions
of all three of rat renins were found to be very similar to that
of hog renin. More recently application of a more elaborate
affinity chromatographic system permitted us to isolate human
renin (Yokosawa et al., 1978). The purification was far more
difficult compared with that of renins from animal tissues. This
was because of the presence of a very strong protease activity and
a far lower concentration of renin compared with rat or hog kidneys.
A special affinity column was devised for the purpose of removing
proteases. Hemoglobin coupled to Sepharose served very well for
this purpose. Although not all of the proteases were removed by
this column, the most destructive ones adhered to the column while
renin did not show much affinity to the column.

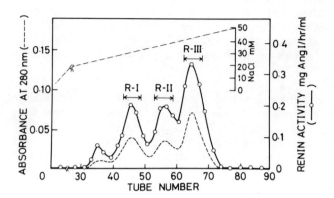

Fig. 2.   Final purification of rat renal renin on a CM-cellulose.
          (Matoba et al., 1978).

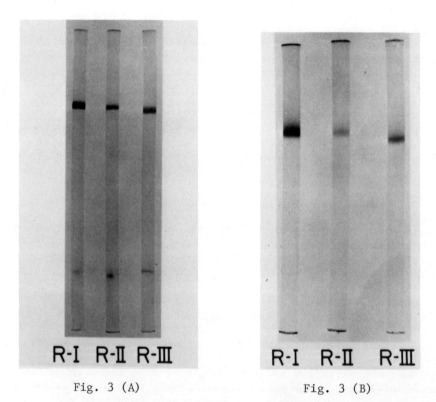

Fig. 3 (A)   Fig. 3 (B)

Fig. 3.   Polyacrylamide gel electrophoresis of rat renal renins
          (A) in the presence of 0.2 % sodium dodecylsulfate (SDS)
          and 0.25 % dithiothreitol(DTT) and (B) in the absence of
          SDS and DTT.   (Matoba et al., 1978)

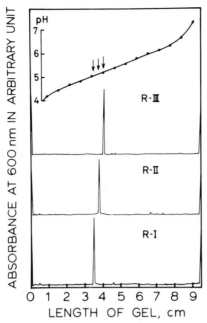

Fig. 4.   Isoelectric focusing of rat renal renin. Isoelectric points
of 5.05 for R-I, 5.15 for R-II and 5.22 for R-III were
estimated. (Matoba et al., 1978)

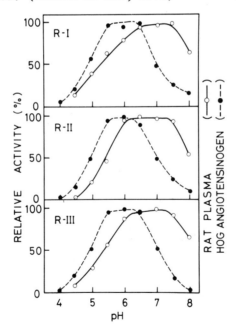

Fig. 5.   pH dependence of the rat renin reaction with different
substrate. (Matoba et al., 1978).

RENIN FROM MOUSE SUBMAXILLARY GLAND

The submaxillary gland of the mouse has been known to contain a large amount of renin-like enzyme. This enzyme was isolated by 5 steps of conventional column chromatographic procedure to five separate isoenzyme peaks (Cohen et al., 1972). All of the components immunologically cross-react and have similar amino acid compositions and molecular weights but slightly different isoelectric points. We believe that these different components arose by different extent of limited proteolysis though other mechanisms cannot be definitively eliminated. The mouse enzyme did not show any protease activity. Furthermore, it cross reacts with anti-hog renin antibodies as stated below. Therefore, we believe the mouse submaxillary gland renin is a true renin though we are completely ignorant about its physiological function in relation to its sex-dependent synthesis. In relation to kallikrein, it is extremely interesting to note that this renin is present in duct cells in the submaxillary gland of mouse as determined by immuno-histochemical method. In view of similar localization of kallikrein in the duct cell of the submandibular gland (Hojima et al., 1977 and Chiang et al., 1968) it is possible that both kallikrein and renin may be located in the same cell area, or at least, in a very close proximity.

ANTIBODY AGAINST RENIN

Antibodies were prepared to the pure hog renin which was insolubilized by various methods. Antibodies produced in one of several rabbits showed strong cross reactivity with rat renin and mouse submaxillary gland renin (Cohen et al., 1972). Direct radioimmunoassay method was developed using the antibody and ^{125}I-labeled renin. Under the optimal conditions, 40-50 pg of hog renin can be detected in hog plasma or extracts from various tissues (Hirose et al., 1977). This method has been very useful for identifying not only the active renin with a regular molecular weight of 40,000 but also to identify higher molecular weight forms of renin. The most useful application of the direct radio-immunoassay method was the distinction of true renin and non-specific renin-like activity by cathepsins. Low levels of angiotensin I generating activity have been reported in various tissues other than the kidney such as adrenals, gut, heart, lung, liver, blood vessel and brain (Ganten et al., 1971). The direct assay method eliminated the activity in most of these tissues such as gut, lung, liver as nonspecific activity of proteases. Further in support of this conclusion the activity in these tissues was not inactivated by the anti-renin antibody.

HIGH MOLECULAR WEIGHT RENIN

Even though the substrate specificity of renin is extremely
specialized and limited, renin is a protease. We have shown that
its active site structure is analogous to that of acid protease
and suggested that it may belong to the family of acid proteases.
As will be published later, numerous evidences supporting this
hypotheses are emerging. Acid proteases are formed from their
respective zymogens. Renins in various tissues such as the kidney,
plasma and amniotic fluid have been found to increase its activity
upon various nonphysiological treatment such as dialysis against
acidic buffers (Boyd, 1974, Leckie and McConnell, 1975, Skinner
et al., 1975),limited proteolysis by pepsin, trypsin (Morris and
Lumber, 1972, Day and Luetscher, 1975) and cathepsin D (Morris,
1978), and exposure to cold temperature without freezing.
Day and Luetscher have demonstrated that a higher molecular weight
($\simeq$ 60,000) form of renin exists in the blood of humans with
Wilms' tumor and diabetics with nephropathy (Day et al., 1976).
This big renin was shown to gain appreciable amount of additional
activity upon dialysis against acidic buffers or trypsin treatment
(Day et al., 1976). We have shown that this high molecular weight
form exists in hog kidney and were able to isolate big renin and
big big renin which possesses molecular weights of 60,000 and
140,000, respectively (Fig. 6). Although these variants of renin
have lower specific activities as shown in Table II and suggest a
possible zymogen-enzyme relationship, it was not possible

$$\text{Big-big renin} \longrightarrow \text{Big renin} \longrightarrow \text{Renin}$$

to demonstrate activation of big big renin nor big renin. At this
point it is not clear whether this was due to technical defect of
the activation technique or due to the loss of the activatable
properties of these high molecular weight forms. Levine and
his associates (Levine et al., 1976), Slater and Haber,and Inagami
et al. were not able to attain the activation of partially
purified preparation of big renin from human or hog kidneys.

REVERSIBLE CONVERSION OF BIG RENIN TO RENIN IN KIDNEY EXTRACTS

We have extracted renins from hog and rat kidneys in the
presence of protease inactivators to eliminate a possible attack
of endogenous proteases against renin in the extracts and found
blockers of sulfhydryl group, sodium tetrathionate of N-ethyl-
maleimide were able to maintain all the renin in the extracts to
big renin (M.W. = 60,000) when the blocker was added to the
extraction buffer. These results suggested that native form of
renin in the kidney is a high molecular weight form and it is
converted by an enzyme or agent requiring sulfhydryl groups to a
low molecular weight (circulating) form (Inagami et al., 1977).

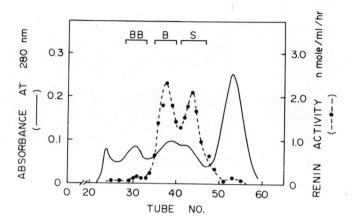

Fig. 6.   Gel filtration on Sephadex G-100 of hog renal renin and
          its high molecular weight forms after pepstatin-amino-
          hexyl agarose column.
          (Inagami & Murakami, 1977(b))
          BB : big big renin, B : big renin, S : regular size renin.

Table II.   Properties of hog renins. (Inagami & Murakami, 1977(b))

	pI	Specific activity* (µg angiotensin I/hr per µg enzyme)		Molecular weight**
Renin	5.2	267	(1,900)	42,500
Big renin	5.6	55	(400)	61,000
Big big renin I		0.5	(3)	140,000
Big big renin II	7.3	0.13	(1)	140,000

*   Determined by radioimmunoassay. Values in parentheses are in
    Goldblatt units/mg estimated in reference to the standard
    renins of Dr. Haas (no. 191, calibrated in March 1976) and
    of Bureau of Biological Standards and Control, London (65/119).

** Estimated by gel filtration.

Very recently, however, we found renin in the hog kidney extracts
was able to be converted to big renin completely with sodium
tetrathionate, when the extracts were incubated at 37°C for 15 min.
This conversion after the incubation was observed partially even
without sodium tetrathionate. Moreover, big renin in human kidney
extracts was converted to renin completely with dithiothreitol
when the extracts were incubated at 37°C for 15 min. Thus, we have
concluded that (1) the conversion of big renin to renin is
reversible (2) sulfhydryl-disulfide interchange plays an important
role in this conversion and (3) a renin binding protein or renin
inhibitor(s) exist in kidney cortex. This interconversion may be
an important role in renin secretion and in blood pressure
regulation.

RENIN ZYMOGEN IN THE PLASMA

     Renin activity in human plasma has been known to undergo
activation as described in the previous section. It has not been
known whether this activation is due to the creation of new
enzyme from completely inactive zymogen which contributes
additional activity to the active renin already present in the
plasma or it is due to the activation of a partially active
enzyme which has a potential for further activation. Boyd (1977),
separated such an enzyme with a partial activity with potential
for further activation. We have constructed a two step affinity
chromatographic system to separate inactive zymogen of renin from
normal human plasma. Since details of the isolation of this
inactive renin are given in another chapter of this volume,
details of the isolation studies are not given here. An
interesting finding associated to this renin zymogen is the fact
that it is activated not only by the nonphysiological enzyme such
as trypsin, but also by human urinary kallikrein, human plasma
kallikrein and hog pancreatic kallikrein when the plasma has been
pretreated by dialysis against pH 3.3. This acidification is
known to destroy plasma kallikrein inhibitors thus permitting
exogenous kallikrein to express its action.

REFERENCES

Aoyagi, T., H. Morishima, R. Nishizawa, S. Kunimoto, T. Takeuchi
    and H. Umezawa, 1972, Biological activity of pepstatins,
    pepstanone A and partial peptides on pepsin, cathepsin D and
    renin, J. Antibiotics 25, 689.
Boyd, G.W., 1974, A protein bound form of porcine renal renin,
    Circ. Res. 35, 426.
Boyd, G.W., 1977, An inactive higher-molecular weight renin in
    normal subjects and hypertensive patients, Lancet 1, 215.

Chiang, T.S., E.G. Erdös, I. Miwa, L.L. Tague and J.J. Coalson, 1968, Isolation from a salivary gland of granules containing renin and kallikrein, Circ. Res. 23, 507.

Cohen, S., J.M. Taylor, K. Murakami, A.M. Michelakis and T.Inagami 1972, Isolation and characterization of renin like enzymes from mouse submaxillary glands, Biochemistry 11, 4286.

Day, R.P. and J.A. Luetscher, 1975, Biochemical properties of big renin extracted from human plasma, J. Cli. Endocrinol. Meta. 40, 1085.

Day, R.P., J.A. Luetscher and P.G. Zager, 1976, Big renin : identification, chemical properties and clinical implication, Am. J. Cardiol. 37, 667.

Haber, E., T. Koerner, L.B. Page, B. Kliman and A. Purnode, 1969, Application of a radioimmunoassay for angiotensin II to the physiologic measurements of plasma renin activity in normal human subjects, J. Clin. Endocrinol. Metab. 29, 1349.

Ganten, D.A., A. Marquez-Julio, P. Granger, K. Hayduk, K.P. Karsunky, R. Boucher and J. Genest, 1971, Renin in dog brain, Am. J. Physiol. 221, 1733.

Hirose, S., T. Inagami and R.J. Workman, 1977, Antibody against pure hog renin and direct radioimmunoassay of renin, Circulation, 55 Suppl. III, 214.

Hojima, Y., B. Maranda, C. Moriwaki and M. Schachter, 1977, Direct evidence for the localization of kallikrein in the striated ducts of the cat's submandibular gland by the use of specific antibody, J. Physiol. 268, 793.

Inagami, T., S. Hirose, K. Murakami and T. Matoba, 1977, Native form of renin in the kidney, J. Biol. Chem. 252, 7733.

Inagami, T. and K. Murakami, 1977(a), Pure renin : isolation from hog kidney and characterization, J. Biol. Chem. 252, 2978.

Inagami, T. and K. Murakami, 1977(b), Purification of high molecular weight forms of renin from hog kidney, Cir. Res. 41,II-12.

Leckie, B. and A. McConnel, 1975, A renin inhibitor from rabbit kidney, Circ. Res. 36, 513.

Levine, M., K.E. Lentz, J.R. Kahn, F.E. Dorer and L.T. Skeggs, 1976, Partial purification of a high molecular weight renin from hog kidney, Circ. Res. 38, II-90.

Morris, B.J., 1978, Activation of human inactive (pro) renin by cathepsin and pepsin, J. Clin. Endocrinol. and Metab. 46, 153.

Morris, B.J. and E.R. Lumber, 1972, The activation of renin in human amniotic fluid by proteolytic enzymes, Biochim. Biophys. Acta, 289, 385.

Matoba, T., K. Murakami and T. Inagami, 1978, Rat renin : purification and characterization, Biochim. Biophys, Acta, 526, 560.

Murakami, K. and T. Inagami, 1975, Isolation of pure and stable renin from the kidney of hog, Biochem. Biophys. Res. Commun. 62, 757.

Reinharz, A. and M. Roth, 1969, Studies on renin with synthetic substrate, European J. Biochem. 7, 334.

Skinner, S.L., E.J. Cran, R. Gibson, R. Taylor and W.A. Walters, 1975, Angiotensin I and II, active and inactive renin, renin substrate, renin activity and angiotensinase in human liquor amnii and plasma, Am. J. Obstet. Gynecol. 121, 626.

Tigerstedt, R. and P.G. Bergman, 1898, Niere und kreislauf, Scand. Arch. Physiol. 8, 223.

Umezawa, H., T. Aoyagi, H. Morishima, M. Matsuzaki, M. Hamada and T. Takeuchi, 1970, Pepstatin, a new pepsin inhibitor produced by actinomycetes, J. Antibiotics. 23, 259.

Yckosawa, H., T. Inagami and E. Haas, 1978, Purification of human renin, Biochem. Biophys. Res. Commun. 83, 306.

PURIFICATION AND BIOCHEMICAL CHARACTERIZATION OF HUMAN URINARY KININASE

G. Porcelli, G.B. Marini-Bettolo, M. Di Jorio,
M. Ranieri, L. Ranalli, L. D'Acquarica

Centro Chimica Recettori C.N.R., Istituto di Chimica,
Fac. Med., Universita Cattolica, Rome, Italy

INTRODUCTION

In order to understand the implication of given kinin levels in the body, it will be necessary to study systematically the various parameters of body physiology and biochemistry that may affect kinin production and destruction (Talamo, 1977). The only information on human urinary kininase was reported by Erdos and Coll, (1964) who established that an ammonium sulfate precipitate of human urine shows carboxypeptidase activity. This activity is probably due to carboxypeptidase N (Kininase I) and peptidase P (kininase II).

Considering that the important kinin-destroying mechanism in man is not really clear at the present time, nor is the effect on this mechanism of various disease states known, we have decided to pursue research on human urinary kininase.

MATERIAL AND METHODS

Normal human urine was collected, covered with toluene, and preserved before treatment in the cold room at 5°C. The following were obtained: Sephadex A-50 from Pharmacia, Bio-gel P-200 from Bio-Rad Laboratories, L-Leucyl-beta-naphthylamide from Serva, Lysozyme from Serva, Ovoalbumin, serum bovine albumin, gamma glo-blulins and trypsin from Sigma, DE-32 and CM-32 from Whatman and hydroxylapatite-SC from Serva. Other chemicals used were reagent grade. Bradykinin (in vials of 0.08 mg/ml) was generously donated by Drs. A. Audibert and Braun of the Sandoz S.A. (Basel, Switzerland). Protein concentration was measured according to the Lowry

et al. method (1951) or estimated in the ultraviolet recorder
spectrophotometer at 280 nm. Molecular weight of human urinary
kininase was estimated by the Andrews method (1964).

A Bio-gel-P-200 column (0.8 x 128 cm) was calibrated with five
proteins of known molecular weight: lysozyme (16,000), Trypsin
(23,000), Ovoalbumin (45,000), serum bovine albumin (64,000) and
bovine gamma-globulins (160,000), using 0.1 M sodium phosphate
pH 7.5 as eluting buffer and reading at 280 nm to locate the protein
peaks. The human urinary kininase was also localized in the eluates
from its enzymatic activity by bioassay on bradykinin and as leu-
cinaminopeptidase (LAP) activity on L-leucine-beta-naphthylamide.
Arylaminopeptidase activity was determined by the method of Lee
et al. (1971).

Peptide derivatives of bradykinin, respectively N-terminal
heptapeptide and C-terminal dipeptide, were hydrolyzed with 6 N
HCl and the aminoacid analyses were performed in an aminoacid
analyzer "C. Erba". Human urinary kininase activity was measured
on the isolated rat uterus by the inactivation of added synthetic
bradykinin, the concentration of which was 0.4 µg. Kininase and
bradykinin were incubated in 0.1 M phosphate buffer at pH 7.5.
Samples were withdrawn from the incubation mixture at specific
intervals, immediately frozen in an ice and NaCl bath (-3°C),
diluted with tyrod solution and then added to the isolated rat
uterus. The decrease in the activity of kinin was determined at
several concentrations to obtain the final and exact concentration
of destroyed kinin.

To 10 lt of human urine sample, dialyzed against running
water for 50-55 hr., after filtration 10 g. of dry A-50 Sephadex
was added and the mixture was stirred for 15 hr in a cold room.
Successively the gel containing the adsorbed enzyme was layered
on the upper part of a column 5 x 10 cm of A-50 Sephadex equilibrated
in H_2O. The final A-50 Sephadex column (5 x 40 cm) was eluted by
buffer obtained by mixing 58.5 g of NaCl; 6.46 g of Na_2HPO_4. $7H_2O$;
0.62 g of $NaH_2PO_4 \cdot H_2O$ in 1 lt of H_2O. On the collected fractions
protein, arylaminopeptidase and kininase activities were determined.
The most active ones were pooled and dialyzed overnight against
running water. After adding 5 g of dry A-50, the enzymatic solution was stirred for 2 hr in a cold room and slowly layered on the
upper part of an A-50 column (3x5 cm) equilibrated in H_2O, obtaining
a final gel column 3x15 cm. This column was eluted by 12% of
buffered 1 M NaCl to the end of elution of kininase activity in
collected fractions. Human urinary kallikrein activity was eluted
from the column by elution with the buffered 1 M NaCl.

The fractions containing the kininase activity were pooled,
dialyzed against running water for 5 hr and treated with 5 ml of
hydroxylapatite. After 2 hr stirring, the hydroxylapatite containing

the adsorbed enzyme was layered to a hydroxylapatite column (2x4 cm), obtaining a final column 2 x 8 cm. This column was eluted by a sodium phosphate gradient as indicated in Table 1. Protein, aryl-aminopeptidase and kininase activity were determined on the collected fractions and the most active ones were pooled and lyophilized. The final product was separated three times on a Bio-gel P-200 column (0.8 x 128 cm) at flow of 0.5 ml/hr (5 fractions/hr).

RESULTS

Sephadex A-50, introduced by Erdos et al. (1974) for human plasma or kidney kininase fractionation, was found to be the best system for concentration of human urinary kininase (from 10 lt to 0.4-0.5 lt). For a partial purification of the enzyme from urinary kallikrein, the same chromatographic system was used again, while hydroxylapatite chromatography permitted the determination in human urine of the presence of three or more kinds of arylaminopeptidases (Fig. 1). The first, eluted from hydroxylapatite, contained a very fast destroying-kinin activity after 30 min. incubation time, and the second showed its kininase power after 45 min. The third arylaminopeptidase peak finally demonstrated a bradykinin-potentiating enzyme with the opposite action on kininase activity (Fig. 2).

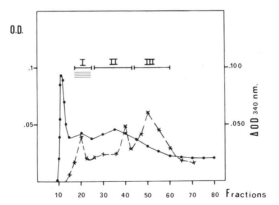

Figure 1. Purification of human urinary kininase activity on hydroxylapatite column. (●—●—●—●) Protein values, and (x--x--x--x) arylaminopeptidase activity in the collected fractions. Kininase activity, indicated by (≡≡≡≡), corresponds to the I peak of aryl-aminopeptidase activity.

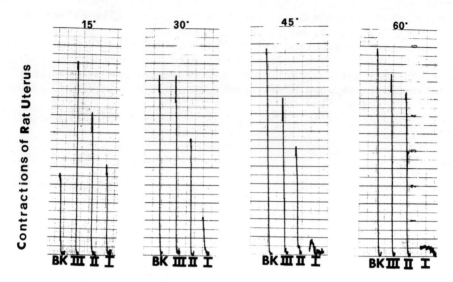

Figure 2.   The arylaminopeptidase components (I, II and III)
            obtained by hydroxylapatite chromatography (see
            Fig. 1), incubated at 37°C with bradykinin, show
            that the I peak corresponds to the human urinary
            kininase activity, the II peak contains a very
            low kininase activity and the III peak a poten-
            tiating effect of bradykinin (BK).

        By three successive separations on Bio-gel P-200 of the first
peak of arylaminopeptidase we obtained the purification of human
urinary kininase (160,000 molecular weight) protein, determined
by the Andrew's method (1964). This final product (0.750 mg of
protein in 3 ml solution) was used for chemical and biological
studies. When 400 ng of bradykinin were incubated with 0.200 ml
of the purified enzyme solution, the biological activity of the
peptide after 5 minutes at 37°C disappears.

        The biological properties of the enzyme in question were
further probed by means of various agents. In the biological
experiments on the inhibition or activation of human urinary
kininase, Co^{++} accelerated the enzyme, while Cd^{++} was an inhibitor.
Chelating agents, such as 1-10-phenantroline or EDTA (ethylendi-
aminetetracetic acid) block the enzyme.

        To determine the hydrolytic properties of human urinary
kininase, mg 0.240 of bradykinin were incubated for 8 hr with the
amount of urinary enzyme corresponding to 3.5 lt of human urine,
in 6 ml of 0.01 M sodium phosphate pH 7.5. After lyophilization
the product was dissolved and separated on Sephadex G-25 fine

column (0.8 x 128 cm) equilibrated and eluted with 0.01 M sodium phosphate at pH 7.5. Two components were separated, as indicated in Fig. 3, corresponding to the elution volumes of bradykinin and phenylalanine previously defined on that column. These components were hydrolyzed in 6 N HCl and then subjected to aminoacid analysis. The results, reproduced in Table 2, are not easily understood. In fact the chromatographic fraction I (Fig. 3), corresponding to the N-terminal heptapeptide derivative of bradykinin, contains more than one Arg residue. Analogously the fraction II (Fig. 3), corresponding to the C-terminal dipeptide derivative of bradykinin (Phe-Arg), shows a lower amount of the Arg residue in respect to the theoretical Phe-Arg C-terminal bradykinin derivative.

TABLE 1

I Cell:	ml 250 H_2O
II Cell:	ml 250 of 0.005 M Sodium phosphate pH 7.5
III Cell:	ml 250 of 0.010 M Sodium phosphate pH 7.5
IV Cell:	ml 250 of 0.050 M Sodium phosphate pH 7.5

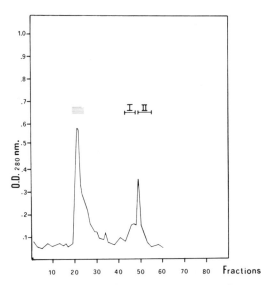

Figure 3.   Separation on Sephadex G-25 fine of human urinary kininase (▬▬▬), N-terminal heptapeptide derivative of bradykinin (I component) and C-terminal dipeptide derivative of bradykinin (II component).

TABLE 2

I Fraction from G-25 (0.8 x 128 cm)

Aminoacid	µMoles	µg	N. of Res.
Ser	0.102 x 2	17.8	1
Pro	0.225 x 2	53.6	3
Gly	0.109 x 2	13.3	1
Phe	0.088 x 2	26.2	1
Arg	0.140 x 2	43.6	> 1

II Fraction from G-25 (0.8 x 128 cm)

Aminoacid	µMoles	µg	N. of Res.
Phe	0.080 x 2	26.2	1
Arg	0.028 x 2	8.7	< 1

Recov. (189.4 µg/240) = 80%

DISCUSSION

Our experiments indicate that in human urine more than one
kininase is present (Fig. 1). The same kininase activity corresponding to the protein fraction obtained by gel filtration on P-200
will include more than a single type of kininase. From our results
human urinary kininase isolated by this procedure is a carboxy-
peptidase-type enzyme, very likely the same enzyme (or enzymes)
found by Erdos et al. (1964). The C-terminal Arg or Phe-Arg ends
of bradykinin attacked by kininase I and kininase II described by
Erdos et al. (1964), correspond to the kininase (or kininases)
described in this article. In fact, the heptapeptide isolated by
gel filtration on G-25 (Fig. 3) and defined by hydrolysis and
aminoacid analysis as the fraction I (Table 2), except for the Arg
residue in excess, corresponds in aminoacid composition to the
heptapeptide derivative of bradykinin. Likewise the dipeptide
Phe-Arg end of bradykinin obtained by gel filtration and defined
by hydrolysis and amino acid analysis as the fraction II reproduced
in Table 2 appears insufficient in Arg residue before the acidic
hydrolysis. The mechanism of this discrepancy may be due to a
free Arg residue obtained by the action of kininase I on bradykinin
and eluted in G-25 with the heptapeptide derivative of bradykinin.

Human urinary kininase can easily be distinguished from proteases like chymotrypsin or carboxypeptidase (A and B - type enzyme), first of all by its molecular weight: 25,000 for chymotrypsin; 45,000 - 50,000 for carboxypeptidases; 160,000 for human urinary kininase. The activity of chymotrypsin is accelerated by calcium, but it is not inhibited. by EDTA or 1-10 phenantroline. Carboxy-peptidases A does not split off basic C-terminal amino acids (Neurat, 1960); the bonds of Arg and Lys are broken by carboxy-peptidase B, which is not inhibited by EDTA (Folk et al., 1960).

This partial purification of human urinary kininase is the first approach to an enzyme which theoretically, destroying the kinins, can influence the biochemical mechanisms of vascular physiology. Through its sensitivity to various agents, the determination of kininase activity presents unquestionable difficulties, which when overcome could provide a key-enzyme for the interpretation of the mechanism leading to hypertension and infarction.

REFERENCES

Andrews, P., 1964. Estimation of the molecular weights of proteins by Sephadex gel filtration. Biochem. J. 91: 222.

Erdos, E.G., Sloane E.M., Wohler, I.M. 1964. Carboxypeptidase in blood and other fluids. J. Biochem. Pharmac. 13: 893.

Folk, J.E., Piez, K.A., Carroll, W.R., Gladner, J.L. 1960. Carboxypeptidase B IV. Purification and Characterization of the porcine enzyme. J. Biol. Chem., 235: 2272.

Lee, H.J., Larue, J.N., Wilson, I.B. 1971. A simple spectrophoto-metric assay for aminoacid arylamidases. Analyt. Biochem. 41: 307.

Lowry, O.H., Rosenbrough, N.J., Farr, A.L., Randall, R.J. 1951. Protein measurement with the folin phenol reagent. J. Biol. Chem., 193: 265.

Neurath, H. 1960. In: The Enzymes, II Edition. P.D. Boyer, H. Lardy, K. Myrback, eds. Vol. IV, p. 11.

Talamo, R.C. 1974. In: Chemistry and Biology of the Kallikrein-Kinin System in Health and Disease. Fogarty Intern. Center Proceeding No. 27, Ed. J.J. Pisano and K.F. Austen. p. 309.

VARIATION OF URINARY KALLIKREIN EXCRETION DURING PREGNANCY AND

THE EFFECTS OF HYPERTENSION

E. Moneta*, G. Porcelli**, S. Bennici*, M. Ranieri**,
and F. Pinca**
* Dept. of Obstetrics and Gynaecology
** Ist. di Chimica, Fac. Med., Universita Catt. Rome
and Centro Chimica Recettori C.N.R., Rome
*** I.P.S.A., Rome

ABSTRACT

In normal pregnant women the excretion of urinary kallikrein diminishes between the second and the third trimester and such reduction is maintained during the first ten days of puerperium.

A comparison between normal women and those suffering from hypertension during the first, second and third trimester of pregnancy shows that, except for the first trimester, there exists a significant net reduction of enzyme excretion in the hypertensive cases. Dividing the patients according to the type of hypertension, it reveals that this phenomenon is unaltered for subjects having essential hypertension, while those affected by secondary hypertension or gestosis do not show any statistically significant variation in enzyme excretion from normal subjects.

During puerperium urinary kallikrein excretion was also found to be normal in women with gestosis, but significantly decreased in women affected by renal hypertension.

INTRODUCTION

Urinary kallikrein excretion in normal pregnant women and in patients developing hypertension in late pregnancy has also been determined. Mean urinary kallikrein was highest in the first trimester and fell significantly in the third trimester to non-pregnant levels. The increase of kallikrein excretion in early pregnancy is

considered unlikely due to the "escape" from the sodium-retaining
effect of the high aldosterone of pregnancy. Reduced kallikrein
excretion has been considered a factor in the development of the
hypertension of gestosis and also noted to resemble the reduced
kallikrein excretion in essential hypertension; Elebute & Mills
(1976). Considering the severe collateral effects of hypertension
in pregnancy, we continued the study of the excretion of kallikrein
in different types of hypertension in pregnancy.

METHODS

Patients and normal subjects: Seventy-six healthy pregnant
women, average age 28.36 yrs (17-42 yrs.), were studied. From
these women 140 urinary samples were taken: 12 samples were collected
between the 6th and 14th week of pregnancy, 24 between the 15th and
27th week, 93 betwee the 28th and 41st week of pregnancy and 11
samples in puerperium. 103 samples were taken from forty-four pregnant women affected by hypertension, with average age 30 years,
(between 21-42 years); 5 were taken between the 6th and 14th week,
20 between the 15th and 27th week, 39 between the 28th and 41st
week of pregnancy and 39 samples were taken in puerperium. Twenty-
one of the 44 women were affected by essential hypertension, 10 by
secondary hypertension (reno-parenchymal) and 13 by hypertensive
gestosis. Blood pressures (systolic and diastolic) were determined
2-4 times daily in the hypertensive hospitalized women during the
period of urine collection.

Urinary samples: 24-hr. urines were obtained from 101 pregnant
women, for a total of 243 samples. The urine samples (100 ml) were
preserved in 5 ml of toluene and stored at 5°C prior to assay.

Urinary kallikrein: The urine samples were assayed for kallikrein esterase activity by a modified version of a previously described method (Porcelli et al., 1976), based on the ability of the
urinary kallikrein to hydrolyze N-benzoyl-L-arginine-ethyl ester.
In the previous method esterase activity was determined by spectrophotometric assay at 253 nm, at pH 8.0, and at 25°C. The treatment
of urine for the measurement of urinary kallikrein, in the present
method, involved only dialysis of the urinary sample in 0.1 M TRIS-
Cl solution at pH 8.0 and at 5°C, instead of the acetone fractionation of urinary proteins and dialysis procedure in running water.
The results were expressed in E.U. (esterase unit) per day (Porcelli
et al., 1974). Urines were routinely examined by bioassay (Porcelli
et al., 1972), and the results of two assay procedures were closely
correlated.

Statistical analysis: Statistical evaluation of urinary kallikrein levels in normal and pathological subjects was obtained by
"variance analysis" with the "F" Fisher test (Fisher and Yates, 1963).

RESULTS

During normal pregnancy kallikrein excretion was markedly decreased between the 28th and 41st week of pregnancy and in puerperium (Fig. 1). The variance analysis with the "F: Fisher test of kallikrein levels from the 6th to the 41st week of normal pregnancy and puerperium was statistically significant. The statistical test applied to compare the following week blocks: 6-14, 15-27, 28-41 and puerperium, showed a highly significant variance between the first trimester block and the third, between the first and puerperium, between the second and third and between the second block and puerperium (Table 1). There was no significant difference in kallikrein excretion (Table 2) from the 6th to 41st week of pregnancy and the puerperium of women affected by essential hypertension, gestosis or secondary hypertension (Fig. 2). A comparison between normal women (Table 3) and those suffering from essential hypertension during the entire pregnancy and puerperium showed a significant net reduction of enzyme excretion in the hypertensive cases, except for the first trimester period. The comparison between normal subjects and those affected by secondary hypertension or by gestosis did not show any statistically significant variation in kallikrein excretion during pregnancy.

During puerperium, urinary kallikrein excretion was also found to be normal with gestosis, but significantly decreased in women affected by renal hypertension.

RESULTS

Our results confirm the findings of Elebute and Mills with regard to the significant reduction of urinary kallikrein excretion during the third trimester of pregnancy, and also indicate that this reduction continues into the first ten days of puerperium.

Sims and Frantz (1958) claim that significant increase in renal blood flow can be measured in the first trimester of pregnancy and a fall in blood flow in the third trimester. Gordon et al., (1975) have shown that plasma renin is high in early pregnancy and falls after the 36th week. The elevation of angiotensin II without increase in blood pressure in normal pregnancy suggests that an antagonism exists between angiotensin II and other substances. Normal blood pressure, despite the high renin activity in normal pregnancy, suggests that angiotensin II may be antagonized also by the action of kallikrein. The comparison of urinary kallikrein excretion in normal and essentially hypertensive pregnant subjects (with the exception of the 1st trimester) showed a significant enzyme reduction in the hypertensive women in the second and third trimester and the puerperium. This phenomenon should not be correlated with the increased diuresis observed in hypertensives relative

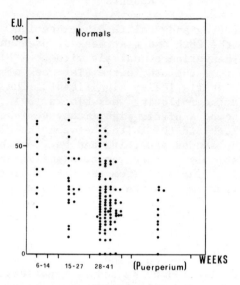

Figure 1

<u>Table 1</u>

Variance analysis of controls calculated by the values (E.U. per day) reproduced in Fig. 1.

Gestation period (in weeks)	Number of urinary samples	variance
6 - 14	13	
15 - 27	24	
28 - 41	93	p 0.001
puerperium	11	
6 - 14	13	P 0.05
15 - 27	24	
15 - 27	24	P 0.05
28 - 41	93	
28 - 41	93	p 0.05
puerperium	11	

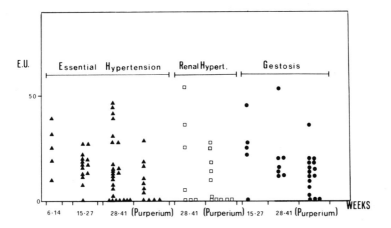

Figure 2

Table 2

Variance analysis of hypertensive subjects, calculated
by the values (E.U./day) reproduced in Fig. 2

Gestation period (in weeks)	Number of urinary samples	variance
Essential hypertension		
6 - 14	5	
15 - 27	16	
28 - 41	27	p 0.05
puerperium	12	
Gestosis		
6 - 14	0	
15 - 27	5	
28 - 41	7	p 0.05
puerperium	16	
Secondary Hypertension		
6 - 14	0	
15 - 27	0	
28 - 41	7	p 0.05
puerperium	11	

Table 3

Variance analysis between controls and hypertensive
subjects calculated by the values (E.U.) reproduced
in Fig. 1 and Fig. 2

Gestation period (in weeks)	Number of urinary samples (Controls/ pathological subj.)	variance	
Controls/Essen-tial Hypertension			
6 - 14	13/5	p	0.05
15 - 27	24/16	p	0.001
28 - 41	93/27	p	0.001
puerperium	11/12	p	0.05
Controls/Secon-dary Hypertension			
28 - 41	93/7	p	0.05
puerperium	11/11	p	0.01
Controls/Gestosis			
15 - 27	24/5	p	0.05
28 - 41	93/7	p	0.05
puerperium	11/16	p	0.05

to normotensives during the first weeks of pregnancy. In comparison
between normotensive pregnancies and women affected by gestosis we
did not find significant variations in urinary levels of kallikrein
excretion. This, in contrast to the results obtained by Elebute
and Mills, would indicate that the kallikrein-kinin system does not
participate in the increased blood pressure observed in these subjects during pregnancy, a phenomenon to be confirmed by more extensive case studies. Lastly, we showed a significant variation in
enzymatic excretion in women affected by renal hypertension relative
to normotensives in the puerperium.

REFERENCES

Elebute, O.A., and Mills, I.H. (1976). in: Hypertension in pregnancy.
    Symposium held at the Univ. of Chicago's Center, Sept. 25/27,
    1975, Ed. New York. p. 329.

Fisher, R.A. and Yates, F. (1963).   Statistical Tables; Ed. Oliver
     and Boyd, London.
Gordon, R.D., Symonds, E.M. and Wilmshurst, E.G. (1975).   Plasma
     renin activity, plasma angiotensin and plasma and urinary
     electrolytes in normal and toxaemic pregnancy including a
     prospective study. Clin. Sci. Mol. Med., 45: 115.
Porcelli, G. (1976). Progress on biochemical urinary kallikrein
     test. Adv. Exp. Med. Biol., 70: 183.
Porcelli, G., Croxatto, H.R. and Porcelli, F. (1972). Clinical
     determination of kallikrein in human urine. Adv. Exp. Med.
     Biol., 21: 135.
Procelli, G., Marini-Bettolo, G.B., Croxatto, H.R. and Di Jorio, M.
     (1974). Purification and chemical characterization of human
     urinary kallikrein. Ital. J. Biochem., 23: 24.
Sims, E.A. and Krantz, K.E. (1958). Serial studies of renal function
     during pregnancy and puerperium in normal women. J. Clin.
     Invest., 37: 1764.

ALTERED URINARY EXCRETION OF HUMAN KININASE ACTIVITY

IN HYPERTENSION

A. Greco, G. Porcelli, M. Di Jorio, M. Ranieri,
L. D'Acquarica, and L. Ranalli

Instituto di Patologia Medica and Instituto di Chimica,
Facolta di Medicina, Universita Cattolica S. Cuore,
Roma - Centro Chimica Recettori C.N.R., Roma, Italy

ABSTRACT

This study describes the levels of urinary kininase activity
in hypertension. Urinary kininase activity in essential and secondary hypertensive patients was higher than in controls ($1010.2 \pm
102.7$ versus 114.4 ± 23.1 ng destroyed bradykinin/min.; $p < 0.001$).
In a group of hypertensive diabetics without nephropathy kininase
activity in urine was decreased (46.0 ± 12.7 ng destroyed brady-
kinin/min.). This investigation shows that in hypertension urinary
kininase activity reaches higher levels. An inverse correlation
was found between urinary kallikrein and urinary kininase activity
from essential hypertensive patients.

INTRODUCTION

As far as we know there are no studies concerning the role of
urinary kininase activity in hypertension. Human urinary kininase
activity was determined by a biological method. The method is
based on the enzymatic properties of the urinary kininase which,
when incubated with bradykinin, destroys it. The amount of destroyed bradykinin/min. is estimated on isolated rat uterus.

MATERIAL AND METHODS

Twenty-one (21) normal male subjects, 21-48 years old, (32.6
± 1.9: mean $\pm$ SE), 6 secondary and 28 essential hypertensive
patients, 17 to 51 years of age (42.5 ± 1.7) were studied.

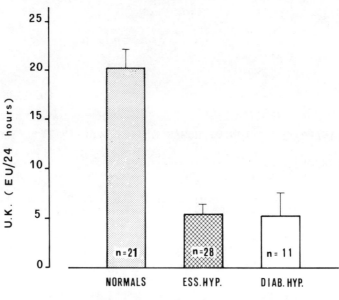

Figure 1

Eleven hypertensive patients with diabetes mellitus, without clinical evidence of diabetic nephropathy, were also studied. Previous to the study, no drug was administered for at least two weeks and were also subjected to a Na+ free diet. Tests of blood creatinine, endogenous clearance, renography, timed intravenous urography with washout test were carried out besides normal routine tests. The urine samples (24 h collection) were kept in toluene at 4°C for not longer than a week for testing the enzymes. Urinary kallikrein activity was assayed by the Porcelli and Marini-Bettolo method (1978), measuring esterase activity upon benzoyl-arginine-ethyl-ester (BAEE). The results are expressed in esterase units (E.U.) excreted per 24 hours. Kininase activity was determined by the Porcelli et al. method (same issue). The results are expressed in ng of destroyed bradykinin (BK) used as substrate in a reaction at 37°C with the urinary enzyme. Student's t test and Pearson's correlation coefficient were used in statistical analyses, the standard error is indicated for all data.

RESULTS

Urinary kallikrein (fig. 1) in apparently normal males ranged from 9.5 to 41.5 E.U./24 hours with a mean value of 20.26 ± 2.11 E.U.; in 28 essential hypertensive patients kallikrein excretion averaged 5.4 ± 1.2 E.U./24 hours P < 0.001), while in secondary

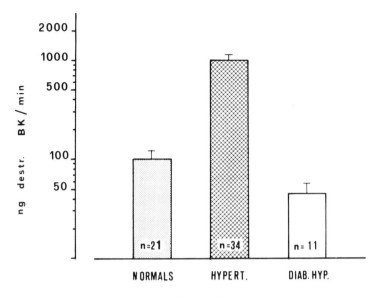

Figure 2

hypertensive patients urinary kallikrein activity was close to
normal values. In diabetics,urinary kallikrein activity was significantly lower than in the controls (5.28 ± 2.4 E.U.; P < 0.001).

Urinary kininase activity (fig. 2) in controls ranged from
0.0 to 380 ng destroyed BK/min. with a mean value of 164.4 ± 23.1;
in 34 hypertensive patients kininase in urine averaged 1013.2 ±
102.7 ng destroyed BK/min. (P< 0.001). In hypertensive diabetics
urinary kininase was 46.0 ± 12.7 with a range from 0.0 to 83 ng
destroyed BK/min. Urinary kallikrein activity and urinary kininase
activity were not directly related with diastolic arterial pressure
in essential hypertensive patients (r = -0.198) while an inverse
correlation was found between urinary kallikrein excretion and
urinary kininase activity from essential hypertensive patients without diabetes(r = 0.596; P < 0.001)(fig. 3).

DISCUSSION

The results of this study confirm that in essential hypertensive
patients urinary kallikrein is lower than in controls (Margolius
et al., 1971), (Greco et al., 1974). The importance of kinin-
inactivating enzymes in man is not yet clear, especially concerning
its role in the imbalance of blood pressure. This study clearly

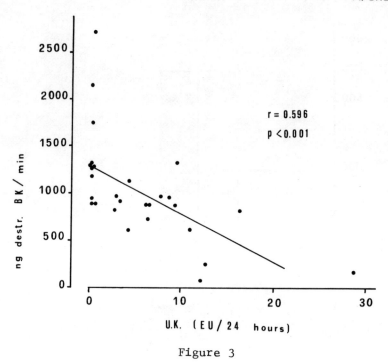

Figure 3

demonstrates that in essential and secondary hypertensive patients
kininase activity in urine reaches higher levels; the same results
have not been detected in diabetic hypertensive patients. Therefore, in understanding the genesis of hypertension further steps
have been done. It may be concluded that this strong capacity for
the destruction of circulating kinins may be responsible for the
high values of blood pressure in primary and secondary hypertensive
patients. Why a decreased kininase activity was detected in the
urine of diabetic hypertensive patients is not clear yet. It is
possible that the metabolic changes of diabetes mellitus have a
negative influence on the kallikrein-kinin system.

REFERENCES

Greco, A., Porcelli, G., Croxatto, H.R., Fedeli, G., Ghirlanda, G.,
    1974. Ipertensione arteriosa e callicreina urinaria. Min.
    Med., 65: 3058.

Margolius, H.S., Geller, R., Pisano, J.J., Sjoerdsma, A., 1971.
    Altered urinary kallikrein excretion in human hypertension.
    Lancet 2: 1063.

Porcelli, G. and Marini-Bettolo G.B., 1978. A simplified method
    to prepare human urinary sample for measurement of kallikrein
    esterase activity. V. National Congress of Soc. Ital. of
    Clinical Biochemistry, October 18-22, Rome.

Porcelli, G., Di Jorio, M., Ranieri, M., Ranalli, L. and D'Acquarica,
    L. (same issue). A method for measurement of human urinary
    kininase activity.

STRUCTURE-ACTIVITY RELATIONSHIPS FOR KININASE II INHIBITION BY LOWER HOMOLOGS OF THE BRADYKININ POTENTIATING PEPTIDE BPP$_{9a}$

George H. Fisher, James W. Ryan, Larry C. Martin, and Guillermo A. Pena

Department of Medicine, University of Miami School of Medicine, Miami, Florida 33101, USA

The bradykinin potentiating peptide BPP$_{9a}$ (<Glu-Trp-Pro-Arg-Pro-Gln-Ile-Pro-Pro) is a potent inhibitor (I_{50}, 28 nM) of kininase II (angiotensin converting enzyme). We have synthesized several N-terminal, C-terminal, and internal lower homologs of BPP$_{9a}$ and determined their potencies as inhibitors of kininase II. Inhibition of kininase II was measured using [^{3}H]-Hip-His-Leu as substrate. Enzyme, partially purified from human urine, was measured in terms of the formation of [^{3}H]-hippuric acid. Three of the lower homologs are as potent as BPP$_{9a}$: the internal hexapeptide Trp^2---Ile^7 (I_{50}, 34 nM), the C-terminal octapeptide Trp^2---Pro^9 (I_{50}, 50 nM), and the N-terminal heptapeptide <Glu^1---Ile^7 (I_{50}, 54 nM). The C-terminal tri- and tetrapeptides show significant inhibitory activities (I_{50}, 330 and 760 nM), whereas the N-terminal di-, tri-, and tetrapeptides are weak inhibitors. <Glu^1 is not necessary for binding but may protect the peptide against enzymic degradation. Trp^2 is critical for binding. Pro^9 facilitates binding, but proline as a penultimate C-terminal residue is generally unfavorable and prevents or greatly reduces binding. Ile^7 as the C-terminal residue of a lower homolog appears to facilitate binding. Arg^4 or a basic side chain at residue 4 is not critical. Pro^3, Pro^5, and Gln^6 do not appear to be important for binding, _per se_, but may affect the overall conformation of the peptide.

INTRODUCTION

The bradykinin potentiating peptide BPP$_{9a}$ (SQ 20,881), isolated from the venom of Bothrops jararaca (Ferreira, 1965; Ferreira et al., 1970; Ondetti et al., 1971) is a potent inhibitor (I_{50}, 28 nM) of kininase II (also known as angiotensin converting enzyme). Prelimi-

inary structure-activity relationships for kininase II inhibition
by BPP_{9a} have been determined by Pluscec et al. (1972) and Cushman
et al. (1973) based on selected lower homologs and analogs of BPP_{9a}.
From these studies, the effects of amino acid replacements on the
inhibitory activity of BPP_{9a} can be summarized as follows:

The pyroglutamic acid residue at the N-terminus can be replaced
with a cyclopentylcarbonyl residue to yield an analog having 5-times
the potency of BPP_{9a}. Aliphatic hydrophobic amino acids are not as
suitable as aromatic amino acids to replace Trp^2 and tryptophan is
preferred to other aromatic amino acids. The basic arginine residue
at position 4 may be replaced by other basic amino acids (Lys, His,
or Orn) or even by glycine with retention of inhibitory activity,
indicating that the basic side chain at residue 4 is not critical.
Changes in the amino acids at positions 6, 7, and 8 that make the
C-terminal tetrapeptide more similar to BPP_{5a} (<Glu-Lys-Trp-Ala-
Pro) lead to an increase of inhibitory potency, e.g., peptides with
phenylalanine in the third position from the C-terminus, such as
Phe^7-BPP_{9a}, are bound more tightly to the enzyme than those having
other residues in this position. A free α-carboxyl group of the
amino acid at the C-terminus is critical for inhibitory activity,
but kininase II does not readily hydrolyze peptides containing a
penultimate amino acid such as proline or a C-terminal dicarboxylic
amino acid such as glutamic acid (Elisseeva et al., 1971).

In efforts to elucidate further the structure-activity relationships of BPP_{9a}, we have begun to synthesize the 40+ possible
lower homologs of BPP_{9a} and to determine their $I50$ values in order
to gain further insights into the structural requirements of BPP_{9a}
and its lower homologs for inhibition of kininase II.

MATERIALS AND METHODS

Syntheses

The lower homologs of BPP_{9a} were synthesized by the Merrifield
solid-phase technique (Merrifield, 1963, 1964; Stewart and Young,
1969; Erickson and Merrifield, 1976) on a Schwarz-Mann automatic
peptide synthesizer. Commercially available protected amino acids
were used. The α-amino functions were protected by the tert-butyl-
oxycarbonyl (Boc) group, with the exception of arginine and pyroglutamic acid, whose α-amino functions were protected by the amyl-
oxycarbonyl (Aoc) and the benzyloxycarbonyl (Z) groups, respectively.

The α-amino protecting group of the amino-protected intermediate
on the resin was removed with 30% trifluoroacetic acid (TFA) in
dichloromethane (CH_2Cl_2), with neutralization of the resulting TFA
salt by 10% triethylamine (TEA) in CH_2Cl_2 to give the free α-amino

group. A 2.5-fold excess of each protected amino acid was used for
each dicyclohexylcarbodiimide (DCC)-mediated coupling with an average
coupling time of 2-4 hours. However, a 5-fold excess of Boc-Gln-
ONP in dimethylformamide (DMF) was used for incorporation of gluta-
mine with an average coupling time of 10-12 hours. Completeness of
each coupling was monitored by the ninhydrin color test procedure
of Kaiser et al. (1970).

Since tryptophan is susceptible to oxidation after incorporation into the peptide, the TFA reagent and solvents used thereafter
contained 1% β-mercaptoethanol. Diketopiperazine formation from a
Pro-Pro or an X-Pro dipeptide resin was avoided by using inverse
addition of DCC and the protected amino acid used for coupling to
the dipeptide resin (Gisin & Merrifield, 1972).

Cleavage of the peptide from the resin with simultaneous
removal of the protecting groups and formation of the terminal
carboxyl group was accomplished with anhydrous (CoF$_3$-dried) liquid
hydrogen fluoride (HF) in the presence of 10% anisole for 60 minutes
at 0° (Sakakibara et al., 1967; Lenard and Robinson, 1967) on a
Toho Kasei HF line. After removal of excess HF in vacuo, the resin
was washed with ethyl acetate-ether (1:1) to remove anisole. The
peptide was extracted from the resin with dilute acetic acid and
then lyophilized. No problems with oxidation of tryptophan have
been encountered during HF cleavage or subsequent purification of
any of the homologs synthesized to date, as evidenced by complete
retention of Trp on amino acid analysis after hydrolysis in 3 N
mercaptoethane sulfonic acid (Penke et al., 1974).

The crude deprotected peptides were purified by combinations
of gel filtration on Bio-Gel P-2 or Sephadex G-10 or G-15 eluted
with 1% acetic acid; partition chromatography on Sephadex G-10,
G-15, or G-25 with the system n-butanol-acetic acid-water (4:1:5);
and finally chromatography on Sephadex LH-20 with 6% n-butanol-water.
The purity of the final peptides was assayed by amino acid analysis
(after hydrolysis in 6 N HCl or 3 N mercaptoethane sulfonic acid,
for Trp-containing peptides, in sealed tubes overnight at 110°),
by thin layer chromatography on silica gel plates in at least 4
systems, by high performance liquid chromatography, and by paper
electrophoresis at pH 2.0 and 5.0.

Kininase II Inhibition Assay

Each of the synthetic lower homologs of BPP$_{9a}$ was assayed for
its ability to inhibit kininase II by the assay techniques developed
in this laboratory (Ryan et al., 1977, 1978). Inhibitory potencies
were measured in terms of the ability of a homolog to inhibit hydrolysis of the substrate p-[^{3}H]-benzoyl-Gly-His-Leu ([^{3}H]-Hip-His-Leu)
by kininase II partially purified from guinea pig lung or human

urine. Essentially identical results are obtained with either
enzyme preparation. A standard amount of the enzyme (taken as the
amount which hydrolyzes 8% of substrate in 15 min) and [3H]-Hip-
His-Leu plus carrier at 100 µM are incubated at 37° C for 15 min
with various concentrations of a given inhibitor in Hepes buffer
containing 0.1 $\underline{M}$ NaCl and 0.75 $\underline{M}$ Na$_2$SO$_4$, at pH 8. The reaction is
terminated by addition of 0.1 $\underline{N}$ HCl, and substrate is separated
from tritiated reaction product, [3H]-hippuric acid, by extraction
of the latter into ethyl acetate. A portion of the organic phase
is submitted to liquid scintillation counting. Enzyme activity is
measured in terms of the rate of formation of [3H]-hippuric acid,
and a plot of enzyme activity of percent inhibition of enzyme
activity vs log concentration of inhibitor is made. That concentration of inhibitor which reduces enzyme activity by half is defined
as the inhibitory potency and is expressed as the I$_{50}$ value.

RESULTS

     Each of the 24 synthetic lower homologs of BPP$_{9a}$ was homoge-
neous, as judged by thin layer chromatography, high performance
liquid chromatography, and paper electrophoresis at pH 2 and 5.
Each homolog was assayed for its ability to inhibit the activity of
kininase II (see Tables 1 and 2).

     Three of the lower homologs are as potent as BPP$_{9a}$ itself:
the internal hexapeptide (II) Trp[2]---Ile[7] (I$_{50}$, 34 nM), the C-
terminal octapeptide (III) Trp[2]---Pro[9] (I$_{50}$, 50 nM), and the N-
terminal heptapeptide (IV) <Glu[1]---Ile[7] (I$_{50}$, 54 nM). Surprisingly,
the C-terminal tripeptide (VI) Ile-Pro-Pro and tetrapeptide (IX)
Gln-Ile-Pro-Pro (Table 4) show significant inhibitory activities
(I$_{50}$, 330 and 760 nM, respectively). The N-terminal di-, tri-, and
tetrapeptides (Table 3), however, are weak inhibitors.

     The pyroglutamic acid residue at position one does not appear
to be necessary for binding; des-<Glu[1]-BPP$_{9a}$ (III) is as potent as
BPP$_{9a}$. The pyroglutamic acid, however, may protect the peptide
against enzymic degradation. Pluscec et al. (1972) have shown that
the pyroglutamic acid residue can be replaced with a cyclopentylcarbonyl residue with a 5-fold increase in inhibitory potency.

     The nature of the last three amino acid residues comprising
the C-terminus of an inhibitor appears to be important for significant interaction with the active site of the enzyme. The presence
of a free α-carboxyl group at the C-terminal residue is necessary
for binding. This binding is most advantageous when the C-terminal
residue is proline (Tables 4 and 5) or isoleucine (Table 6). However, proline as a penultimate C-terminal residue is generally unfavorable and prevents or greatly reduces binding, with the exception
of the C-terminal homologs Trp[2]---Pro[9] (III) and Ile-Pro-Pro (VI)
(Table 4).

Table 1

INHIBITION OF KININASE II BY BPP$_{9a}$ AND SOME OF ITS LOWER HOMOLOGS

Number	Structure	I$_{50}$(nM)
I	<Glu-Trp-Pro-Arg-Pro-Gln-Ile-Pro-Pro (BPP$_{9a}$)	28
II	Trp-Pro-Arg-Pro-Gln-Ile	34
III	Trp-Pro-Arg-Pro-Gln-Ile-Pro-Pro	50
IV	<Glu-Trp-Pro-Arg-Pro-Gln-Ile	54
V	Pro-Arg-Pro-Gln-Ile-Pro	170
VI	Ile-Pro-Pro	330
VII	Pro-Arg-Pro-Gln-Ile-Pro-Pro	350
VIII	Trp-Pro-Arg-Pro-Gln-Ile-Pro	550
IX	Gln-Ile-Pro-Pro	760
X	<Glu-Trp-Pro-Arg-Pro-Gln-Ile-Pro	830
XI	Arg-Pro-Gln-Ile-Pro-Pro	1,100
XII	Pro-Gln-Ile-Pro-Pro	1,500
XIII	<Glu-Trp-Pro-Arg-Pro	2,300
XIV	Trp-Pro-Arg-Pro	6,000
XV	Pro-Arg-Pro-Gln-Ile	7,200
XVI	Arg-Pro-Gln-Ile	7,500
XVII	Pro-Arg-Pro	11,000
XVIII	Arg-Pro-Gln-Ile-Pro	14,000
XIX	<Glu-Trp-Pro	42,000
XX	Pro-Gln-Ile-Pro	62,000
XXI	Pro-Arg-Pro-Gln	65,000
XXII	<Glu-Trp-Pro-Arg-Pro-Gln	71,000
XXIII	Pro-Gln-Ile	110,000
XXIV	<Glu-Trp	290,000
XXV	<Glu-Trp-Pro-Arg	450,000

Tryptophan as residue two of BPP$_{9a}$ appears to be critical for binding. This is particularly evident in the order of potencies of the C-terminal homologs (Table 4); Pro[3]---Pro[9] (VII) is about one tenth as potent as BPP$_{9a}$, whereas Trp[2]---Pro[9] (III), is as potent as BPP$_{9a}$. Table 6 shows the effect of tryptophan even more clearly; Trp[2]---Ile[7] (II) is over 200 times more potent than the next lower homolog Pro[3]---Ile[7] (XV). Tryptophan, however, can be replaced with other aromatic amino acids, such as phenylalanine and tyrosine, with retention of inhibitory activity, but tryptophan is the preferred aromatic amino acid at position two (Cushman et al., 1973).

Arg[4] or a basic side chain at residue 4 is not critical (Plusec et al., 1972). Pro[3], Pro[5], and Gln[6] do not appear to be important for binding, per se, but may affect the overall conformation of the peptide. In related work, we have synthesized analogs of BPP$_{9a}$ containing the amino acid L-3,4-dehydroproline (ΔPro) in place of

Table 2

INHIBITION OF KININASE II BY BPP$_{9a}$ AND SOME OF ITS LOWER HOMOLOGS
(ALIGNED TO PERMIT DIRECT COMPARISON OF THEIR C-TERMINAL RESIDUES)

Number	Structure	I_{50}(nM)
I	\<Glu-Trp-Pro-Arg-Pro-Gln-Ile-Pro-Pro (BPP$_{9a}$)	28
II	Trp-Pro-Arg-Pro-Gln-Ile	34
III	Trp-Pro-Arg-Pro-Gln-Ile-Pro-Pro	50
IV	\<Glu-Trp-Pro-Arg-Pro-Gln-Ile	54
V	Pro-Arg-Pro-Gln-Ile-Pro	170
VI	Ile-Pro-Pro	330
VII	Pro-Arg-Pro-Gln-Ile-Pro-Pro	350
VIII	Trp-Pro-Arg-Pro-Gln-Ile-Pro	550
IX	Gln-Ile-Pro-Pro	760
X	\<Glu-Trp-Pro-Arg-Pro-Gln-Ile-Pro	830
XI	Arg-Pro-Gln-Ile-Pro-Pro	1,100
XII	Pro-Gln-Ile-Pro-Pro	1,500
XIII	\<Glu-Trp-Pro-Arg-Pro	2,300
XIV	Trp-Pro-Arg-Pro	6,000
XV	Pro-Arg-Pro-Gln-Ile	7,200
XVI	Arg-Pro-Gln-Ile	7,500
XVII	Pro-Arg-Pro	11,000
XVIII	Arg-Pro-Gln-Ile-Pro	14,000
XIX	\<Glu-Trp-Pro	42,000
XX	Pro-Gln-Ile-Pro	62,000
XXI	Pro-Arg-Pro-Gln	65,000
XXII	\<Glu-Trp-Pro-Arg-Pro-Gln	71,000
XXIII	Pro-Gln-Ile	110,000
XXIV	\<Glu-Trp	290,000
XXV	\<Glu-Trp-Pro-Arg	450,000

the proline residues at positions 3, 5, 8, or 9 (Fisher et al.,
1978). Two of these analogs, ΔPro^3-BPP$_{9a}$ and ΔPro^5-BPP$_{9a}$, are
approximately 20 times more potent (I_{50}, 0.9 nM) than BPP$_{9a}$ as
kininase II inhibitors, and ΔPro^9-BPP$_{9a}$ is 100 times more potent
(I_{50}, 0.3 nM). The high inhibition potencies of these analogs may
be due to preferential π-π interaction of the deformed electron
cloud of the double bond of the ΔPro residue with binding sites
on the enzyme. Alternatively, the more rigid ΔPro residue at
these positions may alter the overall conformation of the peptide
such that it is more readily recognized by the active site of the
enzyme.

Table 3

INHIBITION OF KININASE II BY AMINO-TERMINAL HOMOLOGS OF BPP$_{9a}$

Number	Structure	I_{50}(nM)
I	<Glu-Trp-Pro-Arg-Pro-Gln-Ile-Pro-Pro (BPP$_{9a}$)	28
X	<Glu-Trp-Pro-Arg-Pro-Gln-Ile-Pro	830
IV	<Glu-Trp-Pro-Arg-Pro-Gln-Ile	54
XXII	<Glu-Trp-Pro-Arg-Pro-Gln	71,000
XIII	<Glu-Trp-Pro-Arg-Pro	2,300
XXV	<Glu-Trp-Pro-Arg	450,000
XIX	<Glu-Trp-Pro	42,000
XXIV	<Glu-Trp	290,000

DISCUSSION

Cushman et al. (1977) have postulated a model for the active site of kininase II for substrates and inhibitors. A positively charged residue at the active site is thought to bind with the negatively charged C-terminal carboxyl group of the peptide substrate or inhibitor. An enzyme-bound zinc ion (Das and Soffer, 1975), which is expected to play a role in the peptide bond cleavage of a substrate, is separated from the positively charged residue by the distance of a dipeptide residue and coordinates with the second amide bond from the C-terminus of a substrate. In addition, it is assumed that the enzyme may also form a hydrogen bond with the carbonyl of the C-terminal amide bond. The enzyme may also have some hydrophobic affinity for the side chains of the two C-terminal residues of a peptide substrate or inhibitor. From the nature of our assay for kininase II, using the acetylated tripeptide substrate Bz-Gly-His-Leu, one can assume that C-terminal binding of substrate

Table 4

INHIBITION OF KININASE II BY CARBOXYL-TERMINAL HOMOLOGS OF BPP$_{9a}$

Number	Structure	I_{50}(nM)
I	<Glu-Trp-Pro-Arg-Pro-Gln-Ile-Pro-Pro (BPP$_{9a}$)	28
III	Trp-Pro-Arg-Pro-Gln-Ile-Pro-Pro	50
VII	Pro-Arg-Pro-Gln-Ile-Pro-Pro	350
XI	Arg-Pro-Gln-Ile-Pro-Pro	1,100
XII	Pro-Gln-Ile-Pro-Pro	1,500
IX	Gln-Ile-Pro-Pro	760
VI	Ile-Pro-Pro	330

Table 5

INHIBITION OF KININASE II BY BPP_{9a} HOMOLOGS HAVING PRO^8 AS C-TERMINUS

Number	Structure	I_{50}(nM)
I	<Glu-Trp-Pro-Arg-Pro-Gln-Ile-Pro-Pro (BPP$_{9a}$)	28
X	<Glu-Trp-Pro-Arg-Pro-Gln-Ile-Pro	830
VIX	Trp-Pro-Arg-Pro-Gln-Ile-Pro	760
V	Pro-Arg-Pro-Gln-Ile-Pro	170
XIX	Arg-Pro-Gln-Ile-Pro	42,000
XX	Pro-Gln-Ile-Pro	62,000
	Gln-Ile-Pro	----

is important, and the characteristics of the hydrolysis that occurs implies such binding. Peptides having C-terminal amides, however, do not bind to the enzyme or inhibit the enzyme. For hydrolysis of a substrate to occur, the C-terminal binding site of the enzyme must be free to interact with the substrate, as also must the zinc ion of the catalytic site of the enzyme.

This information, combined with the present data for inhibition of kininase II by BPP_{9a} and its lower homologs, led us to design the model proposed in Figure 1. Binding of the free α-carboxyl group of the C-terminus may be the first and critical step to enzyme-substrate/inhibitor interaction. This binding appears to be most advantageous when the C-terminal residue is proline or isoleucine (Table 2). Considering the C-terminal lower homologs of BPP_{9a} (Table 4), size, per se, is not a factor in terms of the affinity of binding; in fact, Ile-Pro-Pro (VI) has a higher affinity than any of the higher C-terminal homologs with the exception of Trp^2---Pro^9 (III). Addition of Gln^6, Pro^5, and then Arg^4 does not significantly improve the apparent binding affinity. Pro^3 clearly favors

Table 6

INHIBITION OF KININASE II BY BPP_{9a} HOMOLOGS HAVING ILE^7 AS C-TERMINUS

Number	Structure	I_{50}(nM)
I	<Glu-Trp-Pro-Arg-Pro-Gln-Ile-Pro-Pro (BPP$_{9a}$)	28
III	<Glu-Trp-Pro-Arg-Pro-Gln-Ile	54
II	Trp-Pro-Arg-Pro-Gln-Ile	34
XV	Pro-Arg-Pro-Gln-Ile	7,200
XVI	Arg-Pro-Gln-Ile	7,500
XXIII	Pro-Gln-Ile	110,000
	Gln-Ile	----

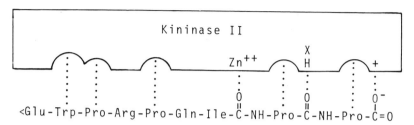

Figure 1.   Proposed model for interaction of BPP$_{9a}$ with kininase II.

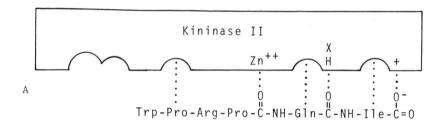

A

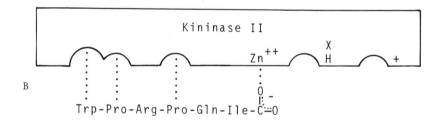

B

Figure 2.   Binding of Trp^2---Ile^7 to kininase II. A. Model for
preferential binding to the carboxyl binding site.
B. Model for preferential binding to the distant
tryptophan binding site.

binding for this series, and the addition of Trp^2 at the N-terminus yields a homolog (III) with virtually the potency of BPP_{9a}. Little advantage, however, is gained by addition of $<Glu^1$. These results, therefore, bespeak the importance of an additional binding site at a distance from the catalytic site of the enzyme, one filled well by an aromatic amino acid, such as tryptophan, at residue 2; a conclusion arrived at independently by Cushman et al. (1973).

BPP_{9a} is bound at least 10-fold more tightly to the enzyme than is its C-terminal tripeptide, Ile-Pro-Pro (VI). However, even the least potent of the lower homologs are bound 100- to 1000-fold more tightly than are substrates commonly employed for the assay of the enzyme (Cheung and Cushman, 1973; Ryan et al., 1978). The extra binding affinity of BPP_{9a} and Trp^2---Pro^9, above and beyond that conferred by the competitive C-terminal tripeptide, argues in favor of an important distant binding site. However, it is still not known whether the distant binding site and the C-terminal carboxyl binding site are competitive or non-competitive; that is, whether the distant binding site can bind those homologs containing tryptophan without invoking interaction of their C-terminal α-carboxyl groups with the carboxyl binding site of the enzyme.

Two of the most potent homologs, Trp^2---Ile^7 (II) and $<Glu^1$---Ile^7 (IV), contain tryptophan. But if one assumes that binding of their free α-carboxyl groups occurs first and is obligatory (Figure 2A), then their tryptophan residues would be misplaced for interaction with the distant binding site. If the C-terminal isoleucine binds preferentially to the C-terminal carboxyl binding site of the enzyme, then the analog Trp^2---Pro^7 should be a superior inhibitor. Conversely, it may be possible that Trp^2---Ile^7 (II) has a greater affinity for the distant binding site, and thus its C-terminus, through steric effects, prevents binding of substrate to the catalytic site (Figure 2B). If the latter model is correct, then a C-terminal peptide amide or ester of Trp^2---Ile^7 might confer greater inhibitory potency. One can not rule out the possibility that both types of binding (2A and 2B) occur. However, if model 2B is correct, in which interaction with the distant binding site predominates and prevents binding of substrate to the C-terminal catalytic site, then there are implications for the development of kininase II inhibitors of a new class, distinct from the type of the new Squibb inhibitor SQ 14,225 (Ondetti et al., 1977).

In addition to the C-terminal binding site and the distant tryptophan binding site shown in our model (Figure 1), the zinc ion of the catalytic site of the enzyme may also interact with the carbonyl group of the third residue from the C-terminus and the enzyme may also form a hydrogen bond with the carbonyl group of the second residue from the C-terminus. Furthermore, the enzyme may also have some hydrophobic affinities for the proline residues at positions 3, 5, 8, and 9. Thus, the nonapeptide inhibitor BPP_{9a} may have as many as 8 potential binding sites for the kininase II enzyme. Although this would appear to be a large number of binding sites, it is not unprecedented in view of the fact that a number of well-characterized enzymes such as papain, elastase, subtilisin, and pepsin have been found to have six to seven subsites (for review, see Walter and Yoshimoto, 1978).

ACKNOWLEDGEMENTS

The authors gratefully acknowledge support of this research by grants from the Florida Heart Association, the John A. Hartford Foundation, Inc., and the Council for Tobacco Research. The authors also thank Dr. Arthur M. Felix, Hoffman-La Roche, Inc., Nutley, N.J. for the generous gift of Boc-L-ΔPro and for assistance in carrying out amino acid analysis of the ΔPro-containing analogs.

REFERENCES

Cheung, H.S. and D.W. Cushman, 1973, Spectrophotometric assay and properties of the angiotensin-converting enzyme of rabbit lung, Biochem. Biophys. Acta, 293, 451.

Cushman, D.W., J. Pluscec, N.J. Williams, E.R. Weaver, E.F. Sabo, O. Kocy, H.S. Cheung, and M.A. Ondetti, 1973, Inhibition of angiotensin converting enzyme by analogs of peptides from Bothrops jararaca venom, Experientia, 29, 1032.

Cushman, D.W., H.S. Cheung, E.F. Sabo and M.A. Ondetti, 1977, Design of potent competitive inhibitors of angiotensin converting enzyme, carboxyalkanoyl and mercaptoalkanoyl amino acids, Biochemistry, 16, 5484.

Das, M. and R.L. Soffer, 1975, Pulmonary angiotensin converting enzyme, J. Biol. Chem., 250, 6762.

Elisseeva, Y.E., V.N. Orekhovich, L.V. Pavalikhina and L.P. Alexeenko, 1971, Carboxycathepsin-a key regulatory component of two physiological systems involved in regulation of blood pressure, Clin. Chim. Acta, 31, 413.

Erickson, B.W. and R.B. Merrifield, Solid phase peptide synthesis, 1976, in: The Proteins, Vol. 2, eds. H. Neurath and R.L. Hill (Academic Press, New York), p. 418.

Ferreira, S.H., 1965, Bradykinin-potentiating factor (BPF) present in the venom of Bothrops jararaca, Brit. J. Pharmacol. Chemother., 24, 163.

Ferreira, S.H., D.C. Bartelt, and L.J. Greene, 1970, Isolation of bradykinin-potentiating peptides from Bothrops jararaca venom, Biochemistry, 9, 2583.

Fisher, G.H., J.W. Ryan, L.C. Martin and A.M. Felix, Superactive analogs of the angiotensin converting enzyme inhibitor BPP9a containing L-3,4-dehydroproline, 176th National Meeting, Amer. Chem. Soc., Miami Beach, Sept. 10-15, 1978 (Abstr. MEDI 26).

Gisin, B.F. and R.B. Merrifield, 1972, Carboxyl-catalyzed intramolecular aminolysis, a side reaction in solid-phase peptide synthesis, J. Amer. Chem. Soc., 94, 3102.

Kaiser, E., R.L. Colescott, C.D. Bossinger, and P.I. Cook, 1970, Color test for detection of free terminal amino groups in the solid-phase synthesis of peptides, 34, 595.

Lenard, J. and A.B. Robinson, 1967, Use of hydrogen fluoride in Merrifield solid-phase peptide synthesis, 89, 181.

Merrifield, R.B., 1963, Solid phase peptide synthesis, I. The synthesis of a tetrapeptide, J. Amer. Chem. Soc., 85, 2149.

Merrifield, R.B., 1964, Solid phase peptide synthesis. IV. The synthesis of methionyl-lysyl-bradykinin, Biochemistry, 3, 1385.

Ondetti, M.A., N.J. Williams, E.F. Sabo, J. Pluscec, E.R. Weaver and O. Kocy, 1971, Angiotensin converting enzyme inhibitors from the venom of Bothrops jararaca: Isolation, elucidation of structure, and synthesis, Biochemistry, 10, 4033.

Ondetti, M.A., B. Rubin and D.W. Cushman, 1977, Design of specific inhibitors of angiotensin converting enzyme: New class of orally active antihypertensive agents, Science, 196, 441.

Penke, B., R. Ferenczi and K. Kovacs, 1974, A new acidic hydrolysis method for determining tryptophan in peptides and proteins, Anal. Biochem., 60, 45.

Pluscec, J., E.R. Weaver, N. Williams, E.F. Sabo and M.A. Ondetti, 1972, Structure-activity relationship of peptidic inhibitors of angiotensin converting enzyme, in: Peptides 1972, Proc. 12th Europ. Pept. Symp., eds. H. Hanson and H.D. Jakubke (North-Holland Publ. Co., Amsterdam) p. 403.

Ryan, J.W., A. Chung, C. Ammons and M.L. Carlton, 1977, A simple radioassay for angiotensin converting enzyme, Biochem. J., 167, 501.

Ryan, J.W., A. Chung, L.C. Martin and U.S. Ryan, 1978, New substrates for the radioassay of angiotensin converting enzyme of
endothelial cells in culture, Tissue & Cell, 10, 555.

Sakakibara, S., The use of hydrogen fluoride in peptide chemistry,
1971, in: Chemistry and Biochemistry of Amino Acids, ed. I.B.
Weinstein, (Marcel Dekker, New York), p. 51.

Stewart, J.M. and J. Young, 1969, Solid-Phase Peptide Synthesis,
(W.H. Freeman Co., San Francisco).

Walter, R. and T. Yoshimoto, 1978, Postproline cleaving enzyme:
Kinetic studies of size and stereospecificity of its active site,
Biochemistry, 17, 4139.

THE SPECIFICITY OF POTENTIATING EFFECT OF GLUTATHIONE ON THE

ACTIONS OF BRADYKININ

Kazumi Takeya and Yoshihiro Hotta

Department of Pharmacology, Aichi Medical University

Nagakute, Aichi-ken 480-11, Japan

ABSTRACT

Potentiating effects of GSH, a physiologic kininase inhibitor
on the bradykinin actions on (a) blood pressure responses of rabbits,
(b) acute inflammatory response in rat's hind paws and (c) the
isolated guinea-pig ileum contractions were examined among the
combinations between various active agents and thiols. The potentiation of the hypotensive response to bradykinin by GSH was highly
specific compared with the other experimental models (B and C).
Throughout these three experiments, specific relation between GSH
and bradykinin was consistently observed.

INTRODUCTION

A large number of compounds belonging to different chemical
classes potentiate the effect of bradykinin. Thiols such as
L-cysteine, dimercaprol, thioglycolic acid are well known to
inhibit enzymatic destruction of bradykinin and to potentiate
the kinin effect (Ferreira and Rocha e Silva, 1962; Erdos and
Wohler, 1963; Aureswald and Doleschel, 1967).

Glutathione, the cysteine-containing tripeptide is a physiologic substance of ubiquitous distribution in the body and present
in high concentration(Boyland and Chasseaud, 1969).

Recently, reduced glutathione(GSH) is widely used clinically
from the biochemical evidences that it participates in essential

665

metabolism and function of the cell(Arias and Jacoby, 1975).

From the pharamacological standpoint , it can be assumed that GSH plays a role of physiologic kininase inhibiter and it regulates the intensity and duration of action of kinin released as local hormone. GSH, pharmacologically a quite inert substance will produce dynamic action with helps of kinin or of angiotensin I. However, the pharmacological information concerning the kinin-potentiation is not available enough and so far reported only fragmentarily (Erdös and Wohler, 1963; Werle et al., 1964; Edery and Grundfeld, 1969; Mita et al., 1978).

In this paper, we compared the specificity of bradykinin-potentiation by GSH in the following three experimental systems:

1. Arterial blood pressure response of rabbits
2. Acute edema response of rat's hind paws
3. - Isolated guinea-pig ileum segments

MATERIALS AND METHODS

Experiment 1.   Arterial blood presure of rabbits.

Albino rabbits of either sex weighing from 1.2 to 2.2 Kg body weight were used. The mean arterial blood pressure in the right cartoid artery of the rabbit anesthetized with urethane(1.2 g/kg, i.m.) was recorded on a paper by means of a straingauge type pressure-electric transducer(Nihonkohden MPU-0.5) and the carrier amplifier with display units. Test substance was injected into either side of ear vein of rabbits at a speed of 0.5 ml/sec. The blood pressure changes was evaluated from both duration and magnitude of the response; As shown in Fig. 1, an area being surrounded by the level 5 mmHg below or above the initial level and the curve of blood pressure was used for the evaluation. The pressor or depressor effect was expressed by mmHg.min. Influence of GSH on the blood pressure responses to various vasoactive substances such as bradykinin and angiotensin I was determined 2 min after GSH injection.

Experiment 2.   Acute edema responses of hind paws of the rat
               (method of Winter et,al. 1962).

Influence of GSH on the inflammatory response to bradykinin and the other phologogens was evaluated by the determination of the volume of hind paws of male rats(Wister strain) weighing in the range between 100-150g.

Test samples were dissolved in 0.9% NaCl solution and injected into the subplantar region of either side of the paws at a vol-

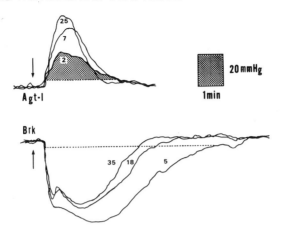

Fig. 1. A method for evaluating the blood pressure response and time course of bradykinin-potentiation and angiotensin-I-inhibition by GSH. The mean arterial blood pressure in carotid artery of a rabbit anesthetized with urethane are shown. Blood pressure responses were evaluated both duration and drop or rise(mmHg. min). A dotted area after angiotensin I(Agt-I) are shown as an example for evaluating the BP response to Agt-I. Time (min) after the injection of GSH (0.1 mM/kg,i.v.) is indicated near the curve of respective response to bradykinin(Brk 1.0 µg/kg) or to angiotensin I(Agt-1, 5 µg). Pressor response to angiotensin I(Agt-I) was inhibited and depressor response to bradykinin(Brk) was augmented by GSH. This effect disappeared gradually within 30 min.

ume of 0.1 ml. A mixture of a phlogogen with GSH or the other related substance as L-cysteine, o-phenanthroline was injected into the corresponding region of the other side.

Fifteen and 60 min after the injection, volume of the paws of a rat was measured by conventional methods using a volume differential meter(Ugo basil) and the difference in volumes of a pair of the paw with swelling was determined and then expressed percent increase or decrease in the volumes comparing one side with the other of the paw of a rat.

Experiment 3.   The isolated guinea-pig ileum.

Terminal ileum segments(1-2 cm), isolated from healthy guinea-pigs were suspended in well oxygenated modified Tyrode solution (NaCl 8.0g; KCl 0.2g; $CaCl_2$ 0.2g; $NaHCO_3$ 1.0g; NaH_2PO_4 0.5g and dextrose 1.0g per 1 of solution, containing atropine sulfate and/or diphenhydramine-HCl each in concentration of 5×10^{-7} g/ml).

Following equilibration at 30°C, several concentrations of
agonists such as bradykinin, histamine, acetylcholine in a volume
smaller than 0.5 ml were added to a 50 ml organ bath. The response of the ileum segment was recorded on a paper by force-displacement transducer under the same resting tension 1.0g. Three
to five cumulative concentration-response curves, at 60 min intervals were determined in each segment for a given agonist. When
used, GSH was added to the bath 10 min prior to the test for concentration-response curve.

From the framework of log-concentration-response curves, the
mode of action and the magnitude of shift of the curve at 50% level
of the maximum response were determined. The shift by thiols was
expressed by a difference in pD_2 values (ΔpD_2) of the two curves
one of which is the control curve and the other that reached in
full extent shift.

The main drugs used were:
bradykinin-3HAc, eledoisin, angiotensin I, angiotensin II(obtained
from Protein Resarch Foundation Minoo Japan); reduced glutathione
GSH(Yamanouchi Pharmac. Co) L-cysteine, o-Phenanthroline(Yoneyama
Yakuhin) λ-carrageenin(Pasco international). The other drugs in
special grade were obtained from the commerical source.

Satistics.

Results are presented as mean values ± S.E and significauce
of differences between means was determined according to the t-
test. Criterion for significance was $p < 0.05$.

RESULTS AND DISCUSSION

Experiment 1. Arterial blood pressure response of rabbits.

The effect of bradykinin on the arterial blood pressure of
anesthetized rabbits was tested and compared before and after the
intravenous injection of GSH(0.1 mmole/kg, = 30.7mg/kg). Bradykinin in doses from 0.1 to 5.0 µmoles/kg body weight produced dose-
dependent drop in blood pressure.

After the administration of GSH, the hypotensive response
to doses of bradykinin became bigger and longer lasting. As shown
in Fig. 2, bradykinin in dose of 1.0 µg/kg caused a drop of the
blood pressure 58.4 ± 17 mmHg. min. While 2 min after GSH, the
same dose of bradykinin caused 288 ± 80 mmHg. min(n=5). The hypotensive response to bradykinin was augmented five times by the
pretreatment of GSH. This finding is in accord with the observation of
Erdös and Wholer(1963) that in guinea pig GSH of 88 mg/kg potentiated 2.5 times increase in drop of pressure.

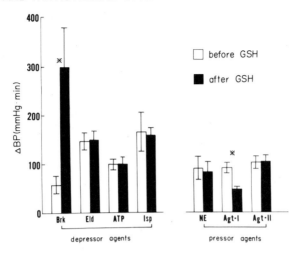

Fig. 2. Influence of GSH on blood presure response of rabbits to various vasoactive agents. Seven groups of 5 rabbits under ureth- ane anesthesia were used. Vasoactive agents were injected into the ear vein just 2 min after i.v. administration of GSH(0.1 mM/kg, 30.7 mg): bradykinin(Brk) 1.0 µg, eledoisin(Eld) 0.5 µg, norepi- nephrine-HCl(NE) 15 µg, angiotensin II(Agt-II) 4.1 µg/ per Kg body weight, respectively. Column and bar: mean ± S.E. n = 5.

GSH did not affect the actions of the other hypotensive agents as eledoisin(0.5 µg/kg), ATP-Na$_2$(1 mg/kg) and isoproterenol. Fig. 2). Pressor responses to norepinephrine and angiotensin II were not influenced by the pretreatment of GSH.

While the development of pressor response to angiotensin I was significantly inhibited (p < 0.01) after GSH. As shown in Fig.1, 2 min after GSH, angiotensin I in dose of 5 µg/kg caused a response of only the half of the control. The blood pressure response to angiotensin I after GSH was characterized by a slow rate of rise and small peak of the response curve.

The inhibitory effect of GSH on the pressor response to ang- iotensin I and the augmentative effects on hypotensive response to bradykinin, both consequently would be interpreted by the in- hibition of kininase II, angiotensin converting enzyme since the two enzymes are assumed to be the same (Dorer et al., 1974).

However the situation is complicated from the evidence that rabbit serum contains no kininase II(Erdös et al.,1968). It is, therefore, assumed that the inhibition of conversion by GSH from angiotensin I to angiotensin II took place at the surface of endo-

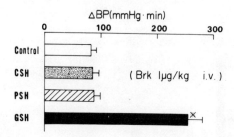

Fig. 3. Influence of equimolar thiols on the hypotensive response
of rabbits to bradykinin. GSH, L-cysteine(CSH), DL-penicillamine
(PSH) in a dose of 0.1 mM/kg were given i.v. just 2 min before
the administration of bradykinin(1.0 µg/kg. Brk). Hypotensive
effect of Brk was increased 4 times by GSH.

thelial cells of pulmonary blood vessels in the rabbit(Ryan et al.,
1975).

Experiment 2. Acute edema response of rat's hind paws.

Fig. 4 shows the effect of GSH on percent difference(ΔS %) in
edema response of rat hind paws 15 min and 60 min after the injection of various phologogens(n=5 $\sim$ 8). In preliminary experiment, single effect of GSH and cysteine was tested: when GSH(1.0
mg) or cysteine (1.0 mg) was injected, they produced a swelling of
such a slight degree that it could not differentiated from changes
in volume of the paw that recieved 0.9% NaCl solution.

The mixed injection of 0.3 µg of bradykinin with GSH(1.0 mg)
caused a marked increase in volume of one side of rat's paw compared with that of the other side which recieved the injection
of bradykinin alone. Percent increments of the volume 15 and 60
min after injections were 14 ± 2.6, 12 ± 2.2(n=8), respectively.

The edema response produced by the injection of 10 µg histamine was also strengthened 4.5 ± 1.0%(n=5, p < 0.05) by GSH.

5-hydroxytryptamine-induced edema was strenghtened 8 $\sim$ 9 %
by GSH after the injection.

Carrageenin-induced edema was not significantly affected by
GSH but it inhibited the swelling later ; i.e., the edema produced
by the mixed injection of carrageenin with GSH disappeared faster
than that by carragenin alone.

The acute edema response of rat's hind paws to formaldehyde
was not affected by GSH.

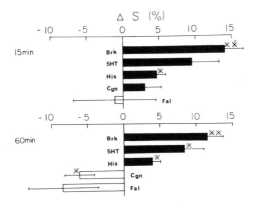

Fig. 4. Influence of GSH on the acute edema response of rat hind paws to bradykinin and the other phologogens. Healthy male rats (Wister strain) weighing in the range between 100 -150 g were used. Test materials in 0.9% NaCl solution was injected into the sub-plantar region of rat's paws. Percent differences in swelling responses produced by phologogen alone and the phologogen plus GSH are illustrated. Dose of phologogen in 0.1 ml volume injected was: bradykinin(Brk) 0.3 µg, 5-hydroxytryptamine(5HT) 0.1 µg, λ-carrageenin(Cgn) 100 µg and formaldehyde(Fahl) 300 µg.

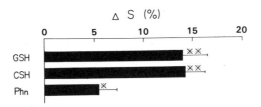

Fig. 5. Influence of kininase inhibitors on the acute edema response of rat hind paws to bradykinin. Bradykinin 0.3 µg, o-phenanthroline(Phn) 5.0 µg, GSH and L-cysteine(CSH) 1.0 mg.

As shown in Fig. 5, kininase inhibiters such as L-cysteine and o-phenanthroline enhanced significantly the edema response to bradykinin as well as GSH(n=5 ∿ 8, p < 0.05 ∿ 0.01).

Influence of thiols on the inflammation is known to be complicated; It has been reported that thiols may be either pro- or anti-inflammatory depending entirely on the model selected for study(Steinetz et al., 1973).

From the present study, it became apparent that GSH, L-cys-

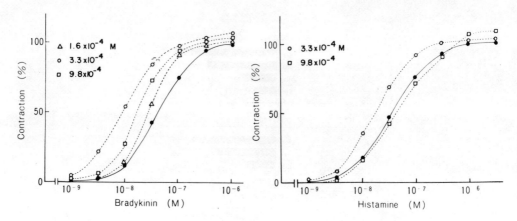

Fig. 6. Influence of GSH on the log-concentration-response curves for bradykinin and histamine. Isolated ileum segments from guinea pigs were used in modified Tyrode sol. of 30°C. Cumulative concentration-response curves were determined in each segment for bradykinin and histamine in the presence and absence of GSH. In the presence of 3.3 x 10^{-4} M GSH, the maximum shift of the curve for bradykinin occured in parallel fashion. At higher concentration of GSH, the shift of the curve for both bradykinin and histamine was inhibited. The magnitude of the shift at 50% response level is summarized in Table 1.

teine and o-phenanthroline promoted the inflammatory state in which kinins participiated.

Increased vascular permeability produced by bradykinin is suggested to be due largely to its venoconstrictor effect(Rowly, 1964).

Contraction of isolated vein from carotid vein of the rabbit was promoted by GSH as shown in Fig. 7.

Experiment 3.   The isolated guinea-pig ileum.

Following equilibration in Tyrode solution containing atropine sulfate and dephenhydramine-HCl each in concentrations of 5 x 10^{-7}g/ml, four cumulative concentration-response curves were determined.

Figure 6. at left hand side shows the log-concentration-response curve for bradykinin. At a low GSH concentration of 1.6 x 10^{-4}M, only the slope of curve increased. This finding accords the observation that GSH potentiated but did not affect the sensitivity of the guinea pig ileum to bradykinin(Edery and Grundfest, 1969).

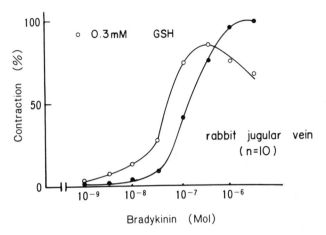

Fig. 7. Influence of GSH upon log-concentration-response curve for bradykinin in isolated strips of jugular vein from rabbits.

However, in the presence of 3.3×10^{-4} M GSH(=1 mg/ml), the log-concentration-response curve shifted to the left in a parallel fashion. This indicates that GSH produced both sensitization and potentiation of the guinea pig ileum for bradykinin. At this concentration, full extent shift of the curve was occured.

GSH at the concentration of 9.8×10^{-4} M, the shift was rather suppressed. It was observed that high concentration of cysteine inhibited the guinea-pig ileum's response to bradykinin (Aureswald, 1967).

The response of the ileum to histamine was tested in Tyrode solution containing only atropine sulfate(5×10^{-7} g/ml). The log-dose-response curve for histamine shifted to the left in the presence of 3.3×10^{-4} M GSH in parallel fashion with slight increase in the maximum response. However, GSH at a higher concentration(9.8×10^{-4} M) did not cause any shift of the log-concentration-response curve to the left.

The log-concentration-response curve for acetylcholine was shifted slightly to the left by the presence of GSH.

The response of the guinea pig ileum to eledoisin was not affected by GSH.

In Table I, the power of 3.3×10^{-4} M GSH on the shift of log-concentration response curve for each agonist was summarized.

Table 1. Influence of GSH on the shift of log-concentration-response curves for various agonists in isolated guina pig ileum. GSH and L-cysteine conc.: 3.3×10^{-4} M.

Combinations		Agonists-concentrations producing 50% response of the maximum effect in absence (A) and presence (B) of thiols		Magnitudes of the LCR-curve shift (ΔpD_2)
Agonists	Thiols	(A)	(B)	
Bradykinin	GSH	4.0×10^{-8} M	0.9×10^{-8} M	0.65
Bradykinin	Cysteine	2.0×10^{-8} M	1.0×10^{-8} M	0.30
Acetylcholine	GSH	10.0×10^{-8} M	5.5×10^{-8} M	0.26
Histamine	GSH	3.6×10^{-8} M	1.6×10^{-8} M	0.35
Eledoisin	GSH	1.4×10^{-8} (g/ml)	1.0×10^{-8} (g/ml)	0.13
Prostaglandin -F$_{2\alpha}$	GSH	14.5×10^{-8} (g/ml)	13.8×10^{-8} (g/ml)	0.02

When the magnitude of the curve shift for a tenfold decrease in agonist concentration was expressed as 1.0, the power of GSH of 3.3×10^{-4} M on the shift of the curve for bradykinin was 0.65.

A potent kiniase inhibiter, o-phenanthroline, did not cause any shift of the curve for bradykinin to the left, showing non-competitive inhibition at higher concentrations than 10^{-5} g/ml. Its pD_2' value was 3.4.

REFERENCES

Aureswald, W. and W. Doleschel, 1967. On the potentiation of kinins by sulfhydryl compound, Arch. int. Pharmacodyn. 168: 188.

Boyland, E. and L. F. Chasseaud. The role of glutathione S-transferases in mercapturic acid biosynthesis, 1969. In: Advances in Enzymology, vol. 32, F.F. Nord, ed. (New York, London) p. 173.

Dorer, F.E., J.R. Kahn, K.E. Lentz, M. Levine and L.T. Skeggs, 1974. Hydrolysis of bradykinin by angiotensin-converting enzyme, Circulation Res. 34: 824.

Erdos, E.G. and J.R. Wohler, 1963. Inhibition in vivo of the enzymatic inactivation of bradykinin and kallidin, Biochem. Pharmacol. 12: 1193.

Edery, H. and Y. Grunfeld, 1969. Sensitization of smooth muscle to plasma kinins: effects of enzymes and peptides on various preparations. Brit. J. Pharmacol. 35: 51.

Ferreira, S.H. and M. Rocha e Silva, 1962. Potentiation of bradykinin by dimercaptopropanol (BAL) and other inhibitors of its destroying enzyme in plasma. Biochem. Pharmacol. 11: 1123.

Mita, I., J. Iwao, M. Oya, T. Chiba and T. Iso, 1978. New sulfhydryl compounds with potent antihypertensive activities. Chem. Pharm. Bull. 26: 1333.

Ryan, U.S., J.W. Ryan and A. Chiu, 1975. Kininase II (angiotensin converting enzyme) and endothelial cells in culture, In: Kinins, Pharmacodynamics and Biological Roles, ed. F. Sicuteri, et al., Plenum Press (New York, London) pp. 217.

Rowly, D.A., 1964. Venous constriction as the case of increased permeability produced by 5-hydroxytryptamine, histamine, bradykinin and 48/80 in the rat. Brit. J. Exp. Pathol. 45: 56.

Steinetz, B., T. Giannina and M. Butler, 1973. The role of sulfhydryl groups in three models of inflammatory disease. J. Pharmacol. Exptl. Therap. 185: 139.

Werle, E., K. HochstraBer, I. Trautschold and G. Leysath, 1964. Wirkung von Thioglykolsaure auf Kininogen und Kininase, Hoppe-Seylers Z. Physiol. Chem. 337: 286.

Winter, C., Risely, E. and G. Nuss, 1962. Carrageenin-induced edema in hind paws of the rat as an assay for anti-inflammatory drugs. Proc. Soc. Exp. Biol. Med. 111: 544.

CATABOLISM OF VASOACTIVE PEPTIDES AND A RAT LIVER ENDOPEPTIDASE*

J.L. Prado**,D.R.Borges,J.A.Guimarães**,E.A.Limãos and
A.C.M.Camargo

Dept.Biochem.&Pharm,Escola Paulista Med. and Dept. of
Pharm., Faculdade Med. Rib. Preto, USP.
Caixa Postal 20372, 01000 São Paulo, SP, Brasil.

There is ample evidence that circulating kinins are inactivated
rapidly by enzymes along the luminal surface of pulmonary endothelial cells (cf. Ryan et al., 1976a and Ryan et al., 1976b). Kinins
may also be hydrolyzed by kinin-converting aminopeptidases found in
human plasma, rat and human liver (cf. Guimarães et al., 1973; cf.
Borges et al., 1974). The last enzymes do not attack bradykinin
(BK) itself, which is the limit product of this hydrolysis.

In experiments designed to demonstrate the occurrence of kinin
conversion in perfused rat preparations, Prado et al. (1975) showed
that in exsanguinated rats with lung bypass considerable amounts of
BK are rapidly inactivated; average recoveries following single
injections of 100 to 200 μg of BK were 20% at 3 minutes and 5% at 6
minutes following the injection. When radioactive bradykinin was
given, around 100% of the radioactivity was recovered within the
same time. Furthermore the kininase activity of the perfusate
itself was found to be about 50- fold less than the kininase
activity of rat plasma. These two observations seem to indicate
that BK was inactivated by enzymes located at the endothelial
surface of the rat preparation used. When similar amounts of BK
were perfused in exsanguinated whole rat preparations with the
lungs, BK recoveries were smaller, that is, 6% at 2 minutes and 0%

* Work supported by grants from Financiadora de Estudos e Projetos
(FINEP), Rio and Fundação de Amparo à Pesquisa do Estado de São
Paulo (FAPESP), São Paulo.

**With fellowship from Conselho Nacional de Desenvolvimento Cientí-
fico e Tecnológico (CNPq), Rio.

at 4 minutes following injection. It may be thus concluded that although the lungs are actually important regarding kinin inactivation, extrapulmonary inactivation of kinins cannot be disregarded.

We had observed, indeed, that perfused rat liver was able to inactivate BK at a relatively rapid rate, although less fast than perfused rat lung (Prado et al., 1975). Several years ago Ferreira and Vane (1967) had observed also that when BK was infused in cat vascular beds of the body below the diaphragm, hind quarters, liver, kidneys and head, it disappeared quickly. We have made further observations on the catabolism of vasoactive polypeptides by perfused rat liver, obtaining the following main results (Borges et al., 1976):

a) the BK inactivation rates, expressed as nmoles of BK per g of liver tissue, depend on the initial BK concentration in the perfusing medium. BK inactivation rates varied between 2.3 to 9.1 for initial BK concentrations between 3.1 to 18.9 x 10^{-6}M. At the highest BK concentration tried, 1 g of liver inactivated 18.2 ± 4.5 (s.e.) nmoles of BK in a single passage through the perfused organ (44 experiments).

b) the total BK inactivation by the liver perfusate itself was the lowest, when compared to inactivation rates of the perfused liver, rat plasma and of a homogenate supernatant obtained from exsanguinated rat liver. The whole perfused liver of a 300 g body weight rat would be able to inactivate about 98 nmoles per minute at the highest BK concentration tried.

c) at the nanogram range, which is probably more physiological, the inactivation of BK was studied superfusing isolated rat uterus with the liver perfusate. It was found that around 90% of injected BK were inactivated by a single passage through the organ.

d) isoleucyl[5]-angiotensin II (AII), similarly to BK, was inactivated by perfused rat liver (4 experiments); at the highest concentration tried (17 x 10^{-6}M) recirculation of AII was followed by an inactivation rate of 15 nmoles x min^{-1} x g^{-1}. At the nanogram range and assaying the liver perfusate on superfused rat uterus, AII was inactivated about 90% following a single passage through the liver.

e) when isoleucyl[5]-angiotensin I (AI) recirculated through perfused rat liver for 8 minutes the recovered activity was around 100% when assayed on the isolated rat uterus. This seemingly high recovery was actually due to a partial conversion of the decapeptide AI into the 20- fold more active octapeptide AII (Carlini et al., 1958); this was shown both by a change in the potency ratio AI:AII, assayed on the superfused rat uterus, before and following one

Table 1.   Inactivation rates of bradykinin, bradykinylamide (BKNH$_2$)
and bradykinylglycylamide (BKGlyNH$_2$) by perfused   rat
liver.

Experiment	Peptide and its initial* concentration x 10^{-6} M		Inactivation nmoles x min^{-1} x g^{-1}		
			BK	BKNH$_2$	BKGlyNH$_2$
1	BK and BKNH$_2$,	3.2	0.8	0.8	–
2	BK and BKNH$_2$,	6.5	3.0	2.9	–
3	BK and BKNH$_2$,	12.9	3.6	3.5	–
4	BK and BKGlyNH$_2$,	11.0	10.2	–	9.4
5	BK and BKGlyNH$_2$,	11.0	8.1	–	9.1

*BK was perfused and its inactivation rate was determined; three
minutes later and following Tyrode change, inactivation-rate of
the indicated amides was measured in the same liver.

single passage of AI through the liver and by separating on
carboxymethylcellulose columns an average of 4.9% AII   from liver
perfusates (3 experiments).

f) addition of the pure bradykinin-potentiating peptide BPP5a (PCA-
Lys-Trp-Ala-Pro) to the perfusing medium reduced both BK-inactiva-
tion and AI-conversion by perfused rat liver.

g) perfusion through liver of 4.70 nmoles of BK per ml for 2 minutes resulted in 75% inactivation of the peptide; the concentrations of free Arg and Phe increased in the perfusate. The
following total corrected values for amino acids and peptides were
found, as nmoles per ml of perfusates: Arg, 4.14; Phe, 6.40; Phe-
Arg, 1.10; Ser-Pro, 1.86 and Gly-Phe, 1.59. The dipeptides were not
found in control perfusates.

The bulk of the evidence then available, both from the literature and from our own results mentioned above, suggested that the
catabolic changes at the C-terminal end of vasopeptides produced
by liver perfusion of BK and AI, and which are more important
pharmacologically, would be explained by one enzyme. This is a
peptidyldipeptide hydrolase (EC 3.4.15.1),which splits dipeptides
at the C-terminal end of peptides; it is trivially known as
angiotensin converting enzyme and as kininase II.

We have lately made new observations regarding the inactivation of BK by perfused rat liver (Borges et al., 1977; Borges
et al., 1978). Table 1 shows that bradykinylamide and bradykinylglycylamide were inactivated by perfused liver at the same

Table 2. Bradykinin inactivation[1] by purified Triton X-100 removed
          liver kininase[2] and formation of the pentapeptide Arg^1-
          Phe^5.

Bradykinin inactivation %	nmoles of Arg^1-Phe^5 [3]	
	Found	Theoretical
40	31	36
55	50	52
75	72	71

[1] 94.3 nmoles of bradykinin in sodium phosphate buffer were
     preincubated with the purified kininase preparation at pH
     7.0, 37° for 10, 20 and 30 minutes and the reaction inter-
     rupted. The remaining activity was bioassayed   on   the
     guinea pig ileum.

[2] Fifteen-fold purified liver kininase, as described in the
     text.

[3] The pentapeptide Arg.Pro.Pro.Gly.Phe was determined   on
     the amino acid analyzer, as described by Oliveira et al.
     (1976).

rate as BK, indicating that the angiotensin converting enzyme,
which requires a free carboxyl group on substrates (Bakhle, 1974),
could not be responsible for this inactivation. Using 0.05% Triton
X-100 in the perfusing Tyrode solution, we were able to remove in
the perfusate, among a few other enzymes, the   liver   kininase
activity, which was purified 15- fold on a DEAE-cellulose column.
The liver kininase activity removed by Triton X-100 corresponded
to only 3.7% of the kininase activity contained in the whole liver
homogenate supernatant. The purified kininase preparation was
essentialy free of angiotensin I converting and angiotensin II
inactivating activities. Table 2 shows that, on hydrolysis of BK
with this purified kininase, stoichiometric amounts   of   the
peptides Arg^1-Phe^5 and Ser^6-Arg^9 were found, indicating that the
new kininase in rat liver is an endopeptidase which splits BK at
the Phe^5-Ser^6 bond. A kininase was found in rabbit brain (Oliveira
et al., 1976) which hydrolyses BK at this same bond.

We suppose that by the combined action of this endopeptidase
and the peptidyldipeptide hydrolase on BK, the tripeptide Arg-Pro-
Pro and the dipeptides Gly-Phe, Ser-Pro and Phe-Arg are finally
obtained; in the perfused liver they may be further   degraded.

REFERENCES

Borges, D.R., E.A. Limãos, J.L. Prado and A.C.M. Camargo, 1976,
    Catabolism of vasoactive polypeptides by perfused rat liver.
    Naunyn-Schmiedeberg's Arch. Pharmacol. 295, 33.

Bakhle, Y.S., 1974, Converting enzyme in vitro. Measurement and pro-
    perties. In: Angiotensin (I.H. Page and F.M. Bumpus, eds.).
    Hand. Exper. Pharmacol. Vol. XXXVII, pp. 41-80. Berlin-
    Heidelberg-New York: Springer.

Borges, D.R., J.L Prado, and J.A. Guimarães, 1974, Characterization
    of a kinin-converting arylamidase from human liver. Naunyn-
    -Schmiedeberg's Arch. Pharmacol. 281, 403.

Borges, D.R., J.A. Guimarães, E.A. Limãos, J.L. Prado and A.C.M.
    Camargo, 1978, Bradykinin inactivation by perfused rat liver:
    role of an endopeptidase. II Regional PAABS Meeting and XIII
    SAIB Meeting, Abstract nQ 26, La Falda, Cordoba, Argentina, 1977.
    Submitted for publication in Biochem. J.

Carlini, E.A., Z.P. Picarelli and J.L. Prado, 1958, Pharmacological
    activity of hypertensin I and its conversion into hypertensin II.
    Bull. Soc. Chim. Biol. 40: 1825.

Ferreira, S.H. and J.R. Vane, 1967, The disappearance of bradykinin
    and eledoisin in the circulation and vascular beds of the cat.
    Brit. J. Pharmacol. 30, 417.

Guimarães, J.A., D.R. Borges, E.S. Prado and J.L. Prado, 1973, Kinin-
    -converting aminopeptidase from human serum. Biochem. Pharmacol.
    22, 3157.

Oliveira, E.B., A.R. Martins and A.C.M. Camargo, 1976, Isolation of
    brain endopeptidases: influence of size and sequence of substra-
    tes structurally related to bradykinin. Biochemistry 15, 1967.

Prado, J.L., E.A. Limãos, J. Roblero, J.O. Freitas, E.S. Prado and
    A.C.M. Paiva, 1975, Recovery and conversion of kinins in exsan-
    guinated rat preparations. Naunyn-Schmiedeberg's Arch.Pharmacol.
    290, 191.

Ryan, J.W., A.R. Day, D.R. Schultz, U.S. Ryan., A. Chung, D.I.
    Malborough and F.E. Dorer, 1976a, Localization of angiotensin
    converting enzyme (Kininase II). I. Preparation of antibody-heme-
    -octapeptide conjugates. Tissue and Cell 8, 11.

Ryan, U.S., J.W. Ryan, C. Whitaker and A. Chiu, 1976b, Localization
    of angiotensin converting enzyme (Kininase II). II. Immunocyto-
    chemistry and immunofluorescence. Tissue and Cell 8, 125.

THE URINARY KALLIKREIN ACTIVITY IN CADMIUM EXPOSURE

A. Iannaccone, G. Porcelli and P. Boscolo

Institutes of Occupational Medicine and Chemistry,
Catholic University, Via Pineta Sacchetti 526, Rome (I)

Urinary kallikrein activity has been found to be reduced not
only in patients suffering from essential hypertension but also in
lead exposed workers (Iannaccone et al., 1975). This alteration
appeared to be more evident in old than in young subjects with the
same period of lead exposure (Boscolo et al., 1978). It has been
suggested that the kidney of older workers may be altered by an accumulation of cadmium, a frequent contaminant in the working environment.

Epidemiological investigations have showm a positive correlation
between cadmium levels in the environment and in the kidney of exposed populations and blood hypertension. Male rats exposed to
various doses of cadmium for a period of five months showed increased
blood pressure and reduced urinary kallikrein activity with a dose-
response effect (Boscolo et al., 1977). The regression analysis
between blood pressure and kallikrein activity was highly significant.

Six male rabbits were receiving 20 µg/ml of cadmium in drinking
water for 150 days. At the end of the exposure their blood pressure
was not increased in comparison with a control group of ten animals.
However, the urinary kallikrein activity, determined in 24-hr urine
of controls was (Mean $\pm$ S.E.) 406 $\pm$ 42 esterase units/g creatinine
and that of exposed rabbits was 221 $\pm$ 32 showing a statistical significant difference ($p < 0.02$).

Urinary kallikrein activity was also determined in 20 male
workers exposed to cadmium and lower quantities of lead. Their mean
age was 29 years and their mean period of cadmium exposure was 3

years; two of them presented labile hypertension and another diabetes; the others were apparently in good health. The kallikrein activity in the morning urine of age-matched controls was (Mean +
S.E.) 18.2 + 2.0 esterase units/g creatinine and that of cadmium-
workers 2.8 + 0.9.

Since no biological screening test is available for early
cadmium exposure, we propose that further studies may be directed
in establishing the validity of the urinary kallikrein activity as
a possible screening test in human population exposed to cadmium.

REFERENCES

P. Boscolo, V.N. Finelli, H. Choudhury and H.G. Petering, 1977
    Kallikrein activity in urine of cadmium exposed rats in relation
    to the development of hypertension, Cadmium-Symposium, Jena,
    1-3 August 1977, in press.
P. Boscolo, G. Porcelli, G. Cecchetti, E. Salimei and A. Iannaccone,
    1978, Urinary kallikrein activity of workers exposed to lead,
    Brit. J. Ind. Med. 35, 226.
A. Iannaccone, G. Porcelli, P. Boscolo and M. Ranieri, 1975,
    Urinary kallikrein excretion in lead intoxication, Life Sciences
    16, 820.

HOMOLOGOUS INSEMINATION WITH THE ADDITION OF PANCREATIC KALLIKREIN

M. Littich and W.-B. Schill

Andrology Unit of the Department of Dermatology,
The Ludwig-Maximilians University of Munich
Munich, FRG.

INTRODUCTION

Hog pancreatic kallikren (EC 3.4.21.8) stimulates sperm motility and sperm migration in vitro (Schill et al., 1976).

These experimental data provide the theoretical basis for the topical use of kallikrein in artificial insemination of semen in order to improve a reduced cervical mucus penetration ability by spermatozoa with low motility.

Before insemination with kallikrein, an in vitro stimulation test should be performed to determine whether or not stimulation of sperm motility by kallikrein is possible.

MATERIAL AND METHODS

A.   Patient Material

52 childless couples suffering from a male factor (reduced sperm motility).

Classification of patients according to sperm count:
37% asthenozoospermia, 63% oligozoospermia

B.   Addition of Kallikrein to Human Semen
                          for Artificial   Insemination

<u>Substance</u>: highly purified kallikrein

<u>Stock solution</u>: 100 KU/ml kallikrein in
                        physiol. saline, stored
                        at 4^0 C up to 3 months

<u>Notice</u>: Use only plastic material or siliconized
                glass ware

<u>Insemination</u>: 2 ml semen + 0.1 ml stock solution

C.   Insemination Technique
                Paracervical insemination by vacuum cap (Semm et al.,
                1976) twice at the time of ovulation (9-11 cycles).

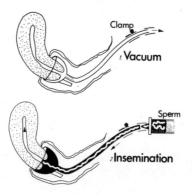

RESULTS

<u>Cervical mucus sperm penetration in vivo</u>

	Sims-Huhner test after paracervical insemination in 8 couples	
Observation time	without kallikrein	with kallikrein (5 KU/ml)
36 hours	negative	positive (5-10 spermatozoa/HPF)

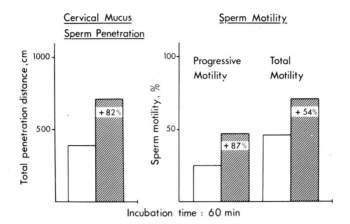

Figure 1.   Correlation between stimulation of sperm motility and
            improvement of cervical mucus sperm penetration by
            Kallikrein (n = 14).   For details see Wallner et al.,
            1975.☐ Control ▨ Kallikrein (1 KU/ml).

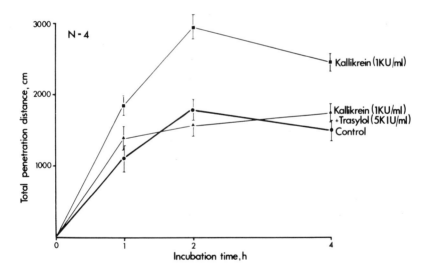

Figure 2.   Kallikrein-induced enhancement of sperm penetration
            through mid-cycle cervical mucus determined by the
            Kremer capillary tube test. Mean values ± SEM of 4
            typical experiments using oligozoospermic semen
            specimens. For details see Schill and Preissler, 1977.

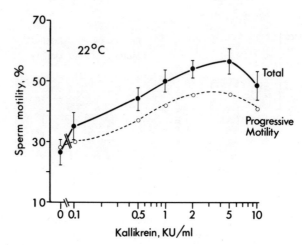

Figure 3.   Dose-response relationship between hog pancreatic
            kallikrein and quantitative and qualitative sperm
            motility. Mean values ± SEM of 6 oligozoospermic
            semen specimens with reduced motility. For experi-
            mental details see Schill and Preissler, 1977.

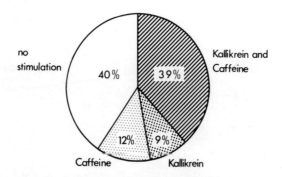

Figure 4.   In vitro sperm stimulation test using kallikrein
            (5 KU/ml) and caffeine (5 mM) as well as both compounds
            simultaneously.   57 ejaculates with reduced motility
            were investigated for their response towards either
            substance concerning the ability to react with a
            stimulation of sperm motility.   For details see
            Schill and Preissler, 1977.

Homologous insemination with addition of kallikrein.

Number of couples	52
Number of conceptions	20
Conception rate	38.5%
Maximum of success	6th – 7th cycle of treatment
Number of abortions	3
Abortion rate	15%

Delivery of 16 healthy babies, one woman in the last trimenon.

Sex ratio of born children: ♀ : ♂   =   11.5

CONCLUSION

Hog pancreatic kallikrein does improve sperm motility and sperm migration in vitro.

Kallikrein can be used for artificial insemination to improve cervical mucus sperm penetration ability of spermatozoa with reduced motility.

Homologous insemination in 52 couples during a period of one year yields a conception rate of 38.5%.

Insemination with kallikrein showed no side effects. Abortion rate with 15% was within the normal range.

All delivered babies were healthy and showed no abnormalities.

REFERENCES

Schill, W.-B., O. Wallner, S. Palm and H. Fritz, 1976. Kinin stimulation of spermatozoa motility and migration in cervical mucus, In: Hafez, E.S.E., (ed.) Human Semen and Fertility Regulation in Man. Mosby Comp., St. Louis, Miss., pp. 442-451.
Schill, W.-B., G. Preissler, 1977. Improvement of cervical mucus spermatozoal penetration by kinins – a possible therapeutical approach in the treatment of male subfertility, In: Insler,V., G. Bettendorf (eds.) The Uterine Cervix in Reproduction, Thieme, Stuttgart, pp. 134-146.
Semm, K., E. Brandl and L. Mettler, 1976. Vacuum insemination cap, In: Hafez, E.S.E. (ed.) Human Semen and Fertility Regulation in Man, Mosby Comp., St. Louis, Miss., pp. 439-441.
Wallner, O., W.-B. Schill, A. Grosser and H. Fritz, 1975. Partici- pation of the kallikrein-kinin system in sperm penetration through cervical mucus-in vitro studies. In: Haberland, G.L.,

J.W. Rohen, C. Schirren and P. Huber (eds.), Kininogenases.
Kallikrein 2, Schattauer, Stuttgart-New York, pp. 63-70.

INHIBITION OF THE CONTRACTILE ACTION OF BRADYKININ ON ISOLATED
SMOOTH MUSCLE PREPARATIONS BY DERIVATIVES OF LOW MOLECULAR WEIGHT
PEPTIDES.

Goran Claeson, Jawed Fareed, Carin Larsson, Gisela
Kindel, Salo Arielly, Roger Simonsson, Harry L. Messmore
and John U. Balis

Kabi AB, Research Department, Molndal and Stockholm,
Sweden, and Depts. of Pathology, Medicine and Pharma-
cology, Loyola Univ. Stritch School of Med., Maywood,
Illinois 60153, and Univ. of South Florida, Tampa,
Florida 33612.

ABSTRACT

The carbonyl terminal tripeptide sequence of bradykinin (Pro-
Phe-Arg) is molecularly manipulated to obtain agents with potent
antagonistic activity towards the smooth muscle contractile activity
of bradykinin. Screening of various peptide derivatives revealed
that heptyl amides or esters of H-D-Pro-Phe-Arg, and H-D-Phe-Phe-
Arg possessed relatively stronger antibradykinin activity on the
isolated smooth muscle preparation. The parent tripeptides, H-D-
Pro-Phe-Arg-OH, and H-D-Phe-Phe-Arg-OH, and their amino acid components, i.e. D-Proline, D-Phenylalanine, L-Phenylalanine and
Arginine, did not possess any antibradykinin activity in concentrations of up to 10^{-4}M. When the heptyl derivatives of these peptides were incubated with either heparinized or citrated whole
blood or plasma, the antibradykinin activity was not lost.
Incubation of these peptide derivatives with either carboxypeptidase
A or B did not result in any loss of the pharmacological effect.
However, pancreatic protease extract produced a significant loss
of the anti-oxytocic action on the isolated rat uterus preparation.
H-D-Pro-Phe-Arg-NH-lauryl derivative also blocked the action of
bradykinin and this effect sustained for a longer period of time
comparative to the blockade with H-D-Pro-Phe-Arg-NH-heptyl derivative. In concentrations of 10^{-7}M and 10^{-8} M and 1 min incubation,
which blocked the contractile action of bradykinin (1 nmole) on
the isolated guinea pig ileum, these peptide derivatives did not
block the action of acetylcholine, histamine, and serotonin.

However, in concentrations of about 10^{-6}M and higher with 5 min.
incubation histamin is also blocked. On the isolated rat uterus
preparation the contractile action of acetylcholine, angiotensin,
oxytocin and vasopressin was blocked at concentrations of 10^{-6}M.
These findings warrant a differential pharmacological evaluation
and in vivo testing of these peptide derivatives to investigate
their therapeutic potential.

INTRODUCTION

    Plasma kallikrein releases (BK) from kininogen, its natural
substrate

K I N I N O G E N

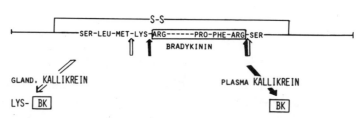

The synthetic chromogenic substrates for plasma kallikrein (1-3)
            H-D-Pro-Phe-Arg-pNA (S-2302) and
            Bz-Pro-Phe-Arg-pNA (Chromozym PK)
mimic the amino acid sequence preceding the one of the bonds split
in kininogen by plasma kallikrein. The amino acid sequence
            Pro-Phe-Arg
of these substrates is thus identical with that of the C-terminal
end of BK.

    Although these substrates have been extensively used for the
analysis of prekallikrein in human and animal plasma, none of these
substrates have been tested for their ability to potentiate or to
antagonize the smooth muscle contractile activity and other actions
of bradykinin. Previous communications from our laboratories have
reported on the antagonism of the responses of the isolated guinea pig ileum and rat uterus preparations (4,5). Our preliminary
studies indicated that substrates which mimic the carboxyl terminal
peptide sequence of bradykinin effectively blocked the bradykinin
induced contractions of the isolated guinea pig ileum and rat
uterus preparations. In addition, we found that the removal of
the p-nitroaniline group from the carboxyl terminal of these
peptides resulted in a total loss of the antagonistic activity.
In order to study the effect of various groups at the carboxyl
end of these peptides, organic synthetic studies were undertaken
and the carboxyl end was derivated to different esters and amides.
Numerous modified forms of the parent tripeptide structure, Pro-
Phe-Arg, containing different amino acids were also synthesized.

To study the structure-activity relationship of these peptides, with particular reference to their bradykinin antagonistic activity on the isolated smooth muscle preparation, and a comparison of their activity with some of the other oligopeptides the present study was undertaken. In addition, the effect of these peptides on the contractile action of other agonists, such as angiotensin, Substance P, serotonin, histamine, acetylcholine and other auto-coids have been investigated.

Review of the Pertinent Literature

While specific antagonists are available for blocking histamine, serotonin, catecholamines and acetylcholine, none has been found to antagonize the action of kinins. Little progress has been made in the development of potentially useful specific inhibitors of kinin action despite the preparation of many structural analogues (6-8). Analgesic and anti-inflammatory agents such as aspirin and indomethacin can effectively reduce the pain and inflammatory action of kinins, but they probably act by blocking the synthesis of prostaglandins, which are the mediators of many kinin actions. Other compounds which block histamine and/or serotonin in isolated organ assay also inhibit bradykinin. They are non-competitive in-hibitors and probably do not act on bradykinin receptors. Rocha e Silva has reviewed this work (9). Butylated hydroxyanisole in concentrations of up to $8 \times 10^{-9}M$ have been shown to inhibit the bradykinin induced contraction of smooth muscles (10). Halopyr-amine, an antihistamine, has also been studied and showed anti-bradykinin activity in both in vivo and in vitro conditions (11). Antibodies to bradykinin have been shown to inhibit the oxytocic and hypotensive activities of bradykinin. In this study the author showed that bradykinin-binding antibodies not only inhibited brady-kinin activity, but also protected the bradykinin against kininase (12). Wilkens and Back have shown the reversal of bradykinin ac-tion by a high molecular weight ethylene oxide polymer (13). Garcia Leme and Rocha e Silva have also investigated a large series of compounds including dibenzodiazpine, thiazanthene, cyclokindole, dihydro-dibenzo-cycloheptane, and benzodiazpine derivatives, besides other phenothiazine, dihydrobenzodiazpine and dibenzocyclo-heptane derivatives, in an attempt to find more potent and more specific antagonists to bradykinin (14). Posati and coworkers showed that Gallic acid and its esters will suppress the brady-kinin induced contractile response of isolated guinea pig ileum (15). Cyproheptadine, an inhibitor of serotonin and histamine, has also been shown to block the contraction of guinea pig ileum caused by acetylcholine, histamine, serotonin and bradykinin (16). This compound also prevents the appearance of the anaphylactic shock in mice sensitized by an α-blocking agent to histamine, serotonin and bradykinin (17). The interference of sandomigram with some of the biological effects of bradykinin has been inves-tigated in the rat (18). In addition, many other agents have been

tested for their possible antagonistic action towards the action
of bradykinin. Numerous peptide analogues of bradykinin have been
synthesized and tested for biological activity (6,8,19-22). Only
a few of these have shown some antibradykinin activity (6,8).
Regoli and coworkers (23,24) have also synthesized a large number
of bradykinin fragments and analogues. They found that replacement
of 8-Phe with aliphatic residues gives antagonists of bradykinin
in rabbit aortae strips. These compounds were, however, found to
be inactive against bradykinin in guinea pig ileum and rat uterus
preparations. Nagase and coworkers have reported on the antibradykinin activity in the crude juice of beet (Beta vulgaris. L.
var rapa Durmot f. rubra) and purified it using chromatographic
methods (25). A synthetic tetrapeptide BPP_{5a} (PCA-Lys-Trp-Ala-Pro)
has been shown to potentiate the action of bradykinin (26,27).
Peptides which block conversion of angiotensin I and the inactivation of bradykinin have been purified from snake venoms and
synthesized (28-30). The C terminal end of most of the potent
ones is prolylproline. Since the N terminal region of bradykinin
contains an arginylprolylproline sequence (Arg-Pro-Pro), Oshima
and coworkers tested Arg-Pro-Pro-tripeptide as an inhibitor of
kininase II; however, no attempt was made to study the inhibition
or potentiation of bradykinin by this peptide (31). Gecse and
coworkers have shown that C-Phenyl-gylcine-n-heptyl ester is a
potent inhibitor of mediators of allergic reactions in both in vivo
and in vitro conditions (32). It is well known that basic amino
acids (Agr, Lys) and amino acids containing aromatic rings are
important in the bradykinin receptor interaction. Heptyl esters
of these two amino acid groups have been synthesized and their
anti-bradykinin effect determined (33).

Synthesis of the Peptides

     The synthesis of the final products was performed by two
different methods:

A.) The aminoterminal dipeptide was coupled with the carboxyterminal
aminoacid derivative as described in example I.
B.) Stepwise method as described in example II.

     Thin layer chromatography (TLC) on silica gel 60 F (E. Merck)
was carried out using the following solvent systems:

P_1 Chloroform:methanol 9:1
Pa   "   "   :water 17:2:2
Pa_6 "   "   "   :acetic acid 34:4:2:9
A n-Butanol:acetic acid:water 6:2:2
M   "   "   "   "   :pyridin 30:6:24:20

The R_f-values stated are the results from separate experiments.

Evaporation of solvents during working up was continuously carried out below 40°C under reduced pressure.

The following abbreviations were used: DMF for N,N-dimethyl-formamide; TEA for triethylamine; HBT for 1-hydroxybenzotiazole; DCC for dicyclohexylcarbodiimide.

Example I H-D-Phe-Phe-Arg-NH-heptyl.2HCl (S-2445)

__Ia.__ Cbo-Arg(NO_2)-NH-heptyl M.W. = 405.5

A solution of Cbo-Arg(NO_2)OH (5.3 g; 15 mmol), heptylamine (2.41 ml; 16 mmol), HBT (2.03 g; 15 mmol) in DMF (30 ml) was mixed at -10°C with DCC (3.71 g; 18 mmol) dissolved in DMF (10 ml). The mixture was stirred overnight at room temperature. The suspension was filtered and the solution evaporated. The residue (oil) was triturated several times with 2% $NaHCO_3$, water, 0.4N HCl and water. The product was crystallized from ethanol-water. Yield 6.5 g (96%).

R_f = 0.31 (P_1)

__Ib.__ Cbo-D-Phe-Phe-OMe   M.W. = 460.5

A solution of Cbo-D-Phe-OpNP (6.2 g; 14.8 mmol), H-PheOMe.HCl (3.25 g; 15 mmol) and TEA (2.1 ml; 15 mmol) in DMF (60 ml) was stirred for 1 h at 0°C and stirred overnight at room temperature. The solution was evaporated, the residue was dissolved in ethyl acetate (200 ml), washed with 2% $NaHCO_3$, 0.4N HCl and water, dried over Na_2SO_4, evaporated and crystallized from ethyl acetate-ether. Yield 5.6 g (82%)

R_f = 0.7 (P_1)

__Ic.__ Cbo-D-Phe-Phe-OH   M.W. = 446.5

The protected dipeptide Ib (5.5 g; 12 mmol) was dissolved in methanol (200 ml) and stirred at room temperature for 3 h with 14 ml 1M NaOH (14 mmol). The solution was evaporated, the residue dissolved in water (300 ml) and the pH adjusted to 2 with diluted HCl. The formed precipitate was filtered and washed with water. Yield: 5 g (93.5%)

R_f = 0.9 (Pa_6)

__Id.__ Cbo-D-Phe-Phe-Arg(NO_2)-NH-heptyl   M.W. = 744.9

To the protected Ia (0.90 g; 2.0 mmol) in glacial acetic acid (4 ml), HBr (2.8 ml; 5.6 M) in acetic acid was added. The mixture was stirred for 30 minutes at room temperature, precipitated with

ether (100 ml) and filtered. The precipitate was washed with ether
and dried in vacuo. The product was dissolved in DMF (4 ml) and
neutralized at -10°C with TEA (0.35 ml; 2.5 mmol). To the mixture
Ic (0.89 g; 2.0 mmol), HBT (2.0 mmol) and DCC (0.45 g; 2.2 mmol)
were added. The reaction mixture was stirred overnight at room
temperature. The suspension was filtered, evaporated and triturated as in example Ia. The crude substance was crystallized
from hot methanol. Yield: 1.15 g (77.5%)

$$R_f = 0.41 \ (P_1)$$

Ie. H-D-Phe-Phe-Arg-NH-heptyl.2HCl   M.W. = 638.7

To 400 mg Id (0.54 mmol), anisol (0.4 mol) and liquid HF
(30 ml) were added. The mixture was stirred for 1 h at 0°C
followed by evaporation of the HF. The residue was dried in vacuo
for several hours. The solid was dissolved in 2% acetic acid
(20 ml) and washed with ether (2x20 ml). The water phase was
applied to a Sephadex G15 column and eluted with 2% acetic acid.
The fraction with the pure product – as acetate salt – was evaporated.
The residue was taken up in a small amount of 0.4 M HCl and evaporated. The last operation was repeated 3 times. Finally the
solution was lyophilized. Yield: 181 mg (53%).

$$[\alpha]_D^{24} = -17.9° \ (c=0.5, \ 50\% \ \text{acetic acid})$$

$$R_f = 0.33 \ (A).$$

Example II H-D-Pro-Phe-Arg-O-heptyl-2HCl (S-2440)

IIa. Cbo-Phe-Arg(NO$_2$)-OMe   M.W. = 514.5

Synthesized as described in Example Ib. Yield 73%.

$$R_f = 0.52 \ (P_1)$$

IIb. Cbo-Phe-Arg(NO$_2$)-OH   M.W. = 500.5

Synthesized as described in Example Ic. Yield 95%.

$$R_f = 0.55 \ (Pa_6)$$

IIc. Cbo-Phe-Arg(NO$_2$)-O-heptyl   M.W. = 598.7

n-Heptanol (10 ml; 71 mmol) and thionylchloride (0.60 ml;
8.3 mmol) were mixed at room temperature. After 1 h IIb (1.0 g;
2.0 mmol) was added and the suspension formed stirred for 3 hr.
The white, viscous reaction mixture was poured in ether (200 ml)

and filtered. The crude substance was crystallyzed from methanol-
water. Yield: 962 mg (80%)

R_f = 0.60 (P_1)

IId. Boc-D-Pro-Phe-Arg(NO_2)-O-heptyl   M.W. = 661.8

IIc (600 mg; 1.0 mmol) in glacial acetic acid (2 ml) and HBr
(1.4 ml)(5.6M in acetic acid) was deblocked as described in Example
Id. The resulting hydrobromide salt was dissolved in DMF (2 ml)
and neutralized at -10°C with TEA (0.18 ml; 1.3 mmol). Boc-D-
Pro-OH (2.15 mg; 1.0 mmol), HBT (135 mg; 1.0 mmol) and DCC (250 mg;
1.2 mmol) were added. The reaction mixture was stirred overnight
at room temperature. The suspension was filtered and the solution
evaporated. The residue was triturated as described in Example 1a.
The crude product was dissolved in methanol (10 ml), applied to a
Sephadex LH 20 column and eluted with methanol. The fraction with
pure product was evaporated. Yield: 570 mg (88%).

R_f = 0.52 (P_1)

IIe.   H-D-Pro-Phe-Arg-O-heptyl.2HCl   M.W. = 589.6

To IId (400 mg; 0.60 mmol) anisol (0.4 ml) and HF (30 ml)
were added and worked up as described in Example I. The chromatographically purified II, as acetate salt, was dissolved in 50%
ethanol (10 ml), applied to a Sephadex QAE-25 (Cl⁻ form) column
and eluted with the same solvent. The pure substance was lyophilized as the hydrochloride salt. Yield: 318 mg (89%).

R_f = 0.29 (A)

$[\alpha]_D^{24}$ = +10.4° (c=0.7, 50% acetic acid)

Structure-Activity Studies

Available chromogenic substrates and some new synthesized
tripeptide derivatives were tested for bradykinin antagonist
activity (Table 1) with the following method:

Isolated Guinea Pig Ileum and Isolated Rat Uterus Assay for Antibradykinin Effect.

These preparations were set according to standard methods.
A 2-3 cm segment of the guinea pig ileum was mounted in a 10 ml
tissue bath and the contractive responses were recorded using a
Beckman Deprograph multichannel recorder.

No.	Product	Mol. weight	Yield %	Method	TLC R_f		$[\alpha]_D^{25}$
Ia	Cbo-Arg(NO_2)NH-heptyl	450.5	96		0.31	(P_1)	
Ib	Cbo-D-Phe-Phe-OMe	460.5	82		0.7	(P_1)	
Ic	Cbo-D-Phe-Phe-OH	446.5	93		0.9	(P_{a6}^1)	
Id	Cbo-D-Phe-Phe-Arg(NO_2)NH-heptyl	744.9	78	A	0.41	(P_1)	
I	H-D-Phe-Phe-Arg-NH-heptyl.2HCl	638.7	53		0.33	(A)	-17.9 (c 0.5, 50%, acetic acid
IIa	Cbo-Phe-Arg(NO_2)-C-Me	514,5	73		0.52	(P_1)	
IIb	Cbo-Phe-Arg(NO_2)-OH	500.5	95		0.55	(Pa_6)	
IIc	Cbo-Phe-Arg(NO_2)-O-heptyl	598.7	80		0.60	(P_1)	
IId	Cbo-D-Pro-Phe-Arg(NO_2)-O-heptyl	661.8	86	B	0.52	(P_1)	
II	H-D-Pro-Phe-Arg-O-heptyl.2HCl	589.6	89		0.29	(A)	+10.4 (c 0.7, 50% acetic acid
IIIa	Cbo-Arg(NO_2)pNA	473.3	67		0.36	(P_1)	
IIIb	Cbo-Phe-Arg(NO_2)pNA	620.6	81		0.29	(P_1)	
IIIc	Cbo-D-Phe-Phe-Arg(NO_2)pNA	767.8	99	B	0.41	(P_1)	
III	H-D-Phe-Phe-Arg-pNA.2HCl	661.6	58		0.47	(A)	-35.1 (c 0.5, 50% acetic acid
IVa	Cbo-Arg(NO_2)-NH_2	352.4	77		0.09	(P_1)	
IVb	Boc-D-Pro-Phe-OMe	376.5	75		0.13	(P_1)	
IVc	Boc-D-Pro-Phe-OH	362.4	74		0.81	(Pa_6)	
IVd	Boc-D-Pro-Phe-Arg(NO_2)-NH_2	562.6	16	A	0.73	(Pa_6)	
IV	H-D-Pro-Phe-Arg-NH_2.2HCl	490.5	72		0.34	(M)	+12.1 (c 0.5,methanol)

No.	Product	Mol. weight	Yield %	Method	TLC R_f		$[\alpha]_D^{25}$
Va	Cbo-Phe-Arg(NO_2)-OMe	514.5	73		0.52	(P_1)	
Vb	Cbo-Phe-Arg(NO_3)-OH	500.5	95		0.55	(Pa_6)	
Vc	Cbo-Phe-Arg(NO_2)-NH-heptyl	597.7	94		0.58	(Pa)	
Vd	Boc-D-Pro-Phe-Arg(NO_2)-NH-heptyl	660.8	69	B	0.35	(P_1)	
V	H-D-Pro-Phe-Arg-NH-heptyl.2HCl	588.6	90		0.27	(A)	+11.6 (0.06, 50% acetic acid)
VIa	Cbo-Arg(NO_2)NH-lauryl	520.7	96		0.41	(P_1)	
VIb	Boc-D-Pro-Phe-Arg(NO_2)-NH-lauryl	731.0	66	A	0.34	(P_1)	
VI	H-D-Pro-Phe-Arg-NH-lauryl.2HCl	658.8	38		0.35	(A)	+10.4 (c 0.5, 50% acetic acid)
VIIa	Cbo-Phe-Arg(NO_2)pNA	620.6	81		0.29	(P_1)	
VIIb	Boc-D-Pro-Phe-Arg(NO_2)pNA	683.7	74	B	0.69	(Pa)	
VII	H-D-Pro-Phe-Arg-pNA	611.5	72		0.33	(A)	+1.7 (c 1, DMF)
VIII	H-D-Pro-Phe-Arg-OH.2HCl	491.5	85	*	0.17	(A)	+22.2 (c 1, 50% acetic acid)
IXa	Cbo-Pro-Phe-Arg(NO_2)pNA	717.8	86	B	0.34	(P_1)	
IX	H-Pro-Phe-Arg-pNA.2HCl	611.5	77		0.23	(A)	-41.3 (c 0.5, 50% acetic acid)
Xa	Cbo-Phe-Phe-Arg(NO_2) pNA	767.8	58	B	0.47	(P_1)	
X	H-Phe-Phe-Arg-pNA.2HCl	661.6	46		0.46	(A)	-6.7 (c 0.6, 50% acetic acid)

No.	Product	Mol. weight	Yield %	Method	TLC R_f		$[\alpha]_D^{25}$
XIa	Cbo-D-Val-Phe-Arg(NO$_2$)pNA	719.8	81	B	0.40	(P$_1$)	
XI	H-D-Val-Phe-Arg-pNA.2HCl	613.6	73		0.32	(A)	-29.3 (c 1, 50% acetic acid)
XIIa	Cbo-D-Pip-Phe-Arg(NO$_2$)pNA	731.7	70	B	0.64	(Pa)	
XII	H-D-Pip-Phe-Arg-pNA.2HCl	625.6	49		0.22	(A)	-24.2 (c 1, 50% acetic acid)
XIIIa	Cbo-pyro-Glu-Phe-Arg(NO$_2$)pNA	731.7	55	B	0.24	(P$_1$)	
XIII	H-pyro-Glu-Phe-Arg-pNA.HCl	589.1	66		0.35	(A)	-22.8 (c 0.6, 50% acetic acid)
XIV	H-Phe-Arg-pNA.2HCl	514.3	75		0.49	(A)	-2.1 (c 0.5, 50% acetic acid
XVa	Bz-Pro-Phe-Arg(NO$_2$)pNA	687.7	65	**	0.29	(P$_1$)	
XV	Bz-Pro-Phe-Arg-pNA.HCl	679.2	80		0.59	(A)	-73.8 (c 0.5, 50% acetic acid)
XVIa	Bz-Phe-Phe-Arg(NO$_2$) pNA	737.7	92	***	0.63	(P$_1$)	
XVI	Bz-Phe-Phe-Arg-pNA.HCl	729.3	68		0.80	(A)	-25.5 (c 0.7, 50% acetic acid)
XVIIa	α Boc-ε Cbo-Lys-pNA	500.5	63		0.65	(P$_1$)	
XVIIb	Boc-Phe-ε Cbo-Lys-pNA	647.7	65		0.78	(P)	
XVIIc	Cbo-D-Pro-Phe-ε Cbo-Lys-pNA	778.9	31	B	0.78	(P)	
XVII	H-D-Pro-Phe-Lys-pNA.2HCl	583.6	39		0.48	(A)	-6.8 (c 0.5, methanol)

No.	Product	Mol. weight	Yield %	Method	TLC R_f	$[\alpha]_D^{25}$
XVIIIa	Cbo-D-Val-Phe-$^\epsilon$Cbo-Lys-pNA	780.9	58	B	0.80 (P₁)	
XVIII	H-D-Val-Phe-Lys-pNA.2HCl	585.6	47		0.19 (A)	-34.6 (c 0.8, 50% acetic acid)
XIXa	Cbo-Tyr(OBzl)-Arg(NO₂)pNA	726.8	97		0.40 (P₁)	
XIXb	Cbo-D-Phe-Tyr(OBzl)-Arg(NO₂)pNA	873.9	82	B	0.32 (P₁)	
XIX	H-D-Phe-Tyr-Arg-pNA.2HCl	677.6	21		0.34 (A)	-28.5 (c 0.4, 50% acetic acid)

*   Obtained by tryptic digestion of VII

**   Obtained by benzoylation of H-Pro-Phe-Arg(NO₂)pNA with benzoic anhydride

***   Obtained by benzoylation of H-Phe-Phe-Arg(NO₂)pNA with benzoic anhydride

For the rat uterus assay, young female rats weighing 120–150 g were injected subcutaneously with 0.1 mg/kg of ethanolic solution of diethylstilboestrol 12–48 hours before each experiment. A 2–3 cm portion of clean uterine horn was mounted in a 10 ml tissue bath containing Dejalon's solution. The water bath was kept at 35°C and aerated with 95% air and 5% CO_2 mixture throughout the course of the experiment. The tissue was stretched by 0.5 g and left to equilibrate for 1/2–1 hour. A dose-response curve for bradykinin (BK) in concentration $10^{-11} - 10^{-6}$M was obtained and a submaximal dose of BK, varying between $10^{-10} - 10^{-8}$M (ED_{70}), was chosen as the agonist dose against which the antibradykinin effect was tested. Each inhibitor was tested for antibradykinin effect at concentrations 10^{-8}, 10^{-7}, 10^{-6} and 10^{-5} M in the tissue bath. At each concentration the inhibitor was incubated with the tissue for 1, 5 and 10 minutes respectively, before addition of BK. The antibradykinin effect was calculated in terms of a direct inhibiting effect of each inhibitor on the BK induced contractions, and expressed as per cent inhibition of the BK response (= 100%). The duration of the antibradykinin effect was expressed as the time taken by the BK response to obtain its original contractive response. The addition of BK, followed by washing, was repeated in three or five minute cycles.

Specificity Studies

To study the specificity of the antagonism to bradykinin the inhibitory effect on bradykinin (BK) (5×10^{-9}M) of one of the more potent inhibitors, S-2455, was compared to its effect on acetylcholine (Ach)(10^{-8} M), histamine (10^{-7} M), serotonin (100 µg/ml) and substance P (1–5 µg/ml) on guinea pig ileum, and on acetylcholine (10^{-6}M) and oxytocin (15 mU/ml) on rat uterus. S-2455 in concentration 10^{-6}M Isubmax.) was incubated with the tissue for 5 min before addition of agonist. Under these conditions bradykinin (5×10^{-9}M) which was included in each experiment to test the activity of the inhibitor, was inhibited around 50%. The antagonist effect was calculated as described above for the antibradykinin effect.

Stability of the Antibradykinin Activity of S-2440 in Human Blood and Plasma

Nine (9) volumes of various blood and plasma were mixed with 1 volume of an 10^{-3}M aqueous solution of the peptide, mixed well and incubated at 37°C for various periods of time. A parallel was run using the Tyrode buffer as control. Whole blood and plasma samples were tested on the isolated rat uterus preparation with a final peptide concentration of 5×10^{-7}M.

Studies on the Susceptibility of S-2302, S-2455, S-2440 and S-2441
by Carboxypeptidase

Carboxypeptidase A (47 u/ml) and carboxypeptidase B (93 u/ml)
were purchased from Worthington Biochemical Corporation (Freehold,
N.J.). Both enzyme preparations were in the form of suspension and
were diluted with Tyrode buffer to a final concentration of 5.0
u/ml. 0.1 ml of a 10^{-3}M of each of the peptide derivatives is
added to 0.9 ml of the pH 7.4 Tyrode buffer which was preincubated
at 37°C. 0.1 ml of 5 units of the carboxypeptidase A and B is
added to the reaction mixture, mixed well and incubated for 15
minutes. After incubation, the mixture was immediately transferred
to an ice bath and the antibradykinin activity was tested using
the isolated rat uterus preparation employing the usual methodology.
A parallel experiment is set where bradykinin (10^{-8}M) is incubated
with the two enzymes in exactly identical conditions and tested
for any contractile activity on the isolated rat uterus.

RESULTS AND DISCUSSION

Screening of various peptide derivatives (some of which are
shown in Table 1) revealed that the substrates with an amino acid
sequence identical with or very similar to the C-terminal tripeptide sequence of bradykinin (BK) gave the best antagonistic
effect. Neither the free peptide acid (H-D-Pro-Phe-Arg-OH) of
S-2302 nor the free pNA could account for the antagonistic effect
of S-2302. Replacement of the free C-terminal pNA group of S-2302
with simple ester or amide groups gave compounds with even better
antagonistic effect than the original substrate. Peptides with
the N-terminal amino acid in unprotected D-form possessed stronger
antibradykinin activity than the same peptide protected with a
benzoyl group. The same peptide with unprotected or benzoylated
N-terminal amino acid in the L-form was also inferior.

The effect of the peptides was further evaluated on the
isolated rat uterus and guinea pig ileum as described before.
Table 2 shows four of the best peptide derivatives in a rat
uterus study, and Fig. 1 give a typical example of the recorded
effect.

The dose response relationship of bradykinin on rat uterus
with and without S-2455 is shown in Fig. 2.

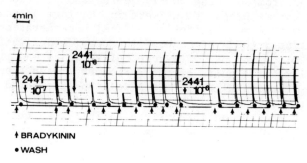

Fig. 1 Effect of S-2441 (H-D-Pro-Phe-Arg-NH-heptyl) at 10^{-7}M and 10^{-6}M concentrations on the BK induced contraction of isolated rat uterus preparation.

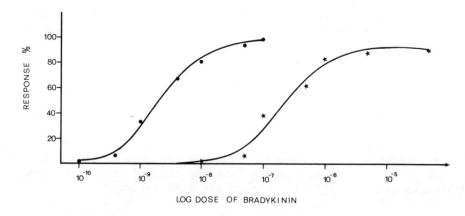

Fig. 2 Dose response curves of rat uterus to bradykinin with and without inhibitor. On the ordinate the percentage response (max. response = 100%) by bradykinin and on the abscissa the log M dose of bradykinin is indicated.

. - . control, without antagonist

* - * pretreatment with S-2455, 5×10^{-6}M, incubated 5 min.

Table 1. Effect of peptide derivatives on the BK induced
contraction of isolated rat uterus preparation

Substrate Structure	Anti BK Activity
H-Phe-Arg-pNA	−
H-Pro- − " −	xxx
H-Phe − " −	xxx
Bz-Pro-Phe-Arg-pNA (Chromozym PK)	xxx
Bz-Phe- − " −	xxx
H-D-Pro-Phe-Arg-pNA (S-2302)	xxxx
H-D-Phe- − " −	xxxx
H-D-Val- − " −	xxxx
H-D-Pip- − " −	xxx
H-Gly- − " −	x
H-D-Pro-Phe-Lys-pNA	xx
H-D-Pro-Phe-Arg-OH	−
pNA	−
H-D-Pro-Phe-Arg-O-heptyl	xxxxx
− " − NH-heptyl	xxxxx
H-D-Phe- − " −	xxxxx

	Inhib.	Incub.	Conc.
xxxxx	100%	10 min	10^{-6}M
xxxx	100-90%	" "	10^{-5}M
xxx	90-60%	" "	"
xx	60-30%	" "	"
x	30-10%	" "	"
−	10-0%	" "	"

Table 2. Effect of tripeptide derivatives on the BK induced
          contraction of isolated rat uterus preparation

Inhibitor structures	Conc.in bath, M	Incubation time, min	% Inhibition of BK response	Dur. of eff.,min.
H-D-Pro-Phe-Arg-O-heptyl	10^{-8}	10	10	15
S-2440	10^{-7}	10	10	15
	10^{-6}	10	100	15
	10^{-5}	5	100	35
	"	10	100	35
H-D-Pro-Phe-Arg-NH-heptyl	10^{-8}	10	15	15
S-2441	10^{-7}	10	15	20
	10^{-6}	5	95	30
	"	10	100	30
	10^{-5}	5	100	30
	"	10	100	45
H-D-Pro-Phe-Arg-NH$_2$	10^{-8}	10	15	15
S-2443	10^{-7}	10	15	15
	10^{-6}	5	100	15
	"	10	100	30
	10^{-5}	5	100	15
	"	10	100	30
H-D-Phe-Phe-Arg-NH-heptyl	10^{-7}	5	20	5
S-24 55	10^{-6}	5	40	15
	5×10^{-6}	5	75	55
	10^{-5}	5	100	70

Specificity studies

In preliminary studies the effect of S-2302 was studied against bradykinin, histamine, oxytocin and acetylcholine on guinea pig ileum and rat uterus (see Fig. 3, Fig. 4 and Table 3). S-2302 $(2.5 \times 10^{-6} - 10^{-5} M)$ was incubated only for one minute before addition of agonist. Under these conditions S-2302 did not inhibit the effect of acetylcholine on guinea pig ileum and on rat uterus. Also the response to histamin remained unchanged. However, in later experiments a more active bradykinin antagonist, S-2455, was tested for specificity as described above. This inhibitor was incubated 5 min before addition of agonist. The results are shown in Fig. 5. Under these conditions S-2455 elicited various degrees of inhibition of all agonists except acetylcholine in guinea pig ileum. The oxytocic action of acetylcholine in uterus may somehow interfere with some mechanism which is inhibited by S-2455 and is not operating in the ileum. More experiments are needed to elucidate this situation.

S-2302 and S-2455 both inhibited the uterine contraction induced by oxytocin. It has been speculated on the fact that these inhibitors may modify the receptor sites for certain non-kinin peptides, among them oxytocin (Fareed et al.)(4).

The response to histamin was not inhibired by S-2302 following 1 min incubation. However, when S-2455 was incubated 5 min the contraction elicited by histamin in ileum was blocked as much as those of bradykinin. The action of histamin on ileum may include some of the bradykinin actions there. The results of this communication are only preliminary and more experiments are needed to elucidate the potency and specificity of these peptides.

The responses to serotonin and substance P on guinea pig ileum were not changed by S-2455.

Stability of antibradykinin activity

The results from the stability studies in human blood and plasma are shown in Table 4, where +++ → + denotes decreasing stability.

The results of the studies with carboxy-peptidase are shown in Table 5. On three separated isolated rat uterus preparations, the antibradykinin action of each of these peptide derivatives was evaluated. None of the peptide derivatives were found to be effected by the action of carboxypeptidase A and B. However, when bradykinin was incubated with these enzymes at $10^{-8}M$ concentration, its contractile action on the isolated rat uterus was completely destroyed by these two enzymes. None of these enzymes

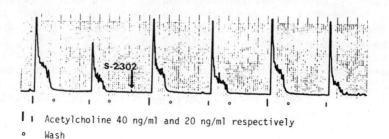

I I   Acetylcholine 40 ng/ml and 20 ng/ml respectively
o   Wash

Fig. 3   Effect of S-2302 (H-D-Pro-Phe-Arg-pNA) at 5.10^{-6}M concentration on the acetylcholine induced contraction of isolated guinea pig ileum.

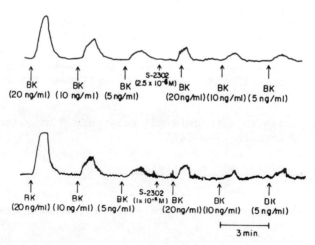

Fig. 4 Effect of S2302 (H-Pro-Phe-Arg-pNA) at $2.5.10^{-6}$ and 1.10^{-5}M concentrations on the BK induced contraction of isolated guinea pig ileum

Table 3

Antagonism of the Oxytocic Action of Various Pharmacologic Agents
by S-2302 as Studied on the Isolated Rat Uterus Preparation

Agent		Antagonism by 10^{-6} M S-2302
Bradykinin	(1.0 ng/ml)	+
Physalaemin	(100 ng)ml)	+
Vasopressin	(0.04 u/ml)	+
Oxytocin	(0.001 u/ml)	+
Acetylcholine	(10 ng/ml)	−

The results of Table 3 are found after incubation of the inhibitor
for one minute. S-2302 also failed to block the contraction induced by acetylcholine, histamine, serotonin and angiotensin on
both isolated guinea pig ileum and rat uterus at a concentration
of $2.5.10^{-6}$M after preincubation of the substrate for one minute
prior to addition of agonist.

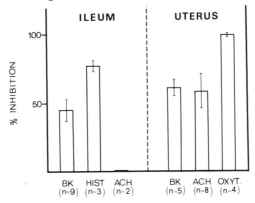

Fig. 5

Effect of S-2455, (10^{-6}M, incubated for 5 min) on the response to
bradykinin (BK; 5×10^{-9}M), histamin (Hist.; 10^{-7}M). acethylcholine
(Ach.; ileum: 10^{-8}M, uterus: 10^{-6}M) and oxytocin (Oxyt.; 15 m U/ml)
on guinea pig ileum and rat uterus , respectively. Mean ± SEM with
numbers of experiments = n in parenteses.

Table 4

Sample	Incubation time, min.				
	0	5	10	20	30
Whole Blood (citrated)	+++	++	++	+	+
Whole Blood (heparinized)	+++	++	++	+	+
Normal Human Plasma (citrated)	+++	+++	+++	+++	+++
Normal Human Plasma (heparinized)	+++	+++	+++	+++	+++
Control (Tyrode buffer)	+++	+++	+++	+++	+++

Table 5

Test material		Carboxypeptidase	
	Control	A	B
(S-2441) H-D-Pro-Phe-Arg-NH-heptyl(10^{-7}M)	++++	++++	++++
(S-2440) H-D-Pro-Phe-Arg-O-heptyl (10^{-7}M)	++++	++++	++++
(S-2455) H-D-Phe-Phe-Arg-NH-heptyl(10^{-7}M)	++++	++++	++++
(S-2302) H-D-Pro-Phe-Arg-pNA (10^{-6}M)	+++	++	++
Control (0.5 u/ml)	– –	– –	– –

produced any measurable antibradykinin action when 10 μl of a 0.5 u/ml (control) solution of each of these enzymes was tested in a 10 ml tissue bath on the contractile action of 1 ng/ml bradykinin on the isolated rat uterus preparation.

10 μl of each of the incubation mixtures was tested for any antibradykinin activity on the isolated rat uterus preparation. Both enzymes, incubated with buffer only, did not produce any antibradykinin activity.

These studies suggest that the peptide derivatives are resistant to the action of carboxypeptidase A and B, and that bradykinin's half life is very susceptible to the action of these enzymes, and that the in vivo half life of these peptide derivatives may be much longer than the vasoactive peptides. The possibility of these peptideases being inhibited by the peptides has to be investigated.

REFERENCES

1. Amundsen, E. and Svendsen, L.: A new assay for plasma kallikrein activity utilizing a synthetic chromogenic substrate in analysis of coagulation. In: I. Witt (Ed.), New Methods for the Analysis of Coagulation Using Chromogenic Substrates. Walter de Gruyter, Berlin/New York, 1977; p. 211.
2. Claeson, G., Aurell, L., Friberger, P., Gustavsson, S., and Karlsson, G.: Designing of Peptide Substrates. Different Approaches Exemplified by New Chromogenic Substrates for Kallikrein and Urokinase. Haemostasis. 7: 62, 1978.
3. Claeson, G., Friberger, P., Knos, M. and Eriksson, E.: Methods for Determination of Prekallikrein in Plasma, Glandular Kallikrein and Urokinase. Haemostasis 7: 76, 1978.
4. Fareed, J., Kindel, G., Messmore, H.L., and Balis, J.U.: Antagonism of the bradykinin induced contractile response of isolated smooth muscle preparation by low molecular weight synthetic chromogenic peptide substrates for serine proteases. In: G. Haberland (Ed)., Progress in Kinin Research. Pergamon Press, London, 1978.
5. Fareed, J., Kindel, G.H., Claeson, G., Larsson, C., Messmore, H.L., and Balis, J.U.: Inhibition of the contractile action of bradykinin on isolated smooth muscle preparations by derivatives of low molecular weight peptides. Fed. Proc. 1979.
6. Stewart, J.M. and Wooley, D.W.: The search for peptides with specific antibradykinin activity. In: E.G. Erdos, N. Back and F. Sicuteri(Eds). Hypotensive Peptides. Springer-Verlag, New York 9L966); p. 23.

7. Stewart, J.M.: Structure activity relationship in bradykinin analogues. Fed. Proc. 27: 63, 1968.

8. Schroder, E.: Structure activity relationship of kinins. In: E.G. Erdos (Ed), Handbook of Experimental Pharmacology, Vol. 25: Bradykinin, Kallidin and Kallikrein. Springer-Verlag New York (1970); p. 324.

9. Rocha e Silva, M. and Garcia Leme, J.: Antagonists of bradykinin. Med. Exp. 8: 287, 1963.

10. Posati, L.P., and Pallansch, M.J.: Bradykinin inhibition by butylated hydroxyanisole. Science 168:121, 1970.

11. Gecse, A., Szekeres, L., and West, G.B.: An antihistamine compound with potent antibradykinin activity. J. Pharm. Pharmac. 21: 544, 1969.

12. Marin Grez, M., Marin Grez, M.S. and Peters, G.: Inhibition of oxytocic and hypotensive activities of bradykinin by bradykinin-binding antibodies. Eur. J. Pharmacol. 29: 35, 1974.

13. Wilkens, H.J. and Back, N.: Reversal of bradykinin act-on by a high molecular weight ethylene oxide polymer. Arch. Int. Pharmacodyn. 209: 305, 1974.

14. Garcia Leme, J. and Rochae e Silva, M.: Competitive and non-competitive inhibition of bradykinin on the guinea-pig ileum. Brit. J. Pharmacol. 25: 50, 1965.

15. Posati, L.P., Fox, K.K. and Pallansche, M.J.: Inhibition of bradykinin by gallates. J. Agr. Food Chem. 18: 632, 1970.

16. Gomazkov, O.A. and Shimkovich, M.V.: Cyproheptadine as an inhibitor of bradykinin effects. Bull. Exp. Bio. Med. 80: 6, 1975.

17. Vargaftig, B.B. and Dao Hai, N.: Paradoxical inhibition of the effects of bradykinin by some sulfhydryl reagents. Experentia 28: 59, 1972.

18. Damas,J.: Sur l'antagonism exerce par le sandomigram (BC 105) sur quelques proprietes de la bradykinine. Arch. Int. Pharmacodyn. Ther. 204: 150, 1973.

19. Safdy, M.E. and Lyons, P.A.: Synthesis and pharmacology of homoarginine bradykinin analogs. J. Med. Chem. 17: 1227, 1974.

20. Bodarszky, M., Ondetti, M.A., Sheehan, J.T. and Lande, S.: Synthetic peptides related to bradykinin. Ann. N.Y. Acad. Sci. 104: 24, 1963.

21. Schroder, E.: Struktur-Aktivitats-Beziehungen bei bradykinin-analogen Polypeptiden. In: L. Zervas (Ed.), Peptides, Proceedings of the 6th European Symposium. Pergamon Press, London; p. 253.

22. Nicolaides, E.D., Dewald, H.A., and McCarty, D.A.: The synthesis of phenylalanine-, 8-p-fluoro-L-phenylalanine-, and 9-p-fluoro-D-phenylalanine-bradykinin. J. Med. Chem. 6: 524, 1963.

23. Regoli, D., Barabe, J. and Park, W.K.: Receptors for Bradykinin in Rabbit aortae. Can. J. Physiol. Pharmacol. 55: 855, 1977.

24. Park, W.K., St-Pierre, S.A., Barabe and Regoli, D.: Synthesis of Peptides by the Solid-Phase Method. III. Bradykinin: Fragments and Analogs. Can. J. Biochem. 56: 92, 1978.
25. Nagase, H., Hojima, Y., Moriwaki, C. and Moriya, H.: Antibradydinin activity found in beet (Beta vulgaris L. var. rapa Dumort. f. rubra DC). Chem. Pharm. Bull. 25: 971, 1975.
26. Ferreira, S.H.: Bradykinin potentiating factor. Br. J. Pharmac. Chemother. 24: 163, 1965.
27. Stewart, J.M., Ferreira, S.H. and Greene, L.J.: Bradykinin potentiating peptide PCA-LCS-TRP-ALA-PRO, an inhibitor of the pulmonary inactivation of bradykinin and conversion of angiotensin I to II. Biochem. Pharmacol. 20: 1557, 1971.
28. Cushman, D.W., Pluscek, J., Williams, N.J., Weaver, E.R., Sabo, E.F., Kocy, O., Cheung, H.S. and Ondetti, M.A.: Inhibition of angiotensin-converting enzyme by analogues of peptides from Bothrops jararaca venom. Experientia 29: 1032, 1973.
30. Bianchi, A., Evans, D.B., Cobb, M., Peschka, M.T., Schaeffer, T.R. and Laffan, R.J.: Inhibition by SQ 20881 of vasopressor response to angiotensin I in conscious animals. Eur. J. Pharmac. 23: 90, 1973.
31. Oshima, G. and Erdos, E.G.: Inhibition of the angiotensin I converting enzyme of the lung by a peptide fragment of bradykinin. Experientia 30: 733, 1974.
32. Gecse, A., Zsilinszky, E., Lonovics, J., West, G.B.: C-phenylglycine-n-heptyl ester as an inhibitor of mediators of allergic reactions. Int. Arch. Allergy 41: 174, 1971.
33. Gecse, A., Zsilinszky, E., Szekeres, L.: Bradykinin antagonism. Adv. Exp. Med. Bio. 70: 5, 1976.
34. Perry, W.L.M., Pharmacological Experiment on Isolated Preparations, E. and S. Livingstone, Ltd., Edinburgh and London, (1968); p. 62-65; 92-93.

SUBJECT INDEX